Thieme

Modern Surgical Management of Chronic Lymphedema

First Edition

Yves Harder, MD
Professor of Plastic Surgery
Head and Medical Director of the Department of Plastic, Reconstructive, and Aesthetic Surgery
Ospedale Regionale di Lugano
Ente Ospedaliero Cantonale (EOC)
Lugano, Switzerland;
Faculty of Biomedical Sciences
Università della Svizzera Italiana (USI)
Lugano, Switzerland

Katrin Seidenstücker, MD
Specialist in Plastic and Aesthetic Surgery
Head of the Department of Plastic and Aesthetic Surgery
Sana Hospital Benrath
Düsseldorf, Germany

Christoph Hirche, MD, FACS
Professor of Plastic Surgery
Head of the Department of Plastic Surgery, Hand Surgery, and Reconstructive Microsurgery
Hand Trauma and Replantation Center
BG Klinik Frankfurt am Main gGmbh
Frankfurt am Main, Germany

Moustapha Hamdi, MD
Professor of Plastic Surgery
Head of the Department of Plastic Surgery and Founder of the Lymph Clinic
Brussels University Hospital
Brussels, Belgium;
Head of the UZ Brussel-Chirec Joint-Network in Plastic Surgery
Brussels, Belgium

320 images

Thieme
Stuttgart • New York • Delhi • Rio de Janeiro

Library of Congress Cataloging-in-Publication Data is available from the publisher.

Important note: Medicine is an ever-changing science undergoing continual development. Research and clinical experience are continually expanding our knowledge, in particular our knowledge of proper treatment and drug therapy. Insofar as this book mentions any dosage or application, readers may rest assured that the authors, editors, and publishers have made every effort to ensure that such references are in accordance with **the state of knowledge at the time of production of the book.**

Nevertheless, this does not involve, imply, or express any guarantee or responsibility on the part of the publishers in respect to any dosage instructions and forms of applications stated in the book. **Every user is requested to examine carefully** the manufacturers' leaflets accompanying each drug and to check, if necessary in consultation with a physician or specialist, whether the dosage schedules mentioned therein or the contraindications stated by the manufacturers differ from the statements made in the present book. Such examination is particularly important with drugs that are either rarely used or have been newly released on the market. Every dosage schedule or every form of application used is entirely at the user's own risk and responsibility. The authors and publishers request every user to report to the publishers any discrepancies or inaccuracies noticed. If errors in this work are found after publication, errata will be posted at www.thieme.com on the product description page.

Some of the product names, patents, and registered designs referred to in this book are in fact registered trademarks or proprietary names even though specific reference to this fact is not always made in the text. Therefore, the appearance of a name without designation as proprietary is not to be construed as a representation by the publisher that it is in the public domain. Thieme addresses people of all gender identities equally. We encourage our authors to use gender-neutral or gender-equal expressions wherever the context allows.

Thieme addresses people of all gender identities equally. We encourage our authors to use gender-neutral or gender-equal expressions wherever the context allows.

Georg Thieme Verlag KG
Rüdigerstrasse 14, 70469 Stuttgart, Germany
+49 [0]711 8931 421,
customerservice@thieme.de

Cover design: © Thieme
Cover image source: the cover image was composed by Thieme using the following images (with permission): Graeme Chambers, Illumina Medical Illustration Ltd. and Mitaka Europe GmbH

Typesetting by TNQ Technologies, India

Printed in Germany by Beltz Grafische Betriebe GmbH 5 4 3 2 1

DOI: 10.1055/b000000221

ISBN: 978-3-13-241428-0

Also available as an e-book:
eISBN (PDF): 978-3-13-241437-2
eISBN (epub): 978-3-13-258238-5

Contents

Section II: Diagnostic Evaluation

Edited by Christoph Hirche

Section III: Modern Management of Chronic Lymphedema

Edited by Yves Harder

Section IV: Non-Surgical Treatment and Techniques

Edited by Christoph Hirche

Section V: Surgical Treatment and Techniques

Edited by Yves Harder

Section VI: Lymphoreconstructive Procedures

Edited by Yves Harder, Christoph Hirche, Katrin Seidenstücker, and Moustapha Hamdi

Acknowledgements

Firstly, we would like to express our special thanks and gratitude to Lewis Enim, who, as the responsible Thieme Managing Editor, put extraordinary personal effort and empathy into this book. We are convinced that he has meanwhile become a lymph-enthusiast and gained all the prerequisites to become a real lymph-expert in the near future. We are really thankful to him. Secondly, we would like to thank Graeme Chambers of Illumina Medical Illustration Ltd. for decisively creating over 70 outstanding illustrations. They bear his personal hallmark of marrying easy-accessibility with attention to detail and represent the spirit of our book well.

Yours gratefully,
The Editors

Foreword

For many years, it has been said that treatment of secondary lymphedema should mainly be conservative, and that surgical options, which have been offered so far, should not be performed, due to their high surgical morbidity and lack of efficacy. Even today, this belief is still strongly held among the community of physiotherapists and lymphologists. That said, conservative treatment cannot cure lymphedema, and both daily compression and nocturnal bandaging of the affected limb are required. Thus, conservative treatment can be quite cumbersome and a heavy burden for the patient, particularly during hot summer days. For many patients, it is often physically and mentally unbearable to adhere to that type of lifelong symptomatic treatment. Accordingly, patients have developed high expectations towards the surgical treatment of lymphedema, since the ultimate goal of lymphedema treatment is ideally to abandon compression therapy altogether.

In 1996, we were able to reveal the dysfunction of lymphatic vessels in patients suffering from lymphedema. We then developed a minimally invasive surgical technique to unify functional lymphatic collectors to neighboring draining veins. Hence, this technique has been described as lymphovenous anastomosis (LVA), which is performed using newly and specifically developed instruments to carry out "supermicrosurgery." Around the same time, surgical techniques describing the transposition or transfer of functional lymphatic vessels or vascularized lymph nodes had been characterized, in order to continuously improve the chronic symptoms of the affected patients.

Meanwhile, it has become common knowledge that surgical treatment cannot only improve lymphedema, but also cure it, in many cases, including severe and advanced instances. Nowadays, it is even possible to prevent lymphedema, by performing specific surgeries in a prophylactic manner during lymph node dissection and/or before radiotherapy.

I have put a lot of personal effort into popularizing LVA for the treatment of lymphedema, and many workshops as well as live surgeries have been held all over the world for the past 25 years to teach lymphatic microsurgeons to quickly spread this technique throughout the world.

Over time, LVA has been increasingly assisted by powerful imaging techniques of the lymphatic vascular system, which has made it possible to easily identify and localize lymphatic vessels and evaluate their functionality.

The ongoing progress of this type of surgery has resulted in an increased number of requests for further information from various professional societies, patient advocate groups, and the media. Currently, there is a common feeling that lymphedema surgery has become one of the hot topics in the field of plastic and reconstructive surgery, which has to be further proven by basic science and scientific evidence in the future.

Many surgeons performing reconstructive surgery of the lymphatic system to treat lymphedema have consistently contributed towards the ongoing development of this surgery in general, and of supermicrosurgical techniques in particular, attending international courses since the late 1990s.

I am confident that this book illustrates the current state of surgical treatment of lymphedema, including diagnostics, conservative treatment, postsurgical treatment, and research. It is an optimal guide for those who want to become experts in lymphatic disease and its treatment.

Isao Koshima, MD
President of the World Symposium of Lymphatic Surgery
International Center for Lymphedema
Hiroshima University Hospital
Hiroshima, Japan
Professor Emeritus
University of Tokyo
Tokyo, Japan

Foreword

A long time ago, a distinguished professor was helping a young medical student with her thesis in surgery. She told him that she had always thought: *"If there are not enough lymph nodes, it could be an idea to implant some!"*

As a young doctor, she performed the implantation of lymph nodes in rats suffering from lymphedema, and the rats fully recovered. The idea did indeed work, but now it was necessary to find sites from where the lymph nodes could be harvested without creating any damage. Accordingly, long-lasting studies in anatomy were performed.

Many years later, the first patients undergoing this surgery felt so much better that the young surgeon decided to dedicate her entire life to treating patients suffering from lymphedema, especially if they were children. A good friend named Christobal helped her to understand the pathophysiology of primary lymphedema in children.

The memories presented above describe my medical career in a nutshell.

With a lot of clinical experience, my aim was to improve the philosophy and the strategy of the surgical treatment of lymphedema in order to describe algorithms to find the best techniques for assessment and treatment.

Further training to improve your own skills is important for successful treatment, but observing and analyzing the patients is the way to continuously improve the quality of the results you achieve. Therefore, also consider performing basic science and reading scientific literature.

Never think that you are the best, that you know everything, but try to achieve perfection...

Modern Surgical Management of Chronic Lymphedema describes all currently used surgical techniques as well as provides a view to the future direction of travel. The book imparts the reader with an irreplaceable overview of imaging and outlines correct surgical procedure by including physiological background information with the goal to defining an individual treatment plan for every single patient.

Corinne Becker, MD
Plastic, Reconstructive, and Microsurgery
Lymphoedema, Hand, and Aesthetic Surgery
American Hospital of Paris (AHP)
Paris, France
Chairman and Board of Trustees
The Corinne Becker Lymphedema Foundation
San Francisco, USA

Preface

Lymphedema, whether primary or secondary, is a chronic and, to date, incurable disease that ensues when the lymphatic system is insufficient to maintain tissue homeostasis. Even though primary lymphedema is rather rare, secondary lymphedema occurs remarkably often also in developed countries, with a conservatively estimated prevalence of ~1 in 1,000 individuals. Secondary lymphedema is usually a consequence of oncological treatment, including surgical excision of lymph nodes and/or radiotherapy of these basins.

Altogether, it has been reported that lymphedema affects as many as 200 million people worldwide. These patients often depend on lifelong conservative therapy—so-called complex decongestion therapy (CDT)—that is only symptomatic and best performed on a regular base to be effective. Unfortunately, treatment delays are common and many patients never receive adequate CDT. Furthermore, no form of systemic drug therapy is available to date. Accordingly, it is not surprising that specific surgical options have been desperately sought after, in order to improve lymph flow respectively decrease edema volume and eventually reduce lymphedema-associated symptoms and complications.

Originally, lymphedema surgery comprised reductive procedures that aimed at decreasing tissue excess resulting from chronic lymphostasis. Unfortunately, these invasive procedures are all associated with a rather high rate of pain, wound healing complications, infection and/or lymph fistulas. Therefore, this type of surgery is nowadays used only occasionally in industrialized countries in very severe cases with advanced lymphedema stages. Lately, suction-assisted lipectomy has been promoted to efficiently remove hypertrophic fat and, fortunately, is associated with far less surgery-associate morbidity compared to reductive procedures. However, this technique requires life-long compression in order to be effective.

Quite recently, microsurgery has successfully gained ground and somehow revolutionized lymphedema surgery, that is lymphatic surgery has become much more sophisticated, offering physiological procedures that aim at reducing the lymphatic fluid burden by improving existing lymphatic outflow and/or establishing alternative outflow pathways. Widespread application of these techniques is based upon newer and more sophisticated diagnostic tools, as well as the continuous improvement of surgical instruments and image magnification up to the level of "supermicrosurgery."

Patients in whom CDT is only able to maintain, rather than reduce the lymphedema stage, seem to be ideal candidates for these surgical procedures, especially if lymphedema has not been present for years and affects the arm rather than the leg. Gradually emerging scientific evidence supports the conclusion that successfully performed physiological procedures may result in the reduced intensity of CDT or even complete cessation of CDT in selected cases of irreversible lymphedema, even in a cost-effective way. Furthermore, patients observe, amongst other things, reduction in edema volume and infection rate, and, eventually, increased quality of life.

Our personal experience is based upon the fact that patients must be always well informed, in order to develop realistic expectations after individual work-up, including pursuing CDT following surgery.

Accordingly, we are particularly proud that several international experts in the field from around the world have contributed to this book and have shared their knowledge and experience, which is addressed not only to surgeons—young or old—involved and interested in the overall surgical management of chronic lymphedema, but to all professionals dealing with lymphedema patients.

The first chapters of this book have been reserved for the understanding of embryology, anatomy and physiology of the healthy lymphatic system. The next chapters focus on diagnosis, preoperative evaluation and treatment indication of chronic lymphedema. Further, conservative treatment is presented in particular as an integral component of surgical lymphedema treatment. Above all, reconstructive procedures, such as lymphovenous and lympho-lymphatic anastomoses as well as autologous lymph vessel and lymph-node transfer are discussed. Finally, teaching and training in reductive and lympho-reconstructive surgery, secondary procedures after reconstructive microsurgery, review of the present literature and outlook on current research in lymphology round off the content.

This textbook is no substitute for what a skilled surgeon should be learning in dedicated courses or at the operation table under the supervision of a surgical teacher. The decisive writing and its consistent illustration are however intended to improve the understanding of the principles and philosophy of modern surgical management of chronic lymphedema.

Enjoy reading, discussing, and improving the outcome of future patients of this striving field!

The Editors
Lugano, Frankfurt am Main, Düsseldorf, Brussels, 2024

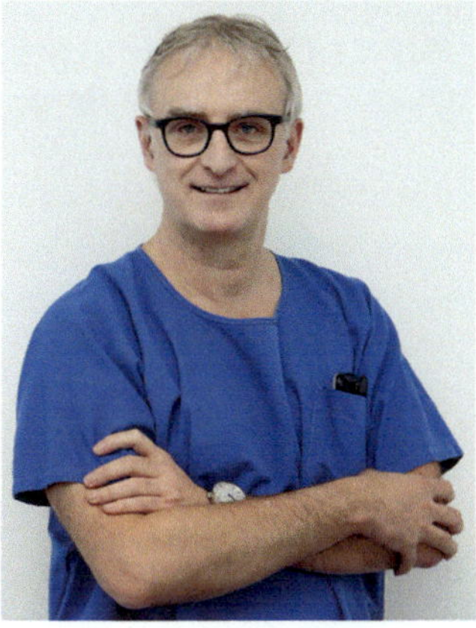

Yves Harder

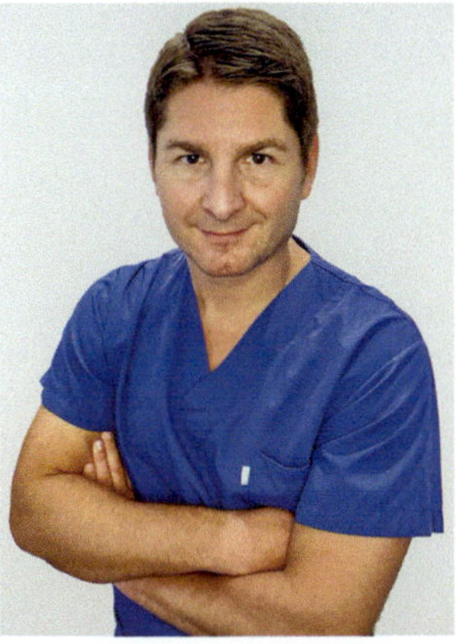

Christoph Hirche

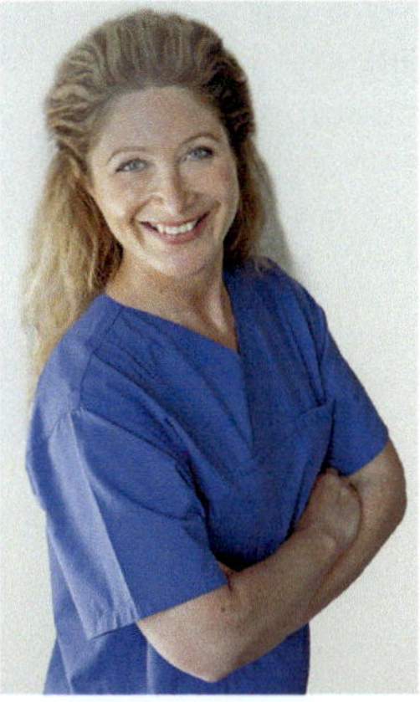

Katrin Seidenstücker

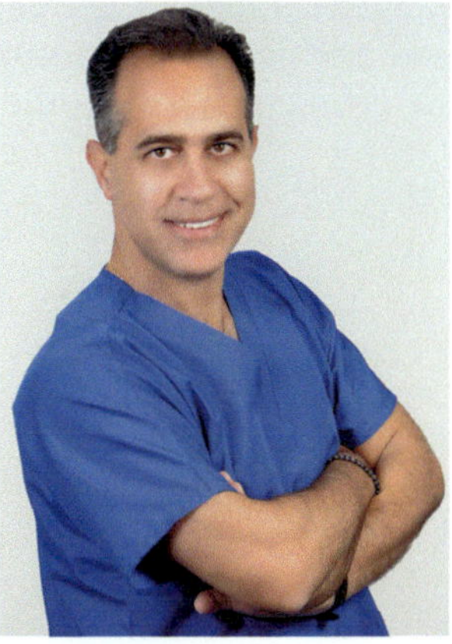

Moustapha Hamdi

Personal Prefaces

It is all about personal curiosity, perseverance, and improving the patient's quality of life...

I first came into contact with reconstructive microsurgery for lymphedema in 2010. After studying the scarce literature available at that time, participating in meetings, in which I shyly initiated discussions about lympho-reconstructive surgery, and visiting Corinne Becker in Paris, my former professor and a surgical colleague gave me the opportunity to participate in the build-up of a lympho-reconstructive unit.

This pioneering work executed in Germany allowed us to gain experience from the first 100 cases in a rather short time. Despite the fascination of this rewarding surgery, at the beginning we obviously suffered some setbacks. Initially, we were too focused on reducing volume and recreating the shape of the affected extremity. It took us some time to understand that the patients were often desperate and therefore more than happy after surgery, especially if they could reduce the number of visits to the physiotherapist or decrease the grade and time of compression of their arm or leg.

Thorough follow-up of the patients and constant inter-professional exchange with physiotherapists, lymphologists and internists allowed me, over time, to better understand not only this chronic and debilitating disease, but also, and foremost, the needs of the patients. These recurrent discussions with professionals also made clear to these “non-surgeons” that the few surgeons performing this type of surgery would never dispossess them of their chronic patients. They are simply far too many!

Nowadays, almost every important meeting in surgery in general, and plastic surgery in particular, dedicates scientific time to discussing standards and progress in this field.

Accordingly, I am happy and proud to have set the stage to bring together friends and colleagues that share their passion for this very specific and yet complex inter-professional and inter-disciplinary medical field that deserves more attention due to its worldwide socio-economic impact.

Yves Harder
Lugano, 2024

It is all about being presented with an opportunity, always...

The lymphatic system and its anatomical-functional structures have long been neglected in all disciplines of medicine as the third vascular system alongside arteries and veins, and little attention was paid to it. It was finally the knowledge of the importance and role of the lymphatic system in tumorigenesis and metastasis that brought the anatomical structures and the lymphatic fluid into the focus of science, which Thomas Mann had described more than two centuries ago as the "very finest, most intimate and most delicate in the whole body."

I experienced something similar myself:

In my doctoral thesis, the lymphatic system was more of a means for obtaining the *Dr. med.* title. By coincidence and through a conversation with my Berlin mentor at the time, a more or less voluntary transfer of a scientific project in my first surgical position meant the continuation of this trajectory. While I was initially able to evaluate ICG lymphangiography for tumor staging and sentinel lymph node biopsy from a general surgical perspective in 2007, over the past 15 years the technique has developed into an indispensable tool for simple, reliable real-time imaging of the lymphatic system. My switch to plastic surgery in 2009 to Ludwigshafen/Germany and the enthusiasm and possibilities in microsurgery have not let go of me since then, and have triggered and imparted a true fascination and passion.

I am grateful and humbled, at the same time, to have met many companions with the same passion and enthusiasm for reconstructive microsurgery of lymphedema and to have found to be valued colleagues, friends and collaborators. Numerous late-night discussions with peers have steadily developed my own perspective on this particular field, which is an ongoing, never-ending process.

Despite the possibilities of lymphatic surgery, lymphedema is and remains the most significant consequence of oncological treatment of malignant tumors and a large infectious burden, and leads to disfigurement, loss of integrity and reduced quality of life, function, form and aesthetics.

I am both grateful and happy to be the co-editor of this book, with many outstanding authors and surgeons, and make a contribution to enabling as many patients as possible to receive the best possible individual, targeted and effective treatment for lymphedema and to encourage and excite young microsurgeons to work in this field, as it continuously excites me.

Christoph Hirche
Frankfurt am Main, 2024

It is all about passion...

I am very fortunate and grateful that my profession is my passion. My favorite place is and has been the OR, where I get to perform surgeries with colleagues who I am able to call my friends. Having happy and thankful patients makes the daily work routine even more enjoyable.

I would like to say thank you to all my teachers—my personal heroes and idols—and to all the valuable companions who share the same dreams. You have, in the meantime, become true friends.

During my education, I have been lucky enough to have had the chance to travel and to visit various pioneers of microsurgery. I started with a fellowship in Ghent (Belgium), with P. Blondeel and M. Hamdi, where they did not only teach me microsurgery, but also passed their passion for it on to me.

In 2010, I visited the first lymphedema meeting in Barcelona, where the definition *supermicrosurgery* was born. The pioneers, Koshima, Becker and Brorson, and the host Masia, talked about this new chapter in microsurgery. Infected by their fascination, I then discovered back home that we also had many patients suffering from breast cancer-related lymphedema–I had not recognized the connection in that way before.

A lot of travelling followed: I went to Corinne in Paris, to Jaume in Barcelona, to Håkan in Malmö and then, step by step, I started lymphedema surgery in Germany and Brussels.

Thank you to all of you who shared your knowledge with me. Thank you, Christoph Andree, for always letting me travel and trusting me to build a lymphedema unit in Düsseldorf.

I would like to advise all young enthusiastic plastic surgeons to visit the masters and to believe in your dreams. In that way, you will gain experience and grow into a coping and responsible person, and, as a positive side factor, you will also gain wonderful friends who share your passion.

Finally, I would like to thank my family. Thank you for understanding that my profession always comes first. Thank you for supporting me on my journey and giving me the "time and the freedom" to focus on my passion.

Katrin Seidenstücker
Düsseldorf, 2024

To the forgotten patients…

It was Gent, 2006. My friends, Koen Van Landuyt, Corrine Becker and I had succeeded in performing the first conjoined free DIEP flap breast reconstruction with a vascularized groin LN flap transfer in history. This was my first contact with such pathology, "Lymphedema."

One year later, Corrine asked me help to organize a VLNT in my motherland, Syria, for an 18-year-old patient with a post-trauma lower extremity lymphedema. There was considerable soft tissue/skin loss with extended scar-tissue, so I decided to harvest a DIEP flap to reconstruct the missing part together with the VLNT. The surgery was successfully carried out. The young patient, "Maha," later became a medical student!

These two cases opened my eyes and mind with respect to extremely challenging surgery.

I also subsequently found out that lymphedema patients do not receive the same attention as breast reconstruction patients:

I named them, "the forgotten patients."

Exchanges and experiences with my international colleagues taught me that surgery is not enough to help those patients, and that a multidisciplinary approach is mandatory, if better outcomes are to be achieved. In 2016, after 10 years of hard work, I succeeded in opening a lymphedema clinic within my plastic surgery department in Brussels. De Lymfklinik is a unique model and magic mixture between surgical activities, clinical research, and patient services. To be sure, this could not have been achieved without a great team. I am so grateful to our nurses, secretaries, physiotherapists, trainees, and mainly to my staff members who built up the European Center of Lymphatic Surgery (Assaf Zeltzer, Katrin Seidenstücker, Randy Debaerdemaeker, and more recently, Alex Nistor).

Moustapha Hamdi
Brussels, 2024

List of Abbreviations

ALND: axillary lymph node dissection
ALVT: autologous lymph vessel transfer
ASIS: anterosuperior iliac spine
CCL21: chemokine ligand 21
CCR7: chemokine receptor 7
CDT: complete decongestive therapy
CNS: central nervous system
COUP-TFII: COUP transcription factor 2
CTA: computed tomography angiography
CXCR4: chemokine receptor 4
DB: dermal backflow
DC: dendritic cell
DIEP: deep inferior epigastric perforator
EGF: epidermal growth factor
ERK1/2: extracellular signal–regulated kinases 1/2
FCI: fasciocutaneous infragluteal
FGF: fibroblast growth factor
FOXC2: forkhead box protein C2
HGF: hepatocyte growth factor
HIF1α: hypoxia-inducible factor 1α
ICG: indocyanine green
IGAP: inferior gluteal artery perforator
IGF-1: insulin-like growth factor 1
ISL: International Society of Lymphology
LAP: lumbar artery perforator
LEC: lymphatic endothelial cell
LN: lymph node
LNU: lymph node unit
LNVA: lymph node to vein anastomosis
LSG: radionuclide lymphoscintigraphy
LV: lymphatic vessel
LVA: lymphovenous anastomosis
LYMPHA: lymphatic microsurgical preventive healing approach
LYVE-1: lymphatic vessel endothelial hyaluronan receptor 1
MALT: mucosa-associated lymphoid tissue
MAPK3: mitogen-activated protein kinase 3
MINORS: methodological index for randomized studies
MLD: manual lymph drainage
MRL: magnetic resonance lymphangiography
NFARc1: nuclear factor of activated T-cells cytoplasmic 1
NRP2: neuropilin 2
PAP: profunda artery perforator
PDGF-B: platelet-derived growth factor B
PROX1: prospero homeobox protein 1
SAPD: suction-assisted protein lipectomy
SCIA: superficial circumflex iliac artery
SCIV: superficial circumflex iliac vein
SFJ: sapheno-femoral junction
SGAP: superior gluteal artery perforator
SIEV: superficial inferior epigastric vein
S1P: sphingosine-1-phosphate
S1PR1: sphingosine-1-phosphate receptor 1
S1PR3: sphingosine-1-phosphate receptor 3
SLNB: sentinel lymph node biopsy
SLO: secondary lymphatic organ
SMC: smooth-muscle cell
SOX18: sex determining region Y box 18
SPECT-CT: single photon emission computed tomography–computed tomography
TGF-β: transforming growth factor β
TI: transport index
T-BAR: total breast anatomy restoration
TMG: transverse myocutaneous gracilis
TUG: transverse upper gracilis
ULL-27: upper limb lymphedema 27
VEGF-C: vascular endothelial growth factor C
VEGF-D: vascular endothelial growth factor D
VEGFR-3: vascular endothelial growth factor receptor 3
VLNT: vascularized lymph node transfer

Contributors

Nele Adriaenssens, PT, PhD
Associate Professor
Department of Physiotherapy
Human Physiology and Anatomy (KIMA)
Faculty of Physical Education and
Physiotherapy–Rehabilitation Research Group
Vrije University Brussels;
Coordinator
Oncological Rehabilitation Program and
Edema Consultation
Medical Oncology Department
Universitair Ziekenhuis Brussel;
President
Belgian Society of Lymphology
Brussels, Belgium

Rüdiger G. H. Baumeister, MD
Former Professor and Head of Plastic, Hand, and
Microsurgery
Ludwig Maximilians University Munich;
Consultant in Lymphology
Urological Clinic Munich Planegg
Munich, Germany

Alessandro Bianchi, MD
Department of Plastic and Reconstructive Surgery
Università Cattolica del Sacro Cuore
Fondazione Policlinico Universitario Agostino
Gemelli IRCSS
Rome, Italy

Amir K. Bigdeli, MD
Department of Hand, Plastic, and
Reconstructive Surgery, Burn Center
BG Klinik Ludwigshafen
Plastic and Hand Surgery, University of Heidelberg
Ludwigshafen, Germany

Anja M. Boos, MD
Senior Physician and Deputy Director
Clinic for Plastic Surgery
Department of Plastic and Hand Surgery
University Hospital RWTH Aachen
Aachen, Germany

Pierre Bourgeois, MD, PhD, MCUH
Professor
Services of Nuclear Medicine, Vascular
Surgery and Dermatology
Institut J Bordet
HIS-IZZ Hospitals and University Hospital Erasme
Université Libre de Bruxelles
Brussels, Belgium

Håkan Brorson, MD, PhD
Senior Plastic Surgeon
Department of Plastic and Reconstructive Surgery
Skåne University Hospital
Malmö, Sweden;
Professor of Plastic Surgery
Department of Clinical Sciences
Lund University
Lund, Sweden;
Professor
Faculty of Medicine
La Escuela de Graduados de la Asociación Médica
Argentina (EGAMA)
Buenos Aires, Argentina

Carola Brussaard, MD
Department of Radiology
Universitair Ziekenhuis Brussel
Brussels, Belgium

Tomke Cordts, MD
Senior Physician
Department of Hand, Plastic, and Reconstructive
Surgery, Burn Center
BG Klinik Ludwigshafen
Plastic and Hand Surgery, University of Heidelberg
Ludwigshafen, Germany

Randy De Baerdemaeker, MD
Professor
Department of Plastic and Reconstructive Surgery
Vrije University Brussels
Brussels, Belgium

Holger Engel, MD, FACS
Professor
Plastic, Reconstructive, and Aesthetic Surgery
ETHIANUM Clinic Heidelberg
Heidelberg, Germany

Andreas Frick, MD
Former Professor Senior Physician
Hand, Plastic and Aesthetic Surgery
University Hospital Munich (LMU)
Munich, Germany

Florian Früh, MD, FEBHS
Head of Hand and Plastic Surgery
Clinic for Plastic Surgery and Hand Surgery
Kantonsspital Aarau (KSA)
Aarau, Switzerland

Emre Gazyakan, MD, MSc, FEBOPRAS, FEBHS
Senior Consultant
Department of Hand, Plastic, and Reconstructive Surgery, Burn Center
BG Klinik Ludwigshafen
Plastic and Hand Surgery, University of Heidelberg
Ludwigshafen, Germany

Jeremy A. Goss, MD
Postdoctoral Research Fellow
Department of Plastic and Oral Surgery
Boston Children's Hospital
Boston, United States

Epameinondas Gousopoulo, MD, PhD
Department of Plastic Surgery and Hand Surgery
University Hospital Zurich
Zurich, Switzerland

Arin K. Greene, MD, MSc
Vascular Anomalies and Pediatric Plastic Surgery Endowed Chair
Department of Plastic and Oral Surgery
Boston Children's Hospital;
Professor of Surgery
Harvard Medical School
Boston, United States

Moustapha Hamdi, MD
Professor of Plastic Surgery
Head of the Department of Plastic Surgery and Founder of Lymph Clinic
Brussels University Hospital
Brussels, Belgium;
Head of UZ Brussel-Chirec Joint-Network in Plastic Surgery
Brussels, Belgium

Yves Harder, MD
Professor of Plastic Surgery
Head and Medical Director of the Department of Plastic, Reconstructive, and Aesthetic Surgery
Ospedale Regionale di Lugano
Ente Ospedaliero Cantonale (EOC)
Lugano, Switzerland;
Faculty of Biomedical Sciences
Università della Svizzera Italiana (USI)
Lugano, Switzerland

Sarah Harnie, PT, MSc
Doctoral Thesis Student
Department of Physiotherapy
Human Physiology and Anatomy (KIMA)
Faculty of Physical Education and Physiotherapy—Rehabilitation Research Group
Vrije University Brussels;
Consultant
Edema Consultation
Universitair Ziekenhuis Brussel
Medical Oncology Department
Brussels, Belgium

Pauliina Hartiala, MD, PhD
Docent for Surgery
Senior Research Fellow, MediCity
Turku University Hospital
Turku, Finland

Akitatsu Hayashi, MD
Plastic Surgeon
Department of Breast Center
Kameda Medical Center
Chiba, Japan

Christoph Hirche, MD, FACS
Professor of Plastic Surgery
Head of the Department of Plastic Surgery, Hand Surgery, and Reconstructive Microsurgery
Hand Trauma and Replantation Center
BG Klinik Frankfurt am Main gGmbh
Frankfurt am Main, Germany

Katja Kilian, MD
Resident
Department of Hand, Plastic, and Reconstructive Surgery, Burn Center
BG Klinik Ludwigshafen
Plastic and Hand Surgery, University of Heidelberg
Ludwigshafen, Germany

Leela Praveen Kumar, MD, MS, MCh
Consultant Plastic Surgeon
Apollo Hospitals
Chennai, India

Min-Seok Kwak, MD
Senior Physician and Deputy Director
Clinic and Polyclinic for Plastic Surgery and Hand Surgery
Technical University of Munich
Rechts der Isar Hospital
Munich, Germany

Nicole Lindenblatt, MD
Professor
Deputy Clinical Director
Department of Plastic Surgery and Hand Surgery
University Hospital Zurich
Zurich, Switzerland

Hans-Günther Machens, MD
Professor and Director
Clinic and Polyclinic for Plastic Surgery and Hand Surgery
Technical University of Munich
Rechts der Isar Hospital
Munich, Germany

Prof. Gurusamy Manokaran, MD, MS, MCh, FICS, FRCS
Professor and Senior Consultant Plastic Surgeon
Apollo Hospitals
Chennai, India;
Chief of Lymphology Services
Department of Plastic and Reconstructive Surgery
Amrita Institute of Medical Sciences
Kochi, India;
Honorary Associate Professor
Macquarie University
Sydney, Australia

Jaume Masià, MD, PhD
Professor of Surgery
Autonomous University of Barcelona
Chief of the Plastic Surgery Department
Sant Pau University Hospital
Chief of the Comprehensive Lymphedema Treatment Unit
Planas Clinic
Barcelona, Spain

Matteo Meroni, MD
Department of Hand- and Plastic Surgery
Luzerner Kantonsspital
Lucerne, Switzerland

Vincenzo Penna, MD
Medical Director
Penna Torio
Clinic for Plastic Surgery
Basel, Switzerland;
Professor of Plastic Surgery
Clinic of Plastic and Hand Surgery
University Medical Center Freiburg
Freiburg, Germany

Claus Christian Pieper, MD
Department of Radiology
University Hospital Bonn
Bonn, Germany

Cristhian D. Pomata, MD, MSc
Attending Plastic Surgeon
Comprehensive Lymphedema Treatment Unit
Planas Clinic
Barcelona, Spain

Elena Rodríguez-Bauza, MD
Plastic Surgery Department
Hospital Universitario Son Espases
Barcelona, Spain

Julia Roka-Palkovits, MD
Senior Physician
Plastic, Reconstructive and Aesthetic Surgery
Krankenhaus Göttlicher Heiland
Vienna, Austria

Anne Saaristo, MD, PhD
Department of Plastic and General Surgery
Turku University Hospital
Turku, Finland

Marzia Salgarello, MD
Professor
Plastic and Reconstructive Surgeon
Department of Surgical Sciences
Università Cattolica del Sacro Cuore
Fondazione Policlinico Universitario Agostino Gemelli IRCSS
Rome, Italy

Mario F. Scaglioni, MD
Department of Hand and Plastic Surgery
Luzerner Kantonsspital
Lucerne, Switzerland;
Zentrum für Plastische Chirurgie
Klinik Pyramide am See
Zurich, Switzerland

Hans Schild, MD
Professor
Department of Radiology
University Hospital Bonn
Bonn, Germany

Katrin Seidenstücker, MD
Specialist in Plastic and Aesthetic Surgery
Head of the Department of Plastic and Aesthetic Surgery
Sana Hospital Benrath
Düsseldorf, Germany

Andreas Spörlein
Medical Student
Department of Hand, Plastic, and Reconstructive Surgery, Burn Center
BG Klinik Ludwigshafen
Plastic and Hand Surgery, University of Heidelberg
Ludwigshafen, Germany

Christiane G. Stäuble, MD
Senior Physician
Department of Anesthesiology and Intensive Care Medicine
Technical University of Munich
Rechts der Isar Hospital
Munich, Germany

Hiroo Suami, MD, PhD
Associate Professor
Australian Lymphoedema Education, Research, and Treatment (ALERT)
Faculty of Medicine, Health, and Human Sciences
Macquarie University
Sydney, Australia

Nestor Torio, MD
Medical Director
Penna Torio
Clinic for Plastic Surgery
Basel, Switzerland;
Professor of Plastic Surgery
Clinic of Plastic and Hand Surgery
University Medical Center Freiburg
Freiburg, Germany

Chieh-Han Tzou, MD
Professor
Specialist in Plastic, Reconstructive and Aesthetic Surgery
TZOU Medical
Plastic, Reconstructive and Aesthetic Surgery
Lymphedema and Facial Palsy Center Vienna
Vienna, Austria

Semra Uyulmaz, MD
Senior Physician for Plastic and Hand Surgery
Clinic for Plastic and Hand Surgery
University Hospital Zurich
Zurich, Switzerland

Ellen Vandyck, PT, MSc
Pedagogic Employee in Educational Development Project Inter-Professional Education
Department of Physiotherapy
Human Physiology and Anatomy (KIMA)
Faculty of Physical Education and Physiotherapy–Rehabilitation Research Group
Vrije University Brussels;
Assistant Research Chair
Universitair Ziekenhuis Brussel
Medical Oncology Department
Brussels, Belgium

Giuseppe Visconti, MD, PhD
Plastic Surgeon
Department of Plastic and Reconstructive Surgery
Università Cattolica del Sacro Cuore
Fondazione Policlinico Universitario Agostino Gemelli IRCSS
Rome, Italy

Mikko Visuri, MD
Department of Plastic and General Surgery
Turku University Hospital
Turku, Finland

Stephan Wagner, MD
Senior Physician
Angiology and Angiological Rehabilitation
Rehabklinik
Bad Zurzach, Switzerland

Karl Waked, MD
Plastic, Reconstructive and Aesthetic Surgeon
Department of Plastic and Reconstructive Surgery
Cirumed Clinic
Marbella, Spain;
Founder and CSO
Augmented Anatomy
Knokke, Belgium

Patrick A. Will, MD, MSc
Senior Surgeon
Department of Plastic and Hand Surgery
Center for Orthopedic, Trauma and Plastic surgery
University Hospital Dresden,
Dresden, Germany

Joerg Wilting, MD
Professor
University Medical Center Göttingen
Center of Anatomy
Department for Anatomy and Cell Biology
Göttingen, Germany

Johnson Chia-Shen Yang, MD, PhD, FACS
Director
International Supermicrosurgical Lymphedema Center;
Associate professor
Plastic and Reconstructive Surgery
Kaohsiung Chang Gung Memorial Hospital
Kaohsiung City, Taiwan

Assaf Zeltzer MD, PhD, FCC(Plast)
Chief of Department Plastic and Reconstructive Surgery
Rambam Health Care Campus
Haifa, Israel

Joachim E. Zuther, PT, MT, CLT
Founder and Education Director
Academy of Lymphatic Studies
Florida, United States

Section I

Lymphology and Clinical Presentation

Edited by Yves Harder and Katrin Seidenstücker

I

1 Lymphatic System

Summary
Throughout the history of vascular biology, the specific and very complex microvascular lymphatic vascular system had not been studied in detail until very recently. A comprehensive understanding only occurred due to tools that guaranteed accurate visualization and allowed for the use of specific cell and tissue markers. Continuous progress of these tools resulted in an increased understanding of the lymphatic vascular system from various perspectives. From an embryological point of view, the lymphatic vascular system depends on a complex interplay of cellular and molecular mechanisms controlling its *de novo* development. Powerful tools that visualize the lymphatic anatomy on a microscopic level have enabled a better understanding of this vascular system not only from a purely anatomical, but also from a physiological point of view, including preservation of tissue fluid balance, absorption of dietary fats, and immunosurveillance, and finally, lymphangiogenesis, which is a complex process of lymphatic cell differentiation, proliferation, migration, sprouting, and eventually tube formation, to create a new microvascular network that occurs not only in early embryological stages, but also in different clinically relevant conditions such as lymphedema, atherosclerosis, cancer, chronic inflammation, dermal infections, fibrosis, hypertension, or obesity. This introductory chapter highlights embryological, anatomical, and physiological issues of the lymphatic vascular system.

Keywords: antigen-presenting cells, chemokine receptor 7 (CCR7), contraction frequency, chemokine receptor 4 (CXCR4), dietary lipid absorption, immune system, immunomodulation, immunosurveillance, lymphatic endothelial cell (LEC), lymphatic drainage, lymph sac, lymphangiogenesis, lymphangion, lymphatic capillary, lymphatic collector, lymphatic pumping, lymphedema, lymphosome, lymphvasculogenesis, mitogen-activated protein kinase 3 (MAPK3), permeability, precollector, prospero homeobox protein 1 (PROX1), sphingosine-1-phosphate (S1P), T cells, tissue fluid homeostasis, vascular endothelial growth factor C (VEGF-C), vascular endothelial growing factor D (VEGF-D), vascular endothelial growth factor receptor 3 (VEGFR-3)

1.1 Embryology of the Lymphatic System

Florian Früh, Patrick A. Will, and Epameinondas Gousopoulos

The lymphatic vascular system has been substantially neglected in the history of vascular biology. Due to the challenge of its visualization and the absence of specific markers, the lymphatic system has been ignored and its anatomy was specified only at the beginning of the 19th century. The identification of specific lymphatic markers in the late 1990s as well as subsequent molecular genetic studies revolutionized our understanding of the mechanisms involved in specification, expansion, and maturation of the lymphatic system.[1]

From a morphological point of view, the murine lymphatic development starts at embryonic day E10.5, corresponding to week 6.5 to 7 in human embryos.[2,3] Endothelial cells of the anterior cardinal vein give rise to the lymphatic primordia, which subsequently form the first primitive lymphatic structures termed lymph sacs. Despite interspecies variabilities of these primordia, the jugular region is generally accepted to be the site of lymphatic induction,[4] and mammalian embryos exhibit eight lymph sacs (▶ Fig. 1.1a,b).[4,5] By the end of the 9th development week in humans, lymphatic vessels connect the lymph sacs. In the fetal period, the lymphatic system already exhibits the asymmetrical condition characteristic of the adult lymphatic system (▶ Fig. 1.1c).

More than 100 years ago, the American anatomist Florence Sabin introduced the now widely accepted centrifugal theory of lymphatic development.[6] She based her theory upon ink-injection experiments in pig embryos and suggested that the peripheral lymphatic system arises from the primary lymph sacs. Then it would spread to the surrounding tissues and organs by endothelial sprouting, where local capillaries are formed. However, in 1910, Huntington and McClure suggested a contradictory centripetal theory, stating that lymphatic vessels arise from peripheral mesenchymal lymphatic endothelial cell (LEC) progenitors, called lymphangioblasts.[7]

Expression studies of the lymphatic-specific marker vascular endothelial growth factor receptor 3 (VEGFR-3) and experiments in mice lacking the homeobox gene PROX1 (prospero homeobox protein 1) confirmed the venous origin of lymphatic vessels.[8,9] Importantly, in PROX1 −/− knockout mice, budding and sprouting of LEC progenitors is arrested without affecting the vasculature of blood vessel development.[9] These landmark studies led to the proposal of a stepwise model for the development of the lymphatic vasculature in mammals.[2,10,11] LEC competence of endothelial progenitor cells in the cardinal veins is achieved around E9.0 by PROX1 expression under the control of the transcription factor gene Sox18 (sex determining region Y box 18).[12] Under the influence of the lymphatic master-regulator gene PROX1, the endothelial progenitors undergo LEC commitment and start budding from the cardinal veins at approximately E10.5.[11] After commitment, cells may give rise to a particular cell type or

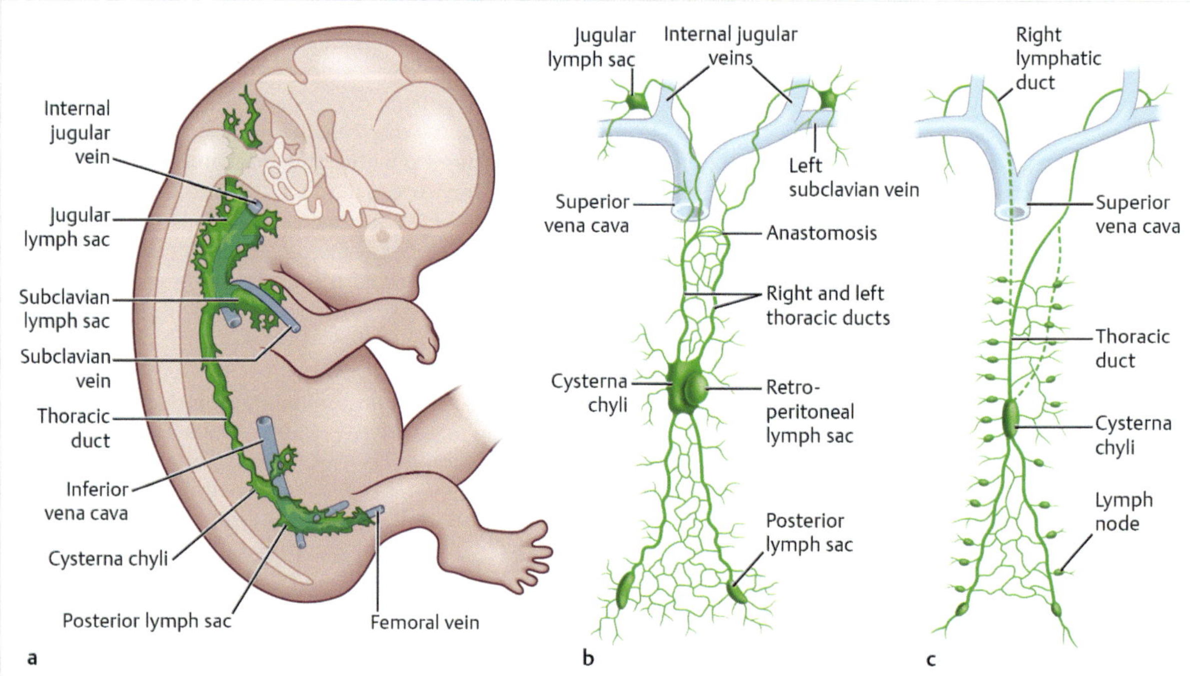

Fig. 1.1 Morphological development of the human lymphatic system. **(a, b)** Illustration of a 9-week-old embryo with a primitive lymphatic system. The paired jugular lymph sacs arise from the anterior cardinal veins. Other lymph sacs: Posterior (paired), subclavian (paired; extension of jugular sac), retroperitoneal, and cisterna chyli. Except for the cisterna chyli, the lymph sacs subsequently differentiate into primary lymph nodes. **(c)** Fetal lymphatic system with asymmetrical anatomy. The thoracic duct drains the majority of the body's lymph into the venous system at the junction of the left internal jugular and subclavian vein. In contrast, the right lymphatic duct only drains the right arm, the upper thorax, and the right side of the face. (Reprinted with permission from Carlson BM. Cardiovascular system. In: Human Embryology and Developmental Biology. 5th ed. Philadelphia: Saunders, 2014.)

structure, depending on the surrounding tissue.[2] Lymphatic vessel sprouting from the embryonic veins is guided by a graded mesenchymal expression of the VEGFR-3 ligand vascular endothelial growth factor C (VEGF-C). Paracrine VEGF-C signaling is crucial for the migration and survival of PROX1-expressing cells from the cardinal veins and for the subsequent formation of lymph sacs.[13] Furthermore, as LEC progenitor cells bud from the embryonic veins into the surrounding mesenchymal tissue, they begin expressing the lymphatic marker podoplanin, indicating lymphatic differentiation and maturation.[14] At around E11.5, PROX1$^+$/VEGFR-3$^+$/podoplanin$^+$ differentiating LECs migrate in interconnected cell groups into the surrounding mesenchyme to form large lymph sacs.[11]

Even though a major part of the lymphatic vasculature develops in a centrifugal manner through lymphangiogenesis (i.e., the growth of new lymphatic vessels from pre-existing capillaries), a dual origin of the lymphatic vasculature has been demonstrated in grafting experiments.[15] This study revealed that the avian lymphatic vasculature possesses both venous and mesenchymal cell contributions. The unequivocal proof of this dual origin came with recent genetic tracing studies in mice, demonstrating that both venous and nonvenous LECs participate in the development of lymphatic vessels.[16,17] LECs were initially observed as isolated cell clusters separate from the sprouting lymphovascular front which subsequently coalesced to form vessels through the process of lymphovasculogenesis.[17,18]

After the establishment of the primitive lymphatic network from E14.5 onward, the lymphatic vessels undergo maturation and remodeling to form a hierarchical tree, characterized by lymphatic capillaries, precollectors, and collecting vessels.[18] Finally, the collecting vessels form lymphatic valves, recruit smooth muscle cells (SMCs), and deposit basement membrane.[11,18]

1.2 Anatomy of the Lymphatic System

Hiroo Suami

Italian anatomist Gasparo Aselli is credited with the discovery of the lymphatic system in 1622.[19] While dissecting live canines, he chanced upon white cords in the mesentery and concluded that these structures were a new anatomic feature related to the absorption of nutrients. To further investigate that new structure, the mercury injection method developed by Anton Nuck was used as the standard technique in the study of cadaver models between the 17th and 20th centuries.[20] Our current anatomical knowledge about the lymphatic system is largely based on the findings that are generated by using the mercury method. However, this method fell out of favor because of the toxicity of mercury and anatomical studies using adult cadavers eventually ceased. A new, safer technique to identify the lymphatics in a cadaver was developed by Hiroo Suami, using hydrogen peroxide to inflate the lymphatic vessel, after which microscope manipulation was used to inject a contrast medium directly into the vessel via needle to allow radiographic demonstration.[21] A further modification was the application of indocyanine green (ICG) lymphangiography to map the superficial lymphatic collectors prior to dissection.[22] These new techniques have allowed us to conduct further anatomical studies of the lymphatics. Precise anatomical knowledge about the normal lymphatics is crucially important because it provides the baseline information required to identify the anatomical changes that occur in lymphedema.

The lymphatic system is divided into superficial and deep systems, separated by the deep fascia (▶ Fig. 1.2). They largely operate independently but converge at the regional lymph nodes (e.g., axillary and inguinal lymph nodes). The superficial lymphatic system originates in the dermal layer of the skin. Blind-ended lymphatic capillaries (initial lymphatics) are located below the epidermis and connect with each other to form a dense, three-dimensional network. The deep lymphatic system originates in the lymphatic capillaries in the muscle fascia and periosteum. The lymphatic collectors of the deep system that run alongside the major arteries are much fewer in number than the collectors in the superficial system.

At the level observed by an electron microscope, endothelial cells in the lymphatic capillaries can be seen to be loosely connected with each other, with each cell connected to the surrounding tissue by an anchoring filament.[23] When the surrounding tissue becomes edematous, the anchoring filaments pull the endothelial cells outwards to open up gaps between them. Thus, in edema, interstitial fluid and macromolecules can move into the lymphatic capillaries more easily. The lymphatic capillaries then connect to precollectors, which are located in the deeper layer of the dermis; however, unlike precollectors, they do not have any valvular structures. The precollectors then merge to form a fewer number of vessels in the deeper layer of the dermis that exit from the dermis and connect to the superficial lymphatic collectors in the subcutaneous tissue (▶ Fig. 1.3). The superficial lymphatic collectors run axially along the limb and centrifugally in the torso toward the regional lymph nodes. Bicuspid valves are present along the lumen of the collectors at short intervals of 2 to 5 mm to regulate the unidirectional flow of lymphatic fluid from distal to proximal in the limbs, and the head and neck region, and from the center to the periphery in the torso. The segment of lymphatic collector between the valves is called a "lymphangion," a functional unit that has an outer lining of SMCs. A chain of lymphangions contracts in a peristaltic manner to propel lymph flow, thus operating as an "intrinsic pump."

In the upper extremity, a medial and lateral pathway of lymphatic vessels has been identified. The dominant

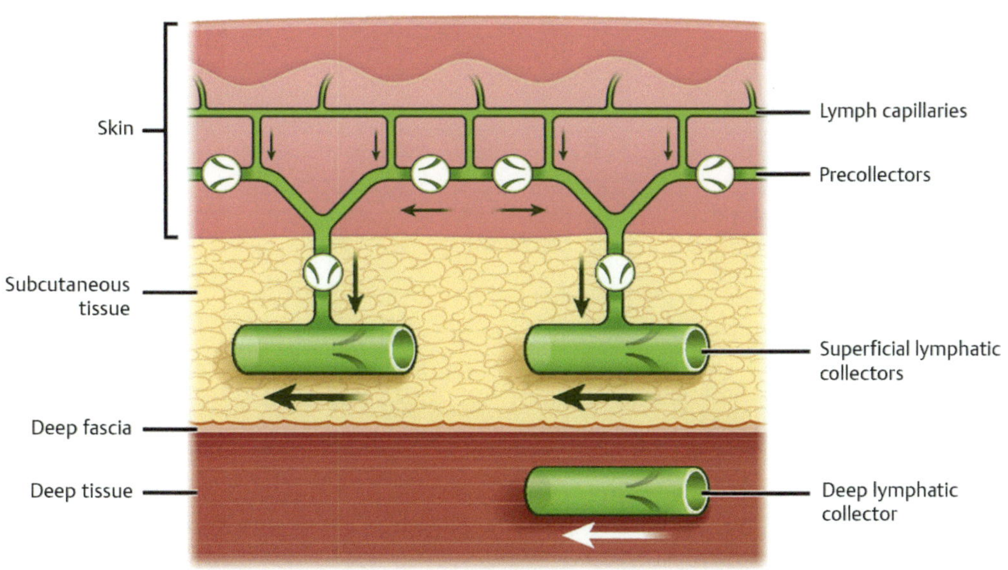

Fig. 1.2 Schematic diagram of the lymphatics. (Redrawn with permission from Hiroo Suami.)

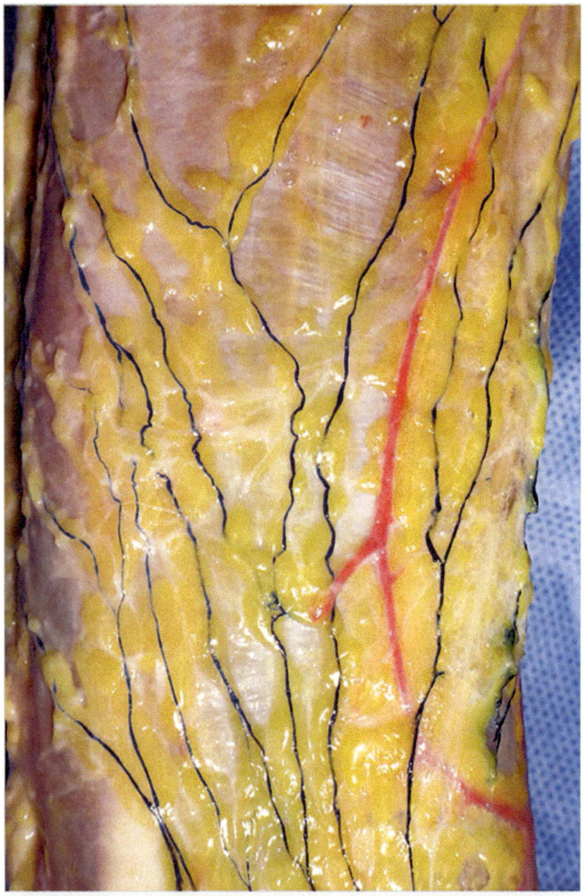

Fig. 1.3 Dorsal forearm of a cadaver showing the superficial lymphatic collectors (blue) and cutaneous vein (red).

medial pathway connects to the axillary lymph nodes, whereas the lateral pathway runs along the cephalic vein to connect to the supraclavicular lymph nodes.[24] The lateral pathway bypasses the axillary lymph nodes and can thus serve as an alternative route in case the medial pathway is compromised following axillary lymph node dissection. Accordingly, two distinct pathways have also been identified in the lower extremity, the medial and the posterior (▶ Fig. 1.4).[25] The dominant medial pathway connects to the superficial inguinal lymph nodes. The posterior pathway runs along the small saphenous vein to connect to the popliteal lymph nodes. The efferent lymphatic vessels of the popliteal nodes go deep at the popliteal fossa to become deep lymphatic collectors that run along the femoral artery in the thigh and connect to the deep inguinal lymph nodes. These deep lymphatic collectors bypass the superficial inguinal nodes, so the posterior pathway may serve as a detour when the medial pathway is obstructed following infection, surgery, or postoperative radiation.

The superficial lymphatic vessels diverge and reconverge, but unlike the blood vascular system, they do not cross over each other or form a three-dimensional vasculature network. This characteristic allowed the author to determine which superficial lymphatic collector connects to which lymph node/s, leading to the development of the concept of "lymphosomes," lymphatic territories in the superficial lymphatic system (▶ Fig. 1.5).

Many new imaging techniques have been developed to visualize the lymphatics (see **Chapter 4**). These include magnetic resonance lymphangiography (MRL), ICG lymphangiography and single-photon emission computed tomography (SPECT-CT). Imaging techniques are

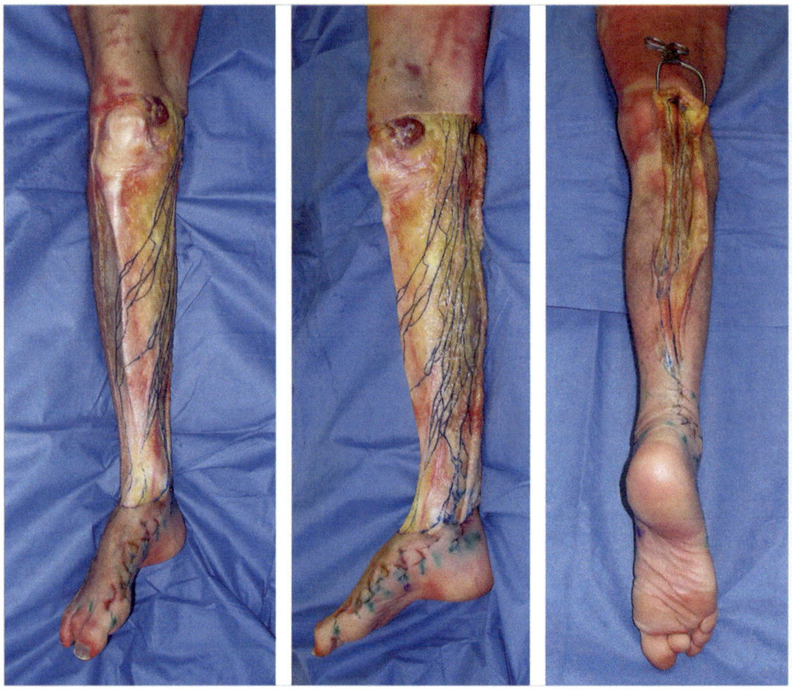

Fig. 1.4 Lower extremity of a cadaver with staining of the superficial lymphatic collectors (blue) showing the medial pathway (left and center) and posterior pathway running along the small saphenous vein (red) (right).

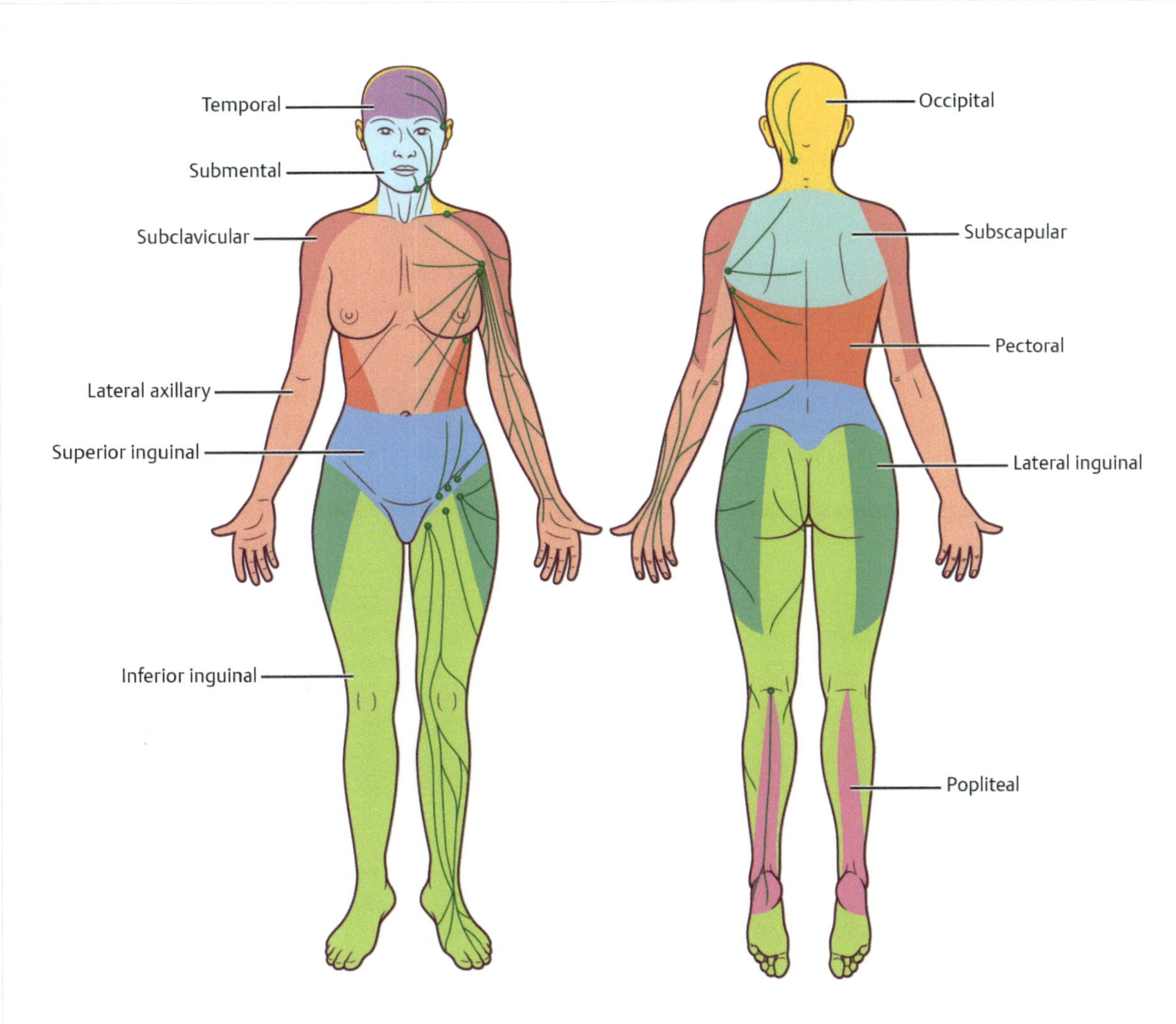

Fig. 1.5 Lymphosomes of the body, that is, the lymphatic territories, are demarcated according to their corresponding lymph nodes. (Redrawn with permission from Hiroo Suami.)

progressing rapidly, providing new information about the lymphatics and lymphedema. To allow accurate reading of this new imaging information, better understanding of the anatomy of the lymphatics has become essential. For example, the presence of dermal backflow (see **Chapter 4**) is one of the imaging criteria used to diagnose lymphedema, as it is never identified in healthy subjects. Anatomically, dermal backflow demonstrates the reflux of lymphatic fluid from the superficial lymphatic collectors to the dermal lymphatics.

1.3 Physiology of the Lymphatic System

Florian Früh, Patrick A. Will, and Epameinondas Gousopoulos

The lymphatic system is unique in higher vertebrates whose complex cardiovascular system and large body size require a secondary vascular system to maintain tissue fluid homeostasis.[26] In contrast to blood vessels, the lymphatic vasculature serves in unidirectional centripetal transport of interstitial fluid, macromolecules, and immune cells back to the blood circulation.[18] Besides maintaining tissue fluid balance, the lymphatic system is crucially involved in the regulation of other biological processes, including immunosurveillance and absorption of dietary fats.

In the villi of the small intestine, specialized lymphatic capillaries, known as lacteals, are responsible for the absorption of long-chain fatty acids and fat-soluble vitamins.[27] After absorption, the molecules are transported toward the systemic circulation by active lacteal contraction. Each lacteal is surrounded by SMCs responsible for contractile dynamics under the control of the autonomic nervous system.[28] In addition, gut lymphatics represent an important route for the transport of microbial antigens and antigen-presenting cells to lymph nodes of the mesentery.

Finally, the lymphatic system is also involved in the drainage of interstitial fluid and macromolecules from the meningeal spaces and the brain parenchyma.[29,30] This is contradictory to older doctrines stating that the central nervous system (CNS) is devoid of a conventional lymphatic system and opens an exciting chapter in lymphatic research.[31]

Understanding the physiology of the lymphatic system provides the basis to appreciate the pathological hallmarks of lymphatic dysfunction. In brief, dysfunction of the lymphatic vasculature is mainly indicated by the appearance of lymphedema, which triggers complex biological alterations in the affected tissues.[32] These include impaired immunity, chronic inflammation, and progressive fibroadipose deposition.[33] The following chapter subparts provide detailed information about the role of the lymphatic system in tissue fluid homeostasis and immune response.

1.3.1 The Lymphatic System to Transport Lymph Fluid (Circulating System)

Florian Früh and Epameinondas Gousopoulos

The blood vascular system is a closed and pressurized circuit, consisting of arteries, veins, and capillaries. It plays a pivotal role in the transfer of oxygen, nutrients, and hormones to peripheral tissues and at the same time collects the produced carbon dioxide and metabolic waste products. Blood pressure causes the extravasation of plasma constituents from the arterial side of the capillary bed into the interstitial space.[34]

The lymphatic vasculature exists in parallel to the blood vasculature and consists of a one-way transport system for fluid, macromolecules, and immune cells, which are collected from the interstitial space to eventually drain back to the central blood circulation.[35] In contrast to the earlier textbook dogma that most of the extravasated fluid is reabsorbed by the venous system, recent studies revealed that the lymphatic system represents the main drainage route for extravasated interstitial fluid, whereas venules reabsorb fluid only under certain conditions.[36] However, there are exceptions, such as the kidney and the intestinal mucosa, where venous fluid absorption is sustained by local epithelial secretions. With an estimated fluid turnover of approximately 8 L per day, where a great majority is transported through the lymphatic system, we can appreciate its major contribution in tissue fluid homeostasis.[37]

Lymphatic fluid is produced at the capillary blind ends of the lymphatic vasculature. The lymphatic capillaries, or alternatively initial lymphatic vessels, consist of a single layer of overlapping, oak-leaf-shaped LECs. The initial lymphatics lack an organized basement membrane and are deprived of pericytes.[38] They are attached to the interstitial tissue via anchoring filaments and adhere to the neighboring endothelial cells via button-junctions.[39] The overlapping LECs form a primary valve, which allows unidirectional flow of lymphatic fluid, macromolecules, and immune cells from the interstitium into the lymphatic capillary space.[40] In instances of high interstitial pressure, lymphatic drainage can be modulated by transmitting tissue pressure to the anchoring filaments. This opens the primary lymphatic valves, thus increasing the paracellular passage of fluid, macromolecules, and immune cells. However, lymph formation may not be a completely passive process. Recent research has revealed that active transcellular mechanisms, via transport of lipids and high-density lipoprotein, could contribute to lymph production.[41]

Lymph flows from the lymphatic capillaries toward the collecting lymphatic vessels, which are lined with a basement membrane and tight zipper-like junctions that interconnect their LECs.[42] Despite the initial belief that collecting lymphatic vessels are "impermeable," it has now been demonstrated that they are indeed permeable to solute and fluid. Their albumin permeability is comparable to that of the postcapillary venules and can be modulated by several signaling pathways, including nitric oxide.[43]

The unidirectional flow of the lymph in the collecting lymphatic vessels is maintained by a combination of intrinsic and extrinsic forces. It is estimated that approximately one-third of lymph transport in the human lower extremities occurs as a result to skeletal muscle contraction (extrinsic pump), whereas the active (intrinsic) pumping of the lymphatic vascular network accounts for the remaining two-thirds.[44] The SMCs covering the collecting lymphatic vessels are the driving force of the robust contractions propelling the lymph against a hydrostatic pressure gradient and one-way valves help to protect against backflow.[45,46]

The functional unit of the lymphatic vasculature is called a lymphangion, which is defined as the segment of the collecting lymphatic vessels between two intraluminal valves. Effective lymph propulsion requires robust spontaneous contractions of the lymphatic SMCs as well as coordination of contraction waves over the length of a lymphangion. As such, active lymphatic pumping results in a net outflow of the collector equal to the centripetal flow due to the contraction minus the reflux through the valves in a contraction cycle.[47]

The lymphatic pump is modulated by four major factors, which are linked to the function of the lymphatic muscle: (i) preload, (ii) afterload, (iii) contraction frequency, and (iv) contractility (i.e., inotropy). Preload and afterload are determined by the end-diastolic pressure and outflow pressure, respectively. An increased filling pressure results in increased pump output. Similarly, increased outflow pressure, as a result of increased central venous pressure or partial outflow obstruction, increases the load against which the pump has to eject.[48,49] The contraction frequency is highly sensitive to such pressure changes and even minute changes in the range of 0.5 cm H_2O can double the contraction frequency. In regard to contractility, this term is commonly used to describe the amplitude or frequency of contractions in response to pressure changes or agonist activation. The term refers to inotropy; increased contractility means positive inotropy, and thus increase in the strength and velocity of the contractual force under constant preload. Other parameters affecting the lymphatic pump include neural influences, coordinated muscle cell contraction (contraction synchrony), and proper lymphatic valve and barrier function.[47]

Any of these parameters affecting lymphatic function may be compromised to a certain extent in a number of pathologies and/or after treatment of diseases (e.g., surgery, radiotherapy) to develop primary (i.e., inherited) or secondary forms of lymphedema.[18]

1.3.2 The Lymphatic System and Its Immunological Function

Patrick A. Will

The immune system is more closely related to the lymphatic system than any other anatomical system or organ in the human body. The thymus, a primary lymphoid organ, develops the T cells from thymocytes of hematopoietic origin and dendritic cells (DC). In a further process, selection and maturation of a tolerogenic T cell repertoire set the foundation of self-tolerance.[50] Failure in this process, called central tolerance, may lead to autoimmune disease or severe immunosuppression.

The lymphatic system comprises a vast network of vessels together with secondary lymphoid tissues all over the body. Immune cells and antigen-carrying particles (i.e., microvesicles, exosomes and apoptotic bodies) circulate from the peripheral tissues to secondary lymphatic organs (SLOs) through the lymphatic vasculature.[51] SLOs include the lymph nodes, the spleen, the tonsils, the Peyer's patches, and the mucosa-associated lymphoid tissue (MALT). Therefore, the lymphatic system represents the first line of contact and defense against environmental pathogens and noxious stimuli.

T cell migration from peripheral tissues takes place via afferent lymphatic vessels. While $CD4^+$ cells seem to crawl out more efficiently via afferent lymphatic vessels, $CD8^+$ cells exhibit only a minimum migration rate and are therefore crucial for tissular immunological memory and defense.[52] Similar to DC and neutrophils, T cells migrate actively from tissue into the lymphatic capillaries under homeostatic and inflammatory conditions.[52] This active crawling is regulated by a fine-tuned microenvironmental chemotactic stimulation, generated not only by macrophages and fibroblasts but also by a molecular crosstalk of LEC with T cells.[53] The interaction of sphingosine-1-phosphate (S1P) with their receptors 1 and 3 (S1PR1 and S1PR3) on T cells represents the main chemotactic pathway for T cell migration since it has been shown that $CD4^+$ and $CD8^+$ cells expressing S1PR1 on the surface migrate faster through the lymphatic system.[54] In contrast, when the S1PR were antagonized on T cells, no active crawling was observed.[54] LEC were identified as the major source of S1 P.[55] Consequently, S1 P level is low in tissue and high in the lymphatic system, creating the described chemotactic gradient for cells expressing S1PR1 and S1PR3. Thus, not only migration but survival, proliferation, and cytoskeletal arrangements of lymphocytes are related to the upregulation of S1PR1.[56]

Since S1 P chemotactic gradient generated by LEC is the main migratory mechanism for T cells during inflammation and homeostatic conditions, a local regulatory process should exist to modulate peripheric immune response. One molecule that crucially promotes internalization and degradation of S1PR1 on resident T cells, and hereby homing of T cells, is CD69. Low expression of CD69 on cells will therefore result in upregulation of S1PR1 and transmigration of immune cells from peripheral tissue into lymphatics and likewise from the afferent lymphatic vessels into the secondary lymphoid organs.[57]

A second key immunomodulatory mechanism of immune cell trafficking is the chemotactic gradient mediated by the expression of C-C chemokine receptor type 7 (CCR7) and complementary C-C-C chemokine receptor 4 (CXCR4). Chemotaxis of CCR7 and CXCR4 have the opposite effect on T cells than the chemotactic gradient of S1RP1 and are mostly secreted by locoregional immune cells. Peripheral immune cells trafficking is regulated by a balance of these two chemotactic mechanisms (▶ Fig. 1.6).

Macrophages and DCs are not only the first line of defense against noxious stimuli, they also represent the main antigen-presenting cells. Only very few naïve T cells are found in the peripheral tissue and blood; hence, an essential function of DC is to carry newly acquired antigens from peripheral tissue into SLOs like lymph nodes where T cell activation and maturation occurs.

In contrast to T cells, where CCR7 inhibits migration from tissue and lymph nodes, DC migration from the skin, lungs, and intestine is dependent on CCR7 interaction.[58] Accordingly, and after decades of research, unequivocal consent exists: when CCR7 is overexpressed in any subpopulation of the mononuclear phagocyte system (i.e., macrophages, DCs, monocytes, and monocyte-derived cells), transmigration occurs.[59] Since the discovery of lymphatic vessels in the CNS, two mechanisms of immune surveillance and antigen presentation have been proposed. Antigens and immune cells first drain from the subventricular and subarachnoid space to the cribriform plate up to the nasal mucosa to the circulatory system

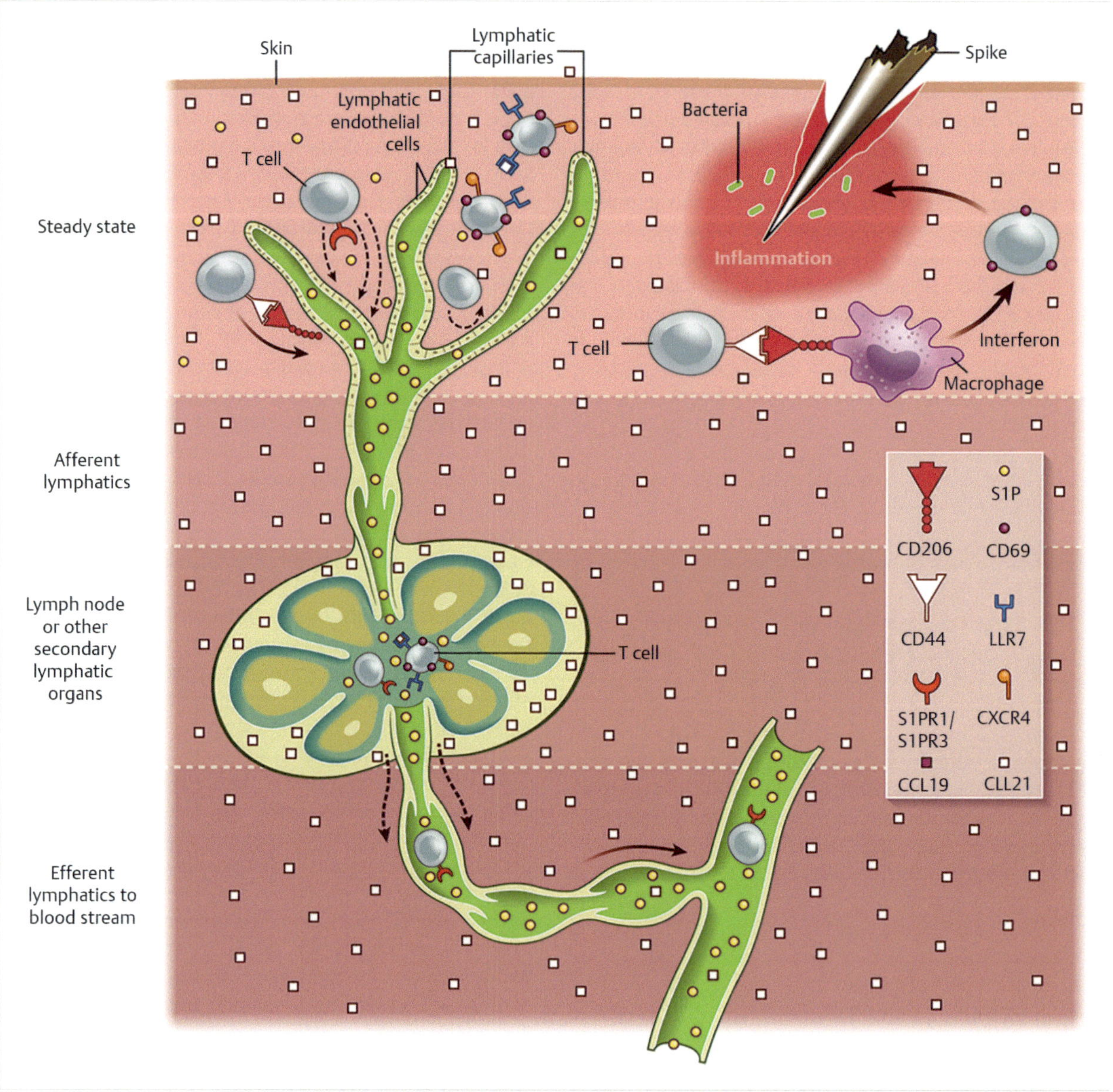

Fig. 1.6 Schematic overview of the main migratory mechanisms of T cells from peripheral tissue to the lymphatic system. (Primordial image development and conception courtesy of Patrick A. Will.)

and second, meningeal lymphatic vessels drain through the venous sinuses.[60] Interestingly, a CCR7-dependent migration of DC and macrophages from the CNS has not been demonstrated yet, whereas S1PR1 and CXCR4-dependent transmigration into the cervical lymph nodes has been suggested.[61] In the remaining organs, no further evidence of any other chemotactic mechanism has been described, suggesting a pivotal monoregulatory role of the CCR7-CCL21 axis for leukocytes and macrophages trafficking.

In order to transmigrate, leukocytes and macrophages require the expression of galectin-1, semaphorins, and integrins on LEC and on themselves, and a simultaneous downregulation of E-cadherins.[53,58] This common immunoregulatory mechanism, shared by all immune cells, is mediated by two phenotypic markers of LEC, podoplanin and lymphatic vessel endothelial hyaluronan receptor 1 (LYVE-1). They play a central immunological role by allowing adhesion and cleavage of immune cells for their migration through the lymphatic monolayers.[62,63] In inflammatory conditions, LEC can upregulate podoplanin and LYVE-1 to increase monocyte migration from the blood into the inflammation site and favor macrophage and leukocytes migration back from the tissue to present the acquired antigens.[58]

Overall, the lymphatic system not only provides a pipeline for immune cell migration but also actively regulates and modulates the peripheral immune response and surveillance. Therefore, a well-adjusted paracrine and autocrine chemotactic gradient is generated by LEC in response to continuous crosstalk between cells and the microenvironment. By regulating migration of immune cells, antigen presentation, immune response, and immunological memory, new therapeutic strategies might be addressed in the future. For example, it has been shown that LEC can be primed by cancer cells to provide local immunotolerance for tumors.[64] Accordingly, immune therapies could be developed to regain homeostasis at the molecular crosstalk between immune cells and LEC in autoimmune, cancer, and chronic inflammatory diseases.

1.4 Lymphangiogenesis

Patrick A. Will

Lymphangiogenesis is a complex process of lymphatic cell differentiation, proliferation, migration, sprouting, and tube formation that occurs not only in early embryological stages but also in different clinically relevant conditions. Besides lymphedema, the dysfunction of the lymphatic system has proven to be involved in numerous pathologic conditions, such as atherosclerosis, cancer, chronic inflammation, dermal infections, fibrosis, hypertension, and obesity.[65]

The microvascular system of the lymphatics develops *in utero* after the blood vessels have been formed. Numerous lymphangiogenic transcription factors such as SRY-Box 18 (SOX 18), PROX1, and COUP transcription factor 2 (COUP-TFII) are involved in the early lymphangiogenesis.[66] Details regarding the embryological development of the lymphatic system are reviewed in **Subchapter 1.1** of this book. In this chapter, the lymphangiogenesis after the embryonic development will be discussed. Of the early transcription factors, only the expression of PROX1 remains necessary for maintaining the lymphatic identity and phenotype. All further lymphangiogenesis and lymphatic sprouting will be chiefly regulated by VEGF-C and its corresponding receptor VEGFR-3.[67]

The interaction of VEGF-C and VEGF-D with its specific receptor VEGFR-3 is the main driver of lymphangiogenesis. VEGFR-3 was one of the first LEC surface molecules to be discovered and exhibits a remarkably similar structure when compared to its homologous receptors VEGFR-1 and VEGFR-2, both of which are involved in angiogenesis.[68] In contrast to them, VEGFR-3 has a minor affinity for the angiogenic factors VEGF-A and VEGF-B, yet a high affinity for VEGF-C and vascular endothelial growth factor D (VEGF-D). The interaction of VEGF-C and VEGF-D with VEGFR3 is the major regulator and promotor in lymphangiogenesis, both in physiological and pathophysiological states.[68] VEGF-C and VEGF-D are not only the key drivers of LEC proliferation, but also central in their migration, tube formation, and survival. Despite the well-known importance of these growth factors and their receptors for lymphangiogenesis, the detailed downstream signaling remains obscured.[70] The most precisely identified intracellular transduction of VEGF-C in LEC is the protein kinase C-dependent activation of the extracellular signal–regulated kinases 1 and 2 (ERK1 and ERK2), followed by a phosphorylation cascade mediated by Akt.[71] According to the latest investigations, the VEGFR-3 co-receptor neuropilin 2 (NRP2) seems to modulate this signal transduction and could be another molecular target of lymphangiogenesis.[72]

In contrast to angiogenesis, where delta-notch signaling has been specifically proposed as the main regulator of lymphatic vascular sprouting, current knowledge implies that sprouting and tube formation in lymphangiogenesis are primarily dependent on a microenvironment with autocrine chemotactic signaling. In inflammatory states, prostaglandins are linked to lymphangiogenesis via VEGF-C.[73]

When locoregional immune cells are activated in the inflammatory tissue, an increased level of different cytokines, enzymes, and chemokines follows. Prostaglandins and leukotrienes will promote the transmigration of more immune cells from the capillary bed to the affected tissue. The immune cell trafficking is guided by a chemokine gradient of cells expressing CCR7 and chemokine ligand 21 (CCL21). In a pro-lymphangiogenic condition, the molecular crosstalk of the immune cells with LEC will neutralize the migration of lymphocytes and macrophages from the tissue into the lymphatic system.[68] Homed immune cells will produce and activate isoforms of VEGF-C and VEGF-D along with a secretion that result in a chemotactic forward loop to attract more immune cells.[74] The perpetuation of this cycle is responsible for lymphatic vessel sprouting and increased lymphatic luminal flow. This is the molecular reason why expression of chemokine receptors in cancer cells is considered a prognostic marker for lymphatic metastasis in breast, colon, liver, and skin cancers.[68] Further, the enzyme involved in the synthesis of prostaglandins (i.e., cyclooxygenase 2) and the prostaglandin receptors expressed by immune cells and tumor cells are currently considered to be the major immunomodulators of lymphangiogenesis in chronic inflammation and cancer.[75]

It is important to remark that many other cytokines have been associated with the induction of lymphangiogenesis through modulation of VEGF-C and VEGF-D expression.[76] Some of them are fibroblast growth factor (FGF-2), epidermal growth factor (EGF), adrenomedullin, S1P, platelet-derived growth factor B (PDGF-B), endothelin-1 (Et-1), angiopoietins, hypoxia-inducible factor 1α (HIF1α), hepatocyte growth factor (HGF), and insulin-like growth factor 1 (IGF-1).[68,77] Paradoxically, the dominant proinflammatory and profibrotic cytokine transforming growth factor β (TGF-β) has been described to be a negative regulator of lymphangiogenesis *in vivo*.[78]

1.4.1 Potential Therapeutic Approaches and Future Perspectives

Current knowledge of lymphangiogenesis has been predominantly gained using *in vitro* experimentation and studies with specific knockout models. Consequently, the complexity of the molecular interactions *in vivo* of the different regulatory mechanisms of lymphangiogenesis is still not fully understood. The details of the downstream pathways of VEGFR-3, the influence of regional immune cells, and specific cytokines during inflammatory states are some topics that remain to be investigated.

References

[1] Alitalo K, Tammela T, Petrova TV. Lymphangiogenesis in development and human disease. Nature. 2005; 438(7070):946–953

[2] Oliver G. Lymphatic vasculature development. Nat Rev Immunol. 2004; 4(1):35–45

[3] Jeltsch M, Tammela T, Alitalo K, Wilting J. Genesis and pathogenesis of lymphatic vessels. Cell Tissue Res. 2003; 314(1):69–84

[4] Sabin FR. The lymphatic system in human embryos, with a consideration of the morphology of the system as a whole. Am J Anat. 1909; 9:43–91

[5] van der Putte SC. The development of the lymphatic system in man. Adv Anat Embryol Cell Biol. 1975; 51(1):3–60

[6] Sabin FR. On the origin of the lymphatic system from the veins, and the development of the lymph hearts and thoracic duct in the pig. Am J Anat. 1902; 1:367–389

[7] Huntington GS, McClure CFW. The anatomy and development of the jugular lymph sacs in the domestic cat (Felis domestica). Am J Anat. 1910; 10:177–312

[8] Kukk E, Lymboussaki A, Taira S, et al. VEGF-C receptor binding and pattern of expression with VEGFR-3 suggests a role in lymphatic vascular development. Development. 1996; 122(12):3829–3837

[9] Wigle JT, Oliver G. Prox1 function is required for the development of the murine lymphatic system. Cell. 1999; 98(6):769–778

[10] Oliver G, Harvey N. A stepwise model of the development of lymphatic vasculature. Ann N Y Acad Sci. 2002; 979:159–165, discussion 188–196

[11] Yang Y, Oliver G. Development of the mammalian lymphatic vasculature. J Clin Invest. 2014; 124(3):888–897

[12] François M, Caprini A, Hosking B, et al. Sox18 induces development of the lymphatic vasculature in mice. Nature. 2008; 456(7222): 643–647

[13] Karkkainen MJ, Haiko P, Sainio K, et al. Vascular endothelial growth factor C is required for sprouting of the first lymphatic vessels from embryonic veins. Nat Immunol. 2004; 5(1):74–80

[14] Yang Y, García-Verdugo JM, Soriano-Navarro M, et al. Lymphatic endothelial progenitors bud from the cardinal vein and intersomitic vessels in mammalian embryos. Blood. 2012; 120(11):2340–2348

[15] Wilting J, Aref Y, Huang R, et al. Dual origin of avian lymphatics. Dev Biol. 2006; 292(1):165–173

[16] Martinez-Corral I, Ulvmar MH, Stanczuk L, et al. Nonvenous origin of dermal lymphatic vasculature. Circ Res. 2015; 116(10):1649–1654

[17] Klotz L, Norman S, Vieira JM, et al. Cardiac lymphatics are heterogeneous in origin and respond to injury. Nature. 2015; 522 (7554):62–67

[18] Aspelund A, Robciuc MR, Karaman S, Makinen T, Alitalo K. Lymphatic system in cardiovascular medicine. Circ Res. 2016; 118 (3):515–530

[19] Aselli G. De Lactibus Sive Lacteis Venis. Milan, Italy: J.B. Bidellius; 1627

[20] Nuck A. Adenographia curiosa et uteri foeminei anatome nova. Lugduni Batavorum: P. vander Aa; 1692

[21] Suami H, Taylor GI, Pan WR. A new radiographic cadaver injection technique for investigating the lymphatic system. Plast Reconstr Surg. 2005; 115(7):2007–2013

[22] Scaglioni MF, Suami H. Lymphatic anatomy of the inguinal region in aid of vascularized lymph node flap harvesting. J Plast Reconstr Aesthet Surg. 2015; 68(3):419–427

[23] Leak LV. Electron microscopic observations on lymphatic capillaries and the structural components of the connective tissue-lymph interface. Microvasc Res. 1970; 2(4):361–391

[24] Kubik S. The role of the lateral upper arm bundle and the lymphatic watersheds in the formation of collateral pathways in lymphedema. Acta Biol Acad Sci Hung. 1980; 31(1–3):191–200

[25] Suami H, Scaglioni MF. Anatomy of the lymphatic system and the lymphosome concept with reference to lymphedema. Semin Plast Surg. 2018; 32(1):5–11

[26] Alitalo K, Tammela T, Petrova TV. Lymphangiogenesis in development and human disease. Nature. 2005; 438(7070):946–953

[27] Bernier-Latmani J, Cisarovsky C, Demir CS, et al. DLL4 promotes continuous adult intestinal lacteal regeneration and dietary fat transport. J Clin Invest. 2015; 125(12):4572–4586

[28] Choe K, Jang JY, Park I, et al. Intravital imaging of intestinal lacteals unveils lipid drainage through contractility. J Clin Invest. 2015; 125 (11):4042–4052

[29] Louveau A, Smirnov I, Keyes TJ, et al. Structural and functional features of central nervous system lymphatic vessels. Nature. 2015; 523(7560):337–341

[30] Aspelund A, Antila S, Proulx ST, et al. A dural lymphatic vascular system that drains brain interstitial fluid and macromolecules. J Exp Med. 2015; 212(7):991–999

[31] Da Mesquita S, Louveau A, Vaccari A, et al. Functional aspects of meningeal lymphatics in ageing and Alzheimer's disease. Nature. 2018; 560(7717):185–191

[32] Rockson SG. Causes and consequences of lymphatic disease. Ann N Y Acad Sci. 2010; 1207 Suppl 1:E2–E6

[33] Dayan JH, Ly CL, Kataru RP, Mehrara BJ. Lymphedema: pathogenesis and novel therapies. Annu Rev Med. 2018; 69:263–276

[34] Choi I, Lee S, Hong YK. The new era of the lymphatic system: no longer secondary to the blood vascular system. Cold Spring Harb Perspect Med. 2012; 2(4):a006445

[35] Adams RH, Alitalo K. Molecular regulation of angiogenesis and lymphangiogenesis. Nat Rev Mol Cell Biol. 2007; 8(6):464–478

[36] Levick JR, Michel CC. Microvascular fluid exchange and the revised Starling principle. Cardiovasc Res. 2010; 87(2):198–210

[37] Wiig H, Swartz MA. Interstitial fluid and lymph formation and transport: physiological regulation and roles in inflammation and cancer. Physiol Rev. 2012; 92(3):1005–1060

[38] Tammela T, Alitalo K. Lymphangiogenesis: molecular mechanisms and future promise. Cell. 2010; 140(4):460–476

[39] Leak LV, Burke JF. Ultrastructural studies on the lymphatic anchoring filaments. J Cell Biol. 1968; 36(1):129–149

[40] Trzewik J, Mallipattu SK, Artmann GM, Delano FA, Schmid-Schönbein GW. Evidence for a second valve system in lymphatics: endothelial microvalves. FASEB J. 2001; 15(10):1711–1717

[41] Lim HY, Thiam CH, Yeo KP, et al. Lymphatic vessels are essential for the removal of cholesterol from peripheral tissues by SR-BI-mediated transport of HDL. Cell Metab. 2013; 17(5):671–684

[42] Baluk P, Fuxe J, Hashizume H, et al. Functionally specialized junctions between endothelial cells of lymphatic vessels. J Exp Med. 2007; 204 (10):2349–2362

[43] Scallan JP, Hill MA, Davis MJ. Lymphatic vascular integrity is disrupted in type 2 diabetes due to impaired nitric oxide signalling. Cardiovasc Res. 2015; 107(1):89–97

[44] Engeset A, Olszewski W, Jaeger PM, Sokolowski J, Theodorsen L. Twenty-four hour variation in flow and composition of leg lymph in normal men. Acta Physiol Scand. 1977; 99(2):140–148

[45] Davis MJ, Rahbar E, Gashev AA, Zawieja DC, Moore JE, Jr. Determinants of valve gating in collecting lymphatic vessels from rat mesentery. Am J Physiol Heart Circ Physiol. 2011; 301(1):H48–H60

[46] von der Weid PY, Zawieja DC. Lymphatic smooth muscle: the motor unit of lymph drainage. Int J Biochem Cell Biol. 2004; 36(7):1147–1153
[47] Scallan JP, Zawieja SD, Castorena-Gonzalez JA, Davis MJ. Lymphatic pumping: mechanics, mechanisms and malfunction. J Physiol. 2016; 594(20):5749–5768
[48] Davis MJ, Davis AM, Lane MM, Ku CW, Gashev AA. Rate-sensitive contractile responses of lymphatic vessels to circumferential stretch. J Physiol. 2009; 587(1):165–182
[49] Davis MJ, Scallan JP, Wolpers JH, Muthuchamy M, Gashev AA, Zawieja DC. Intrinsic increase in lymphangion muscle contractility in response to elevated afterload. Am J Physiol Heart Circ Physiol. 2012; 303(7):H795–H808
[50] Humbert M, Hugues S, Dubrot J. Shaping of peripheral T cell responses by lymphatic endothelial cells. Front Immunol. 2017; 7:684
[51] Gerner MY, Torabi-Parizi P, Germain RN. Strategically localized dendritic cells promote rapid T cell responses to lymph-borne particulate antigens. Immunity. 2015; 42(1):172–185
[52] Gebhardt T, Whitney PG, Zaid A, et al. Different patterns of peripheral migration by memory CD4+and CD8+T cells. Nature. 2011; 477(7363):216–219
[53] Hunter MC, Teijeira A, Halin C. T cell trafficking through lymphatic vessels. Front Immunol. 2016; 7:613
[54] Matloubian M, Lo CG, Cinamon G, et al. Lymphocyte egress from thymus and peripheral lymphoid organs is dependent on S1P receptor 1. Nature. 2004; 427(6972):355–360
[55] Pham THM, Baluk P, Xu Y, et al. Lymphatic endothelial cell sphingosine kinase activity is required for lymphocyte egress and lymphatic patterning. J Exp Med. 2010; 207(1):17–27
[56] Schwab SR, Cyster JG. Finding a way out: lymphocyte egress from lymphoid organs. Nat Immunol. 2007; 8(12):1295–1301
[57] Rosen H, Goetzl EJ. Sphingosine 1-phosphate and its receptors: an autocrine and paracrine network. Nat Rev Immunol. 2005; 5(7): 560–570
[58] Permanyer M, Bošnjak B, Förster R. Dendritic cells, T cells and lymphatics: dialogues in migration and beyond. Curr Opin Immunol. 2018; 53:173–179
[59] Worbs T, Hammerschmidt SI, Förster R. Dendritic cell migration in health and disease. Nat Rev Immunol. 2017; 17(1):30–48
[60] Louveau A, Smirnov I, Keyes TJ, et al. Structural and functional features of central nervous system lymphatic vessels. Nature. 2015; 523(7560):337–341
[61] Hatterer E, Touret M, Belin M-F, Honnorat J, Nataf S. Cerebrospinal fluid dendritic cells infiltrate the brain parenchyma and target the cervical lymph nodes under neuroinflammatory conditions. PLoS One. 2008; 3(10):e3321
[62] Acton SE, Astarita JL, Malhotra D, et al. Podoplanin-rich stromal networks induce dendritic cell motility via activation of the C-type lectin receptor CLEC-2. Immunity. 2012; 37(2):276–289
[63] Johnson LA, Banerji S, Lawrance W, et al. Dendritic cells enter lymph vessels by hyaluronan-mediated docking to the endothelial receptor LYVE-1. Nat Immunol. 2017; 18(7):762–770
[64] Stacker SA, Williams SP, Karnezis T, Shayan R, Fox SB, Achen MG. Lymphangiogenesis and lymphatic vessel remodelling in cancer. Nat Rev Cancer. 2014; 14(3):159–172
[65] Tammela T, Alitalo K. Lymphangiogenesis: molecular mechanisms and future promise. Cell. 2010; 140(4):460–476
[66] François M, Caprini A, Hosking B, et al. Sox18 induces development of the lymphatic vasculature in mice. Nature. 2008; 456(7222): 643–647
[67] Johnson NC, Dillard ME, Baluk P, et al. Lymphatic endothelial cell identity is reversible and its maintenance requires Prox1 activity. Genes Dev. 2008; 22(23):3282–3291
[68] Stacker SA, Williams SP, Karnezis T, Shayan R, Fox SB, Achen MG. Lymphangiogenesis and lymphatic vessel remodelling in cancer. Nat Rev Cancer. 2014; 14(3):159–172
[69] Visuri MT, Honkonen KM, Hartiala P, et al. VEGF-C and VEGF-C156S in the pro-lymphangiogenic growth factor therapy of lymphedema: a large animal study. Angiogenesis. 2015; 18(3): 313–326
[70] Tammela T, Enholm B, Alitalo K, Paavonen K. The biology of vascular endothelial growth factors. Cardiovasc Res. 2005; 65(3): 550–563
[71] Shibuya M. Vascular endothelial growth factor and its receptor system: physiological functions in angiogenesis and pathological roles in various diseases. J Biochem. 2013; 153(1):13–19
[72] Caunt M, Mak J, Liang W-C, et al. Blocking neuropilin-2 function inhibits tumor cell metastasis. Cancer Cell. 2008; 13(4):331–342
[73] Abouelkheir GR, Upchurch BD, Rutkowski JM. Lymphangiogenesis: fuel, smoke, or extinguisher of inflammation's fire? Exp Biol Med (Maywood). 2017; 242(8):884–895
[74] Jeltsch M, Jha SK, Tvorogov D, et al. CCBE1 enhances lymphangiogenesis via A disintegrin and metalloprotease with thrombospondin motifs-3-mediated vascular endothelial growth factor-C activation. Circulation. 2014; 129(19):1962–1971
[75] Zhang X-H, Huang D-P, Guo G-L, et al. Coexpression of VEGF-C and COX-2 and its association with lymphangiogenesis in human breast cancer. BMC Cancer. 2008; 8:4
[76] Karpanen T, Alitalo K. Molecular biology and pathology of lymphangiogenesis. Annu Rev Pathol. 2008; 3:367–397
[77] Adams RH, Alitalo K. Molecular regulation of angiogenesis and lymphangiogenesis. Nat Rev Mol Cell Biol. 2007; 8(6):464–478
[78] Clavin NW, Avraham T, Fernandez J, et al. TGF-beta1 is a negative regulator of lymphatic regeneration during wound repair. Am J Physiol Heart Circ Physiol. 2008; 295(5):H2113–H2127

2 Epidemiological, Clinical, and Pathophysiological Aspects

Summary
Lymphedema is an inefficiency of the lymphatic system which leads to, clinically, swelling and fibroadipose tissue deformation. Primary lymphedema ensues from a disorder during the development of the lymphatic system. This genetic mutation could be inheritable or occur sporadically. There is a separate group known as lymphatic malformations. Secondary lymphedema constitutes the main reason of lymphedema. Worldwide, most frequently, it is caused by filarial nematodes infection. In high-income countries lymphedema is primarily due to surgical interventions like lymphadenectomy, oncological therapies, and trauma. Prevalence and incidence of primary and secondary lymphedema are discussed in this chapter. The pathophysiological changes of lymphedema are caused by the hyaluronan-rich interstitial fluid accumulation in the interstitium. This activates a complex inflammatory response. Another pathological process in late-stage lymphedema is adipose tissue deposition. Recurrent infections of the lymphedema-affected extremity are a common side effect of lymphedema. This often indicates severity of lymphedema. Long-term tissue changes are thickening of the cutis and subcutis due to accumulation of fatty tissue, and development of fibrosis, lymphatic cysts, and fistulae. Trophic changes in the epidermis are variable. Hyperplasia, hyperkeratosis, hyperpigmentation, minor papillomatosis, and verrucous protuberances may appear.

Keywords: etiology of lymphedema, lymphatic malformations, prevalence and incidence, pathophysiology

2.1 Etiology including Lymphatic Malformations

Stephan Wagner and Jörg Wilting

Lymphedema is attributed to an inefficiency of the lymphatic system which implies, clinically, swelling and subsequent fibroadipose tissue deformation.[1] The cause of this chronic disease is the dysfunction of lymphatic transport and subsequent accumulation of lymphatic fluid. As a result, the transportation of interstitial fluid, immune cells, and lipids is disturbed.[2] The etiology of lymphedema is lymphatic damage of primary or secondary origin. Primary lymphedema is often induced congenitally while secondary lymphedema occurs due to a variety of different diseases, trauma, and inflammation.[3]

Primary lymphedema ensues from a disorder during the development of the lymphatic system. This results in a dysfunctionality which is determined at birth or more frequently in adolescence.[1] Primary lymphedema is attributed to genetic mutation caused inheritably or sporadically. The known gene mutations reveal a diversity of molecular changes affecting growth and transcription factors, membrane receptors, intracellular messengers, enzymes, and motor and proteins of the extracellular matrix.[4] The genetic mutation is often a part of a congenital syndrome such as Nonne-Milroy or Hennekam syndrome.[3] Influence on the structure of lymphatic system is common in all the disorders described. They either show an aplasia/hypoplasia or a hyperplasia of the lymphatic vessels. Additionally, the lymph nodes can be affected in terms of fibrosis or agenesis.[3]

A separate group emerges from the abnormalities of the lymphatic system during embryogenesis known as lymphatic malformations or lymphangiomas. They are described as congenital hamartomatous tumors and occur principally in head and neck or oral cavity.[5] Rarely, lymphatic malformations occur in adulthood due to trauma or infections.[5] Lymphatic malformations are suspected to originate from an inadequate sequestration of lymphatic tissue from the lymphovenous sacs. The resulting miscommunication of the lymphovenous sacs with the lymphatic or venous system leads to development of cystic bulges and consequently fluid accumulation.[5]

Secondary lymphedema constitutes the main cause of lymphedema. Worldwide, secondary lymphedema is induced most frequently by filarial nematodes infection.[6,7] Filariasis patients show gigantism of the extremities and genitals caused by direct lymphatic vessel obstruction by to the parasites.[1] Podoconiosis is another disease resulting in lymphedema in low- to middle-income countries. In this disease, mineral particles from red clay soils are incorporated while walking barefoot and block the lymphatic system.[8]

However, in low- to middle-income countries, lymphedema is primarily a consequence of surgical interventions like lymphadenectomy, oncological therapies (including radiotherapy rather than chemotherapy), infection and trauma. Often cancer-related lymphedema may develop in patients with breast cancer, melanoma, as well as gynecologic and urologic cancer.[1] Especially, patients with gynecological and urological as well as breast cancer (see **Chapter 11**) may be affected by undergoing lymph node extirpation and/or radiotherapy.[3,6] In general, patients with an excision of the pelvis, para-aortal, inguinal, or femoral lymph nodes often suffer from lymphedema.[3] The onset of secondary lymphedema is unpredictable and varies from immediately (following surgery and/or radiotherapy) to late onset, 30 years after treatment. Factors that determine the initial manifestation are scarcely known.[6]

Despite the foregoing, cancer can be the cause of lymphedema itself by invading the lymphatic vessels or lymph nodes during metastasis. Therefore, lymphedema should always be considered as carcinogenic—so-called lymphangiosis carcinomatosa.[3] Furthermore, obesity and advanced stages of chronic venous insufficiency may lead to secondary lymphedema.[3]

2.2 Prevalence

Katja Kilian

Generally speaking, the condition of lymphedema is assumed to be underreported as a result of an insufficiently reliable epidemiologic record and a lack of correct diagnosis. Consequently, it is difficult to review a valid statement on the global prevalence of chronic lymphedema.[9]

The international study "Lymphedema Impact and Prevalence International" (LIMPRINT) indicates a point-prevalence of chronic edema by evaluating patients admitted in hospital for any reason in five different countries (Denmark, France, United Kingdom, Ireland, and Australia). It predicts a prevalence of more than 38% of patients with chronic swelling. To define an edema as chronic a duration of 3 months is obligatory. Hence, the etiology or existing comorbidities were not taken into consideration.[9]

An insight of the demographics shows there is no gender difference. A majority of patients with chronic edema is older than 45 years with a mean age of 73 years.[9] The edema is mostly manifested in the lower extremity, especially below the knee. The upper limb is the second most affected area, whereby the edema is sparsely located in the head and neck and genital regions. The edema lasts from 6 months (25%) to more than 10 years. Main side effects are cellulitis and infections; the former was the leading reason for hospitalization.[9]

According to the LIMPRINT study, the main etiology of chronic edema is a venous disease. Cancer constitutes under 10% of the main cause. In addition, it is induced more by cancer treatment than by metastasis. Less than 5% of the patients with chronic edema have a primary lymphedema.[9] Taking the prevalence of risk factors into consideration about 30% of the patients are obese. Moreover, there is association with heart failure (35%), diabetes mellitus (22%), neurological deficiency (18%), and peripheral arterial disease (5.6%).[9] This study focuses on chronic edema on the whole. A closer look at the epidemiological numbers of lymphedema is taken in the following.

In general, secondary lymphedema is the most common condition of lymphedema and, therefore, it is the most thoroughly investigated one. Globally, the parasitic infectious disease filariasis is mainly responsible for developing lymphedema affecting millions of patients (see **Chapter 3**).[6] The estimation of the prevalence varies greatly (see **Subchapter 3.2**). According to the World Health Organization (WHO),[7] about 120 million people were infected in 2000. It is predicted that filariasis is the main cause of permanent disfigurement in the world and the second most common reason for long-term disability. Worldwide, 40 million people with filariasis infection show disfigurement and disability.[7]

Filariasis occurs predominantly in the tropical countries of Africa, Asia, and Central and South America. It is transmitted by mosquitos and will be influenced by the prevalence of parasitic diseases due to climate change. The global warming and the following weather changes may result in spread of endemic areas and new countries will be affected. Additionally, traveling, international trade, and migration to bigger cities will cause increasing spread of parasitic infectious diseases. To conclude, filariasis remains an issue for the future, although the WHO declared filariasis as eradicable in 1997 and its elimination was aimed by 2020.[7]

Podoconiosis is a further condition of secondary lymphedema in low-income countries. The prevalence is between 1 and 80 per 1,000 depending on the country described. It is mostly found in Africa and in some parts of Asia and Latin America.[8]

Secondary lymphedema due to infectious lymphangitis is also an issue in developed countries. Streptococci infections are often responsible for the destruction of the lymphatic vessels. The involved fibrosis and thrombosis of the lymphatic vessels lead subsequently to lymphedema. A precise prevalence for that condition is not mentioned in literature.[10]

In the developed countries, secondary lymphedema is mostly a consequence of surgical interventions such as lymphadenectomy and/or radiotherapy.[6] It is reported that around 2 to 5 million Americans suffer from secondary lymphedema.[6] The reason for the procedures is mainly cancer. In 2007, Brayton et al determined a prevalence of 0.95%, constituting patients with all kinds of cancers. Furthermore, they observed an increase in the prevalence to 1.24% in 2013.[11]

Lymph node dissection and radiotherapy are often indicated and therefore performed for the treatment of melanoma, as well as head and neck, genitourinary, gynecological, and breast cancer. One out of 6 patients with a solid tumor are assumed to develop lymphedema after treatment.[1] However, breast cancer is the most common cause for secondary lymphedema in developed countries.[6] Thus, secondary lymphedema of the upper extremities has been researched relatively well.[1]

Apart from the cancer-related lymphedema, secondary lymphedema can be a consequence of trauma and iatrogenic circumstances. Primarily, it is related to an influence of non-lymphatic vasculature. In peripheral arterial disease, 30% of stage II and 80% of stages III and IV show lymphedema. About 0.5% of patients with varicose vein surgery are also affected. In saphenous vein harvesting for a bypass operation the risk is calculated to be 10%.

In addition, severe burn is a potential cause of lymphedema. The prevalence amounts to 1% in a burn unit. Patients who undergo a noncancer-related penile surgery may develop a lymphedema as a post-surgical complication. Other medical interventions such as intrathecal infusions for analgesia and sirolimus administration after organ transplantation increase the risk of lymphedema as well.[10]

Primary lymphedema is a rare disease so its prevalence can only be estimated. Smeltzer et al reckon a prevalence of 1:87,000 for under 20-year-olds.[12] This constitutes about 1% of all lymphedema patients.[4] Often primary lymphedema is caused by heritable diseases. If the lymphedema is due to a congenital disorder, autosomal dominant transmission like in the lymphedema-distichiasis syndrome will be found in the majority.[10]

Approximately 12% of vascular anomalies in pediatrics are ascribed to lymphatic malformations. Additionally, mixed, low-flow lymphatics venous malformations account for about 10%. In general, occurrence of lymphatic malformation is assessed to be 1 in 500 live births.[13] Mainly, the diagnosis is made at young age—from prenatal to the first few years of life. Nevertheless, it can appear at any age.[14] There is no gender predilection, and it is accompanied by infection or local trauma.[13,14]

2.3 Incidence

Katja Kilian

The incidence rate of primary lymphedema is supposed to be low. Dale et al calculated a probability of 1:6,000 of developing primary lymphedema at birth.[15] In contrast, Smeltzer et al. described an incidence rate of 1.15/100,000 related to the diagnosis of primary lymphedema in adolescents under 20 years of age.[12] About 10% of the patients with primary lymphedema present the disease in adulthood.[16] Various studies indicate a higher appearance in women by a factor of three[15] to four[12] times.

In secondary lymphedema, it is difficult to determine the incidence precisely and the variation depends on the country. The incidence is estimated to be between 0.13% and 2% in developed countries.[3] In secondary lymphedema, the incidence rate is rising due to the increase of the risk factors such as obesity, cancer treatment, and aging.[3] The older the patients are the higher is the risk of secondary lymphedema. Malignant tumors, however, and their treatment represent the highest risk. Hence, lymphadenectomy in the inguinal region tends to develop lymphedema more often than the excision of axillary lymph nodes.[17]

Secondary lymphedema of the upper extremities occurring as a result of tumor therapy has been quite well researched. Cancer-related secondary lymphedema can be a consequence of several different cancer formations. Indeed, some 20% of patients with advanced cancer suffer from lymphedema.[18] Metastatic lymphadenopathy, venous compression, and hypoalbuminemia are the main reasons for developing lymphedema. If a lymphedema is present, it will predict a poor outcome. Thus, it is one of the prognostic factors in "Prognosis in Palliative Care Study" (PiPS).[18]

In two big meta-analysis the incidence of arm lymphedema after axillary lymphadenectomy was assessed to be approximately 21%[19] to 24%.[17] Worldwide approximately 295,000 new cases of upper extremity lymphedema are diagnosed annually.

Perusing the literature of cancer-related lymphedema, breast cancer is one of the most prominent causes. With rise in the breast cancer incidence rate, the relevance of secondary lymphedema subsequently comes to the fore.[19] After a sentinel lymph node biopsy around 5.6% of patients with breast cancer develop a lymphedema 12 to 24 months postoperatively. Breast cancer patients with further excision of axillary lymph nodes are affected in 19.9%.[19] Dayan et al even mentioned a lymphedema risk of 20% to 50% after complete axillary lymph node dissection.[1] The recent preference of sentinel lymph node biopsy to the total lymphadenectomy consequently reduces the risk of lymphedema.

Rupp et al. looked at the breast cancer-related lymphedema, performing a long-term observation. They determined that patients with breast cancer have a high risk for lymphedema: About 35% of breast cancer patients have lymphedema after a mean observation time of 10 years independently of the duration and severity. Around 4% of them have a complete reversibility of the lymphedema within the first year after radiotherapy which complies with stage 0 lymphedema. Approximately 7.5% present a reversible (stage 1) but recurrent lymphedema stage. A majority (23.5%) of the affected patients shows stage 2 to 3 lymphedema. If lymphedema occurs, about 90% are affected during the first year after radiotherapy.[20]

Breast cancer-related lymphedema is influenced by adjuvant chemotherapy as a risk factor.[20] Other risk factors are indicated in the literature. Obesity at the time of cancer diagnosis raises the risk of lymphedema significantly.[3] Radiotherapy, type of surgical intervention, physiotherapeutic treatment, and number of lymph nodes removed also increase the probability of lymphedema.[21]

Mostly, the data on cancer-related lymphedema is gathered from high-income countries.[21] Low- to middle-income countries are underrepresented. Besides the low number of these studies, the differences in measurement methods and treatment cause a high heterogeneity.[21] Thus, no prediction of the sociodemographic impact of cancer-related lymphedema can be determined.

Secondary lymphedema in the lower leg after lymphadenectomy of aortal, iliacal, or inguinal lymph nodes appears on average in about 16/100 patients.[17] However, there can be an incidence of 50% depending on how radical the operation is. Lymphedema of the lower leg is often a result of gynecological cancer. Preoperatively, the incidence of lymphedema amounts to 27%.[18] Regarding lymph node excision in gynecological tumors, a high variety exists.[3] An incidence of between 20%[3] and 60%[22] after a gynecological surgical procedure is reported. The different outcome is due to the fact that there are no official diagnostic criteria. Furthermore, diversity in treatment, surgical intervention, and measurement produces the variation.[23]

If lymphedema follows after gynecological cancer therapy, 40% of the developed lymphedema will occur only once after the treatment. Thus, in the majority of cases, the lymphedema remains.[18] The general risk factors for a patient with a gynecological cancer are similar to the ones in breast cancer. Extensive lymph node dissection, chemotherapy, radiation, and comorbidity of vulvar or vaginal cancers are known. As modifiable risk factors, a high body mass index and a low level of physical activity are mentioned. Interestingly, cancer of the gynecological tract also affects the lymphatic system in another way: in about 20% to 30% of cases, a lymphocele is reported. Often it is diagnosed during postoperative imaging by accident.[23]

Lymphedema as a risk of surgical treatment of patients with melanomas has a high impact. After the excision of the melanoma-related lymph nodes, lymphedema is a frequent postoperative complication. Hence, the type of surgical intervention is essential. Single excision of the sentinel lymph node in the axilla shows an incidence of 5%. If all the lymph nodes are removed in the axilla, the incidence will be about 31%. Interventions in the inguinal region have even a higher risk. About 25% of the patients have a lymphedema after a sentinel lymph node biopsy in the groin. After a whole dissection of inguinal lymph nodes, about 83% of the patients suffer from lymphedema.[18]

In cancer of the head and neck, lymphedema is also reported as a common result of the treatment. Surgical treatment, radiation, or combination of both may lead to lymphedema. It can appear externally in the region of the face and neck or internally in the larynx or pharynx. In more than 90% of cases, lymphedema develops internally, externally, or in both regions during the first 18 months after treatment. External occurrence is more often than internal. A combination of both exists least of all.[18]

2.4 Pathophysiology

Katja Kilian

Pathophysiological changes in lymphedema cause fluid stasis in the interstitium. This can be due to two reasons: a higher fluid inflow from the blood vessels into the interstitium or a lower fluid output from the interstitium in the lymphatic vessel system.[3] The fluid accumulates in the subcutaneous and subfascial tissues. As a result, symptoms of heaviness, tightness, and pitting edema occur.[1] Despite this, fluid accumulation in the interstitium is not the only origin of lymphedema. In the following the different events of complex tissue changes will be described. However, the chronological order still remains unknown.[24]

If the accumulation of hyaluronan-rich interstitial fluid remains, the initial destruction of the collateral lymphatics will follow. During this process, an inflammatory response is activated. CD4 + T cells play an essential part. It is shown that in lymphedema tissue about 70% of the inflammatory cells are CD4 + T cells.[2] Moreover, a high number of CD4 + T cell is correlated with a more severe lymphedema. On the other hand, a lack of CD4 + T cells and inhibition of their proliferation or differentiation prevents development of lymphedema.[1]

CD4 + T cells in lymphedema consist of a mixture of T regulatory (Treg) cells, and T helper cells type 1 (Th1) and type 2 (Th2). The activation of Th2 cells contributes to progression of the lymphatic dysfunction by initiating fibrosis, inhibition of collateral lymphatic vessel formation, and dysfunction of the lymphatic pumping function.[1] Consequently, the inhibition of Th2—but not Th1—cell differentiation shows a reduction in lymphedema.[1] As the effect of Th2 cells is mediated by interleukin (IL)-4, IL-13, and transforming growth factor (TGF)-β, the blockage of these factors results in lymphedema prevention.[1]

In contrast, presence of Treg cells counteracts lymphedema progression. Inhibition of these cells leads to exacerbation of edema and fibrosis. Conversely, a higher number of Treg cells attenuates tissue inflammation in lymphedema.[24]

Macrophages play an essential role as their number rises in lymphedema.[24] It is supposed that the T cell inflammation triggers the macrophage migration and proliferation in lymphedema. Additionally, abnormal adipose deposition enhances the migration of the macrophages. It is induced either indirectly by the adipose inflammation or directly by the released free fatty acids from necrotic adipocytes.

Looking at the different kinds of macrophages an antifibrotic function of the M2 phenotype is assumed.[24] Furthermore, M2 macrophages regulate lymphangiogenesis, tissue remodeling by VEGF-C production, and composition of extracellular matrix proteins. Compared to healthy controls M2 macrophage content is lower in lymphedema. Following this, the M1 to M2 macrophage balance is changed which contributes to the pathological remodeling of lymphedema.[24]

During a transcriptional profiling of lymphedematous tissue, an upregulation of 5-lipoxygenase (5-LO) was identified. The 5-LO metabolite leukotriene B4 (LTB4) is an inflammatory mediator and plays a crucial part in the inflammatory reaction. Secreted by endothelial cells, LTB4 attenuates the function of the lymphatic endothelial cells (LECs). Also, in inflamed tissue it mediates the CD4+and CD8+cell recruitment.[18]

Inflammatory cytokines—particularly from T cell like IL-4, IL-13, TNF-α, and IFN-γ—are increased in lymphedema. They have an antilymphangiogenic effect by impairing the proliferation, tubule formation, and migration of the LECs.[1] In addition, T cell-related cytokines reduce the sensitivity of LECs to lymphangiogenic growth factors. The consequence is ineffectiveness of the vascular endothelial growth factor (VEGF)-C on LECs even if a high amount of VEGF-C is recognizable.[25] In the VEGF family VEGF-C and VEGF-D are essential for the development and postnatal growth of the lymphatic system. As lymphangiogenic growth factors, they bind to VEGF receptors on LECs.[26] In lymphedema tissue high VEGF-C expression is plausible because the lymphatic vessels are less responsive.[1]

Histologically, a change of the lymphatic vessels is visible, i.e., enlargement of the lymphatic capillaries.[24] This is due to chronic fluid accumulation which induces morphological and structural changes in the lymphatic vessels.[27] The higher pressure flattens the smooth muscle cells and makes them slimmer. Additionally, the dermal capillary lymphatic vessels become hypertrophic.[24]

Mihara et al. determined four different types of collecting lymphatic vessels considering the morphology: normal, ectasis, contraction, and sclerosis types.[27] The normal type shows collagen fibers and smooth muscle cells in the medial layer. This is the physiological condition. The ectasis type is typically identifiable by a dilated lymphatic vessel wall. The collagen fibers appear elongated. A thick layer of smooth muscle cells which enhance the growth of collagen fibers is found in the contraction type resulting in narrowing of the lymphatic vessel lumen. In the sclerosis type, the fibrous elements are found to be the main components of the lymphatic vessel wall. The ability to transport and concentrate the lymphatic fluid is lost and the lumen is partly or totally obstructed. In the early stage of lymphedema, the normal and ectasis types are most common. The more severe the lymphedema progresses, the more the contraction and sclerosis types are present. Notably, the sclerosis type is associated with an end stage of lymphedema due to a fibrotic remodeling.[27]

Th2 cells mediate a fibrotic remodeling by secreting profibrotic cytokines like IL-13 or IL-4.[18] Fibrosis is generally an end-organ failure effected by extracellular matrix deposition.[2] Fibroblasts have a key role during fibrosis. They differentiate into myofibroblasts and are mainly responsible for the extracellular matrix protein production.[28]

A progressive development of fibrosis appears during chronic lymphedema whereby collecting vessels are affected and become obliterated.[2] Hence, in skin from clinical and experimental lymphedema, the collagen content is increased.[24] The diameter of the collagen fibers expands, and more long-spacing collagen can be found.[3] Predominantly, collagen types I and III are augmented, followed by thickening of the dermis.[3]

The fibrosis takes place mainly in the dermis, but it is also present in subcutaneous tissue involving the adipose tissue.[24] The collagen accumulation contributes to an induration of the lymphedematous tissue which is clinically described as nonpitting edema.[24] It is mentioned that fibrosis influences the lymphatic flow and lymphangiogenesis negatively. As a result, swelling and dysfunction of fluid transport and lymph drainage occur.[24]

The TGF-β is a key regulator of fibrosis and its level is increased in lymphedema tissue. Decrease in fibrosis by blocking the TGF-β1 receptor confirms the profibrotic effect. The blockade of TGF-β1 receptor also reduces the Th2 cell migration and the expression of profibrotic Th2 cytokines.[2] However, the effect of TGF-β in lymphedema is even more extensive. TGF-β is described as an inhibitor of the lymphatic vessel formation.[3] Furthermore, the TGF-β signal pathway is responsible for an increased epithelial hyperplasia leading to hyperkeratosis of the skin.[29]

Another pathological process in late-stage lymphedema is an adipose tissue deposition. Different studies have shown that a change in adipose tissue is induced by the lymphatic fluid stasis. Fatty acids in the lymph fluid are a potential cause. Various approaches have been proposed that fatty acids directly augment the adipose deposition.[2] Some adipose differentiation markers such as adiponectin and CCAAT/enhancer-binding protein-alpha have been identified. They are increased following the destruction of the lymphatic system. Although IL-6 is highly expressed in lymphedema tissue, it is a negative regulator of adipose deposition. Its loss results in a progress of adipose deposition concluding that IL-6 is essential for the homeostasis of the adipose tissue.[2]

Interestingly, obesity is revealed as a risk factor for secondary lymphedema. Therefore, it is reasonable that adipogenesis is incidental to lymphatic dysfunction.[2] Recent findings reported that in obese mice impairment of lymphatic function including fibrosis and inflammatory response is present.[2] In human, several authors outlined that patients can suffer from lower extremity lymphedema due to obesity without any trauma.[2] Inflammatory cells contribute to the cellular mechanism of the lymphedema development in obese patients. This is substantiated by the fact that an inhibition or deficiency of CD4+T cell prevents lymphedema in obese patients.[2]

Recurrent infections of the affected part of the body are a common side effect of lymphedema. This often implies the severity of lymphedema. Consequently, an infection induces an injury of the lymphatic vessels.[2] On the other hand, infections can trigger the development of lymphedema itself, as bacteria generate a lymphatic dysfunction. Jones et al. reported that the number of lymphatic muscle cells which are essential for the contraction of the lymphatic vessels is reduced in mouse lymphedema model.[30] Apart from this, Tregs seem to diminish the inflammatory process. By occurring in large number in lymphedema tissue they prevent the lymphatic dysfunction during an infection. To summarize, the relation between the lymphatic system and infections is ambivalent—microorganisms can cause a damage of the lymphatic system while lymphedema can weaken the immunological response.[2]

All in all, the described causative effects of lymphedema lead to typical tissue changes. Thickening of the cutis and subcutis is due to the accumulation of fatty tissue, and development of fibrosis, lymphatic cysts, and fistulae. Trophic changes in the epidermis are variable. Hyperplasia, hyperkeratosis, hyperpigmentation, minor papillomatosis, and verrucous protuberances may appear. Erysipelas and mycotic infection may be a result of an abnormal immune response of the affected tissue.[3]

Describing the pathology of lymphedema shows the complexity of its nature. Further investigation is still necessary to understand the whole mechanism and its modulation by genetic and environmental factors.

2.5 Stages and Classification of Lymphedema

Stephan Wagner and Katja Kilian

There are various classification systems in staging lymphedema. Mostly, the staging of the International Society of Lymphology (ISL) is commonly used.[1] It determines different stages of lymphedema by taking clinical criteria such as limb swelling and the occurrence of pitting edema into consideration.[1] This clinical classification ranges from zero with no visible swelling to three further stages with changes in interstitial edema, tissue hypertrophy, and adipose tissue deposition.[18] In the following the different stages are described in detail.

Stage 0 is a latent lymphedema. The patients complain about symptoms of lymphedema, but no swelling is evident.[1] On the contrary, technical tests such as lymph scintigraphy show an impaired lymph transport. For instance, it may exist after a lymph node extirpation and can last for months to years before an apparent lymphedema swelling occurs.[31]

Stage I represents a daily swelling with hyaluronan-rich edema. It disappears overnight or by elevation of the involved body part. At this stage, there is usually no tissue change visible.[31] However, a pitting edema (pressure to the skin leads to an indentation of the skin) may exist.

In stage II, the lymphedema will not reduce completely by elevation of the involved body part. At this stage the tissue is more fibrotic.[31] As a consequence, the pitting edema is less evident.[18]

Stage III encompasses not only very voluminous extremities (the term elephantiasis is no longer used), but also trophic skin changes.[31] The skin changes in terms of its character and skin acanthosis, lichenification, and verrucae may be recognizable. A pitting edema is not present anymore. The thickening of the skin is owing to the extensive proliferation of the subcutaneous connective and adipose tissue. This results in loss of skin flexibility and in cobblestone formation. Moreover, the appearance of the skin reminds of an orange peel which is clinically described as *peau d'orange*. During clinical examination, a positive Stemmer's sign can be evoked at the lower extremity. Here, the skin at the base of the second toe cannot be pinched anymore.[18]

In each stage, the severity of the edema can be additionally classified by the level of volume increase. It is subdivided into minimal (less than 20% increase), moderate (between 20% to 40% increase), or severe (over 40% increase in volume).[31] Additionally, as mentioned above, lymphedema is classified into primary or secondary, according to the origin of the condition (see **Subchapter 2.2**).[31]

References

[1] Dayan JH, Ly CL, Kataru RP, Mehrara BJ. Lymphedema: pathogenesis and novel therapies. Annu Rev Med. 2018; 69:263–276

[2] Li CY, Kataru RP, Mehrara BJ. Histopathologic features of lymphedema: a molecular review. Int J Mol Sci. 2020; 21(7):E2546

[3] Koller M, Baumeister R, Döller W, Földi E, et al. Guideline report on the S2k guideline "Diagnostics and therapy of lymphoedema" (Registry no. 058-001 of the Association of the Scientific Medical Societies in Germany - Arbeitsgemeinschaft der Wissenschaftlichen Medizinischen Fachgesellschaften e.V., AWMF). AWMF. https://www.awmf.org/fileadmin/user_upload/Leitlinien/058_Ges_D_Lymphologen/058-001me_S2k_Diagnostics_and_therapy_of_lymphoedema_2019-07-abgelaufen.pdf. Published May 2017

[4] Wilting J. Genetische Ursachen des primären Lymphödems. LymphForsch. 2014; 1:26–30

[5] Ramashankar CP, Shah NK, Giraddi G. Lymphatic malformations: a dilemma in diagnosis and management. Contemp Clin Dent. 2014; 5 (1):119–122

[6] Yuan Y, Arcucci V, Levy SM, Achen MG. Modulation of immunity by lymphatic dysfunction in lymphedema. Front Immunol. 2019; 10: 76–76

[7] Lourens GB, Ferrell DK. Lymphatic filariasis. Nurs Clin North Am. 2019; 54(2):181–192

[8] Deribe K, Cano J, Trueba ML, Newport MJ, Davey G. Global epidemiology of podoconiosis: a systematic review. PLoS Negl Trop Dis. 2018; 12(3):e0006324

[9] Quéré I, Palmier S, Noerregaard S, et al. LIMPRINT: estimation of the prevalence of lymphoedema/chronic oedema in acute hospital in inpatients. Lymphat Res Biol. 2019; 17(2):135–140

[10] Rockson SG, Rivera KK. Estimating the population burden of lymphedema. Ann N Y Acad Sci. 2008; 1131:147–154

[11] Brayton KM, Hirsch AT, O Brien PJ, Cheville A, Karaca-Mandic P, Rockson SG. Lymphedema prevalence and treatment benefits in cancer: impact of a therapeutic intervention on health outcomes and costs. PLoS One. 2014; 9(12):e114597

[12] Smeltzer DM, Stickler GB, Schirger A. Primary lymphedema in children and adolescents: a follow-up study and review. Pediatrics. 1985; 76(2):206–218

[13] Manning SC, Perkins J. Lymphatic malformations. Curr Opin Otolaryngol Head Neck Surg. 2013; 21(6):571–575

[14] Elluru RG, Balakrishnan K, Padua HM. Lymphatic malformations: diagnosis and management. Semin Pediatr Surg. 2014; 23(4):178–185

[15] Dale RF. The inheritance of primary lymphoedema. J Med Genet. 1985; 22(4):274–278

[16] Goss JA, Maclellan RA, Greene AK. Adult-onset primary lymphedema: a clinical-lymphoscintigraphic study of 26 patients. Lymphat Res Biol. 2019; 17(6):620–623
[17] Brenner E, Kröll A, Neuhüttler S. Aetiology of secondary lymphoedema with non-oncologic origin. Phlebologie. 2006; 35(2):67–74
[18] Rockson SG, Keeley V, Kilbreath S, Szuba A, Towers A. Cancer-associated secondary lymphoedema. Nat Rev Dis Primers. 2019; 5(1):22
[19] DiSipio T, Rye S, Newman B, Hayes S. Incidence of unilateral arm lymphoedema after breast cancer: a systematic review and meta-analysis. Lancet Oncol. 2013; 14(6):500–515
[20] Rupp J, Hadamitzky C, Henkenberens C, Christiansen H, Steinmann D, Bruns F. Frequency and risk factors for arm lymphedema after multimodal breast-conserving treatment of nodal positive breast cancer—a long-term observation. Radiat Oncol. 2019; 14(1):39
[21] Torgbenu E, Luckett T, Buhagiar MA, Chang S, Phillips JL. Prevalence and incidence of cancer related lymphedema in low and middle-income countries: a systematic review and meta-analysis. BMC Cancer. 2020; 20(1):604
[22] Carlson JW, Kauderer J, Walker JL, et al. Gynecologic Oncology Group. A randomized phase III trial of VH fibrin sealant to reduce lymphedema after inguinal lymph node dissection: a gynecologic oncology group study. Gynecol Oncol. 2008; 110(1):76–82
[23] Biglia N, Zanfagnin V, Daniele A, Robba E, Bounous VE. Lower body lymphedema in patients with gynecologic cancer. Anticancer Res. 2017; 37(8):4005–4015
[24] Azhar SH, Lim HY, Tan BK, Angeli V. The unresolved pathophysiology of lymphedema. Front Physiol. 2020; 11:137
[25] Savetsky IL, Ghanta S, Gardenier JC, et al. Th2 cytokines inhibit lymphangiogenesis. PLoS One. 2015; 10(6):e0126908
[26] Shin WS, Rockson SG. Animal models for the molecular and mechanistic study of lymphatic biology and disease. Ann N Y Acad Sci. 2008; 1131:50–74
[27] Mihara M, Hara H, Hayashi Y, et al. Pathological steps of cancer-related lymphedema: histological changes in the collecting lymphatic vessels after lymphadenectomy. PLoS One. 2012; 7(7): e41126
[28] Jiang X, Nicolls MR, Tian W, Rockson SG. Lymphatic dysfunction, leukotrienes, and lymphedema. Annu Rev Physiol. 2018; 80:49–70
[29] Torrisi JS, Joseph WJ, Ghanta S, et al. Lymphaticovenous bypass decreases pathologic skin changes in upper extremity breast cancer-related lymphedema. Lymphat Res Biol. 2015; 13(1):46–53
[30] Jones D, Meijer EFJ, Blatter C, et al. Methicillin-resistant Staphylococcus aureus causes sustained collecting lymphatic vessel dysfunction. Sci Transl Med. 2018; 10(424):eaam7964
[31] Executive Committee. The diagnosis and treatment of peripheral lymphedema: 2016 Consensus Document of the International Society of Lymphology. Lymphology. 2016; 49(4):170–184

3 Lymphatic Filariasis

Gurusamy Manokaran and Leela Praveen Kumar

Summary

In low-income countries, the most common cause of lymphedema is lymphatic filariasis. It is a neglected tropical disease. Here, the lymphedema is caused by an abnormal or defective lymphatic function, resulting in the accumulation of lymph in the tissue spaces. LF is caused by an infection of a nematode of the family Filarioidea, *W. bancrofti*, *Brugia malayi* (India), or *Brugia timori* (Africa). All these nematodes infecting humans have a complex life cycle involving an insect vector (mosquito). The mosquito deposits the larva, which is the infectious stage, at the time a bite occurs. The larvae enter into the lymphatics, and then into the lymph nodes, settle there, and grow into adult worms. Following mating, the live microfilariae circulate in the bloodstream. The mosquito ingests the microfilariae while ingesting blood and these larvae undergo development in the mosquito. Adult worms nest in the lymphatic vessels and disrupt the normal function of the lymphatic system.

Keywords: diethyl carbamazine (DEC), vector control, Wucheraria Bancrofti, Wolbachia

3.1 Prevalence

Lymphatic filariasis (LF) is a public health problem in India despite the existence of National Filaria Control Program since 1955. It is prevalent in 17 states and 6 union territories. India accounts for 40% of the world's LF burden. Currently, there may be up to 31 million microfilaraemics, 23 million cases of symptomatic filariasis, and about 500 million individuals potentially at risk of contracting the disease in the country (2017).

The World Health Organization data reveals that 1 billion people (20% of the world's population) in over 54 countries are at a risk of developing this disease. India, Indonesia, Nigeria, and Bangladesh contribute to 70% of the infections worldwide. India had set the ambitious goal of eradicating filariasis by the year 2020, but in the current scenario it seems unlikely.

Each year nearly 120 million people become infected with filariasis, over 40 million get severely disfigured and disabled, and nearly 76 million have hidden damage to the lymphatic and renal system while remaining symptomless.

Although filariasis does not kill, it causes frailty and imposes a severe social and economic burden on the affected individuals, their families, and the endemic communities. The painful and profoundly disfiguring visible manifestations of the disease—lymphedema, voluminous extremities, and scrotal swelling that occur can later—lead to permanent disability. These patients are not only physically disabled, but suffer mental, social, and financial losses contributing to stigma and poverty. Eliminating lymphatic filariasis can prevent unnecessary suffering and contribute to the reduction of poverty.

Prevention and elimination of this disease is vital. However, it will take a long time, as low-income countries are still struggling with providing basic human needs such as drinking water, food, and shelter.

3.2 Pathophysiology

LF is a chronic debilitating parasitic disease caused by *Wuchereria bancrofti*, *Brugia malayi*, and *Brugia timori* (▶ Fig. 3.1). This is transmitted to humans via the culex mosquito.

Filariasis is a neglected mosquito-borne tropical disease. These human-infecting nematodes have a complex life cycle involving an insect vector (mosquito). The mosquito deposits the larva when it bites. The larvae enter into the lymphatics and then into the lymph nodes where they settle and grow into adult worms. This process usually takes 2 to 4 years and sometimes up to 6 to 8 years. After mating, the living microfilariae circulate in the bloodstream. The mosquito ingests the microfilariae

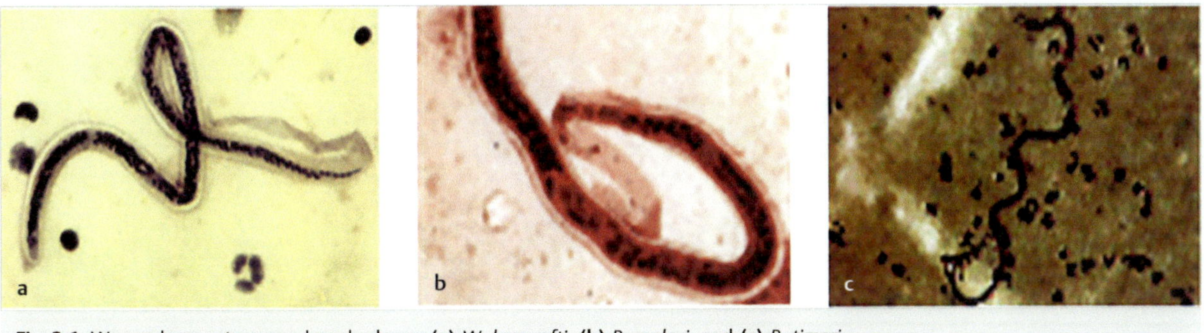

Fig. 3.1 Worms known to cause lymphedema: **(a)** *W. bancrofti*, **(b)** *B. malayi*, and **(c)** *B. timori*.

while ingesting blood and these larvae undergo development in the mosquito.

Adult worms nest in the lymphatic vessels and disrupt the normal function of the lymphatic system. The worms can live for approximately 6 to 8 years and, during their lifetime, produce millions of microfilariae (immature larvae) that circulate in the blood. Mosquitoes are infected with microfilariae by ingesting blood when biting an infected host. Microfilariae mature into infective larvae within the mosquito. When infected mosquitoes bite people, mature parasite larvae are deposited in the skin from where they can enter the body. The larvae then migrate to the lymphatic vessels, where they develop into adult worms, thus continuing a cycle of transmission. The adult worm prefers to live in the scrotum in males, and in the genital area or the axillae in females.

3.2.1 Pathology

Infection is usually acquired during childhood. The effects are not seen immediately, but it slowly causes hidden damage to the lymphatic system. Once the organism settles in the lymph nodes, it lives for 2 to 4 years, producing millions of new microfilariae during its lifetime. LF does not produce any obstruction or discontinuity of the lymphatics. When the adult worm dies, it releases an endotoxin which damages the lymphatic vessels, leading to dilatation of vessels and deformation of valves. This reduces the efficiency of the pumping mechanism of the lymphatics.[1,2,3] Also, with the loss of lymphatic pumping capacity, there is an increase in the risk of infection, as the transport of bacteria to lymph nodes is impaired. This causes the acute manifestations that we see in lymphedema such as acute adenolymphangitis, acute dermato-lymphangitis, hydrocele, acute epididymo-orchitis, funiculitis, abscess formation, acute abdominal lymphadenitis, hematuria, etc.

The accumulation of the lymphatic fluid increases the size of the limbs and over time leads to the hypertrophy of the tissue. There can be recurrent episodes of lymphangitis, especially in patients who have dental caries (focus of sepsis) or foot lesions like intertrigo. Recurrent episodes of lymphangitis can cause more lymphatic damage

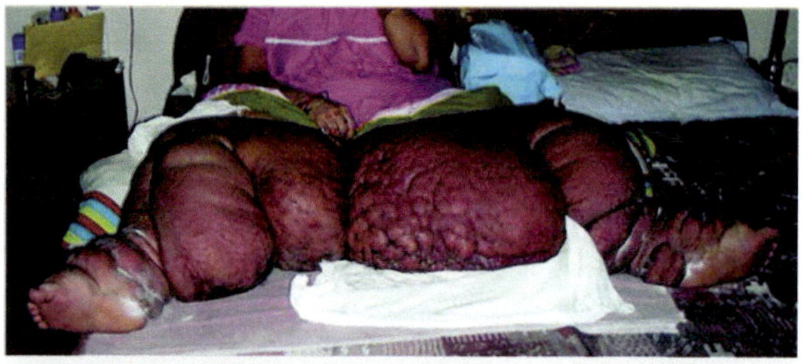

Fig. 3.2 Female patient with bilateral lymphedema due to lymphatic filariasis (massive voluminous extremities).

3.3 Clinical Manifestations

Acute manifestations that we see in lymphedema are acute adenolymphangitis, acute dermato-lymphangitis, hydrocele, acute epididymo-orchitis, funiculitis, abscess formation, acute abdominal lymphadenitis, hematuria, etc.

The most common chronic presentations of LF are hydroceles and lymphedema of both upper and lower limbs, and some less common presentations include chylothorax, chyluria, and chylascitis.

Other presentations include genital manifestations (filarial scrotum, cutaneous horn of the penis [ram's horn], genital vesicles, etc.) and atypical LF in the form of fleeting joint pains and lymphangitis (string sign). It can also affect the breast, gluteal region, abdomen, and suprapubic region in the form of isolated lesions. The lower limb is the most common manifestation, and women are more frequently affected than men[4,5,6,7,8,9] (▶ Fig. 3.2 and ▶ Fig. 3.3).

In an endemic area like India, lymphatic filariasis may present completely asymptomatically, with acute symptoms, or with chronic infection.

3.3.1 Diagnosis

When diagnosing a case of filarial lymphedema, it is very important to look into the history of the patient as it provides an indication regarding the cause of the lymphedema. The immunochromatographic test (ICT)[10,11] card test gives a bedside test for LF, which is highly sensitive for *W. bancrofti* at 90% to 95%.

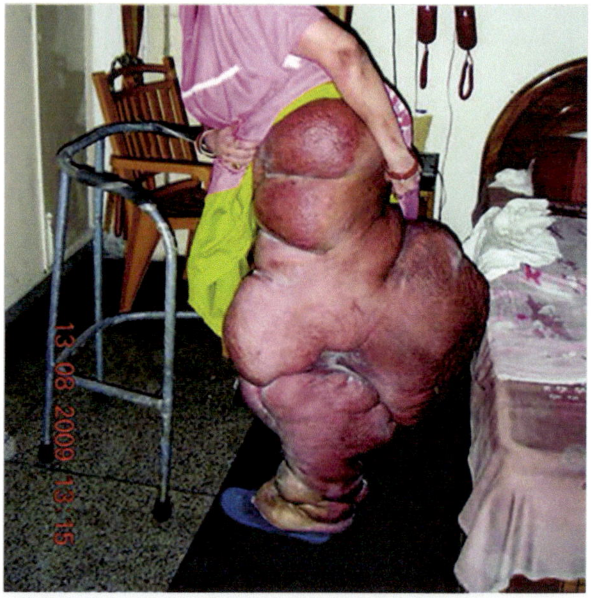

Fig. 3.3 Lateral view of the same patient as ▶ Fig. 3.2.

In endemic areas, ultrasound[12,13,14,15] is used as a screening test. When performing an ultrasound, it can sometimes show *dancing adult worms* in the scrotum in men and in the breast in women. Patients positive for adult worms on ultrasound may not have had any clinical signs or symptoms, thus removing the adult worms surgically from these patients will prevent the occurrence of LF.

Lymphoscintigraphy[6,16,17,18,19,20] is the single most useful examination in establishing diagnosis, grading, and etiology. This investigation can tell us about the outcome of this treatment both after chemotherapy and postsurgical results.

3.3.2 Clinical Classification of Filarial Lymphedema

For practical purposes we divide filarial lymphedema into seven clinical stages (▸ Table 3.1).[21]

Table 3.1 Gerusa Dreyer classification system for lymphoedema

Seven Stages of Filarial Lymphedema of the Lower Extremity	
Stages	**Symptoms**
Stage I	Swelling reverses at night Skin folds: Absent Appearance of skin: Smooth, normal
Stage II	Swelling not reversible at night Skin folds: Absent Appearance of skin: Smooth, normal
Stage III	Swelling not reversible at night Skin folds: Shallow Appearance of skin: Smooth, normal
Stage IV	Swelling not reversible at night Skin folds: Shallow Appearance of skin: Irregular, knobs, nodules
Stage V	Swelling not reversible at night Skin folds: Deep Appearance of skin: Smooth or irregular
Stage VI	Swelling not reversible at night Skin folds: Absent, shallow, deep Appearance of skin: Wart-like lesions on foot or top of toes
Stage VII	Swelling not reversible at night Skin folds: Deep Appearance of skin: Irregular Needs help for daily activities: Walking, bathing, using bathrooms, dependent on family or health care systems

3.4 Management

Management of LF can be divided into three parts:
- Prevention of spread/eradication of parasite (chemotherapy)
- Management of the lymphedema (MLD; bandaging and surgeries which include bypass shunts and debulking procedures)
- Vector control

The chemotherapeutic management[22] of these problems is either with diethyl carbamazine (DEC) alone or in the following combinations: DEC + albendazole, DEC + ivermectin, along with periodic antibiotics like penicillin, doxycycline, and sulfonamides. DEC, ivermectin, and albendazole are antiparasitic drugs. Penicillins and doxycycline are very effective antibiotics and are very useful against the symbiotic bacteria called *Wolbachia*,[23,24,25,26,27] which reside inside the parasite and cause resistance to antifilarial drugs.[28,29,30,31,32] Presently, we are using doxycycline as our preferred antibiotic as it has been noted that it helps in reducing limb edema and the patients using it have better skin quality as compared to the group using penicillin.

Vector control: Mosquito control is a supplemental strategy supported by the WHO. It is used to reduce transmission of LF and other mosquito-borne infections. Depending on the parasite vector species, measures such as insecticide-treated nets, indoor residual spraying, or personal protection measures may help protect people from infection. The use of insecticide-treated nets in areas where *Anopheles* is the primary vector for filariasis enhances the impact on transmission during and after mass drug administration (MDA).

3.4.1 Management of Filarial Lymphedema

The flowchart shown in ▸ Fig. 3.4, which has been designed based on our observations over a period of more than 35 years, provides a brief outline of how lymphedema can be managed.

For all the seven stages of lymphedema, the recommendations below should be followed.

Stages I and II of LF lymphedemas are totally reversible, which has been demonstrated by lymphoscintigraphy before and after treatment.

3.4.2 Management of Stage I and II

- Foot care
- Avoiding injury and injections to the affected limb
- Elimination of the focus of sepsis, teeth with caries, and intertrigo (fungal infection)

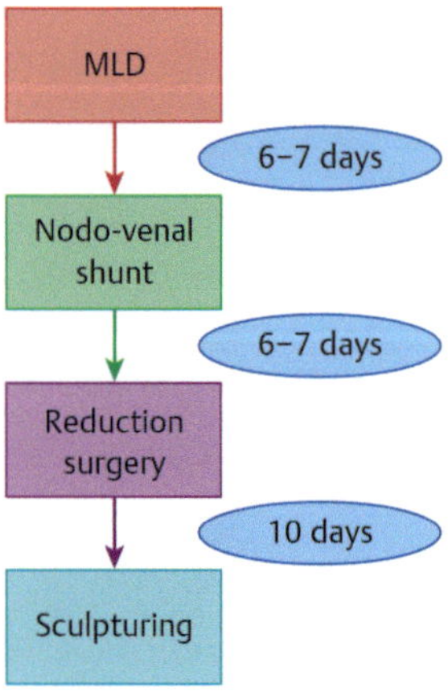

Fig. 3.4 Protocol for the management of filariasis-induced chronic lymphedema.

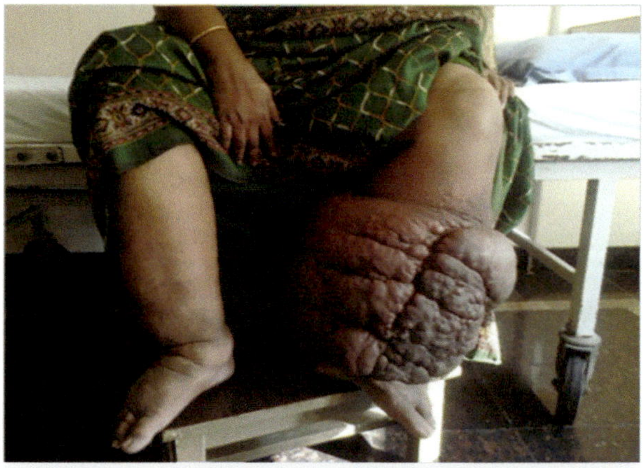

Fig. 3.5 Before management of the lymphedema.

- Complete decongestive therapy (CDT) with bandaging followed by
  - pressure garments;
  - elevation of the affected extremity
- Cyclical chemotherapy (antibiotics and antifilarials, as described above) to prevent secondary infections and spreading of the disease

3.4.3 Management of Stage III and IV

In stage III and IV, there is gross edema, but not many skin changes. Apart from the basic recommendations listed earlier, surgical correction needs to be undertaken. For these stages complete decongestive therapy (CDT) or manual lymphatic drainage (MLD) + bandaging is done for 5 to 7 days, followed by a physiological surgery like a lymph node–venous anastomosis (LNVA) with or without a reduction surgery. In stage III, just a physiological bypass procedure may be sufficient. But in stage IV, immediately after the shunt, it is followed by an excisional procedure (without skin grafting) (see **Chapter 14**).

In our experience of 35 years, we have evolved the technique where the functional and aesthetic aspects of the limb are preserved. Although microvascular surgeries like free lymphatic channel transfer, lymph node transfer, and omental transfer and supramicrovascular surgery like lymphatico-lymphatic anastomosis are useful in congenital and postsurgical lymphedemas, they however do not play as much of a role in filarial lymphedemas.

3.4.4 Management of Stage V, VI, and VII

For stage V cases, a single stage of debulking may not be sufficient to get a good reduction in size. Such cases may be taken up for another stage of debulking, after a period of 6 to 8 weeks. The same medial incision used in the previous debulking surgery is used.

Stage VI and VII cases, which have developed mossy or warty lesions, will need additional surgical procedure called sculpturing. Here, the lesions are excised tangentially, like harvesting a skin graft, up to the level of the dermis (which is generally thickened in these cases). Then it is dressed like a skin graft donor site, and a bulky compression dressing is given. It is opened after a week and then redressed in the same manner again to be opened after another week. It generally heals in 2 to 3 weeks, just like any other skin graft donor site.

After the surgeries, the patients need to strictly follow the recommendations, which been followed even preoperatively, i.e., periodic antifilarial and antibiotic medications, protection/prevention of entry lesions (foot care to prevent intertrigo, oral hygiene and preventing dental caries), wearing of pressure garments, auto-massage, leg elevation, and consistent, periodic follow-up consultations.

More details with regard to reconstructive and reductive procedures to treat chronic lymphedema are described in **Chapters 8–14**.

3.5 Clinical Case

The amount of laxity that can be achieved with MLD and bandaging can be seen in the pictures shown in ▶ Fig. 3.5 and ▶ Fig. 3.6.

3.6 Conclusions

It can be said that LF is not just another lymphedema (and it cannot be treated like other types of lymphedemas) because

- it is one of the major causes of lymphedema, especially in the tropical regions;

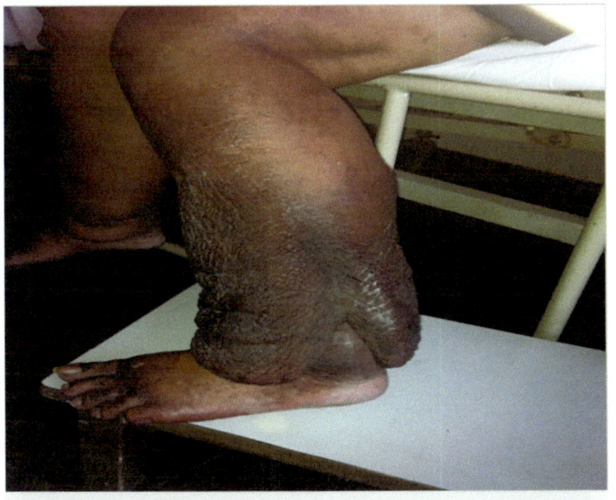

Fig. 3.6 Same patient, after management of the lymphedema. The skin has become lax and is now convenient to do limb reduction by excision of the redundant skin.

- the ways it manifests are also variable, and it can affect any organ, unlike other types which are seen only distal to the site of trauma/surgery;
- the pathology in LF causing the problems is not obstruction or loss of continuity (as in post lymph node resection/trauma/post radiotherapy but loss of efficiency of pumping the lymph due to dilatation of the lymphatics. The pathology is different, therefore, so is the treatment;
- the cases of LF that present to the clinic are generally of a higher stage where surgical procedures like lymphovenous anastomosis (LVA: see **Chapter 8**) or lympholymphatic anastomois do not give satisfying long-term results. The treatment protocol that has been described above has been applied on patients and modified to continuously evolve over 35 years in order to show promising results nowadays.

References

[1] Figueredo-Silva J, Norões J, Cedenho A, Dreyer G. The histopathology of bancroftian filariasis revisited: the role of the adult worm in the lymphatic-vessel disease. Ann Trop Med Parasitol. 2002; 96(6):531–541

[2] Connor DH, Palmieri JR, Gibson DW. Pathogenesis of lymphatic filariasis in man. Z Parasitenkd. 1986; 72(1):13–28

[3] von Lichtenberg F. The Wellcome Trust lecture. Inflammatory responses to filarial connective tissue parasites. Parasitology. 1987; 94 Suppl:S101–S122

[4] Ottesen EA. The Wellcome Trust Lecture. Infection and disease in lymphatic filariasis: an immunological perspective. Parasitology. 1992; 104 Suppl:S71–S79

[5] Dreyer G, Ottesen EA, Galdino E, et al. Renal abnormalities in microfilaremic patients with Bancroftian filariasis. Am J Trop Med Hyg. 1992; 46(6):745–751

[6] Freedman DO, de Almeida Filho PJ, Besh S, Maia e Silva MC, Braga C, Maciel A. Lymphoscintigraphic analysis of lymphatic abnormalities in symptomatic and asymptomatic human filariasis. J Infect Dis. 1994; 170(4):927–933

[7] Norões J, Addiss D, Amaral F, Coutinho A, Medeiros Z, Dreyer G. Occurrence of living adult Wuchereria bancrofti in the scrotal area of men with microfilaraemia. Trans R Soc Trop Med Hyg. 1996; 90(1): 55–56

[8] Pani SP, Yuvaraj J, Vanamail P, et al. Episodic adenolymphangitis and lymphoedema in patients with bancroftian filariasis. Trans R Soc Trop Med Hyg. 1995; 89(1):72–74

[9] Ottesen EA, Nutman TB. Tropical pulmonary eosinophilia. Annu Rev Med. 1992; 43:417–424

[10] Schuetz A, Addiss DG, Eberhard ML, Lammie PJ. Evaluation of the whole blood filariasis ICT test for short-term monitoring after antifilarial treatment. Am J Trop Med Hyg. 2000; 62(4):502–503

[11] Weil GJ, Lammie PJ, Weiss N. The ICT Filariasis Test: a rapid-format antigen test for diagnosis of bancroftian filariasis. Parasitol Today. 1997; 13(10):401–404

[12] Amaral F, Dreyer G, Figueredo-Silva J, et al. Live adult worms detected by ultrasonography in human Bancroftian filariasis. Am J Trop Med Hyg. 1994; 50(6):753–757

[13] Dreyer G, Santos A, Noroes J, Amaral F, Addiss D. Ultrasonographic detection of living adult Wuchereria bancrofti using a 3.5-MHz transducer. Am J Trop Med Hyg. 1998; 59(3):399–403

[14] Homeida MA, Mackenzie CD, Williams JF, Ghalib HW. The detection of onchocercal nodules by ultrasound technique. Trans R Soc Trop Med Hyg. 1986; 80(4):570–571

[15] Leichsenring M, Tröger J, Nelle M, Büttner DW, Darge K, Doehring-Schwerdtfeger E. Ultrasonographical investigations of onchocerciasis in Liberia. Am J Trop Med Hyg. 1990; 43(4):380–385

[16] Shelley S, Manokaran G, Indirani M, Gokhale S, Anirudhan N. Lymphoscintigraphy as a diagnostic tool in patients with lymphedema of filarial origin—an Indian study. Lymphology. 2006; 39(2):69–75

[17] Szuba A, Shin WS, Strauss HW, Rockson S. The third circulation: radionuclide lymphoscintigraphy in the evaluation of lymphedema. J Nucl Med. 2003; 44(1):43–57

[18] Sherman AI, Ter-Pogossian M. Lymph-node concentration of radioactive colloidal gold following interstitial injection. Cancer. 1953; 6(6):1238–1240

[19] Nawaz K, Hamad MM, Sadek S, Awdeh M, Eklof B, Abdel-Dayem HM. Dynamic lymph flow imaging in lymphedema. Normal and abnormal patterns. Clin Nucl Med. 1986; 11(9):653–658

[20] Werner GT, Scheck R, Kaiserling E. Magnetic resonance imaging of peripheral lymphedema. Lymphology. 1998; 31(1):34–36

[21] G Dreyer, A Coutinho, R Albuquerque. Clinical manifestations of lymphatic bancroftian filariasis. AMB Rev Assoc Med Bras. 1989; 35(5):189-96.

[22] Molyneux DH, Bradley M, Hoerauf A, Kyelem D, Taylor MJ. Mass drug treatment for lymphatic filariasis and onchocerciasis. Trends Parasitol. 2003; 19(11):516–522

[23] Bosshardt SC, McCall JW, Coleman SU, Jones KL, Petit TA, Klei TR. Prophylactic activity of tetracycline against Brugia pahangi infection in jirds (Meriones unguiculatus). J Parasitol. 1993; 79(5): 775–777

[24] McCall JW, Jun JJ, Bandi C. Wolbachia and the antifilarial properties of tetracycline. An untold story. Ital J Zool (Modena). 1999; 66:7–10

[25] Bandi C, McCall JW, Genchi C, Corona S, Venco L, Sacchi L. Effects of tetracycline on the filarial worms Brugia pahangi and Dirofilaria immitis and their bacterial endosymbionts Wolbachia. Int J Parasitol. 1999; 29(2):357–364

[26] Hoerauf A, et al. Targeting of Wolbachia in Litomosoidessigmodontis: comparison of tetracycline with chloramphenicol, macrolides and ciprofloxacin. Trop Med Int Health.

[27] Townson S, et al. The activity of rifampicin, oxytetracycline and chloramphenicol against Onchocercalienalis and O. gutturosa. Trans R Soc Trop Med Hyg. 1999; 93:123–124

[28] Zug R, Hammerstein P. Still a host of hosts for Wolbachia: analysis of recent data suggests that 40% of terrestrial arthropod species are infected. PLoS One. 2012; 7(6):e38544

[29] Taylor MJ, Cross HF, Bilo K. Inflammatory responses induced by the filarial nematode Brugia malayi are mediated by lipopolysaccharide-like activity from endosymbiotic Wolbachia bacteria. J Exp Med. 2000; 191(8):1429–1436

[30] Brattig NW, Büttner DW, Hoerauf A. Neutrophil accumulation around Onchocerca worms and chemotaxis of neutrophils are dependent on Wolbachia endobacteria. Microbes Infect. 2001; 3(6):439–446

[31] Tamarozzi F, Halliday A, Gentil K, Hoerauf A, Pearlman E, Taylor MJ. Onchocerciasis: the role of Wolbachia bacterial endosymbionts in parasite biology, disease pathogenesis, and treatment. Clin Microbiol Rev. 2011; 24(3):459–468

[32] Debrah AY, Mand S, Marfo-Debrekyei Y, et al. Reduction in levels of plasma vascular endothelial growth factor-A and improvement in hydrocele patients by targeting endosymbiotic Wolbachia sp. in Wuchereria bancrofti with doxycycline. Am J Trop Med Hyg. 2009; 80 (6):956–963

Section II

Diagnostic Evaluation

Edited by Christoph Hirche

II

4 Diagnostics and Stage-Dependent Preoperative Evaluation

Summary
Modern surgical management of chronic lymphedema requires a subtle diagnostic workup to address the clinical lymphedema stage, tissue characteristics, and functionality of the lymphatic system. The workup aims at an individualized, targeted surgery, which is as less invasive as possible. Several clinical and image-based parameters are available to gain an all-encompassing evaluation of the lymphedema stage. The modern approach involves not defining one stage per extremity, but rather approaching the alterations of the lymphatic system individually within the extremity—"one size does not fit all." Ultrasound and magnetic resonance imaging are indicated to define the amount of free tissue water, fibrosis, and adipogenetic tissue changes, or even aggravating diseases such as chronic venous insufficiency. ICG lymphangiography has evolved into a safe screening tool for the lymphatic system providing intraoperative reverse mapping. Magnetic resonance imaging and functional magnetic resonance lymphangiography are complex procedures to provide high spatial resolution of the functionality of the lymphatic vessels in relation to veins and reference points. Conventional high-frequency ultrasound has been used as a substitute for ICG lymphangiography for the detection of lymphatic vessels even in the limbs severely affected by lymphedema in a region masked by dermal backflow pattern or in patients with allergic reactions to ICG.

Keywords: diagnostic workup, personal history, volume measurement, circumference, water displacement, ultrasound, scintigraphy, indocyanine green (ICG), near-infrared imaging, reversed mapping, conventional magnetic resonance imaging (MRI), magnetic resonance lymphangiography (MRL), conventional high-frequency ultrasound (CHFUS)

4.1 Medical History

Tomke Cordts

Careful assessment of the patient's medical history is crucial for appropriate and stage-dependent treatment of chronic lymphedema. Basic questions should include age of onset, family history, and course of the condition to preliminarily characterize the disease and patient complaints. As primary lymphedema is derived from congenital lymphatic dysplasia,[1] these patients often report about similarly affected relatives. Some of the genetic alterations have been characterized (see ▸ Table 4.1) but a great number remains elusive. The primary form accounts for only 1% of all lymphedema cases,[2,3,4] and in this group, heterozygote mutations of the gene *VEGFR-3*, which alter the tyrosine kinase function of the vascular endothelial growth factor receptor-3 (VEGFR-3), are most common.[5] Patients may also present with complex, congenital syndromes (i.e., Klippel-Trenaunay-Weber syndrome, Turner syndrome) in which lymphedema is just one characteristic in a long list of symptoms.

In contrast to the primary form, secondary lymphedema develops after an acquired anatomical obliteration of the lymphovascular system.[1] It can result from various etiologies and stimuli (see ▸ Table 4.2).

Common extrinsic causes are trauma, surgery, infection, or oncologic treatment, such as axillary lymphadenectomy or radiation following breast cancer,[17] neck dissection,[18] or removal of para-aortic, inguinal, or femoral lymph nodes.[19,20] A detailed list of potentially relevant, previous surgeries and procedures (vascular, oncologic, orthopedic, etc.) needs to be assessed. Infections and skin alterations may also lead to chronic edema—questions should therefore include preceding erysipelas, tick or insect bites, and travel to tropical regions.[21] Common intrinsic pathologies are obesity[22] and chronic venous insufficiency, where venous hypertension exceeds lymphatic transport capacity.[23] The long list of risk factors requires a broad and exceptionally thorough investigation by the treating physician (see checklist in ▸ Table 4.3). Whenever possible, underlying diseases need to be addressed first. For example, in patients with chronic heart failure, lower leg edema can be predominantly caused by decreased cardiac output; hence, it should be treated by a cardiologist.

4.2 Clinical Examination

Tomke Cordts

Whenever lymphedema is suspected, a thorough and comprehensive physical examination is invaluable. Step 1, *inspection*, is always performed with the patient undressed. Localization of swelling and the corresponding changes in circumference are evaluated and quantified. When located at the center, whether symmetrical or asymmetrical, lymphedema is rather unlikely and a condition originating from adipose tissue should be suspected instead. Corresponding skin changes, such as alterations in color, texture, pigmentation, vasculature, etc., need to be carefully assessed to fully characterize the underlying pathology (see ▸ Table 4.4).[6,24,25]

Table 4.1 Genetic alterations associated with primary lymphedema (adapted from Wilting et al.[6])

Gene	Locus	Disease	OMIM®	Molecule/Mutation	Reference
FLT4 = VEGFR-3	5q35.3	Primary congenital lymphedema, Nonne-Milroy disease	153100	Tyrosine kinase	Karkkainen et al.[7]
FOXC2	16q24.3	Lymphedema-distichiasis syndrome + others	153400	Winged-helix transcription factor, nonsense or frameshift mutation	Fang et al,[8] Finegold et al.[9]
VEGF-C	16q24.3	Milroy-like disease	615907	Growth factor	Balboa-Beltran et al.[10]
GJC2	1q41–42	Arm and leg lymphedema	613480	Connexin 47	Ferrell et al.[11]
GATA2	3q21	Leg and genital lymphedema	614028	Transcription factor	Ostergaard et al.[12]
SOX18	20q13.33	Hypotrichosis-lymphedema-telangiectasia	607823	SRY-type HMG-box transcription factor, missense mutation	Irrthum et al.[13]
PTPN14	1q41	Leg lymphedema and choanal atresia	613611	Tyrosine phosphatase (nonreceptor type)	Har-El et al.[14]
CCBE1	18q21	Hennekam syndrome	235510	Secreted protein	Alders et al.[15]
KIF11	10q23.33	Microcephaly, lymphedema and chorioretinopathy	152950	Motor protein	Ostergaard et al.[16]

Table 4.2 Known causes of primary and secondary lymphedema (adapted from Wilting et al.[6])

Primary lymphedema	Secondary lymphedema
Aplasia/atresia Hypoplasia Hyperplasia/dysplasia Lymph node fibrosis Lymph node agenesia	Surgery Adipositas Advanced chronic venous insufficiency Infectious/postinfectious (scars) Iatrogenous Lymphadenectomy Malignant tumors Radiation Traumatic/posttraumatic (scars)

In step 2, *palpation*, lymph nodes are manually examined in terms of size, consistency, mobility, and tenderness. Local arteries and veins are palpated and the swelling is characterized by its consistency (soft, elastic, hard/fibrotic). Visible scars in relation to the lymphatic system are examined and assessed. A standardized evaluation of the possible range of motion should also be performed to assess any accompanying movement limitations (see ▶ Table 4.5).[6,24,25]

4.2.1 Tissue Resistance

Special attention needs to be given to the appearance and characteristics of the edematous extremity or body part. In the early stages of lymphedema, edema will be pitting (indention stays for some time after pressure release) (▶ Fig. 4.1) until the accumulation of excess extravascular fluid has led to fibrosis, fat deposition, and cutaneous and subcutaneous thickening (▶ Fig. 4.2).[24] As tissue resistance increases, the edema becomes nonpitting. "Stemmer's sign"[26] is used to detect an accompanying hardening of tissue and is performed by pinching and lifting up the skin on the proximal phalanx of the second or third finger or the toes. It is considered positive if the tissue cannot be lifted and negative if it is possible to lift the tissue normally.

4.3 Nonapparative Volume Measurement

Tomke Cordts

To determine the extent of the swelling, some form of measurement is required. Today, different methods, apparative and nonapparative, are available. They all vary in terms of cost, accuracy, maintenance, and practicability. While perometry—the use of infrared light to estimate limb volume—and bioelectral spectroscopy—measurement by resistance to a painless electrical current—require expensive, specialized devices, circumferential measurement and water displacement are used most commonly.[27] Whatever method is chosen, because measurements need to be repeated and compared at different time points, special emphasis should be put on standardization and consistency.

Table 4.3 Checklist for patient history (adapted from Wilting et al.[6])

- Family
  - Family history of lymphedema or chronic extremity swelling?
- BMI
- Waist-to-hip-ratio
  - Weight increase?
- Surgeries
  - Vascular, oncologic, orthopedic, etc.
- Pre-existing conditions
  - Metabolic
  - Hormone imbalances
  - Kidney
  - Liver
  - Cardiac
- Venous or arterial diseases
- Previous infections
  - Erysipelas
  - Erythema
  - Tick or insect bites
- Travels in the past months/years? Tropical regions?
- Oncologic history
  - Cancer type
  - TNM classification
  - Histology
  - Therapy
  - Course of disease (relapses)
- Immobilization
  - Times of immobilization due to orthopedic or neurological diseases?
- Injuries
  - Tissue damage
  - Fractures and associated surgeries
- Medications
  - Diuretics
  - Chemotherapy
  - Neurologic medications (i.e., dopamine or GABA antagonists)
  - Hormones (steroids, estrogen, progestogens, rGH)
  - Calcium antagonists
  - Glitazones (possible in combination with insulin)
  - Others
- Additional questions
  - History of weight gain or loss (cyclic increases? days? months?)
  - Association with menstruation?

Abbreviations: BMI, body mass index; GABA, gamma-aminobutyric acid; rGH, recombinant growth hormone; TNM, tumor (T), nodes (N), and metastases (M) staging system

4.3.1 Circumference

Circumferential measurement is the easiest of all techniques.[28] A flexible, nonstretchable tape is used to measure and compare limb circumference at fixed points on the affected and the contralateral extremities. These points can either be at incremental distances (i.e., every 4 cm) from the middle fingertip or at fixed anatomic landmarks, such as the acromion or patella, with the latter method being more accurate.[29] Even though not directly measured, the volume can be calculated from

Table 4.4 Checklist for inspection (adapted from Wilting et al.[6])

- Unilateral or bilateral swelling
- Symmetrical or asymmetrical swelling
- Difference in extremity length (hemihypertrophy)
- Localization of swelling
  - Symmetrical, truncal swelling
    - Shoulders, neck, breast—painful (Dercum's disease)
    - Shoulders, neck, breast—nonpainful (Madelung's disease)
  - Asymmetrical, truncal swelling
    - Lipohypertrophy
  - Asymmetrical extremity swelling
- Skin
  - Color
  - Trophic changes, hair growth
  - Ulcers
  - Pigmentation
  - Scars
  - Papillomatosis cutis lymphostatica
  - Erythema (erysipelas, erythroderma, dermatoses, dermatitis)
  - Hyperkeratosis
  - Lymphectasia
  - Lymphatic cysts
  - Lymphatic fistulas
  - Coarsening of skin texture
  - Signs of dermatomycosis
  - Deepening of skin folds
  - Blunt, "squared off" appearance of toes (▶ Fig. 4.2)
  - Syndactyly
  - Venous changes (varicose veins, phlebitis, corona phlebectatica)

Table 4.5 Checklist for palpation (adapted from Wilting et al.[6])

- Lymph nodes
  - Enlarged
  - Soft
  - Rubbery
  - Hard
  - Tethering to other structures
  - Tender
- Arterial status
  - Pulses palpable
  - Frequency
  - Rhythm
- Venous status
  - Venous filling, varicose veins, corona phlebectatica
  - Signs of phlebitis (pain or burning, hardening, warmth, thrombosis?)
- Edema
  - Soft, pitting
  - Rubbery, elastic, nonpitting
  - Fibrotic, nonpitting
  - Hard, nonpitting
- Subfascial edema (pain on calf compression)
- Lymphatic cysts
- Skin temperature
- Elevation of skin folds, Stemmer's sign
- Thigh pinch test (pressure/pain)
- Range of motion
  - Shoulders, arm, hand
  - Hip, knee, foot

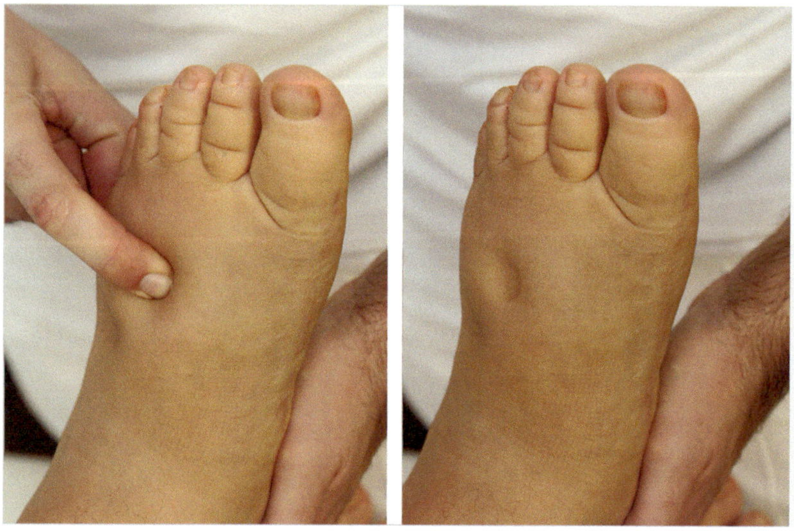

Fig. 4.1 Soft pitting edema.

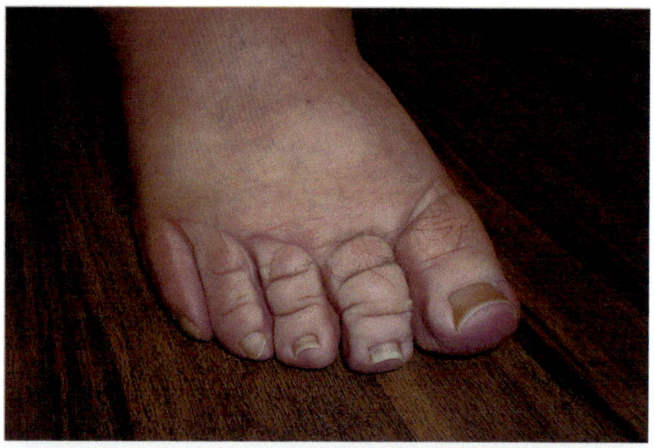

Fig. 4.2 "Squared off" appearance of toes with a positive "Stemmer's sign" by pinching and lifting up the skin.

Table 4.6 Suggested five-point circumference measurement system for edematous upper and lower extremity.

Lower extremity
1. Acromion
2. Mid upper arm
3. Olecranon
4. Mid forearm
5. Mid ulnar styloid
Upper Extremity
1. Anterior iliac spine
2. Mid upper leg
3. Patella
4. Mid lower leg
5. Lateral malleolus

circumference by using a geometrical model consisting of a series of truncated cones (frustums) which are found to approximate the edematous extremity most closely.[30] The arm or leg is divided into a series of corresponding segments, which are then separately calculated by using the formula[29]:

$$V = h(C_1^2 + C_1C_2 + C_2^2)/12\pi$$

V = volume of the segment, C_1 and C_2 = circumferences at the ends of the segment, h = segment length.

A measurement interval (h) of 6 cm was found to produce the smallest standard error of measurement (SEM) compared to water displacement,[30] which is considered "gold standard" by some authors[31,32] but not convenient for routine clinical use[29].

If only circumference is to be used, we suggest the widely practiced protocol of measuring the affected extremity at the most proximal, middle, and most distal anatomical landmark (leg: anterior iliac spine–patella–lateral malleolus; arm: acromion–olecranon–mid ulnar styloid). Between these three points, additional two measurements are taken halfway in between (leg: mid upper leg–mid lower leg; arm: mid upper arm–mid forearm), giving each extremity a set of 5 data points (see ▶ Table 4.6, ▶ Fig. 4.3 and ▶ Fig. 4.4). We consider this method to be fast, reliable, and easy to reproduce, therefore minimizing interobserver variance.

4.3.2 Water Displacement

Volumes are most accurately measured by water displacement.[29,30,33] By Archimedes' principle, when the affected extremity is lowered into a special water tank equipped with an overflow tube (see ▶ Fig. 4.5), the displaced amount of water resembles the volume of the extremity (see ▶ Fig. 4.6). As with any technique, measurement protocol should be followed as closely as possible to achieve comparable results. Hand volumeters usually have a stopping point, which should be placed between the third and fourth digits (see ▶ Fig. 4.5). For the

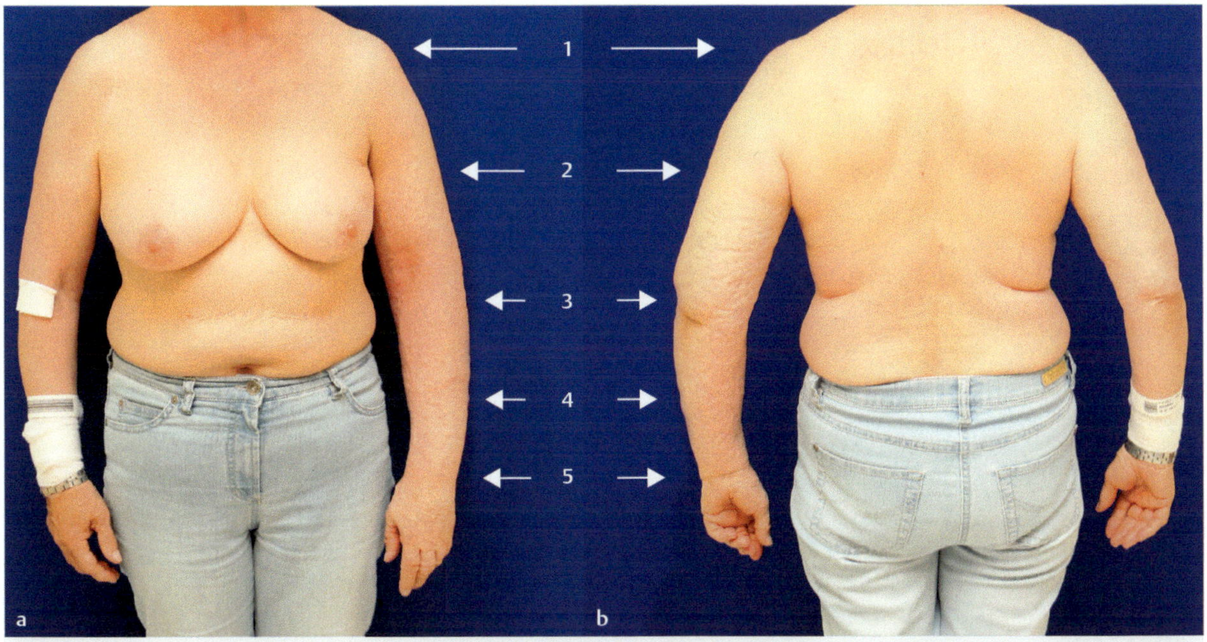

Fig. 4.3 Suggested levels for basic circumferential measurements on the upper extremity: 1, acromion; 2, mid upper arm; 3, olecranon; 4, mid forearm; 5, mid ulnar styloid. (a) frontal view, (b) dorsal view. (Courtesy of Yves Harder.)

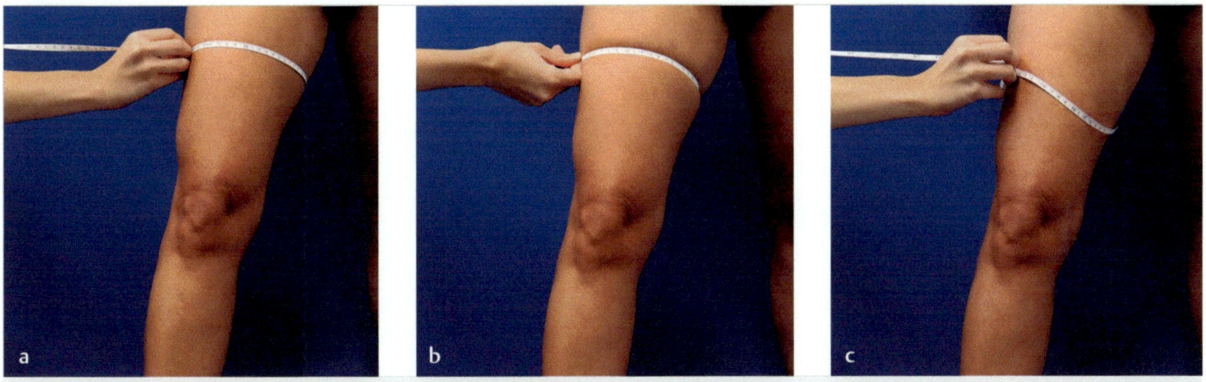

Fig. 4.4 **(a)** How to measure circumference of the lower extremity in a "model" patient at the level of the mid-thigh: **(a)** correct use of measuring tape, **(b)** measuring tape too tight, **(c)** measuring tape too loose. (Courtesy of Yves Harder.)

upper extremity, one way is to instruct the subjects to lower the affected arm slowly into the volumeter and to stop when the top of the volumeter comes in contact with the axilla. The arm is to be held in the water until the outflow reduces to a rate of less than 1 drop per second.[33,34] To achieve an even higher level of standardization, the water temperature should be maintained between 28° and 32 °C[30] as the skin temperature of the extremities is found to be in that area.[35]

However, this method also has relevant disadvantages. In end-stage lymphedema, the grossly enlarged extremity may be too bulky to fit into the water tank. The whole procedure is time consuming, not portable, cannot be used for patients with open wounds, possibly unhygienic, and may be difficult for patients who are less mobile or have reduced limb mobility. Because of these issues and drawbacks, many researchers choose not to use this measurement technique.[29,34,36]

4.4 Ultrasound Imaging

Giuseppe Visconti, Alessendro Bianchi, Marzia Salgarello, and Akitatsu Hayashi

In early stages of lymphedema, enhancement of the lymphatic pathways by using ICG to evaluate an extremity

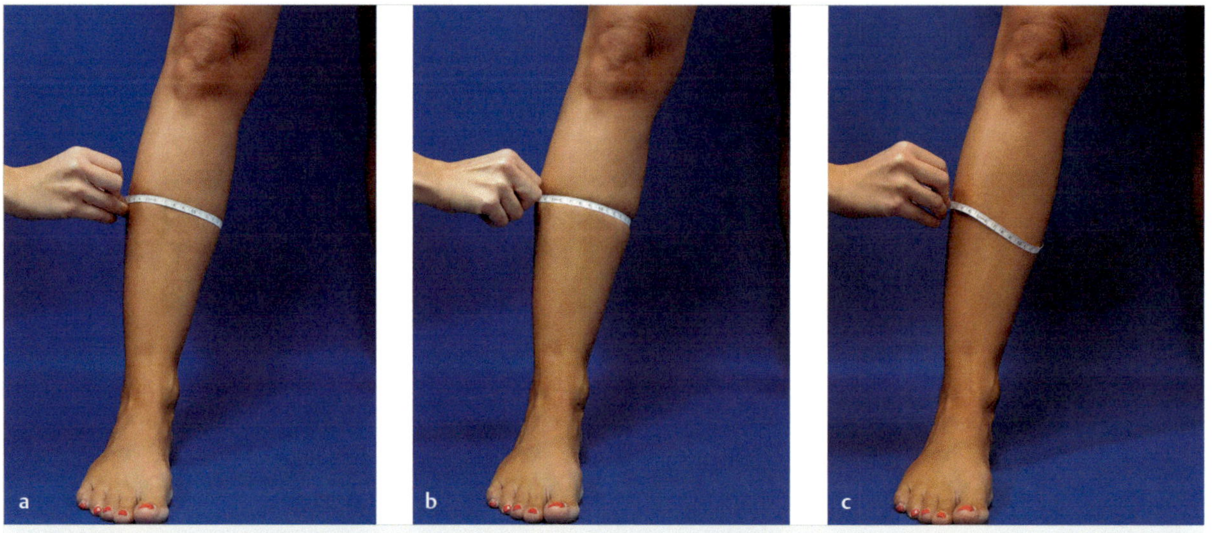

Fig. 4.4b **(b)** How to measure circumference of the lower extremity in a "model" patient at the level of the mid lower leg: **(a)** correct use of measuring tape, **(b)** measuring tape too tight, **(c)** measuring tape too loose. (Courtesy of Yves Harder.)

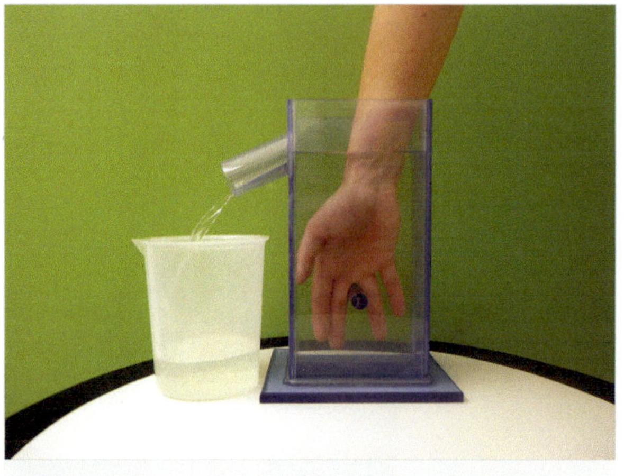

Fig. 4.5 Volume measurement of hand by overflow water tank.

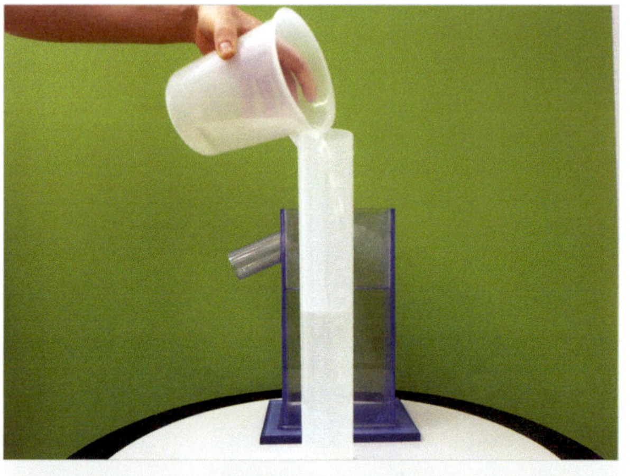

Fig. 4.6 The amount of the displaced water resembles the volume of the extremity.

for functional lymphatic collectors is quite common and feasible.

In advanced cases, International Society of Lymphology (ISL) II to III stage and/or lymphedema patients with active lymphorrea, the imaging modalities based on contrast enhancement of lymphatic channels may fail in visualizing functional lymphatic channels for various technical reasons. Considering one of the most used examinations, ICG lymphangiography, this tool will probably fail in locating linear pattern in such advanced cases for two main reasons: fast spreading of dermal backflow and depth-limited visualization. In advanced cases, one more technical side effect is the contrast-based technology itself. These images will show the lymphosome superimposed by the fluorescence by the injection itself. If that lymphosome is damaged, it does not mean that there are no collateral compensatory pathways still working—but they are not visualized.

Ultrasound may "bring light to the invisible".

In this perspective, *ultrasound technology* should be considered as a further helpful tool for evaluating lymphedema patients, as this technology is based on the direct visualization of lymphatic channels, and not those related to the lymphosome only.

In our opinion, ultrasound represents a quintessence in lymphatic surgery and should be considered as a further standard in lymphatic surgery[37,38,39,40,41,42,43] (▶ Fig. 4.7 and ▶ Fig. 4.8).

In 2016, Hayashi et al. demonstrated that it is possible to identify lymphatic channels in the lower limb by using high-frequency ultrasound (UHF-US) technology.[37] Later, we demonstrated that UHF-US gives clearer and

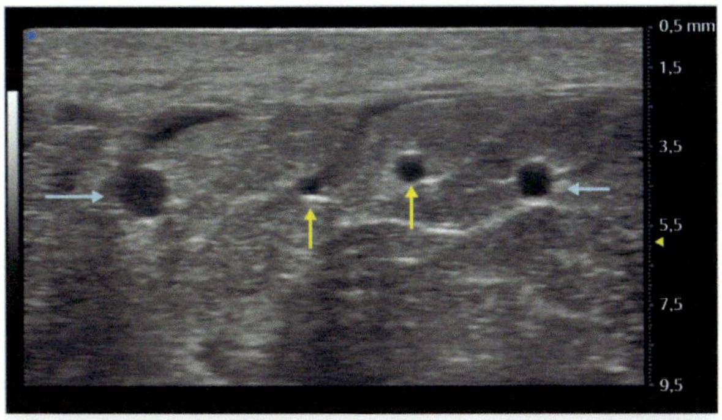

Fig. 4.7 High-frequency ultrasound scan of upper extremity lymphedema. Two functional lymphatic channels (yellow arrows) and two nearby favorable recipient venules (blue arrows) are located. Finally, two lymphovenous anastomosis were thus planned at this incision point in the presented case.

more preoperative information on lymphatic channels, especially by the use of 48 and 70 MHz probes, which have resolutions of 50 and 30 µm, respectively.[39]

UHF-US should not be seen as an alternative to other imaging modalities for visualizing lymphatic channels, but rather as a second level examination and helpful adjunct. In fact, it can be used to further analyze the "linear patterns" enhanced by ICG lymphangiography.

The UHF-US examination includes the:

- position
- number
- degeneration status
- caliber

of lymphatic channels along the linear pattern and can be determined preoperatively. When ICG lymphangiography fails to detect lymphatic channels, the limb can be scanned in search of functional lymphatic channels.

This examination requires ultrasound skills that should be mastered by the operating surgeon rather than delegating it to other specialists. In fact, the operating surgeon will define and personally mark the operative planning during the study based on her/his findings.

Note:

Lymphatic channels show peculiar static and dynamic ultrasound images:

- In B mode, lymphatic channels appear as misshapen, specular, hypoechoic structures surrounded by a hyperechoic texture.
- In color-doppler mode, they show no color signal.
- There is a tendency to maintain a similar caliber in their course and no convergence with vein, artery, and/or nerves.
- Expandability is achieved after constant pressure is exerted with the probe.

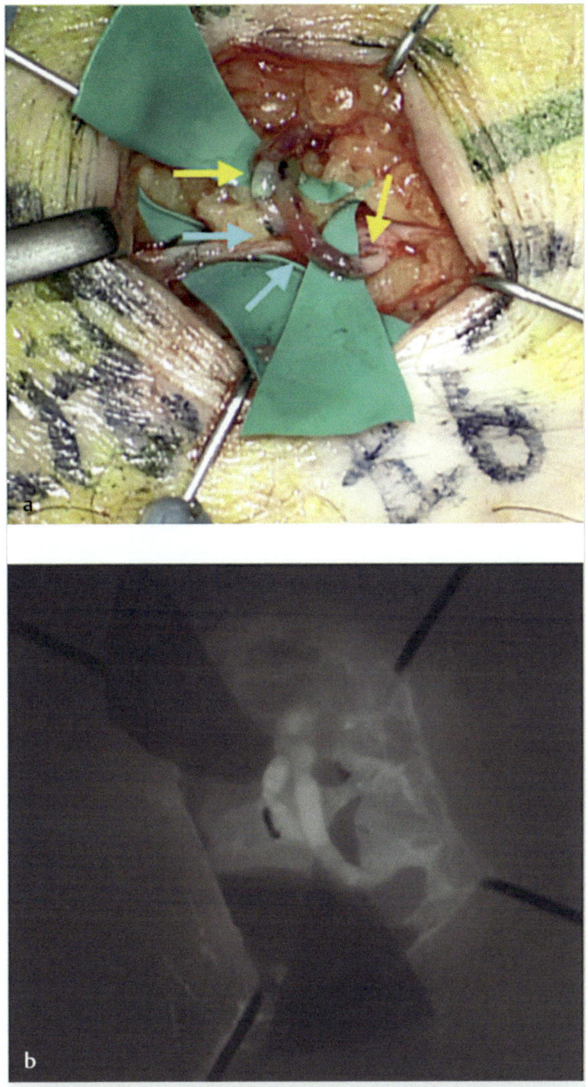

Fig. 4.8 Intraoperative situs of two lymphovenous anastomoses. **(a)** The surgeon needs to dissect the vessels and perform the lymphovenous anastomosis. In the image, patent lymphovenous anastomoses are shown (venule, blue arrows; lymphatic channel, yellow arrows). **(b)** Patency is controlled using ICG imaging. This image shows a high level of accuracy achieved after lymphovenous reconstruction, representing the benefits of preoperative planning conducted with high-frequency ultrasound.

4.4.1 Advantages of Technology in Preoperative Planning of Lymphovenous Anastomoses

Evaluation of a Recipient Venule nearby the Selected Lymphatic Collector

This is paramount to obtain functional, patent, and reflux-free lymphovenous anastomoses (LVA), as recipient venules play an independent but important role in the efficacy of the procedure. For this purpose, UHF-US is sufficient in evaluating both the recipient venule and lymphatic collector.

Recipient venule should be evaluated in B-mode and color-doppler mode for position, caliber, and presence of competent valve with no blood reflux.[44,45]

Evaluation of Lymphatic Channels

For this purpose, UHF-US with 48 and 70 MHz probes is recommended. Ultrasound can be used to further explore a linear pattern found at ICG lymphangiography. In addition, it is recommended for locating lymphatic channels not seen at ICG lymphangiography such us in dermal backflow areas.

UHF-US has been demonstrated to provide details of lymphatic channels comparable to histology, allowing the surgeon to select functional lymphatic collectors which enables to obtain consistent results with LVA.[41]

Preoperative Planning in Patients with Iodine Allergy or Hyperthyroidism

ICG should not be administered in patients with an iodine allergy or significant hyperthyroidism. Different from drug washout when used intravascularly, ICG used for lymphangiography (intradermal/subcutaneous injection), especially in lymphedematous limb, can remain within the tissue for up to 1 to 2 months. This may represent a real challenge where there is a risk anaphylaxis. In patients with iodine allergy, ICG lymphangiography should be avoided and preoperative planning can be performed by using a hybrid or pure ultrasound methods.[40]

Intraoperative Selection of Lymphatic Collectors

It is quite common to find more than one lymphatic collector at the same incision site during exploration for LVA, which can be limited by the availability and physiology of good and numerous recipient venules. Although an end-to-side anastomosis can always be considered in these cases, the surgeon may use UHF-US to select the best functional lymphatic channels to bypass before cutting them. Intraoperative UHF-US helps to evaluate the quality of the lymphatic channel and thus select the most functional vessel for the bypass.[42]

Preoperative and Intraoperative Planning of Venule Rerouting

Ultrasound technology helps to locate favorable recipient venule for LVA. However, in some cases, no favorable recipient venule can be located nearby a functional lymphatic collector. In this scenario, a venule rerouting should be planned preoperatively, or intraoperatively, to be able to bypass the lymphatic channel in an efficient and effective way.[43]

4.4.2 Advantages of Ultrasound in Preoperative Planning of Vascularized Lymph Node Transfer

Ultrasound technology

- aids the study of the number and type of lymph nodes to be included in the flap (either preoperatively, or intraoperatively after the harvest);
- aids the study of the microvascular pedicle anatomy of the flap (not intrabdominal);
- aids the study of the lymph nodes anatomical relation to perforator vessels for a skin island to be included;
- aids the mapping and locating of the recipient vessel.

UHF-US is used to study lymph node efferent lymphatic collectors to perform additional efferent LVA after traditional revascularization.

To conclude, ultrasound technology is a quintessence in lymphatic surgery, especially for LVA.

It facilitates very detailed preoperative planning, which improves surgical efficiency by:

- reducing time for exploration and dissection;
- reducing time for decision-making (already done preoperatively);
- avoiding useless incisions (devoid of lymphatic channels and/or recipient venule);
- reducing the length of the incision;
- allowing to perform LVA with a good lymphatic collector in the absence of valid recipient venule (venule rerouting).

Overall, ultrasound in lymphatic surgery may address reduction of operative time, reduction of operation-related costs, more predictive results, higher patient compliance, satisfaction, and adherence to postoperative protocols.

4.5 Scintigraphic Lymphangiography

Pierre Bourgeois

Lymphoscintigraphy has been the standard diagnostic device for imaging of the lymphatic system including lymph node and lymphatic vessels for decades and now has been successfully complemented by ICG and magnetic resonance lymphangiography (MRL). It has been applied both for oncologic staging and for evaluating the lymphedema stage with measurement of the transport index.

In the 1980s, a three-phase protocol for scintigraphic investigation and imaging of the superficial lymphatic system in lymphedema staging after the subcutaneous injection of 99mTc-labeled nanosized colloids of human serum albumin (one-tenth of one vial in 0.2 ml) in the first interdigital space of each limb was developed. The protocol was then refined over time.[46,47] These three phases correspond to image acquisitions as follows:

- **Phase 1.** Images are acquired during (dynamic) and after a resting period (whole body imaging and/or static images), with the patient lying on the examination table for 30 minutes.
- **Phase 2.** With the patient lying on the examination table, the images are acquired during (dynamic) and after (whole body imaging and/or static images) performing a standardized exercise (5 minutes of tiptoeing or 15 minutes of hand gripping).
- **Phase 3.** Images (whole body imaging and/or static imaging: now, SPECT-CT is also quite systematically done) are acquired after the patient performs normal activities for 1 hour. In cases with lower limb edema, the images should be acquired after walking, making sure that the patient does not remain sitting in the waiting room prior to imaging (▶ Fig. 4.9). In cases with upper limb edema, the images should be acquired after the patient performs movements with the fingers, hands, and limbs in ways that would be part of normal daily activity (one study is under way evaluating if 30 minutes of normal activities are not enough to give the useful information). These delayed images can also be obtained after longer periods of normal activity, but normal values for the extractions of the tracer will have to be obtained.

Note:

One hour is usually convenient both for patients and for imaging scheduling at a nuclear medicine service.

The information provided by these images is important for the surgeons in many ways:

- They represent the anatomical basis for the choice of the surgery to be performed, for example, LVA if intact lymph vessels are detected.
- They represent response of the lymphatic system to the lifestyle activities that precede the appearance of lymphedema (latent stage 0), more precisely of the lymphatic flows in resting conditions (phase 1) and with exercise conditions (phase 2).
- The planar imaging provides anatomical localization of the lymphatic vessels and of the lymph nodes (these can be marked on the skin) and, with SPECT-CT, the depth of these lymphatic structures and their relationships with the surrounding structures (veins, arteries) can also be obtained.

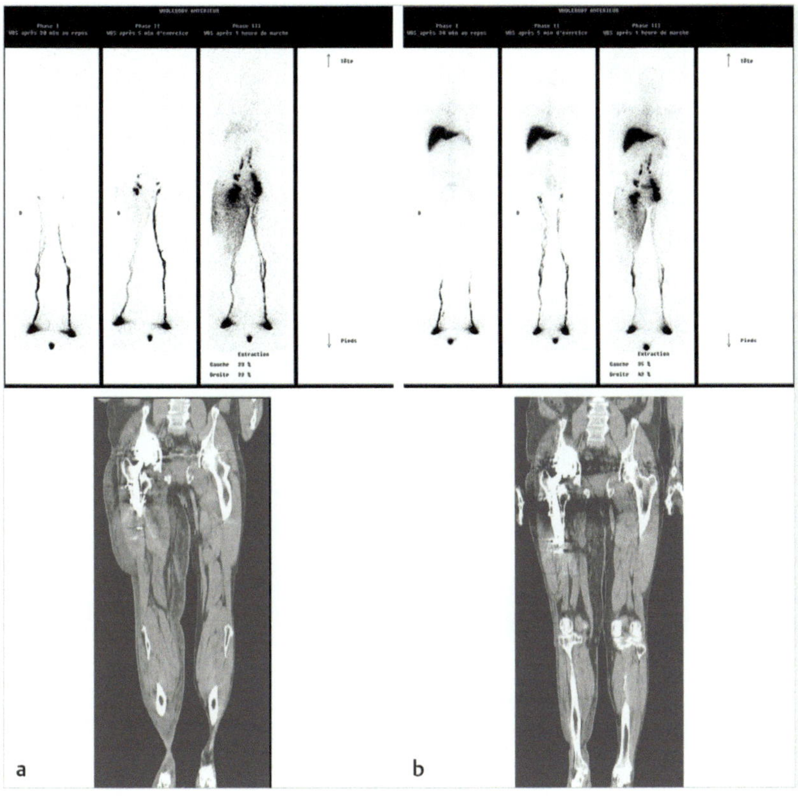

Fig. 4.9 Anterior whole-body scan images obtained in one patient with one right lower limb post-traumatic lymphedema before surgery ([**a**] from left to right, whole-body scan after 30 minutes in resting condition, after 5 minutes of tiptoeing, and after 60 minutes of walking) and after one lymph node to vein anastomosis performed at the inguinal level ([**b**] whole-body scan after 60 minutes of walking). Before surgery, the tracer reached the first inguinal lymph node (arrow 1 in [**a**]). With exercise, the lymph flow (the activity in the inguinal lymph nodes) appears higher in the right lymph node than in the left lymph node (arrow 2 in [**a**]). After 1 hour of walking, the lymphatic fluid flows back from the right inguinal lymph node in the superficial collateralizing dermal lymphatic network of the thigh (arrow 3 in [**a**]). After surgery, the dermal backflow appears less pronounced than before surgery (**b**).

- The lymphoscintigraphic pictures are inherently quantitative, and several parameters can be calculated (▶ Table 4.7).
- Postoperatively, lymphoscintigraphy can be used to evaluate the patency of LVA or rearrangement of the lymphatics after vascularized lymph node transfer (VLNT) surgery (▶ Fig. 4.10).

One transport index has been proposed by Kleinhans et al.[48] It represents one way to analyze the lymphoscintigraphic imaging and to classify these pictures. This transport index has unfortunately been used indiscriminately and in technical situations that did not correspond to the conditions in which it was initially established (another radiotracer is used which influences the kinetics and distribution; another site of injection and/or another kind of injection, for instance, intradermal and not subcutaneous).

Table 4.7 Quantitative and functional parameters of lymphoscintigraphic investigations

- Extraction of the tracer by the lymphatic system at the level of the injected site(s)
- Dynamics/speed of lymphatic flows in the lymphatic vessels
- Activity remaining in the lymphatic vascular structures
- Time taken by the tracer to reach the first lymph nodes (for instance, from the foot to the first inguinal lymph nodes)
- Activity in the lymph nodes
- Time to reach half of the maximum activity in the lymph nodes
- Activity in the liver
- Ratio of the activity in the lymph nodes versus the activity in the liver

The dynamic and/or static acquisitions will sometimes have to be adapted to answer specific questions:

- To study the patency of the thoracic duct
- To precisely determine the region and level of the lymphatic leakage
- To demonstrate the patency and functionality of the LVA or lymphatic vessel transplantation
- To investigate edema at the level of the face, of the breast, or (limited to part) of the genitals
- In patients with lymphangioma, lymphangiomatosis, or lymphoceles, to show the arrival and accumulation of the tracer in the lymphatic space

4.6 Indocyanine Green Near-Infrared Imaging

Emre Gazyakan

4.6.1 Indocyanine Green

ICG is a water-soluble tricarbocyanine dye and the only near-infrared (NIR) excited fluorophore used clinically in various applications. ICG was discovered by the Kodak Research Laboratories in 1955 and first approved for

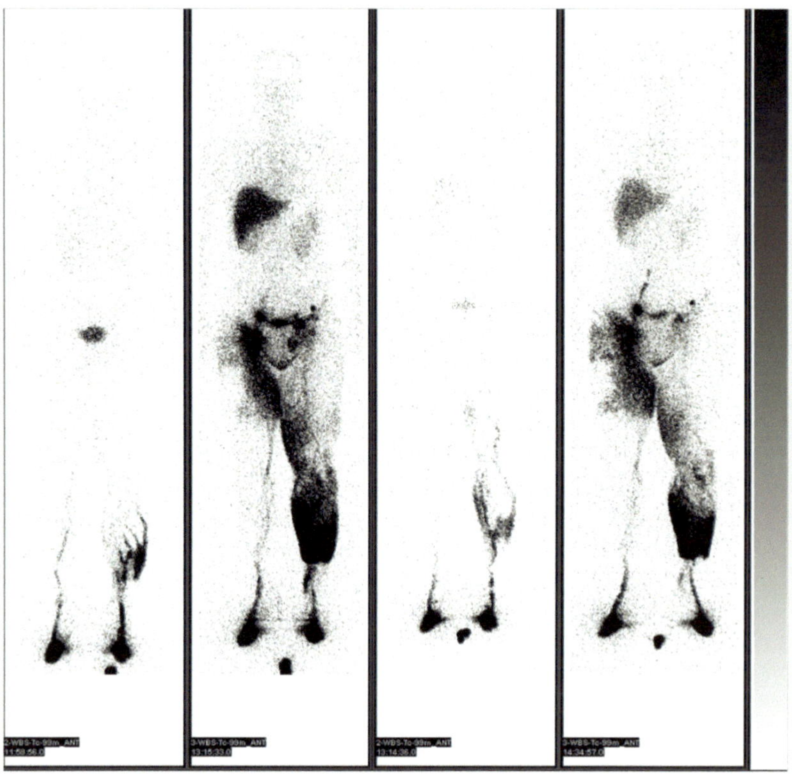

Fig. 4.10 Anterior whole-body scan obtained in one patient with bilateral lower limb lymphedema and penoscrotal edema secondary to surgery and radiotherapy for prostate cancer (from left to right, whole-body scan after 5 minutes of tiptoeing and after 60 minutes of walking) before and after one lymphovenous anastomosis performed at the inguinal level. After surgery, the dermal backflow appears less pronounced than before surgery.

clinical use in 1956.[49] However, it took many years before ICG was routinely used, first in angiography and later in retinal angiography.[50,51]

The fluorescent dye rapidly binds to plasma proteins, of which apolipoprotein B is the main carrier. ICG has a plasma half-life time of 2.4 minutes. Hepatic metabolism begins just shortly after injection, and ICG is secreted in its unconjugated form entirely into the bile. There is no significant extrahepatic or enterohepatic circulation.[52]

Absorption and fluorescence of ICG occurs in the NIR range with maxima of 805 and 835 nm, respectively, which ranges near the isosbestic point of hemoglobin and oxyhemoglobin.[53] The spectrum depends on the dilution medium, the ICG concentration, and the temperature among others.[54] Correct application aids deep penetration of the skin with fluorescence induced from blood vessels, mainly within the deep dermal plexus and subcutaneous fat. The fluorescence dye is invisible to the human eye. An infrared-sensitive charge-coupled device (CCD) camera can detect the fluorescence emission of the excited dye and visualize on a monitor (▸ Fig. 4.11).

The use of ICG is safe and shows rates of adverse effects comparable to other types of contrast media, with frequencies of 0.05% for severe side effects, such as arrhythmia, hypotension, or, more rarely, anaphylactic shock, to 0.2% for moderate and mild side effects, such as syncope, nausea, pruritus, or skin eruptions.[55] In this context, exposure to blue dye showed severe allergic reaction and anaphylaxis in 1% to 3% of patients during sentinel lymph node biopsy.[56] ICG is contraindicated in patients with allergy and intolerance to sodium iodide and iodine. Relative contraindications are thyroid disorders such as hyperthyroidism and thyrotoxicosis.

ICG dye is present in powder form and can be dissolved in various solvents. However, it is advised to dissolve it in distilled water for its spectral stabilization. It is not recommended to dissolve it in isotonic saline because of precipitation.[57] ICG is unstable in aqueous solution and when exposed to light and should be used within 6 to 10 hours. The storage of ICG solution should be at low temperature (4 °C) to prevent decomposition.

ICG has been successfully applied for many years in liver surgery, vascular surgery, coronary surgery, and sentinel lymph node biopsy among others.[58,59] Another recent application of ICG fluorescence imaging is the evaluation of the lymphatics in lymphovascular disorders. Lymphoscintigraphy has long been considered as the main approach for lymphedema evaluation.[60] However, it is not providing the degree of fine anatomical detail, real-time characterization, and carries the risk of radiation exposure. Here, ICG fluorescence imaging displays its advantages of being nonionizing, nontoxic, high contrast, and easy to use in real-time.

For this application, ICG needs to be **administered as an off-label use for subcutaneous or intradermal injections in many countries** at varying doses for mapping the lymphatic vasculature or assessing LVA surgery. Several ICG fluorescence imaging devices are available on the market such as the photodynamic eye Neo II (PDE; Hamamatsu Photonics Co., Hamamatsu, Japan), the SPY Elite (Stryker Corporation, Kalamazoo, Michigan, USA), Fluobeam (Fluoptics, Grenoble, France), Hyper Eye Medical Systems (HEMS, Mizuho Medical Co., Ltd., Tokyo, Japan), IC-Flow™ Imaging System (Diagnostic Green GmbH, Aschheim-Dornach, Germany), and Surgical Microscopes (Carl Zeiss AG, Oberkochen, Germany; Leica, Wetzlar, Germany).

4.6.2 Lymphangiography

Unno et al. used ICG for the first time in 2007 to evaluate the lymphatic vasculature in patients with secondary lymphedema.[61] Ogata et al. also emphasized the easy detection of functional lymphatic vessels for LVA in patients with lymphedema.[62] Since then a series of clinical studies has been performed to establish ICG lymphangiography for pre-, peri-, and postoperative assessments.[63,64,65,66] After completing the workup and before the procedure, obtaining a patient-centered informed consent for the surgical treatment and, where applicable, for the "off-label use" of ICG is advisable.

ICG lymphangiography can be performed without any special preparation by administrating it into the region of interest. An insulin syringe (1 ml; scale value 0.01 ml) is loaded with ICG solution and a 30-gauge syringe needle is used for injection. Under aseptic conditions, 0.05 to 0.2 ml

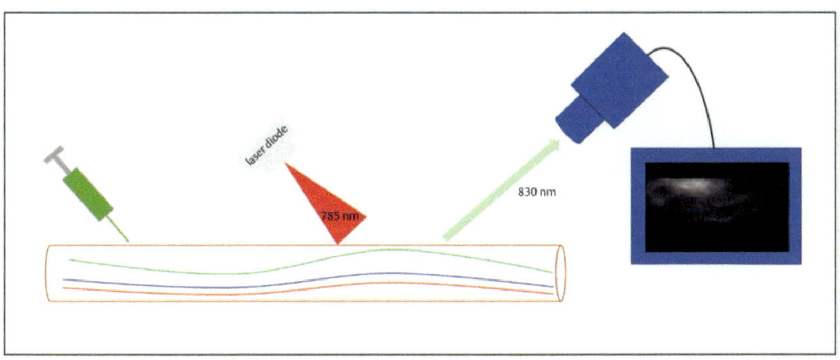

Fig. 4.11 Basic principle of ICG near-infrared imaging: After intravenous or intradermal injection, the region of interest is excited with near-infrared light (785 nm). The fluorescence emission is detected 1 to 2 cm beneath the skin by a charge-coupled device camera system.

of the ICG solution is injected intradermally or subcutaneously. The ICG dosage for lymphangiography ranges from 0.03 to 0.25 mg.[67] For the lower extremity, injections can be performed either into the first and second web space of the foot or into the first web space of the foot and the posterior region of the lateral malleolus. For the upper extremity, injections can be performed either into the second and third web spaces of the hand or into the second web space of the hand and at the ulnar border of the palmaris longus tendon at the level of the wrist.

With the fluorescence imaging system, dermal and subdermal lymphatics (collectors, precollectors, and capillary plexus) can be identified to an approximate depth of 15 mm. Immediately after ICG injection, the observation begins at the injection site, where a wipe contamination of the skin with a superimposed fluorescence image should be prevented. Real-time lymphatic flow is observed and captured with the fluorescence imaging system. After 3 to 5 minutes, patients are allowed to move freely, but are instructed to present immediately in case of any intolerance. Because the period to visualize the lymphatic system takes approximately 6 hours to plateau, patients are encouraged to move their extremities abundantly for about 1 to 1.5 hours. This enables an earlier achievement of the plateau after ICG injection. In terms of evaluation of lymphatics, Yamamoto et al. differentiate between static and dynamic protocols.[68,69] However, feasibility in a daily setting in the hospital and in private practice demonstrated that patients receive their dye injection and after a waiting period ICG lymphangiography is performed.

ICG lymphangiography reveals various flow patterns regarding the pathophysiologic severity. Lymphographic pattern can be linear and demonstrate a regular function and directed flow via the lymphatic collectors: Lymphatic function is normal. ICG lymphographic patterns change with the progression of lymphedema. A variety of nondirected, dermal backflow patterns are observed with it.[64] Changes are reflected in splash, stardust, and ultimately diffuse lymphographic patterns (▸ Fig. 4.12). The history of these lymphographic findings depends in the disease progression. With injury to the lymphatics, lymphatic hypertension occurs, thus changing the lymphodynamic conditions of lymph vessels from normal to ectasia to vessel wall hyperthrophy to fibrotic changes and stenosis.[70] These changes are partially evident on ICG lymphographic studies. Dilated lymphatic capillaries and precollectors are seen in the splash pattern, while in the stardust pattern, lymph extravasation takes place because of collaterals failing to compensate lymph flow overload. This is observed through multiple bright spots during ICG lymphangiography. In the final stage, the diffuse pattern, ICG is widely distributed representing a distinct pooling and diffuse, nondirected flow. In obstructive lymphedema, the dermal backflow pattern extends from proximal to distal. ICG lymphangiography facilitates the assessment of the affected and unaffected regions of interest and may require further modalities as ultrasound or MRI as an adjunct. With dermal backflow pattern staging, a structured categorization enables the surgeon to choose the correct lymphedema management and therapy (▸ Table 4.8).[64,64,71,72] All these patterns can be correlated to morphological changes of the soft tissue, the lymphatic collectors and the ISL stage (see **Chapter 3, 4** and **Fig. 18.1**).

In the operative, setting ICG lymphangiography is used for strategic incision placement for LVA. In addition to marking the lymphatic vessels, smaller veins also need to be identified, mostly during dissection. A more targeted and advanced approach is the ultrasound or NIR vein visualization (see **Subchapters 4.5** and **8.4.5**). Superficial venules can be mapped which are in close proximity or better intersecting nearby lymphatic vessels (▸ Fig. 4.13). This guided approach could increase the possibility of successful vessel mapping thus increasing successful LVA.[73]

Even without guided mapping, ICG lymphangiography can be used intraoperatively for navigation during surgery. With a sterile, draped, handheld device, the surgeon can find adequate lymphatic vessel even in deeper layers of the subcutaneous tissue which might be suitable for LVA after incision. Intraoperative ICG lymphangiography works better in the early stages. Due to lymphosclerosis with concomitant absence of flow in severe stage dermal

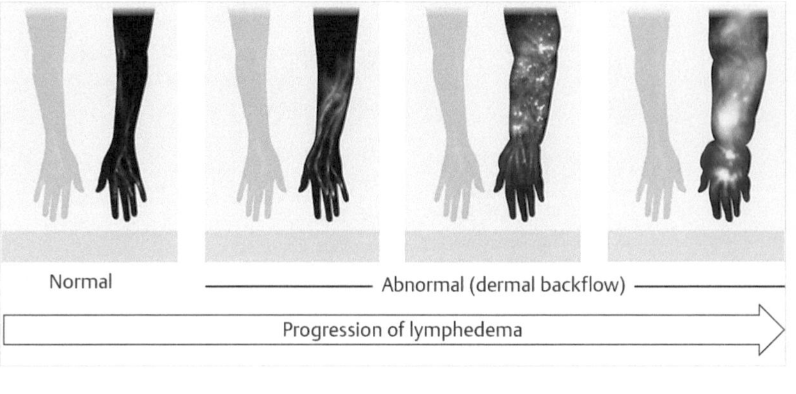

Fig. 4.12 Different patterns and images of ICG lymphangiography. The progression of lymphedema becomes apparent with changes in lymphographic findings from linear to splash, stardust, and diffuse pattern, reflecting the pathophysiological changes (see also **Chapter 18** and Fig 18.1).[64]

Table 4.8 Dermal backflow pattern staging for the upper and lower extremities (adapted from Yamamoto et al.[63,64])

Stage	Upper Extremity	Lower Extremity
0	No dermal backflow pattern	No dermal backflow pattern
I	Splash pattern around the axilla	Splash pattern around the groin region
II	Stardust pattern limited between the axilla and the olecranon	Stardust pattern extended proximal to the superior border of the patella
III	Stardust pattern exceeding the olecranon	Stardust pattern extended distal to the superior border of the patella
IV	Stardust pattern observed throughout the limb	Stardust pattern extended to the whole limb
V	Diffuse pattern and stardust pattern observed throughout the limb	Existence of diffuse pattern with stardust pattern in the background

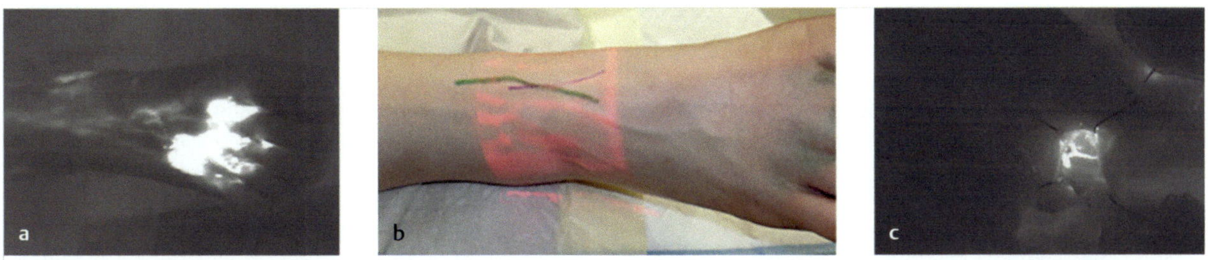

Fig. 4.13 Strategic incision placement for lymphovenous anastomosis with ICG lymphangiography for lymphatic vessel mapping **(a)** and near-infrared vein visualization **(b)** for superficial venule mapping. Intersection of the vessels were marked **(b)**, and intraoperative confirmation of successful lymphovenous anastomosis through ICG lymphangiography is performed **(c)**.

backflow pattern, visualization of lymphatic vessels can be difficult. However, Yang et al. could demonstrate in their study that even non-ICG enhanced but lymphatic flow-positive could be considered for a functional LVA.[74] (**Chapter 8**) Post-LVA patency can also be detected intraoperatively with ICG lymphangiography.

There have been reports on ICG lymphangiography being an effective postoperative tracking modality after lymphatic reconstructions such as LVA.[75,76] The evaluation was performed at 1 month for up to 12 months postoperatively demonstrating high correlation with the clinical outcome.

Another potential diagnostic use of ICG lymphangiography is predictive lymphatic mapping. It was first described by Mihara and colleagues in the preoperative assessment of patients with severe unilateral lymphedema.[77] ICG lymphangiography was unable to detect any linear lymphatics for LVA because of advanced dermal backflow pattern. Instead of just operating along the anatomical landmarks, Mihara and colleagues used the anatomy of the healthy contralateral lower extremity and transferred lymphatic mapping patterns from the unaffected to the affected extremity in those patients. By using fixed lines and scaling the results to the affected limb they were able to perform LVA successfully with a 2-cm incision. This preliminary study was refined in a current study of lymphatic mapping of the upper limb by mirroring of the healthy limb.[78] Predictive lymphatic mapping was performed in 16 patients with unilateral upper limb lymphedema showing stardust or diffuse dermal backflow pattern. They were able to find at least three incision sites each carrying a minimum of one lymphatic vessel suitable for LVA. In this way, the patients received approximately three anastomoses. Predictive lymphatic mapping appears to be a good alternative in preoperative mapping of lymphatics in severe dermal backflow patterns. However, further studies are needed with a long follow-up to prove its efficacy.

4.6.3 Reversed Lymphatic Mapping

Free vascularized lymph node transfer (VLNT) is applied more and more in the treatment of lymphedema.[79] (see **Chapter 10** and **11**) Even though the results are promising, the risk of iatrogenic lymphedema at the donor site should be not underestimated.[80,81,82,83,84,85]

For this reason, Dayan and colleagues modified the hitherto concept of axillary reverse mapping (ARM) by Klimberg.[86,87] The idea behind mapping the lymphatic drainage of the arm and the breast region is the reduction of potential disruption of lymphatics during lymphadenectomy, thus minimizing the risk of subsequent lymphedema. For this, blue dye is injected into the arm to display and to preserve the lymphatics, and technetium is administrated to map the drainage of the breast. Dayan and colleagues basically used this mapping technique for VLNT in order to minimize the risk of iatrogenic lymphedema.[88] Instead of blue dye, they used ICG to visualize the lymphatic drainage pattern and especially the lymph nodes for VLNT. The injection of technetium to the limb help identify and thus avoid the lymph nodes draining the extremity. Reverse lymphatic mapping can be applied for groin lymph node, axillary lymph node, and supraclavicular lymph node harvest.

For the axilla, ARM is applied for harvesting a vascularized thoracodorsal artery or lateral thoracic artery-based lymph node transfer (▶ Fig. 4.14). Technetium is injected into the first and second web spaces of the ipsilateral hand of lymph node harvest about 2 hours before the surgery.

ICG is injected into about four to five areas transversely to the chest and back about 15 to 20 cm inferior to the axillary fold. Gamma probe identification of the axillary nodes allows them to be spared from flap dissection or incidental injury. ICG lymphangiography identifies the vascularized lymph nodes at the lateral chest wall that can be harvested safely. This procedure is done pre- and intraoperatively. For the groin, technetium, or an alternative tracer (e.g., blue dye) is injected into the first and second web spaces of the foot and drained to lymph nodes that drain the lower leg. Usually these are the lymph nodes below the groin crease. These nodes can be identified with the gamma probe and hence be avoided. Injection of ICG to the lower abdomen identifies the lymph nodes in the groin area that can be safely harvested.

A retrospective review of 35 patients undergoing VLNT using reverse lymphatic mapping demonstrated no observed cases of donor-site lymphedema.[88] Demiri and colleagues showed in their meta-analysis of 189 patients in 11 clinical studies a rate of donor-site lymphedema of 1.6%.[84] This is the only clinical study using ICG for antegrade and technetium for reverse lymphatic mapping. Shortcomings of this study are lack of long-term follow-up, ranging only from 1 to 30 months, and further clinical experience.[89] A newer approach is reverse lymphatic mapping without radioisotope.[90] The idea behind is avoiding the adverse effects of the radioisotope technetium, thereby improving patient safety. In addition, reverse lymphatic mapping can be applied in more institutions that are lacking nuclear medicine and are resource limited. By combining ICG lymphangiography and blue dye injections coupled with anatomical expertise, the surgeon should be able to harvest lymph nodes flaps safely (▶ Fig. 4.15).

In a preliminary study, Aliotta and Schwarz followed up on 17 patients with this technique demonstrating no iatrogenic lymphedema in the extremity associated with the lymph node harvest.[90] They reported one case of skin necrosis from subdermal injection of methylene blue that required surgical therapy. This new approach to reverse lymphatic mapping seems to be a real alternative. It appears to be safe, cost effective, and can be performed in institutions without nuclear medicine. However, further studies are necessary to prove its long-term outcome.

4.6.4 Conclusions

ICG lymphangiography is a necessary basic tool for preoperative diagnostics, intraoperative navigation or reverse mapping, and postoperative follow-up after LVA or VLNT to visualize the lymphatic rearrangement. It is considered to be safe and reliable and to offer real-time presentation, although it still must be regarded as an off-label use. ICG lymphangiography facilitates the evaluation and staging of

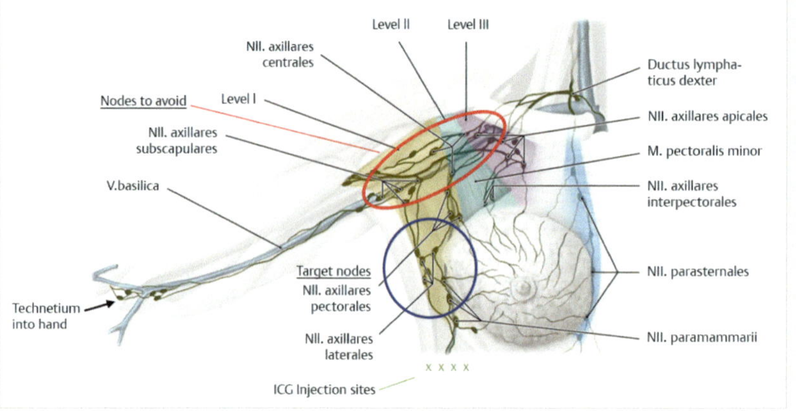

Fig. 4.14 Target lymph nodes for a vascularized lymph node flap based on the thoracodorsal artery or lateral thoracic artery. Lymph nodes in the axilla should be avoided. Injection of technetium or an alternative tracer into the first and second web spaces of the hand. Indocyanine green injections transversely cross the chest and back to identify includable lymph nodes. (Reproduced with permission from Schünke M, Schulte E, Schumacher U, Voll M, Wesker K. Prometheus LernAtlas: Innere Organe. 5th ed. Thieme; 2018.)

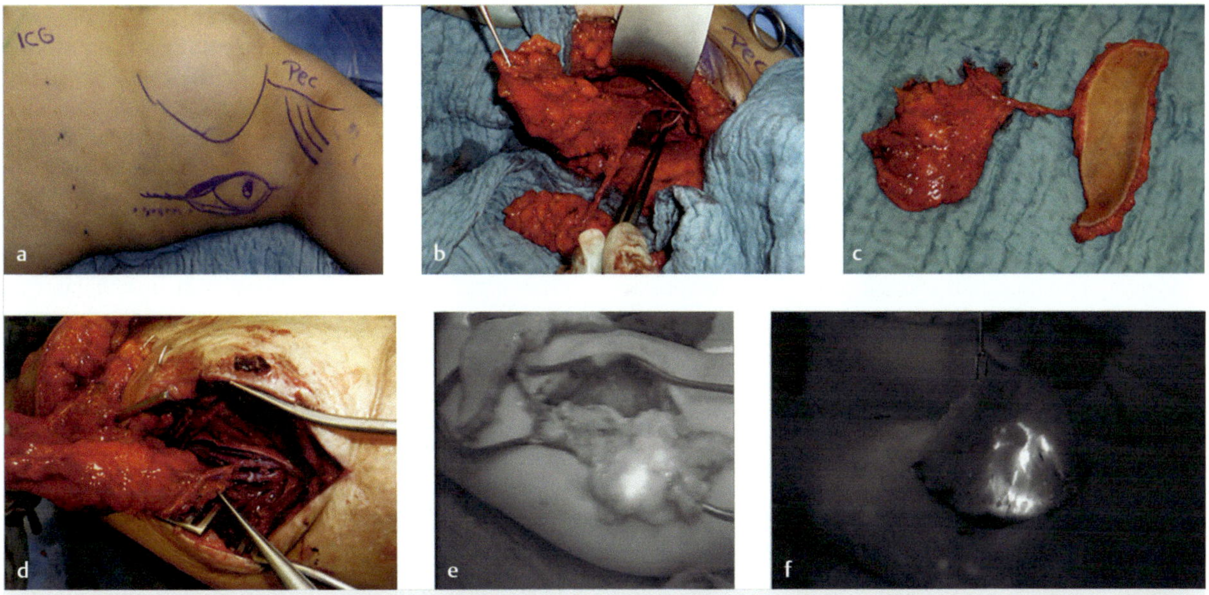

Fig. 4.15 Intraoperative markings (anterior edge of latissimus dorsi and inferior edge of pectoralis major muscle) for vascularized lymph node transfer based on the thoracodorsal vessels **(a)**. Lymph node flap with skin island based on the thoracodorsal vessels and with preservation of the thoracodorsal nerve **(b)**. The harvested lymph node flap with a perforator-based skin island **(c)** is anastomosed to the anterior tibial vessels **(d)**. Indocyanine green is injected intraoperatively into the skin island to demonstrate uptake of the lymph nodes **(e)** and again, 2 years after the initial surgery, during a flap thinning procedure **(f)**.

the lymphatics. The characteristic flow patterns lead to the corresponding lymphedema management. In the preoperative assessment strategic markings of lymphatics for LVA can lead to good outcome. It can also be applied intraoperatively to detect lymphatics more quickly, thus concentrating the surgical field for reliable LVA.

Reverse lymphatic mapping appears to be a promising tool for safer lymph node harvest to reduce donor-site morbidity, especially donor-site lymphedema. Further clinical experience and long-term follow-up is necessary, especially without radioisotopes, to underline its efficacy.

4.7 Magnetic Resonance Imaging

Carola Brussaard

The success of treating lymphedema is strongly related to choosing the most appropriate and individual therapeutic option for the patient. The delicate composition of the subcutaneous tissue and the functionality and accessibility of lymph collectors primarily determine the therapeutic options.

Conventional MRI provides additional diagnostic information to clinical tests to evaluate the amount of free movable fluids as a stage parameter with detailed mapping of the exact location, whether or not already complicated by the occurrence of hypertrophy of subcutaneous adipose tissue as part of stage progression.

With or without the additional use of contrast agents with intra-/subdermal injection, MRL offers additional insight into the lymphatic vasculature, allowing a high spatial resolution of the lymphatics, including the venules. Nonfunctional MRL imaging is based on the three-dimensional T2 and visualizes stasis of fluid or slow-moving fluid (but stasis of fluid in a widened, nonfunctional lymph vessel is also highlighted). Functional MRL injection of gadolinium into the web spaces facilitates imaging of the transit of the contrast agent in lymph vessels (three-dimensional T1 Volumetric interpolated breath-hold examination [VIBE] with fat suppression).

Unfortunately, MRI is an expensive technique that is not widely available. Moreover, the available scanning time should be distributed equally among all colleagues. So, it is essential to consider the clinical question for a patient with lymphedema to use the most tailored sequence(s). The surgeon should be aware that an MRL taken at different time points may last up to 2 hours.

4.7.1 Conventional Magnetic Resonance Imaging: Detection of Free Movable Fluid, Fat Deposition as Stage Parameter, and Volumetry

The application of conventional MRI in lymphedema patients provides the opportunity to **detect movable free**

fluids in the affected area. Using the short tau inversion recovery (STIR) sequence, free movable fluid will be detected. This MR sequence uses fat-suppression technique. As a result, a low signal intensity (SI) is obtained from the fat in the subcutis. The fluid in the subcutaneous fat retains a high SI on this sequence (▸ Fig. 4.16). As fat suppression is not complete, the skin, the subcutis, the muscles, the bone marrow, and the delineation of the bony structures are still seen. The STIR sequence has a moderate resolution, not enough to visualize lymphatic vessels. This sequence has numerous applications in orthopedics, and so it is widely available. The MR sequence takes place in a reasonable time frame of approximately 8 minutes per scan station. Two scan stations are needed to cover an arm and three stations to cover a leg. The STIR sequence is useful for selecting those patients who would benefit from an initial conservative therapeutic approach by complete decongestive therapy (CDT) to diminish the free fluid load in their limbs, e.g., prior to a surgical approach (see **Chapter 6** and **Subchapter 7.3**). Slotting a conventional MRI ahead of a lymphangiography when in clinical doubt of the presence of free fluid or where there is an excess of movable fluid is advisable. Excess of free fluid load interferes with the ability to visualize lymphatic vessels by MRL as described below.

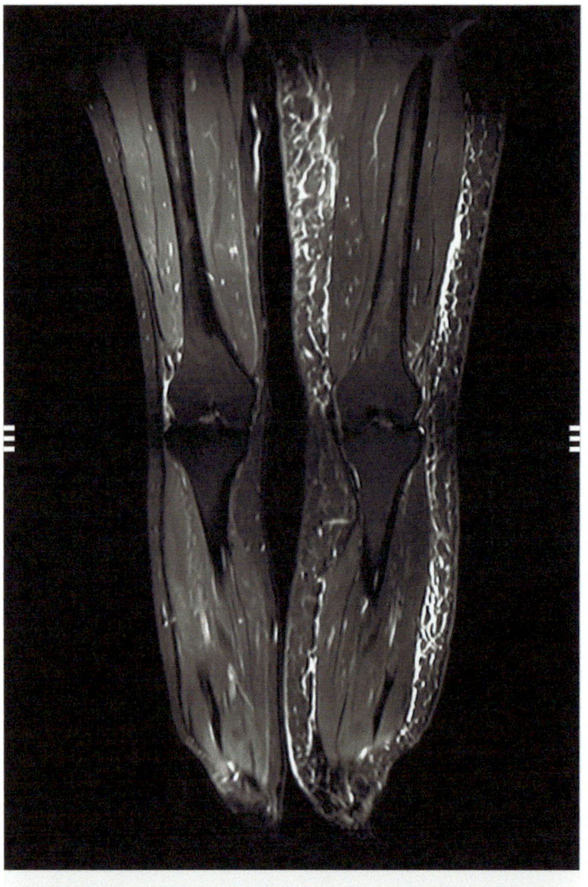

Fig. 4.16 Conventional magnetic resonance imaging short tau inversion recovery sequence of both legs: Note the apparent increase in volume of the left leg compared with the right one due to an increase in the left side's subcutaneous fat layer. The strings with high signal intensity in the subcutis on the left side (bright) are mainly caused by lymphedema. The other line-shaped hyperintensities visible on the left- and right-hand sides in both subcutis and muscles are caused by slow-moving fluid in veins.

The application of conventional MRI in lymphedema patients may add the opportunity to **detect the degree of fat deposition**, another parameter of stage migration, and to evaluate benefit from suction-assisted lipectomy (▸ Fig. 4.17).

The application of conventional MRI in lymphedema patients may add the opportunity to include **volumetry** to a scheduled MRI, e.g., on the T2-sequence with fat suppression. For the volumetry of a limb, the limb, or a part of the limb, with some surrounding air is roughly circumscribed (three-dimensional). The software calculates the number of encircled voxels. The histogram displays the SI in the voxels. Air is always hypointense on each MR sequence due to the lack of protons. On the T2 sequence with fat suppression, water has a high SI. With a slider, the reasonable minimum threshold for water's signal intensity is determined per patient. In a histogram, the number of voxels originating from the air (low SI), water (high SI), and other structures such as muscles/ blood vessels (intermediate SI) are displayed. The software calculates the limb's water content (voxels with high SI) and the actual limb volume (voxel with high plus intermediate SI). As the voxel volume is known, the percentage of water and the volume of water in the limb can be calculated. At this moment, the optimal sequence and parameters to divide the three subgroups (low SI, intermediate SI, and high SI) are part of scientific work to clarify the clinical relevance of the numeric MR-volumetry relative to the subjective visible fraction of water and fat in the subcutis as demonstrated in ▸ Fig. 4.16 and ▸ Fig. 4.17.

Conventional MRI with the STIR sequence for the assessment of free fluid load, degree of fat deposition, and for volumetry can be performed during one acquisition sequence. The postprocessing may take 5 to 10 minutes but summarizes all relevant information that conventional MRI may deliver.

4.7.2 Magnetic Resonance Imaging of Lymphatic Vessels

MRL offers additional **insight into the physiological and pathophysiological lymphatic vasculature** compared with conventional MRI. It is indicated to evaluate the most individual and preferred approach for patients prior to lymphedema surgery.

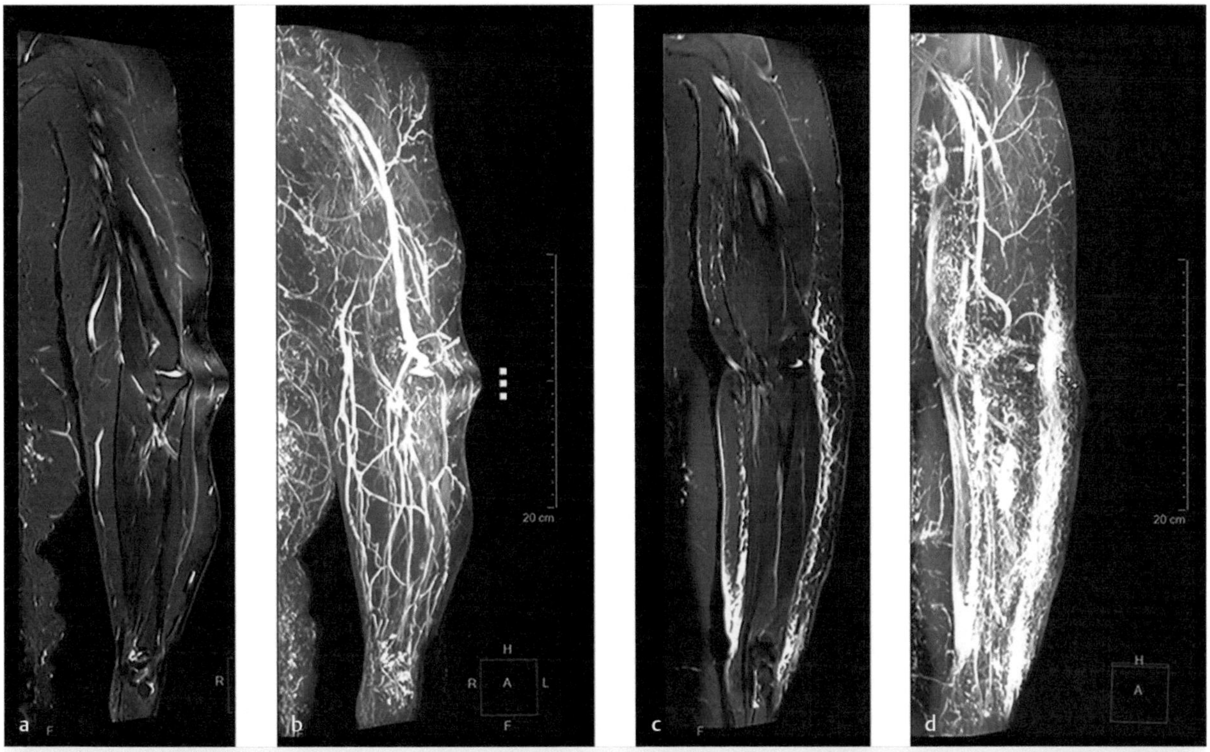

Fig. 4.17 (a, b) On the left side, the short tau inversion recovery sequence and maximum intensity projection maximum intensity projection of the same short tau inversion recovery series show a swollen left arm after surgery in the axilla after breast cancer treatment. The short tau inversion recovery sequence shows no hyperintense strings in the subcutis. The maximum intensity projection reconstruction of the short tau inversion recovery sequence show linear hyperintensities representing the larger veins in the arms. The thickened subcutis is due to abundant fat deposition. **(c, d)** On the right side, images, with the same technique, of another patient with a swollen arm after surgery, with clinically pitting edema. The images show hyperintense strings in the subcutis in the forearm, the elbow region, and the medial side of the upper arm, representing lymphedema. The maximum intensity projection reconstruction **(d)** provides an excellent overview of the location of the lymphedema. Only the patient displayed on the right side will benefit from a therapeutic approach focused on reducing edema.

Technically, it has been differentiated into noncontrast (nonfunctional) and contrast-enhanced (functional) MRL.

Noncontrast

In *noncontrast MRL*, a heavily weighted, high-resolution, three-dimensional T2 sequence is used, performed for visualization of both standing fluid and slow-moving fluid. The sequences used for noncontrast MRL are the same as those used for magnetic resonance cholangiopancreaticography (MRCP). In the noncontrast MR lymphangiography, both the lymph vessels and fluid accumulation are documented in one image (▶ Fig. 4.18). This MR sequence is 50% more time consuming than the STIR sequence, resulting in an acquisition time of approximately 12 minutes per station. The interpretation of the lymphatics position is challenging. In the MRCP sequence, (almost) complete fat suppression is programmed. The result is that no SI is present from the fat in the subcutis, nor from the bone marrow. The bones themselves always have a low SI on each MR sequence due to the lack of protons in the cortex. The lack of SI of the described tissues compromises the possibilities for the description of the position of lymphatic vessels in relation to landmarks. Besides, a description of the position of lymph vessels can be compromised due to abundant dermal backflow since the MR signal of fluid in lymph vessels and those of fluids due to dermal backflow are of the same high SI intensity on the MRCP sequence.

Contrast-Enhanced Magnetic Resonance Lymphangiography

In the procedure of contrast-enhanced MRL (CE-MRL), depots of gadolinium are injected very superficially in to the dermis and/or superficial subcutaneous tissue in all

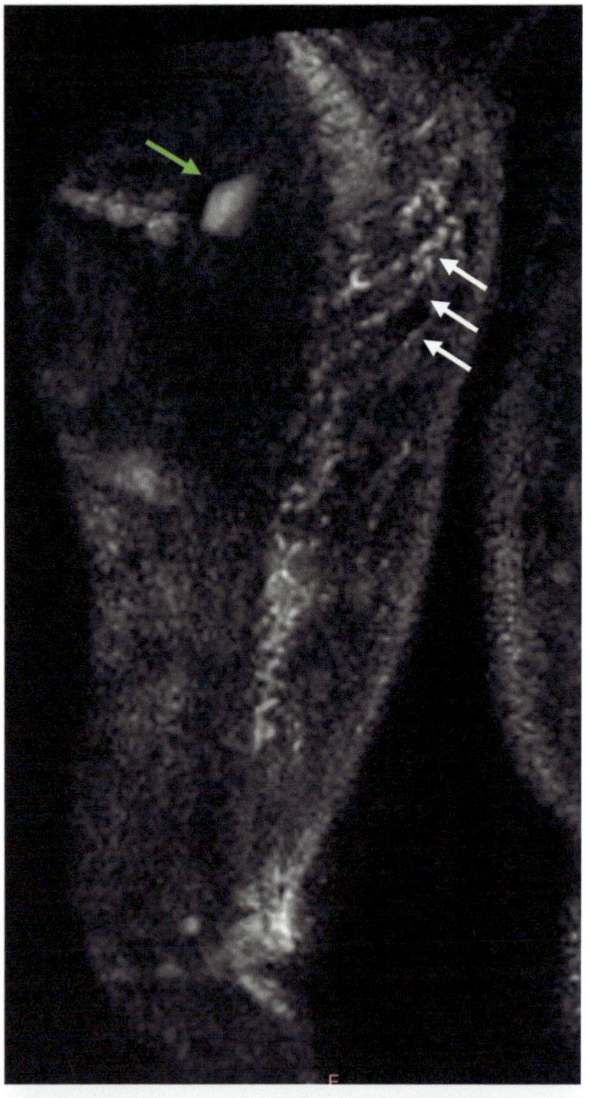

Fig. 4.18 Thin maximum intensity projection reconstruction (5 mm) of a high-resolution, three-dimensional T2 sequence of a right underarm. The lymphatic vessels are indicated by the white arrows and are recognized as a cord of beads with a limited meandering gradient. The localization of the lymphatic vessels in relation to bony landmarks is difficult as due to precise fat suppression no signal intensity derived from the subcutaneous fat or the fat of the bone marrow remains. The fluid (high signal intensity) in the olecranon fossa is indicated by the green arrow.

web spaces of the hand or foot. As gadolinium contrast agents are developed for intravascular use.

Note:

Gadolinium contrast for MRL is currently considered off-label use in most countries. Consequently, the use of gadolinium contrast for MRL is currently unregulated in most countries.

However, as the gadolinium contrast products were developed initially for intravascular use, its extravasates side effect is extensively tested. Despite the side effects ranging from irritation to in the worst-case scenario of tissue necrosis, gadolinium products are approved by various inspection authorities.

The injected gadolinium contrast for CE-MRL in the interstitial space (up to four web spaces) is resorbed not only by the lymph collectors, but also by venules. High-resolution, three-dimensional T1 sequences, taken with an interval of 15 minutes (15–30 minutes and when necessary 45 minutes), show small and large venous structures and functional lymphatic vessels in the subcutis, no matter their depth from the skin, and their proximity in the same image. The sequence is also available in standardized form on MR equipment as it is also used for imaging of other structures, e.g., the liver. The technique also requires postprocessing with maximum intensity projection (MIP) reconstructions. Postprocessing of a sequence usually requires 15 to 20 minutes (▶ Fig. 4.19).

The additional goal of the CE-MRL procedure is to visualize functional lymphatic vessels in close relation to small venules in one image. Association of regions of interest to relevant anatomical landmarks should reduce LVA procedure time in the operating room. The interpretation of CE-MRL might be compromised by dermal backflow. Nevertheless, drawbacks for MRI remain its availability, costs, and time-consuming acquisition of interpretable sequences. Further evaluation in prospective studies should address the following issues in this promising field of lymphedema diagnostics.

Contrast-enhanced magnetic resonance lymphangiography (CE-MRL)—how to do it?

The procedure starts with proper skin disinfection. In CE-MRL, small extravasates of up to 0.8 ml are injected into web spaces, resulting in a burning sensation and a little redness. The inconvenience of the burning sensation is overcome by the subcutaneous injection of a local anesthetics, e.g., 0.2 ml of Xylocaine 1%, into web spaces 1 minute before the injection of gadolinium. The redness disappears in the next few hours and is not painful. The patient is fully informed about the gadolinium's off-label use before the examination and the expected inconvenience. After the contrast depots are created, the patient is asked whether they still experience any burning sensation. If that is the case, 0.1 ml supplementary local anesthesia is given at the designated sites. The contrast is drained to both the functional lymphatics and the capillary system. The time delay between the start of the injection outside the MR room and positioning on the MR table is about 10 minutes. The patient is carefully braced overall to achieve a moderate homogeneous pressure on the limb. The bracing prevents the patient from trembling during the examination, as the overall scan time is long. The arm is positioned along the body with the thumb pointing ventrally. The legs are fixated so that the toes face ventrally. ▶ Fig. 4.20 shows the technical set-up for a CE-MRL of an arm. The first three-dimensional T1 sequence covers the region from the midpoint of the hand to the upper third of the underarm. Next, two stations are scanned with the STIR sequence and spliced, covering the whole arm. Finally, a second three-dimensional T1 sequence is performed covering the region from 10 cm above the elbow, mostly until the distal two-thirds of the underarm. The overall scanning time for an arm is about 20 minutes. Scanning of legs is more time consuming as they are longer and have a larger transverse diameter, so more voxels must be scanned. The three-dimensional T1 sequence for legs takes about 7 minutes. The STIR sequence needs three scan stations to cover the region from the feet to the midpoint of the small pelvis and lasts 29 minutes. Patients are advised to wear no support stocking after the examination for the rest of the day to give the resorption of contrast agent every chance. Detailed information on each moment of the examination reduces the patient's stress. The examination is well tolerated.

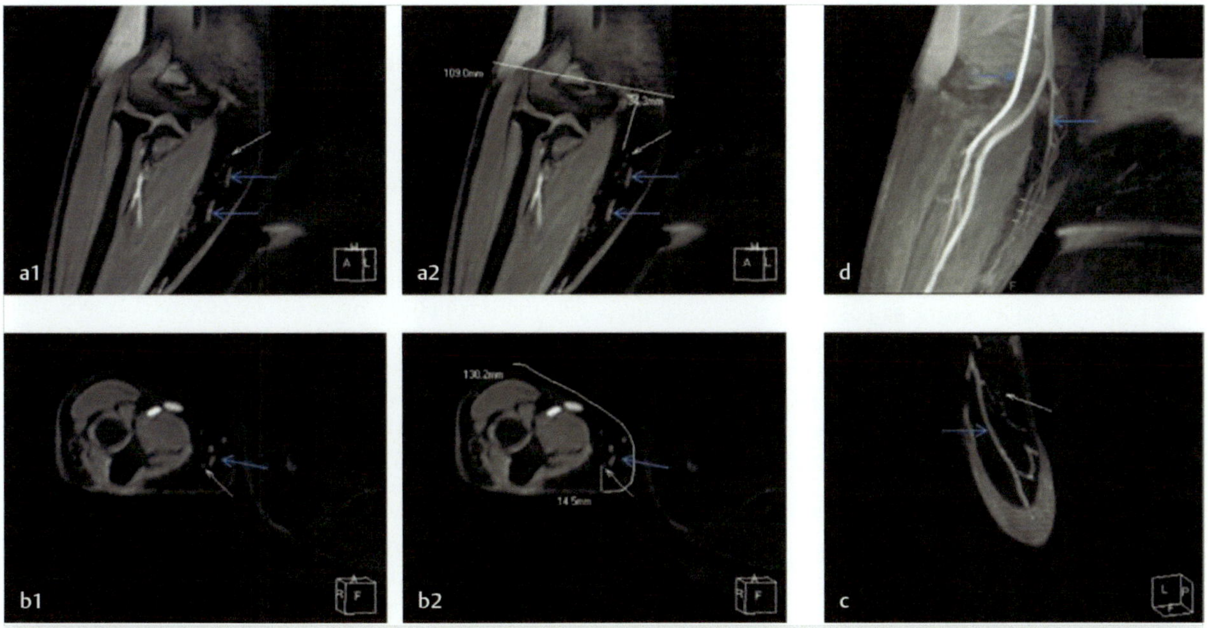

Fig. 4.19 (a1) Coronal, **(b1)** axial, and **(c)** sagittal thin maximum intensity projection reconstructions (5 mm) of a three-dimensional T1 sequence (VIBE, Siemens Skyra, Erlangen, Germany) of the forearm, performed 30 minutes after injection of gadolinium into the web spaces of the right hand. Functional lymphatic vessels are visible at the ulnar side as a cord of beads (white arrow). The smooth structures represent nearby small venous vessels (blue arrows). **(a2, b2)** Annotation of lymph vessels (and small venous structures) relative to an anatomical landmark (in this case the olecranon fossa). (Reproduced with permission from Zeltzer et al.[96])

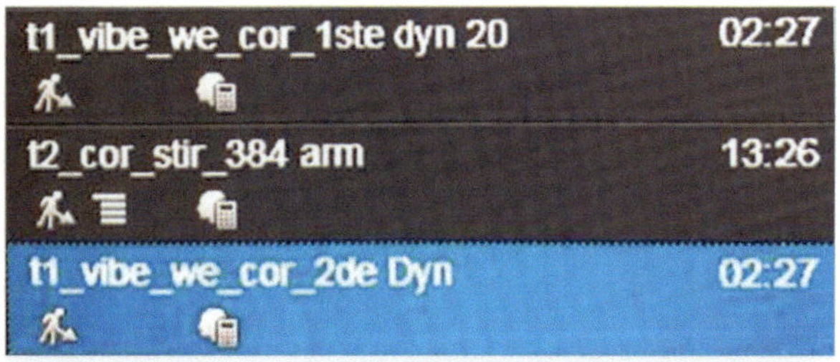

Fig. 4.20 Screenshot for planning of contrast-enhanced magnetic resonance lymphangiography sequences of the arm (Siemens Skyra, Erlangen, Germany).

4.7.3 Tips and Tricks

The clinical success of MRL and its usage for improved patient care depend on close cooperation and mutual understanding between radiologists and plastic surgeons. Surgeons should, however, be aware of the limitations of the examination itself, e.g., MRL imaging is hindered by dermal backflow. Thus, when employing ICG lymphangiography, the following is recommended:

- MRL imaging should be scheduled 1 day after manual lymph drainage (MLD).
- Compression garments should be worn until just before the examination.

Radiologists must show interest to the surgeons' demand to understand the surgical anatomical landmarks and questions desired for LVA. In this way, radiologists identify relevant positions for the planned procedure in the operating room, addressing both functional lymphatic vessel (LV) and venules in proximity. Regular multidisciplinary meetings with imaging discussions including patients' follow-up add a significant value.

Finally, in the radiology department itself, one or two dedicated radiologists are needed to spend time for and with patients with lymphatic pathologies. Patients fear injection to limbs affected with lymphedema, as they are said to be vulnerable to infection. They must be convinced that extensive skin disinfection will prevent this type of possible complication. In cooperation with motivated technologists, MRL can be regarded as a standardized procedure, resulting in predictable quality.

4.8 Functional Magnetic Resonance Lymphangiography

Carola Brussaard, Hans Schild, and Claus Christian Pieper

Functional MRL must be regarded as the royal discipline of MRL, providing dynamic information for the surgeon. Visualizing functional lymphatics with MRI in a swollen extremity with lymphedema is still challenging and further evaluation of the technique is in continuous progress.

4.8.1 Technique

The procedure starts with a sub- or intradermal injection of gadolinium-based contrast products in web spaces of toes or fingers. We prefer to inject a local anesthetic (0.3 ml) in the web spaces first followed by 0.8 ml of gadolinium-based contrast medium. Undiluted gadolinium-based contrast medium in the extravascular space causes an irritating effect with occasional redness in the injection site. By injecting the anesthetic first, the procedure is well tolerated. Patients are told that the redness will disappear in the following hours. With three-dimensional, T1-weighted images with fat suppression, the tract of the contrast in the functional lymphatics is followed from the distal to the proximal part of the limb. After the gadolinium enters the interstitial space, the product will be absorbed primarily by the lymphatic or the venule capillary system, causing venous enhancement as well. Therefore, some of the gadolinium will end soon in the blood circulation system and will subsequently be excreted, mostly by the urinary tract.[92,96]

The veins are well visible in the source images of the three-dimensional, TI-weighted sequence (thin slices). The functional lymphatics become visible after postprocessing of the image. For visualization of functional lymphatics, again the principle of the MIP is used. In MIP images the maximum intensity of a position in an image is depicted in a slice with thickness suitable for the purpose. For visualization of functional lymphatics, slice thickness of the MIP between 3 and 8 mm are useful (▶ Fig. 4.21).

For LVA, accurate localization of the exact position of the functional lymphatics in relation to small veins or venules by a coordinate system is useful and improves dissection time and success. With functional MRI, on T1 sequences with fat suppression, the functional lymphatics can be described relative to any point that is of clinical interest. Images for localization are provided in three orthogonal planes for the surgeon. The depth of the functional lymphatic vessel can be described as well, indicating whether it will be visible subcutaneously with the technique of ICG lymphangiography (see **Subchapter 4.7**). An example in which those lymphatics are labelled relative to reference points is shown in ▶ Fig. 4.19.

For identifying functional lymphatics, series enhanced with gadolinium contrast agents are required. A three-dimensional T1 sequence with fat suppression can demonstrate functional lymphatics nicely. The time from contrast injection to optimal imaging depends on the velocity of the lymph flow. A huge variation according to the condition of the patients exists. Therefore, it is difficult to predict the optimal imaging time with the maximal signal intensity of the lymphatics. Furthermore, the postprocessing of the images performed at different time points is very time consuming. A close interaction between the surgeon and the radiologist is necessary to benefit from the advantages of standardization and postprocessing with a coordinate system by MRI for techniques such as LVA or lymph vessel transfer.

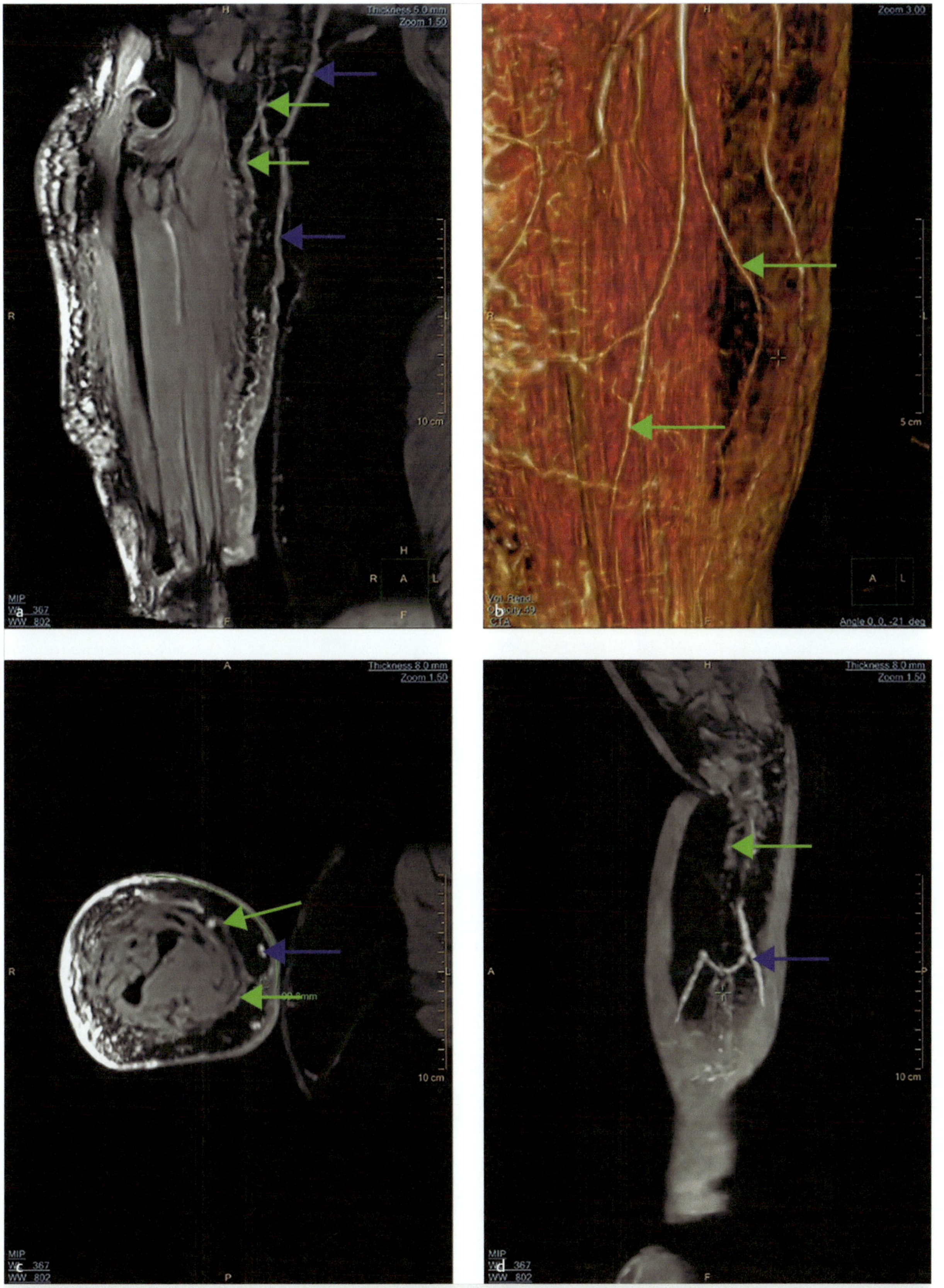

Fig. 4.21 (a-d) Axial, transversal, and sagittal maximum intensity projection reconstructions of a three-dimensional T1-weighted sequence (VIBE, Siemens Skyra, Erlangen, Germany) of a right/left upper extremity with lymphedema stage 2/3. At the ulnar side, a band with lymphatics parallel to the forearm is visible (green arrows). They show a lower signal intensity than the straighter course of the veins (blue arrows).

4.8.2 Diagnosis of Peripheral Lymphatic Leakage

Various surgical procedures, such as lymph node biopsy, or trauma involving the lymphatic vessels of an extremity can not only lead to secondary lymphedema, but may also result in lymphatic leakage due to direct injury and development of a lymphocutaneous fistula. Although rare, lymphatic leakages are a severe complication associated with a delay of necessary (oncologic) therapies as well as infectious, dermatological, and psychosocial sequelae. Initially conservative treatment (e.g., immobilization and pressure bandage) is pursued, but may fail in several patients due to permanent leakage.[94]

In such cases imaging is often necessary to guide further treatment options, such as surgical or—more recently—interventional-radiological measures.[95,96,97] Conventional imaging techniques like MRI, CT, or ultrasound can depict the location of subcutaneous fluid collections but can neither differentiate between a postoperative seroma and a true lymphocele due to lymphatic leakage nor show the exact location, course, and number of leaking lymphatic vessels. Lymphoscintigraphy can demonstrate lymphatic flow and leakage but has insufficient anatomical resolution to depict individual lymphatic vessels. ICG lymphangiography may be able to differentiate between leaking lymphatic vessels and seroma, but also has its limitations due to two-dimensional resolution. Direct (transpedal) lymphangiography with iodized oil can be used for exact anatomical evaluation of the leaking lymphatics and has also been described to have a therapeutic effect.[98] However, it is technically difficult, time consuming, and associated with severe complications (e.g., anaphylaxia, pedal lymphatic leakage, pulmonary oil embolization) and thus regarded to be obsolete.

Therefore, functional MRL is increasingly used in the pretherapeutic workup of patients with lymphatic leakages to determine the optimal treatment strategy. MRL can be performed at 1.5 T and 3.0 T. Typically, fat-suppressed, T2-weighted images are acquired to evaluate subcutaneous fluid collections as well as extremity edema (▶ Fig. 4.22a). Although heavily T2-weighted three-dimensional sequences can be used to delineate lymphatic vessels,[98] the mainstay of MR evaluation for lymphatic leakages is contrast-enhanced transpedal MRL.[99] Contrast injection is performed in a similar way as for lymphedema evaluation. After contrast application, dynamic (preferably three-dimensional), T1-weighted, fat-suppressed images should be acquired for at least 30 to 45 minutes until contrast medium is observed at the

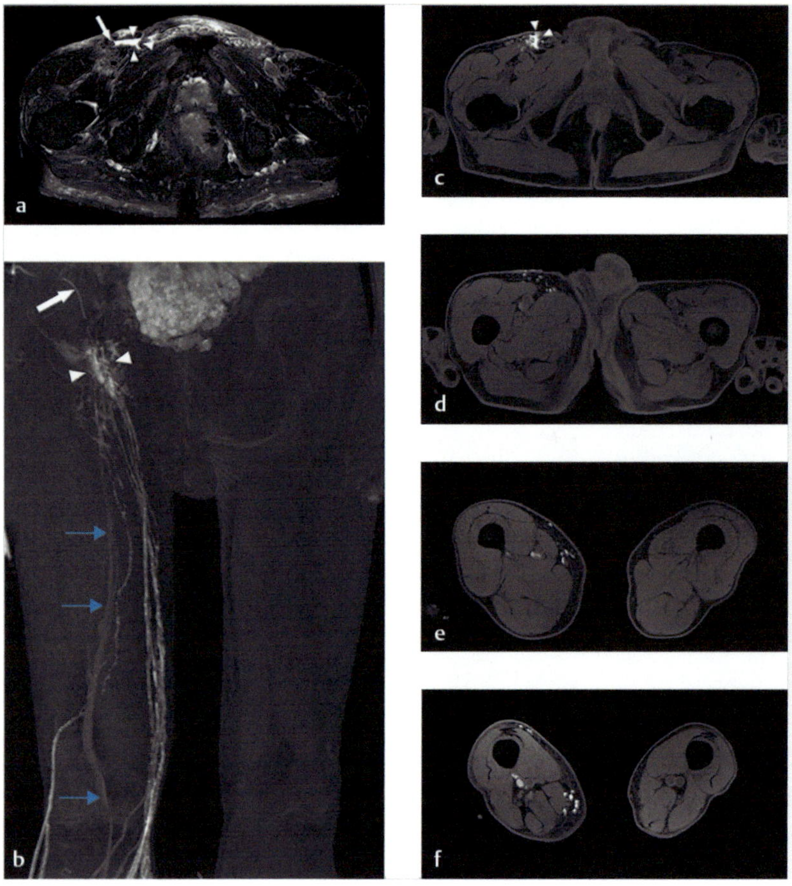

Fig. 4.22 (a–f) A 75-year-old male patient with inguinal lymphatic leakage after inguinal lymph node dissection. The axial, fat-suppressed, T2-weighted image **(a)** demonstrates a small fluid collection/ lymphocele in the right groin (white arrowheads) with an indwelling drainage catheter (white arrow). The maximum intensity projection of a fat-suppressed, three-dimensional, T1-weighted sequence after pedal indirect lymphangiography subdermal contrast injection **(b)** and the corresponding axial images **(c–f)** show continuous contrast-enhancement of ventromedial lymph collectors as well as leakage from several of these collectors in the right groin (white arrowheads in **c**). Contrast medium is also drained via the indwelling catheter (white arrow in **b**). Notice also contrast enhancement within the veins (blue arrows).

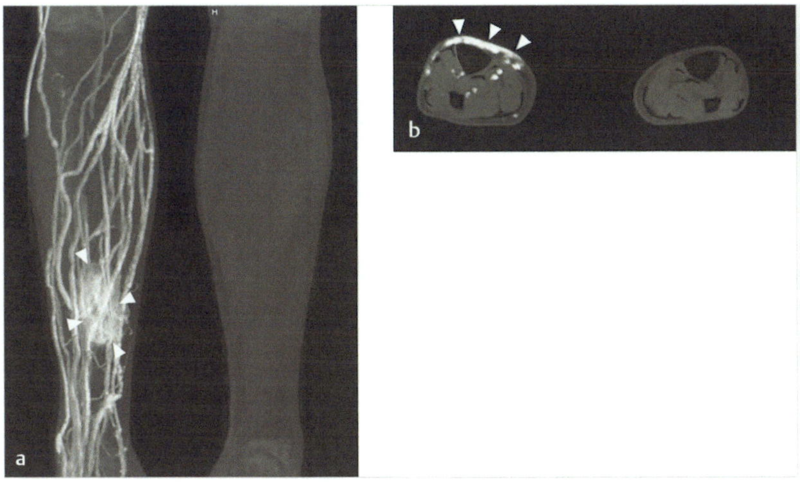

Fig. 4.23 (a, b) The same patient as in ▸ Fig. 4.22. Magnetic resonance lymphangiography (**a**: coronal plane maximum intensity projection, **b**: single axial plane) demonstrating dilated ventromedial lymphatic vessels in the lower right leg and an area of focal dermal backflow (white arrowheads) as a sign of lymphedema associated with the inguinal lymphatic leakage.

leakage site, in inguinal lymph nodes, or in lymph vessels and nodes above the suspected level of leakage (▸ Fig. 4.22b–f). In cases with severe lymphedema the patients can be asked to move their legs between image acquisitions to propagate lymph flow.

Contrast-enhanced images should then be evaluated concerning the presence and site of leakage, the location, course, and number of lymphatic vessels supplying the leakage, the location and enhancement of adjacent lymph nodes as well as signs of associated lymphoedema (▸ Fig. 4.23).

Results of MRL in inguinal lymphatic leakage have so far only been published in small case series.[100] In one report on 16 patients with iatrogenic/traumatic inguinal lymphatic leakage, the leakage site/the leaking vessels could be identified in 15/16 cases. Interestingly these 15 patients also presented with lower extremity lymphedema of the respective leg. These patients subsequently underwent successful surgical treatment. The patient without a detectable lymphatic leakage or edema subsequently responded to continued conservative treatment.

MRL is a clinically helpful imaging technique in the pretherapeutic workup of patients with therapy refractory lymphatic leakage and can guide further treatment strategy based on its high degree of spatial resolution and local accuracy.

4.9 Pearls and Pitfalls

Tomke Cordts

Lymphedema patients require an extra amount of attention from the consulting physician and no fateful standard of care treatment. A thorough and extensive examination is as vital as a careful assessment of the individual personal history. Moreover, selecting the appropriate patients for the right surgery can be difficult. In the general population, the term "lymphedema" is often used synonymously for all kinds of diseases involving unilateral or bilateral swelling. This includes adipose disorders, such as "lipedema," which occurs almost exclusively in women. Its prevalence is estimated to be as high as 10% in adult Caucasian women,[101] much higher than the 0.001% prevalence generally attributed to primary and the 0.1% attributed to secondary lymphedema.[102] Therefore, as per our own experience, finding actual presentations of lymphedema can be quite challenging. During consultation, these few cases must be carefully filtered out of the large number of other patients.

Another common cause of error involves edema quantification. Using a nonstretch tape to measure extremity circumference is considered a quick and easy method.[103] But as therapeutic decisions are often based on these numbers (i.e., conservative treatment vs. surgical intervention), special care must be taken in obtaining them. When patients are seen at follow-up examinations, variances of only a few centimeters can mean a considerable difference. Therefore, measurement should be as standardized as possible in order to keep interpersonal variances to a minimum. Finally, the available imaging modalities of ICG lymphangiography, lymphoscintigraphic lymphangiography, and magnetic resonannace lymphangiography have to be chosen with reference to their advantages and disadvantages, summarized in ▸ Table 4.9.

Table 4.9 Imaging modalities to evaluate lymphedema

	Imaging Modality		
Evaluation	**LSG**	**ICG Lymphangiography**	**MRL**
Information about anatomy	Poor resolution	Excellent resolution of superficial lymphatics	Excellent resolution of lymphatic vessels, lymph nodes, venules, and interstitial tissues
Information about function	Excellent information regarding lymphatic vessel and lymph node function	Shows only functional state of superficial lymphatics	Rather poor to assess lymphatic function
Exposure to radiation	Yes	No	No
Can be performed in outpatient clinic and/or operating room	No	Yes	No

Abbreviations: ICG, indocyanine green; LSG, lymphoscintigraphy; MRL, magnetic resonance lymphangiography.

References

[1] International Society of Lymphology. The diagnosis and treatment of peripheral lymphedema: 2013 Consensus Document of the International Society of Lymphology. Lymphology. 2013; 46(1):1–11

[2] Mattonet K, Wilting J, Jeltsch M. Die genetischen Ursachen des primären Lymphödems: Erkrankungen Des Lymphgefäßsystems 2015;2013:in-press

[3] Radhakrishnan K, Rockson SG. The clinical spectrum of lymphatic disease. Ann N Y Acad Sci. 2008; 1131:155–184

[4] Witte MH, Bernas MJ, Martin CP, Witte CL. Lymphangiogenesis and lymphangiodysplasia: from molecular to clinical lymphology. Microsc Res Tech. 2001; 55(2):122–145

[5] Evans AL, Bell R, Brice G, et al. Identification of eight novel VEGFR-3 mutations in families with primary congenital lymphoedema. J Med Genet. 2003; 40(9):697–703

[6] Wilting J, Bartkowski R, Baumeister R, Földi E, Stöhr S, Strubel G, et al. S2k Leitlinie Diagnostik und Therapie der Lymphödeme AWMF Reg.-Nr. 058-001 2017. https://www.awmf.org/uploads/tx_szleitlinien/058-001l_S2k_Diagnostik_und_Therapie_der_Lymphoedeme_2019-07.pdf

[7] Karkkainen MJ, Ferrell RE, Lawrence EC, et al. Missense mutations interfere with VEGFR-3 signalling in primary lymphoedema. Nat Genet. 2000; 25(2):153–159

[8] Fang J, Dagenais SL, Erickson RP, et al. Mutations in FOXC2 (MFH-1), a forkhead family transcription factor, are responsible for the hereditary lymphedema-distichiasis syndrome. Am J Hum Genet. 2000; 67(6):1382–1388

[9] Finegold DN, Kimak MA, Lawrence EC, et al. Truncating mutations in FOXC2 cause multiple lymphedema syndromes. Hum Mol Genet. 2001; 10(11):1185–1189

[10] Balboa-Beltran E, Fernández-Seara MJ, Pérez-Muñuzuri A, et al. A novel stop mutation in the vascular endothelial growth factor-C gene (VEGFC) results in Milroy-like disease. J Med Genet. 2014; 51(7): 475–478

[11] Ferrell RE, Baty CJ, Kimak MA, et al. GJC2 missense mutations cause human lymphedema. Am J Hum Genet. 2010; 86(6):943–948

[12] Ostergaard P, Simpson MA, Connell FC, et al. Mutations in GATA2 cause primary lymphedema associated with a predisposition to acute myeloid leukemia (Emberger syndrome). Nat Genet. 2011; 43(10): 929–931

[13] Irrthum A, Devriendt K, Chitayat D, et al. Mutations in the transcription factor gene SOX18 underlie recessive and dominant forms of hypotrichosis-lymphedema-telangiectasia. Am J Hum Genet. 2003; 72(6):1470–1478

[14] Har-El G, Borderon ML, Weiss MH. Choanal atresia and lymphedema. Ann Otol Rhinol Laryngol. 1991; 100(8):661–664

[15] Alders M, Hogan BM, Gjini E, et al. Mutations in CCBE1 cause generalized lymph vessel dysplasia in humans. Nat Genet. 2009; 41 (12):1272–1274

[16] Ostergaard P, Simpson MA, Mendola A, et al. Mutations in KIF11 cause autosomal-dominant microcephaly variably associated with congenital lymphedema and chorioretinopathy. Am J Hum Genet. 2012; 90(2):356–362

[17] Quirion E. Recognizing and treating upper extremity lymphedema in postmastectomy/lumpectomy patients: a guide for primary care providers. J Am Acad Nurse Pract. 2010; 22(9):450–459

[18] Cormier JN, Askew RL, Mungovan KS, Xing Y, Ross MI, Armer JM. Lymphedema beyond breast cancer: a systematic review and meta-analysis of cancer-related secondary lymphedema. Cancer. 2010; 116 (22):5138–5149

[19] de Vries M, Vonkeman WG, van Ginkel RJ, Hoekstra HJ. Morbidity after inguinal sentinel lymph node biopsy and completion lymph node dissection in patients with cutaneous melanoma. Eur J Surg Oncol. 2006; 32(7):785–789

[20] Füller J, Guderian D, Köhler C, Schneider A, Wendt TG. Lymph edema of the lower extremities after lymphadenectomy and radiotherapy for cervical cancer. Strahlenther Onkol. 2008; 184(4):206–211

[21] Földi M, Földi E, Kubik S, eds. Lehrbuch der Lymphologie für Mediziner, Masseure und Physiotherapeuten. 6. Munich: Urban und Fischer; 2005

[22] Mehrara BJ, Greene AK. Lymphedema and obesity: is there a link? Plast Reconstr Surg. 2014; 134(1):154e–160e

[23] Eberhardt RT, Raffetto JD. Chronic venous insufficiency. Circulation. 2014; 130(4):333–346

[24] International Society of Lymphology. The diagnosis and treatment of peripheral lymphedema: 2013 Consensus Document of the International Society of Lymphology. Lymphology. 2013; 46(1):1–11

[25] Grada AA, Phillips TJ. Lymphedema: diagnostic workup and management. J Am Acad Dermatol. 2017; 77(6):995–1006

[26] Stemmer R. Ein klinisches Zeichen zur Früh- und Differential-diagnose des Lymphödems [A clinical symptom for the early and differential diagnosis of lymphedema]. Vasa. 1976; 5(3):261–262

[27] Gerber LH. A review of measures of lymphedema. Cancer. 1998; 83 (12) Suppl American:2803–2804

[28] Caban ME. Trends in the evaluation of lymphedema. Lymphology. 2002; 35(1):28–38

[29] Taylor R, Jayasinghe UW, Koelmeyer L, Ung O, Boyages J. Reliability and validity of arm volume measurements for assessment of lymphedema. Phys Ther. 2006; 86(2):205–214

[30] Sander AP, Hajer NM, Hemenway K, Miller AC. Upper-extremity volume measurements in women with lymphedema: a comparison of measurements obtained via water displacement with geometrically determined volume. Phys Ther. 2002; 82(12):1201–1212
[31] Stanton AW, Badger C, Sitzia J. Non-invasive assessment of the lymphedematous limb. Lymphology. 2000; 33(3):122–135
[32] Perrin M, Guex JJ. Edema and leg volume: methods of assessment. Angiology. 2000; 51(1):9–12
[33] Kaulesar Sukul DM, den Hoed PT, Johannes EJ, van Dolder R, Benda E. Direct and indirect methods for the quantification of leg volume: comparison between water displacement volumetry, the disk model method and the frustum sign model method, using the correlation coefficient and the limits of agreement. J Biomed Eng. 1993; 15(6): 477–480
[34] Megens AM, Harris SR, Kim-Sing C, McKenzie DC. Measurement of upper extremity volume in women after axillary dissection for breast cancer. Arch Phys Med Rehabil. 2001; 82(12):1639–1644
[35] Stranden E. A comparison between surface measurements and water displacement volumetry for the quantification of leg edema. J Oslo City Hosp. 1981; 31(12):153–155
[36] Bernas M. Assessment and risk reduction in lymphedema. Semin Oncol Nurs. 2013; 29(1):12–19
[37] Hayashi A, Yamamoto T, Yoshimatsu H, et al. Ultrasound visualization of the lymphatic vessels in the lower leg. Microsurgery. 2016; 36(5): 397–401
[38] Visconti G, Yamamoto T, Hayashi N, Hayashi A. Ultrasound-assisted lymphaticovenular anastomosis for the treatment of peripheral lymphedema. Plast Reconstr Surg. 2017; 139(6):1380e–1381e
[39] Hayashi A, Giacalone G, Yamamoto T, et al. Ultra high-frequency ultrasonographic imaging with 70 MHz scanner for visualization of the lymphatic vessels. Plast Reconstr Surg Glob Open. 2019; 7(1):e2086
[40] Visconti G, Hayashi A, Tartaglione G, Yamamoto T, Bianchi A, Salgarello M. Preoperative planning of lymphaticovenular anastomosis in patients with iodine allergy: a multicentric experience. J Plast Reconstr Aesthet Surg. 2020; 73(4):783–808
[41] Bianchi A, Visconti G, Hayashi A, Santoro A, Longo V, Salgarello M. Ultra-high frequency ultrasound imaging of lymphatic channels correlates with their histological features: a step forward in lymphatic surgery. J Plast Reconstr Aesthet Surg. 2020; 73(9):1622–1629
[42] Hayashi A, Visconti G, Yamamoto T, et al. Intraoperative imaging of lymphatic vessel using ultra high-frequency ultrasound. J Plast Reconstr Aesthet Surg. 2018; 71(5):778–780
[43] Visconti G, Bianchi A, Hayashi A, Salgarello M. Ultra-high frequency ultrasound preoperative planning of the rerouting method for lymphaticovenular anastomosis in incisions devoid of vein. Microsurgery. 2020; 40(6):717–718
[44] Visconti G, Salgarello M, Hayashi A. The recipient venule in supermicrosurgical lymphaticovenular anastomosis: flow dynamic classification and correlation with surgical outcomes. J Reconstr Microsurg. 2018; 34(8):581–589
[45] Bianchi A, Salgarello M, Hayashi A, Yang JC, Visconti G. Recipient venule selection and anastomosis configuration for lymphaticovenular anastomosis in extremity lymphedema: algorithm based on 1,000 lymphaticovenular anastomosis. J Reconstr Microsurg. 2021. Epub ahead of print.. DOI: 10.1055/s-0041-1735836
[46] Bourgeois P, Munck D, Becker C, Leduc O, Leduc A. Evaluation of a three-phase lymphoscintigraphic investigation protocol of the lower limbedemas. Eur J Lymphol. 1997; 21:22–28
[47] Bourgeois P. Radionuclide lymphoscintigraphies. In: Lee BB, Rockson SG, Bergan J, eds. Lymphedema: A Concise Compendium of Theory and Practice. Springer International Publishing AG; 2018:257–313
[48] Kleinhans E, Baumeister RGH, Hahn D, Siuda S, Büll U, Moser E. Evaluation of transport kinetics in lymphoscintigraphy: follow-up study in patients with transplanted lymphatic vessels. Eur J Nucl Med. 1985; 10(7–8):349–352
[49] Fox IJ, Brooker LG, Heseltine DW, Essex HE, Wood EH. A tricarbocyanine dye for continuous recording of dilution curves in whole blood independent of variations in blood oxygen saturation. Proc Staff Meet Mayo Clin. 1957; 32(18):478–484
[50] Flower RW. Injection technique for indocyanine green and sodium fluorescein dye angiography of the eye. Invest Ophthalmol. 1973; 12 (12):881–895
[51] Kogure K, Choromokos E. Infrared absorption angiography. J Appl Physiol. 1969; 26(1):154–157
[52] Hollins B, Noe B, Henderson JM. Fluorometric determination of indocyanine green in plasma. Clin Chem. 1987; 33(6):765–768
[53] Yoneya S, Saito T, Komatsu Y, Koyama I, Takahashi K, Duvoll-Young J. Binding properties of indocyanine green in human blood. Invest Ophthalmol Vis Sci. 1998; 39(7):1286–1290
[54] Alander JT, Kaartinen I, Laakso A, et al. A review of indocyanine green fluorescent imaging in surgery. Int J Biomed Imaging. 2012; 2012: 940585
[55] Hope-Ross M, Yannuzzi LA, Gragoudas ES, et al. Adverse reactions due to indocyanine green. Ophthalmology. 1994; 101(3):529–533
[56] Liang MI, Carson WE, III. Biphasic anaphylactic reaction to blue dye during sentinel lymph node biopsy. World J Surg Oncol. 2008; 6:79
[57] Landsman ML, Kwant G, Mook GA, Zijlstra WG. Light-absorbing properties, stability, and spectral stabilization of indocyanine green. J Appl Physiol. 1976; 40(4):575–583
[58] Hirche C, Murawa D, Mohr Z, Kneif S, Hünerbein M. ICG fluorescence-guided sentinel node biopsy for axillary nodal staging in breast cancer. Breast Cancer Res Treat. 2010; 121(2):373–378
[59] Hirche C, Mohr Z, Kneif S, et al. Ultrastaging of colon cancer by sentinel node biopsy using fluorescence navigation with indocyanine green. Int J Colorectal Dis. 2012; 27(3):319–324
[60] Executive C, Executive Committee. The diagnosis and treatment of peripheral lymphedema: 2016 Consensus Document of the International Society of Lymphology. Lymphology. 2016; 49(4): 170–184
[61] Unno N, Inuzuka K, Suzuki M, et al. Preliminary experience with a novel fluorescence lymphography using indocyanine green in patients with secondary lymphedema. J Vasc Surg. 2007; 45(5): 1016–1021
[62] Ogata F, Narushima M, Mihara M, Azuma R, Morimoto Y, Koshima I. Intraoperative lymphography using indocyanine green dye for near-infrared fluorescence labeling in lymphedema. Ann Plast Surg. 2007; 59(2):180–184
[63] Yamamoto T, Matsuda N, Doi K, et al. The earliest finding of indocyanine green lymphography in asymptomatic limbs of lower extremity lymphedema patients secondary to cancer treatment: the modified dermal backflow stage and concept of subclinical lymphedema. Plast Reconstr Surg. 2011; 128(4):314e–321e
[64] Yamamoto T, Yamamoto N, Doi K, et al. Indocyanine green-enhanced lymphography for upper extremity lymphedema: a novel severity staging system using dermal backflow patterns. Plast Reconstr Surg. 2011; 128(4):941–947
[65] Chang DW, Suami H, Skoracki R. A prospective analysis of 100 consecutive lymphovenous bypass cases for treatment of extremity lymphedema. Plast Reconstr Surg. 2013; 132(5):1305–1314
[66] Rosian K, Stanak M. Efficacy and safety assessment of lymphovenous anastomosis in patients with primary and secondary lymphoedema: a systematic review of prospective evidence. Microsurgery. 2019; 39 (8):763–772
[67] Cornelissen AJM, van Mulken TJM, Graupner C, et al. Near-infrared fluorescence image-guidance in plastic surgery: a systematic review. Eur J Plast Surg. 2018; 41(3):269–278
[68] Yamamoto T, Narushima M, Yoshimatsu H, et al. Indocyanine green velocity: lymph transportation capacity deterioration with progression of lymphedema. Ann Plast Surg. 2013; 71(5):591–594
[69] Yamamoto T, Narushima M, Yoshimatsu H, et al. Dynamic indocyanine green (ICG) lymphography for breast cancer-related arm lymphedema. Ann Plast Surg. 2014; 73(6):706–709
[70] Olszewski WL. Contractility patterns of normal and pathologically changed human lymphatics. Ann N Y Acad Sci. 2002; 979:52–63, discussion 76–79

[71] Yamamoto T, Iida T, Matsuda N, et al. Indocyanine green (ICG)-enhanced lymphography for evaluation of facial lymphoedema. J Plast Reconstr Aesthet Surg. 2011; 64(11):1541–1544

[72] Yamamoto T, Yamamoto N, Yoshimatsu H, Hayami S, Narushima M, Koshima I. Indocyanine green lymphography for evaluation of genital lymphedema in secondary lower extremity lymphedema patients. J Vasc Surg Venous Lymphat Disord. 2013; 1(4):400–405.e1

[73] Mihara M, Hara H, Kikuchi K, et al. Scarless lymphatic venous anastomosis for latent and early-stage lymphoedema using indocyanine green lymphography and non-invasive instruments for visualising subcutaneous vein. J Plast Reconstr Aesthet Surg. 2012; 65(11):1551–1558

[74] Yang JC, Wu SC, Chiang MH, Lin WC, Hsieh CH. Intraoperative identification and definition of "functional" lymphatic collecting vessels for supermicrosurgical lymphatico-venous anastomosis in treating lymphedema patients. J Surg Oncol. 2018; 117(5):994–1000

[75] Chen WF, Zhao H, Yamamoto T, Hara H, Ding J. Indocyanine green lymphographic evidence of surgical efficacy following microsurgical and supermicrosurgical lymphedema reconstructions. J Reconstr Microsurg. 2016; 32(9):688–698

[76] Shih HB, Shakir A, Nguyen DH. Use of indocyanine green-SPY angiography for tracking lymphatic recovery after lymphaticovenous anastomosis. Ann Plast Surg. 2016; 76 Suppl 3:S232–S237

[77] Mihara M, Seki Y, Hara H, et al. Predictive lymphatic mapping: a method for mapping lymphatic channels in patients with advanced unilateral lymphedema using indocyanine green lymphography. Ann Plast Surg. 2014; 72(6):706–710

[78] Gentileschi S, Servillo M, Albanese R, De Bonis F, Tartaglione G, Salgarello M. Lymphatic mapping of the upper limb with lymphedema before lymphatic supermicrosurgery by mirroring of the healthy limb. Microsurgery. 2017; 37(8):881–889

[79] Basta MN, Gao LL, Wu LC. Operative treatment of peripheral lymphedema: a systematic meta-analysis of the efficacy and safety of lymphovenous microsurgery and tissue transplantation. Plast Reconstr Surg. 2014; 133(4):905–913

[80] Azuma S, Yamamoto T, Koshima I. Donor-site lymphatic function after microvascular lymph node transfer should be followed using indocyanine green lymphography. Plast Reconstr Surg. 2013; 131(3): 443e–444e

[81] Vignes S, Blanchard M, Yannoutsos A, Arrault M. Complications of autologous lymph-node transplantation for limb lymphoedema. Eur J Vasc Endovasc Surg. 2013; 45(5):516–520

[82] Pons G, Masia J, Loschi P, Nardulli ML, Duch J. A case of donor-site lymphoedema after lymph node-superficial circumflex iliac artery perforator flap transfer. J Plast Reconstr Aesthet Surg. 2014; 67(1): 119–123

[83] Ciudad P, Manrique OJ, Date S, et al. A head-to-head comparison among donor site morbidity after vascularized lymph node transfer: pearls and pitfalls of a 6-year single center experience. J Surg Oncol. 2017; 115(1):37–42

[84] Demiri E, Dionyssiou D, Tsimponis A, et al. Donor-site lymphedema following lymph node transfer for breast cancer-related lymphedema: a systematic review of the literature. Lymphat Res Biol. 2018; 16(1):2–8

[85] Scaglioni MF, Arvanitakis M, Chen YC, Giovanoli P, Chia-Shen Yang J, Chang EI. Comprehensive review of vascularized lymph node transfers for lymphedema: outcomes and complications. Microsurgery. 2018; 38 (2):222–229

[86] Klimberg VS. A new concept toward the prevention of lymphedema: axillary reverse mapping. J Surg Oncol. 2008; 97(7):563–564

[87] Ochoa D, Korourian S, Boneti C, Adkins L, Badgwell B, Klimberg VS. Axillary reverse mapping: five-year experience. Surgery. 2014; 156 (5):1261–1268

[88] Dayan JH, Dayan E, Smith ML. Reverse lymphatic mapping: a new technique for maximizing safety in vascularized lymph node transfer. Plast Reconstr Surg. 2015; 135(1):277–285

[89] Halvorson EG, Orgill DP. Discussion: reverse lymphatic mapping: a new technique for maximizing safety in vascularized lymph node transfer. Plast Reconstr Surg. 2015; 135(1):286–288

[90] Aliotta RE, Schwarz GS. Reverse lymphatic mapping without radioisotope in the surgical treatment of lymphedema. J Plast Reconstr Aesthet Surg. 2018; 71(5):766

[91] Arrivé L, Derhy S, El Mouhadi S, Monnier-Cholley L, Menu Y, Becker C. Noncontrast magnetic resonance lymphography. J Reconstr Microsurg. 2016; 32(1):80–86

[92] Lohrmann C, Foeldi E, Langer M. Indirect magnetic resonance lymphangiography in patients with lymphedema preliminary results in humans. Eur J Radiol. 2006; 59(3):401–406

[93] Mitsumori LM, McDonald ES, Wilson GJ, Neligan PC, Minoshima S, Maki JH. MR lymphangiography: how I do it. J Magn Reson Imaging. 2015; 42(6):1465–1477

[94] Twine CP, Lane IF, Williams IM. Management of lymphatic fistulas after arterial reconstruction in the groin. Ann Vasc Surg. 2013; 27(8): 1207–1215

[95] Pieper CC. [Thoracic lymphatic pathologies with chylous leakages—imaging and interventional treatment]. Röfo Fortschr Geb Röntgenstr Nuklearmed. 2018; 190(8):674–679

[96] Pieper CC, Hur S, Sommer CM, et al. Back to the future: lipiodol in lymphography—from diagnostics to theranostics. Invest Radiol. 2019; 54(9):600–615

[97] Gruber-Rouh T, Naguib NNN, Lehnert T, et al. Direct lymphangiography as treatment option of lymphatic leakage: indications, outcomes and role in patient's management. Eur J Radiol. 2014; 83(12):2167–2171

[98] Arrivé L, Derhy S, Dahan B, et al. Primary lower limb lymphoedema: classification with non-contrast MR lymphography. Eur Radiol. 2018; 28(1):291–300

[99] Pieper CC, Schild HH. Interstitial transpedal MR-lymphangiography of central lymphatics using a standard MR contrast agent: feasibility and initial results in patients with chylous effusions. Röfo Fortschr Geb Röntgenstr Nuklearmed. 2018; 190(10):938–945

[100] Lu Q, Bui D, Liu NF, Xu JR, Zhao XH, Zhang XF. Magnetic resonance lymphography at 3T: a promising noninvasive approach to characterise inguinal lymphatic vessel leakage. Eur J Vasc Endovasc Surg. 2012; 43(1):106–111

[101] Wollina U. Lipedema—an update. Dermatol Ther (Heidelb). 2019; 32 (2):e12805

[102] Grada AA, Phillips TJ. Lymphedema: pathophysiology and clinical manifestations. J Am Acad Dermatol. 2017; 77(6):1009–1020

[103] Caban ME. Trends in the evaluation of lymphedema. Lymphology. 2002; 35(1):28–38

Section III

Modern Management of Chronic Lymphedema

Edited by Yves Harder

III

5 Establishment of an Interprofessional and Multidisciplinary Lymphedema Network

Holger Engel

Summary

The adequate treatment of lymphedema depends on a multimodal approach that includes all available options, such as conservative therapy, specific lymphatic surgery, and, eventually in the future, specific anti-inflammatory drugs and regenerative medicine (see **Chapter 19**). The basis for lymphedema treatment is still considered to be conservative therapy, i.e., integrative, multiprofessional conservative treatment, whereas lymphatic surgery predominantly aims at reconstructing lymph flow (e.g., lymphovenous anastomosis and/or autologous lymph node transfer) and reducing extra fat deposit (e.g., suction-assisted lipectomy). To coordinate this spectrum of treatment modalities, a single physician or patient manager is barely sufficient. A patient should, therefore, be treated in an interprofessional and multidisciplinary national lymphedema network to ensure the provision of structured and evidence-based therapy.

Keywords: conservative treatment, interprofessional collaboration, lymphoablative surgery, multidisciplinary lymphedema network, multimodal treatment, reconstructive surgery, surgical treatment

5.1 Presentation of the Concept

Health care systems around the world can differ from one another. They vary in terms of their financial coverage of patient therapy, compensation of health care providers, and availability of therapeutic modalities, e.g., lymphatic therapists, medical supply stores, chiropodists, general practitioners, microsurgeons, etc. The establishment of a functioning lymphedema network should be regional or ideally "national" (national lymphedema network [NLN]) and should take into consideration each health care system's peculiarities (▶ Fig. 5.1).

5.2 Goals

An NLN should have both a clear framework and purpose that define its level of ambition.[1] First, an NLN should create awareness of lymphedema among the medical community, the patients, and the general public by disseminating information, providing education, organizing conferences, and constituting patient advocacy group (patient support group) professionals. Prediction and prevention of lymphedema are the most critical issues to be addressed initially.

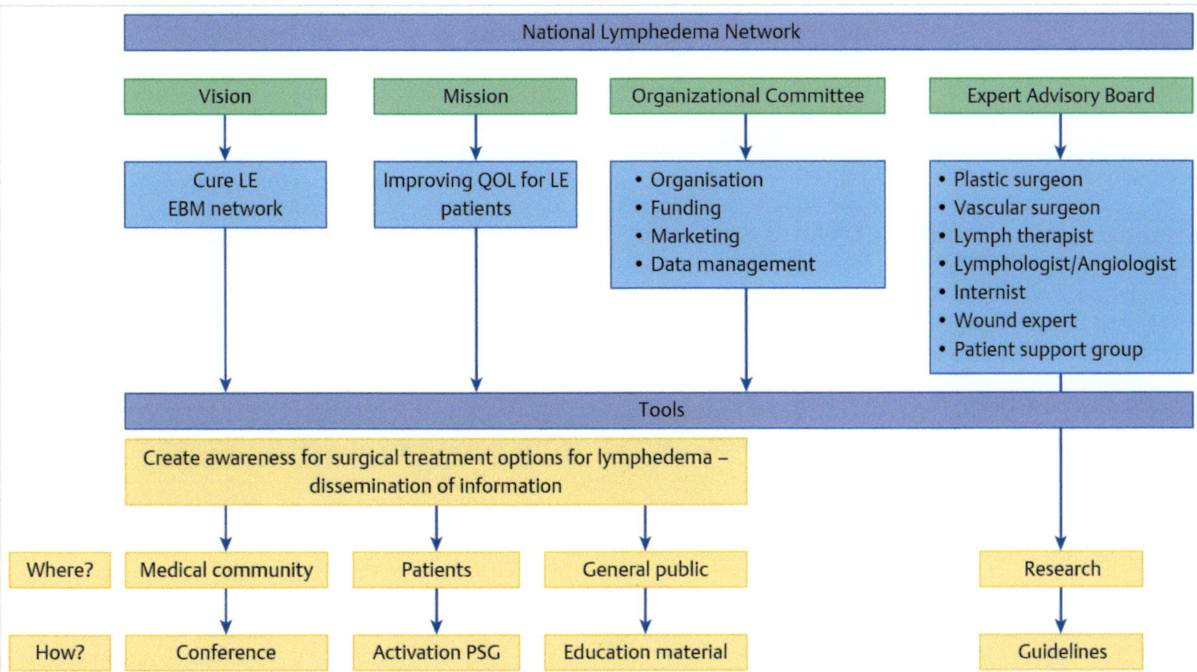

Fig. 5.1 Composition of a national lymphedema network. EBM, evidence-based medicine; LE, lymphedema; PSG, patient support group (patient advocacy); QoL, quality of life.

Second, an NLN should provide points of contact for patients and relatives, involved health care providers such as physicians, medical supply stores, and hospitals, as well as for insurance companies to increase the quality of diagnosis and therapy. Centralizing these services on an evidence-based practice is crucial to ensure predictable patient outcomes. Therefore, recording performance data regarding each activity is essential.

Third, the NLN should also support research groups, raise funds, and provide scholarships.[2] These aims can be most effectively accomplished in cooperation with national and international societies of lymphology and lymphatic surgery.

5.3 Organizational Structure and Involved Personnel

An absolute prerequisite to achieving the aforementioned aims begins with the finding of dedicated people who share the same vision and passion for delivering the best specific and individualized care to the patient. If only a few people begin networking, other people will soon join in support. Unfortunately, due to an under-compensation of treatment involving lymphedema, this work is not attractive enough to potential caregivers, eventually leading to an undersupply in most areas. However, this does not mean that individuals and organizations lack interest in this field. For example, medical supply stores and companies earn money by selling compression garments, so they have a financial interest in joining lymphedema networks. It is, therefore, essential to be familiar with every party's interest when establishing such a network. Finding the "right" people requires the involvement of physicians and nonmedical health care providers as well as persons with the expertise in bylaws, juridical issues, marketing, and event organization, among other things. Members of an NLN should meet regularly.

For each meeting, different topics should be included in a given agenda. It is advisable to discuss organization-related issues separately from those involving specific patient issues and medical education. In particular, an accredited continuing medical education (CME) program attracts other physicians and experts in the field to participate in such a meeting.

Structuring an NLN as a nonprofit organization that operates independently best fits the purpose and allows for tax advantages in many countries. The organization should have a committee as well as an advisory board of experts. The resumes, certificates, and proof of training held by the experts must meet high standards in the field of lymphedema treatment. It is advisable if these standards are precise and partially case-load guided (e.g., a lymphatic therapist with practical experience of 5 years of weekly practice of 10 treatments; a plastic surgeon with practical experience of 5 years, 250 free tissue transfers, and 50 LVAs). Different types of potential membership could allow an NLN to grow and to ensure its financial sustainability. These memberships could be differentiated between experts and laypersons in the field and active and passive members both with and without the right to vote. The standards should also implement a transparent declaration for the executive committee, stating that they have no conflict of interest.

5.4 Funding

Membership fees and donations should be the basis of the financing of such an organization. The establishment of national conferences in which sponsoring fees are charged for industry exhibition offers another source of income. As the popularity of an NLN increases, it could become possible for the organization to provide specific and foremost certified educational activities to physicians, lymphatic therapists, nurses, and eventually patients, including online webinars, live chats, etc. Later on, and after having achieved a standard of patient care using evidence-based practices, there will also be the possibility of obtaining support directly from the health care system or the government.

5.5 Marketing

The establishment of an NLN has been shown to lead to a significant improvement in patient care.[2,3,4] However, it is crucial that such an organization disseminates information and becomes well known, not only to fulfill its own goals but also to establish a solid financial foundation from which to act. Lymphedema networks should utilize all the marketing tools today available, including branding, corporate identity and design, search engine optimization (SEO), flyers, posters, business cards, Facebook, TikTok, and Instagram. Online performance marketers could create funnels that subsequently create leads, new members, and followers. Additionally, nonmember health care providers could be certified by NLNs, thus demonstrating their high-quality standards. However, the certification process costs money but provides prestige to the health care provider.

5.6 Expert Group/Lymphedema Board and Patient Advocacy

In the medical curriculum of most universities, there is still a lack of information with regard to lymphology. In Europe, to date there is no board-certified specialist in lymphology, which complicates the selection of an ideal specialist.

Therefore, patients should be seen and reviewed by a group of specialists, namely, a "lymphedema board." These board members should include a general practitioner, an internist, a plastic surgeon, and a vascular surgeon who all have profound knowledge and practical experience in the field of lymphology. Plastic surgeons should be trained in the field of supermicrosurgery and microvascular tissue transfer. Further and ideally, these boards need to include lymphatic therapists trained in complete decongestive therapy (CDT: also known as complete decongestive therapy), health care providers working with compression garments (e.g., medical supply stores), chiropodists trained in infection prevention, psychologists, wound experts, and other skincare-related providers. Finally, a patient advocacy should be included as well.

5.7 Evidence-Based Medical Care

The expert advisory board has to establish the evidence-based standard for each diagnosis and treatment modality, which should be eventually published and updated on a regular base in guidelines. Every involved health care provider needs to adhere to the NLN to guarantee the implementation of the standards, recommendations, and guidelines.[5,6]

To monitor the quality of patient care, a registry for data acquisition and a system for data assessment is crucial. Basically, a personalized diagnostic and treatment plan should be defined for every patient, including the monitoring during follow-up, and eventually objectively registered in specific data bases. Although most probably institution-specific, data should be electronically available to all health care professionals of the network. Therefore, informed consent of the patients which declares their agreement to share sensitive data is necessary.

The monitored outcome parameters can be qualitatively assessed using measurements related to circumference, volume (water displacement vs. perometer [see www.pero-system.de]), tissue quality (tonometry, bioimpedance), and functionality of the lymphatic system (lymphoscintigraphy, ICG lymphangiography, CT or MRL, and ultrasound) (see **Chapter 4**). The number of infectious events including cellulitis and erysipelas should also be recorded. Further, it is essential to monitor the patient's quality of life before and after treatment, which can be accomplished using a wide array of available quality of life questionnaires (e.g., LYMQOL, Lymph-ICF, SF36 a.o.).[7,8]

Since indication for surgery is diverse, for example, for LVA (see **Chapter 8**), autologous lymph vessel transfer (see **Chapter 9**), autologous lymph node transfer (see **Chapter 10** and **11**), nod-venal shunt (see **Chapter 12**), suction-assisted lipectomy, lymphoablative surgery (see **Chapter 13**), and lympho-ablative procedures (see **Chapter 14**), as well as secondary procedures (see **Chapter 15**), it is essential to document each intervention accurately.

5.8 Future of Lymphedema Networks and Data-Driven Medicine

Currently, data acquisition in the health care sector is continuously and progressively shifting from handwritten paper-based to electronic paper-free form registry databases. Accordingly, the volume of "virtual" medical data increases at a rate of 50% per year. These data are linked with each other to demonstrate correlations and causalities that have not been previously visible.[9,10] Additionally, in the future artificial intelligence (AI) could be implemented for retrospective analyses used to detect lymphedema.[11] For example, deep learning systems could be employed to implement new algorithms that predict lymphedema treatment outcomes. In the future, lymphedema networking will also change dramatically, resulting in a new "partner AI" that will further improve the care of lymphedema patients.[12,13]

5.9 Pearls and Pitfalls

- When creating an NLM, the crucial element is to find the right fellow companions who share the same vision and passion.
- An NLN should exemplify professionalism similar to any other successful company.
- An NLN needs time to grow such an organization.
- Possible short-term accomplishments are generally overestimated.
- Standards of treatment quality should not be lowered.
- The network should ideally unite the experts in the field, guarantee specialist independence irrespective of personal interests and political issues.

References

[1] Friett K. Lymphoedema Support Network update. Br J Community Nurs. 2019; 24 Sup4:S38

[2] Underwood E, Woods M, Riches K, Keeley V, Wallace A, Freeman J. Lymphedema research prioritization partnership: a collaborative approach to setting research priorities for lymphedema management. Lymphat Res Biol. 2019; 17(3):356–361

[3] Omidi Z, Kheirkhah M, Abolghasemi J, Haghighat S. Effect of lymphedema self-management group-based education compared with social network-based education on quality of life and fear of cancer recurrence in women with breast cancer: a randomized controlled clinical trial. Qual Life Res. 2020; 29(7):1789–1800

[4] Thomas MJ, Morgan K. The development of Lymphoedema Network Wales to improve care. Br J Nurs. 2017; 26(13):740–750

[5] O'Donnell TF, Jr, Allison GM, Iafrati MD. A systematic review of guidelines for lymphedema and the need for contemporary intersocietal guidelines for the management of lymphedema. J Vasc Surg Venous Lymphat Disord. 2020; 8(4):676–684

[6] O'Donnell TF, Jr, Allison GM, Melikian R, Iafrati MD. A systematic review of the quality of clinical practice guidelines for lymphedema, as assessed using the Appraisal of Guidelines for Research and Evaluation II instrument. J Vasc Surg Venous Lymphat Disord. 2020; 8 (4):685–692

[7] Borman P, Yaman A, Denizli M, Karahan S. The reliability and validity of Lymphedema Quality of Life Questionnaire-Leg in Turkish patients with lower limb lymphedema. Lymphat Res Biol. 2020; 18(1):42–48
[8] Wedin M, Fredrikson M, Ahlner E, et al. Validation of the Lymphoedema Quality of Life Questionnaire (LYMQOL) in Swedish cancer patients. Acta Oncol. 2020; 59(3):365–371
[9] Roski J, Bo-Linn GW, Andrews TA. Creating value in health care through big data: opportunities and policy implications. Health Aff (Millwood). 2014; 33(7):1115–1122
[10] Vayena E, Dzenowagis J, Brownstein JS, Sheikh A. Policy implications of big data in the health sector. Bull World Health Organ. 2018; 96 (1):66–68
[11] Fu MR, Wang Y, Li C, et al. Machine learning for detection of lymphedema among breast cancer survivors. mHealth. 2018; 4:17
[12] Briganti G, Le Moine O. Artificial intelligence in medicine: today and tomorrow. Front Med (Lausanne). 2020; 7:27
[13] Vougas K, Almpanis S, Gorgoulis V. Deep learning: shaping the medicine of tomorrow. Mol Cell Oncol. 2020; 7(3):1723462

Section IV

Non-Surgical Treatment and Techniques

Edited by Christoph Hirche

IV

6 Integrative, Multiprofessional Conservative Treatment

Joachim E. Zuther

Summary

The conservative approach to the management of lymphedema is essential for all lymphedema patients and remains a mainstay for all patients scheduled for the modern surgical management of lymphedema. Conservative treatment is indicated for a minimum of 6 months, and needs to include verification of the patient's compliance to this treatment. This is a prerequisite, particularly for patients who will undergo lymphoreconstructive surgery, such as lymphovenous anastomosis or vascularized lymph node transfer, or lymphoablative surgery. This may help identify suitable candidates and best prepare these patients for optimal postoperative results. In addition, it is recommended to be continued after surgery—lifelong after lymphoablative surgery and with a stepwise reduction after reconstructive microsurgery.

This chapter discusses the techniques and concepts of the conservative approach to the management of lymphedema and provides a comprehensive explanation of the internationally recognized gold-standard treatment known as complete decongestive therapy, a noninvasive, multicomponent approach. It helps the reader of this surgical textbook to understand the mechanisms and strategies of complete decongestive therapy alone and in conjunction with lymphatic surgery. Finally, it aims to successfully embed the surgical techniques into an integral, multiprofessional therapeutic concept.

Keywords: bandages, complete decongestive therapy (CDT), compression therapy, conservative treatment, exercises, garments, manual lymph drainage (MLD), self-management, skin care, two-phase approach, wound care

6.1 Background

Successful treatment of lymphedema requires the coordination of integrated, multiprofessionally qualified health care providers specialized in lymphology. Various surgical, especially microsurgical, procedures for reconstructive treatment of lymphedema have been practiced for over a century and continue to be refined and improved. Recent advancements have led to increased discussion of the role of surgical treatment for lymphedema. Despite these recent improvements there is a broad consensus among clinicians that surgical procedures do not eliminate the need of nonsurgical conservative treatment regimens preoperatively as well as postoperatively.[1,2] Noninvasive conservative lymphedema therapy remains the first-line standard of care for lymphedema and should always be explored prior to consideration for surgery as an effective and low-cost treatment option for lymphedema, despite its limited availability for continuous outpatient treatment in some countries worldwide. Current surgical procedures can be highly successful for a select group of patients affected by lymphedema with individualized indications; however, achieving optimal and long-term results requires a coordinated team effort between the surgical team, the lymphedema therapists, and the patient. The specific timing and protocols of complete decongestive therapy (CDT), manual lymph drainage (MLD), compression therapy, exercises, and skin care in the perioperative setting are addressed in **Subchapter 6.3** (in which the basic techniques are described).

6.2 Complete Decongestive Therapy

Complete Decongestive Therapy (CDT) is a noninvasive, multicomponent approach to symptomatically treat lymphedema and related conditions.[3] Numerous studies have proven the scientific basis and effectiveness of this therapy, which has been well established in European countries since the 1970s and has been practiced in the United States in one form or another since the 1980s. CDT consists of a combination of integrated treatment modalities that include MLD, compression therapy, patient-tailored exercises, and skin care. Each component will be discussed in this chapter.

6.2.1 Goals of Complete Decongestive Therapy

The main goal of CDT is to return the body part affected by lymphedema to a normal or near-normal size with improved function and quality of life, that is, to achieve a subclinical stage of lymphedema and to prevent reaccumulation of lymphatic fluid in the affected body part.

Decongestion is achieved by manually rerouting stagnated lymphatic fluid around blocked or insufficient areas with injured collectors or lymph node basins, utilizing remaining healthy lymphatic vessels and other lymphatic pathways, into more centrally located and sufficient lymphatic vessels, which drain into the venous system. To maintain the reduction, compression is applied on the affected area following the manual rerouting techniques, either with padded short-stretch bandages or compression garments.

Secondary goals include the maintenance and improvement of the decongestive results, prevention of infections, patient education, as well as prevention of progressive stage changes such as fat deposition or fibrotic tissue.

History and pioneers of complete decongestive therapy

Early developments of CDT can be traced back to Alexander von Winiwarter (1848–1917), a surgeon from Austria who successfully treated swollen limbs with elevation, compression, and a special manual massage-like technique. After Winiwarter's death, his treatment approach was not developed further.

The evolution of MLD can be attributed to Emil Vodder (1896–1986), a PhD from Denmark, who lived and worked in France between 1928 and 1939. Vodder "intuitively" manipulated the swollen lymph nodes of some of his patients who suffered from chronic colds and sinus infections. He reported that his manual therapy was successful and individuals who were treated with his techniques felt better. He continued to develop his treatment method and moved to Paris to do further research on the lymphatic system. Vodder called his technique "lymph drainage massage" and introduced it during an international health fair as *le drainage lymphatique.*

In 1963, Johannes Asdonk (1910–2003), a German physician, learned about Vodder's technique while working in Essen, Germany, and decided to meet personally with Vodder. Impressed with the results Vodder achieved, Asdonk decided to study his hands-on technique and established the first school for MLD in Germany in 1969, with Emil Vodder and Vodder's wife, Astrid, as instructors.

With a more detailed knowledge about the anatomy and physiology of the lymphatic system and the expanding list of indications for this treatment, it was necessary to add new procedures to modify Vodder's existing techniques. Vodder and Asdonk had differing opinions regarding the technical aspects of the MLD strokes and subsequently ended their partnership in 1971. Vodder moved to Austria to start his own school, and Asdonk remained in Germany, where he continued his extensive research on the effectiveness of MLD and its impact on the lymphatic system.

Based on Asdonk's work, MLD as a treatment for lymphedema became reimbursable by national health insurance in Germany in 1974. In cooperation with other researchers, namely, Eberhard Kuhnke, Etelka Földi, Anton Gregl, and others, Asdonk founded the German Society of Lymphology in 1976. The cooperation between these scientists within the society led to the development of a new therapy concept, which enabled the successful treatment of edemas of different geneses with the addition of various and new intervention techniques. The combination of these techniques is known today as "complete decongestive therapy".

Kuhnke's work in the development of limb volume measurement techniques helped to provide evidence of the effectiveness of CDT and offered valuable support to further establish this therapy in the treatment of lymphedema and other related conditions. Most schools providing lymphedema training throughout the world today teach all components of CDT, which includes the advanced version of Vodder's MLD.

6.2.2 Components of Complete Decongestive Therapy

Manual Lymph Drainage

Manual Lymph Drainage (MLD) is a gentle manual treatment technique, which is often confused with traditional massage. The word *massage,* meaning "to knead" (from the Greek *masso/massain*), is used to describe such techniques as effleurage, petrissage, vibration, etc. Massage techniques are traditionally applied to treat ailments in muscle tissues, tendons, and ligaments; to achieve the desired effect, these techniques are generally applied with considerable pressure. MLD, on the other hand, consists of very gentle manual techniques, designed to influence the fluid components and lymphatic structures located in superficial tissues, such as the skin and the subcutis where lymphedema almost exclusively manifests itself. The sole common denominator between MLD and "traditional massage" is that both techniques are administered manually. The techniques, applied pressures, and indications for which these two therapeutic measures are used are significantly different, and it is important to recognize that traditional massage should not regarded as effective to treat lymphedema. Therefore, the term *massage* should never be used to describe MLD. The effects of traditional massage generally result in an increase of blood flow in those areas. An increased blood flow in the skin results in more water leaving the blood capillaries into the subcutaneous tissues. This increased amount of water, for the most part, must be removed by the lymphatic system, which, in the case of lymphedema, is not working properly. Additional blood flow not only overloads an already stressed or impaired lymphatic system but can seriously worsen the swelling associated with lymphedema. There are several reasonable explanations why MLD and massage are often confused with each other. One is that there is a tendency to call any hands-on manual therapeutic technique a form of massage; the other is that massage can be very helpful if applied to treat edema. Lymphedema and edema, however, are two very different conditions; it is important to understand that, although both conditions involve swelling, different treatment approaches are required.

The four basic strokes of manual lymph drainage by Vodder

The techniques of MLD are based on the four basic strokes developed by Vodder, namely the "stationary circle" and the "pump," "rotary," and "scoop" techniques. The common denominator in all strokes is the working phase and the resting phase. In the working phase of each stroke, stretch stimuli are applied to the subcutaneous tissues, resulting in the manipulation of anchoring filaments attached to lymph capillaries and the smooth musculature in the wall of lymphangions. The light directional pressure in the working phase also serves to move lymphatic fluid in the appropriate direction. The pressure in this phase should be sufficient to stretch the subcutaneous tissue against the underlying fascia to its elastic capacity; it is not necessary to apply high pressure to achieve this goal. In fact, too much pressure may damage anchoring filaments and other lymphatic structures, or cause spasm of the lymphangions in lymphatic collectors. The pressure should also be light enough to avoid vasodilation; the amount of pressure is sometimes described as the pressure applied while stroking a newborn's head. However, more pressure may be necessary in certain conditions, such as long-standing and sluggish lymphedema, or the presence of fibrotic tissue.

The pressure is released during the resting phase in which the elasticity of the skin moves the therapist's hand passively back to the starting position. In this pressure-free phase, initial lymphatic vessels absorb tissue fluid from the interstitial spaces.

To achieve maximum results, each working phase should last about 1 s and should be repeated five to seven times in the same area using either a stationary or a dynamic pattern.

In the treatment of lymphedema, MLD techniques are applied on healthy lymph nodes and lymphatic vessels, which are generally located adjacent to the area with insufficient lymphatic drainage, i.e., lymphedema. The resulting increase in lymphatic vessel activity (lymphangiomotoricity) in the healthy areas creates a "suction effect," which enables accumulated lymphatic fluid to move from an area with insufficient lymph flow into an area with normal lymphatic drainage. To stimulate the return of lymphatic fluid into the venous system via the cervical venous angles, the lymph nodes on the neck are manipulated. Depending on the location of the damage to the lymphatic system, the thorax, abdominal area, and ipsilateral and contralateral axillary or inguinal lymph node groups may be included in the treatment. The extremity itself is treated in segments; the proximal aspect of the affected extremity is decongested prior to expanding the treatment to the more distal aspects.

Effects of manual lymph drainage

The principal effects of MLD include:

- *Increase in lymph production:* The manual stretch applied to the anchoring filaments of lymph capillaries stimulates the intake of lymphatic loads into the lymphatic system.
- *Increase in lymphangiomotoricity:* Mild stretches applied perpendicular to the smooth musculature located in the wall of lymphatic collectors result in an increased contraction frequency of lymphangions. In addition, the increased lymph production results in an elevated volume of transported lymphatic fluid; the subsequently elevated intralymphatic pressure produces an increased contraction frequency of lymphangions.
- *Reverse of lymph flow:* In the treatment of lymphedema, MLD techniques enable lymphatic fluid to move against its natural flow patterns utilizing superficial lymphatic vessels. Lymphatic fluid is rerouted around blocked or insufficient areas using collateral lymphatic collectors, lymphatic anastomoses, or tissue channels.
- *Increase in venous return:* The directional pressure in the working phase of MLD strokes elevates the venous return in the superficial venous system. Deeper and more specialized techniques of MLD, especially in the abdominal area, affect the venous return in the deep venous system.
- *Soothing:* The light pressures applied in MLD decrease the sympathetic mode and promote the parasympathetic response.
- *Analgesic:* Accelerated drainage of nociceptive substances from the tissues promotes pain control.

Basic Strokes of Manual Lymph Drainage

Stationary Circles

Characteristic for this technique are oval-shaped stretches of the skin, which are applied with the palmar surfaces of the fingers or the entire hand. Stationary circles may be applied with one hand or bimanually (alternating or simultaneously), and are used on the entire body surface, but predominantly on the large lymph node groups, the neck, and the face.

In the working phase, the pressure increases and decreases gradually in the direction of lymphatic drainage for about half of a circle, achieved by either radial or ulnar deviation in the wrist. In the first part of the working phase, the stretch is applied perpendicular to the lymphatic collectors, in the second part, parallel to the lymphatic collectors. The full elasticity of the skin should be used to apply the stretch.

The working hand relaxes in the resting phase of this technique, during which the therapist's hand maintains contact with the patient's skin. The pressure is completely released, and the elasticity of the skin moves the therapist's hand passively back to the starting position (▸ Fig. 6.1a).

For the application on smaller surfaces, such as the hand and foot, in the area of joints, and in the treatment of infants, stationary circles are applied with the palmar surface of the thumb (▸ Fig. 6.1b).

Pump Technique

The entire palm and the proximal phalanges are used in this technique, which are applied in a circular-shaped pressure operating within almost the full range between the ulnar and radial deviation. Pumps are dynamic strokes (i.e., the working hand moves from distal to proximal), and can be applied with one hand or bimanually (alternating); this technique is applied primarily on the extremities.

At the beginning of the working phase, the hand is placed on the skin with ulnar deviation and wrist flexion, the fingers are extended, and the thumb is in opposition to the fingers. In this starting position, the radial aspect of the thumb and index finger, as well as the web space between these two phalanges, is in contact with the skin. The pressure increases and decreases gradually during the transition to radial deviation and wrist extension and reaches its maximum stretch when the entire palm has made contact. Pressure is applied in the drainage direction (▸ Fig. 6.2a,b).

When the skin is stretched to its maximum elasticity and the hand is in radial deviation, the transition to the resting phase begins in which the elasticity of the skin carries the therapist's hand back to the starting position. To reach the starting point of the next working phase, the hand glides without pressure, approximately half a hand width in the proximal direction.

Scoop Technique

This stroke is applied predominantly on the distal parts of extremities and consists of a spiral-shaped movement; this dynamic stroke is administered with one hand or bimanually (alternating). A transitional movement between ulnar deviation with forearm pronation, moving into radial deviation with forearm supination, is used in the application of this technique.

At the beginning of the working phase, the hand is placed in ulnar deviation and pronation onto the skin (perpendicular to the pathway of lymphatic collectors). The web space between the index finger and the thumb is in contact with the body surface at this point. The working phase starts with the hand gliding over the skin in a spiral-shaped movement in the proximal direction. During the gliding (working) phase, the pressure increases gradually, and the palm and the palmar surfaces of the fingers get in contact with the skin. The pressure reaches its maximum when the palm is in complete contact with the surface of the skin. With the palm in contact, the fingers glide over the skin in a fanlike pattern until they are aligned parallel with the extremity. During this phase, the pressure gradually decreases again (▸ Fig. 6.3a,b).

The resting phase begins once the hand and fingers are parallel with the extremity. The hand does not return to the starting position, but returns to ulnar deviation and

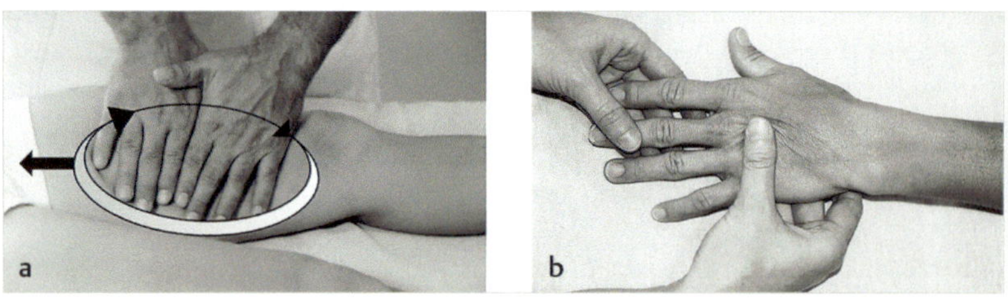

Fig. 6.1 **(a)** Stationary circles working phase (white half circle) and resting phase of stationary circles; **(b)** Thumb circles on the dorsum of the hand.

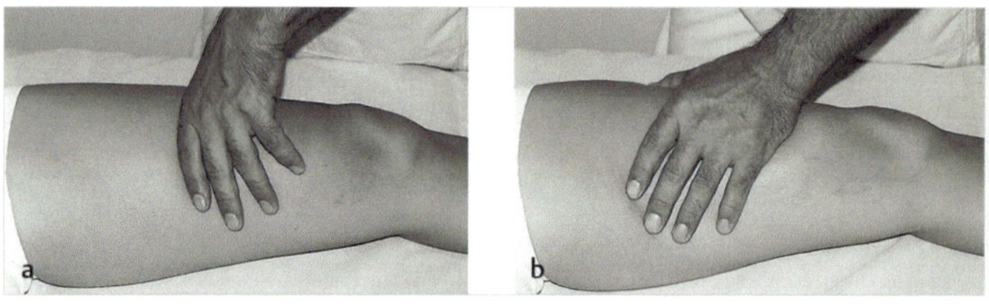

Fig. 6.2 **(a)** Pump stroke at the beginning of the working phase. **(b)** Pump stroke at the end of the working phase.

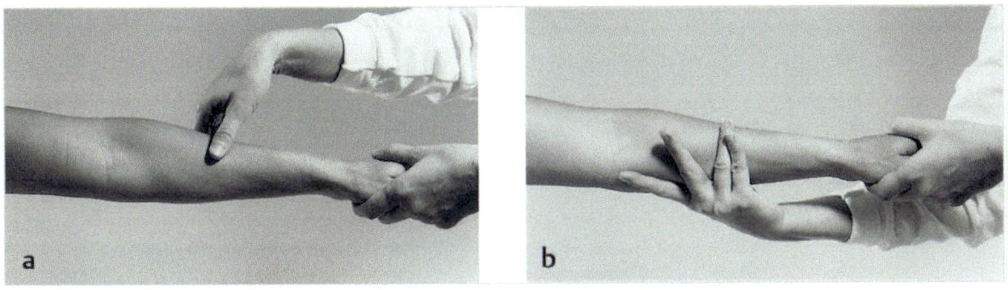

Fig. 6.3 **(a)** Scoop at the beginning of the working phase. **(b)** Scoop during the working phase.

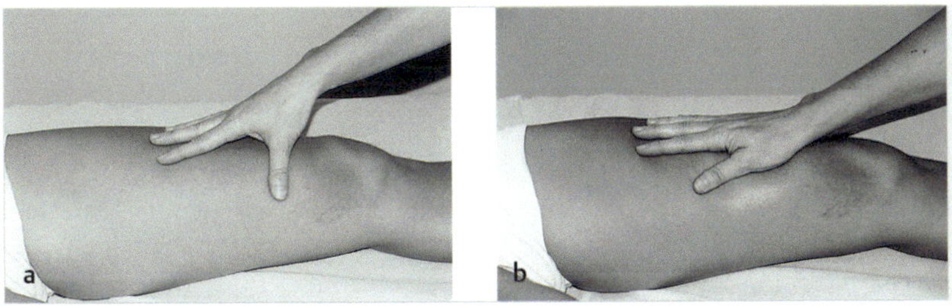

Fig. 6.4 **(a)** Rotary at the beginning of the working phase. **(b)** Rotary at the end of the working phase.

pronation, approximately one hand width further proximal where the next working phase starts.

Rotary Technique

This dynamic technique can be applied with one hand or bimanually (at the same time or alternating) and is used not only on large surface areas, primarily on the trunk, but also on lymphedematous extremities.

The hand is placed on the body surface in an elevated position and parallel to the pathway of the lymphatic collectors at the beginning of the working phase. The wrist is in flexion, the finger joints (except the thumb) are in a neutral position, and the thumb is in approximately 90 degrees of abduction; all fingertips are in contact with the skin. The working phase is initiated as the palm is placed on the skin in an elliptical movement (over the ulnar side). At the same time, the thumb slides into abduction. In this phase, the subcutaneous tissues are stretched against the fascia and perpendicular to the flow of lymph. When contact is established with the full hand and palmar surface, the skin is stretched toward the drainage area with gradually increasing pressure. While the hand stretches, the thumb is adducted until aligned with the hand. The pressure decreases again, the elasticity of the skin moves the hand back to the starting position, and the hand relaxes (▶ Fig. 6.4a,b).

During the resting phase, the hand moves back into wrist flexion until it is elevated again, with the fingers sliding without pressure (but in contact with skin) in the drainage direction, until the thumb reaches approximately 90 degrees of abduction. The sequence continues in this position in the next working phase.

During the working and the resting phases, the fingers remain in the neutral position.

Additional Techniques of Manual Lymph Drainage

Deep Abdominal Technique

The goal of this technique is to stimulate deep lymphatic structures, such as the cisterna chyli, the abdominal part of the thoracic duct, lumbar trunks and lymph nodes, pelvic lymph nodes, and certain organ systems with their lymphatic systems. Manipulation of these lymphatic structures, particularly the thoracic duct, accelerates lymph transport toward the venous angles. This results in improved lymphatic drainage from structures distal to the thoracic duct, including the lower extremities. The manipulation of deep veins located in the same area also improves the venous return to the heart.

The considerable decongestive effects on the lymphatic and the venous systems make deep abdominal techniques a valuable tool in the treatment of lower extremity swelling.

More pressure than those associated with the basic MLD strokes are necessary to reach the deeper structures of the lymphatic system; therefore, the following cautionary measures must be observed:

This technique is applied on five different locations (for a total of nine applications). The therapist coordinates the technique with the patient's diaphragmatic breathing rhythm. The flat and soft hand follows the patient's exhalation into the abdominal cavity, where it remains until the next inhalation (at this point, it is important to note the patient's response to the pressure). A brief period of moderate resistance is applied during the initial inhalation phase. The resistance is released to allow full inhalation. The hand is moved to the next placement on the abdomen during the pause between inhalation and the next exhalation phase. To avoid discomfort, the therapist's hand remains soft and passive; pressure is applied with the top hand, which rests on the working hand (▶ Fig. 6.5).

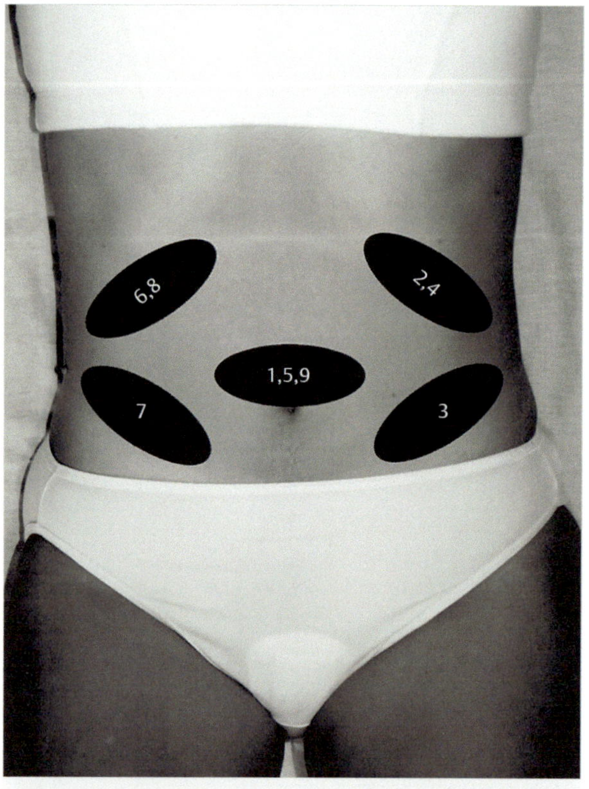

Fig. 6.5 The deep abdominal technique: A sequence of five different hand placements is applied to the abdominal area. Ideally, the placements on the thoracic cage and in the center of the abdomen are repeated during the full sequence. There is a total of nine manipulations (1–9), depending on the patient's reaction.

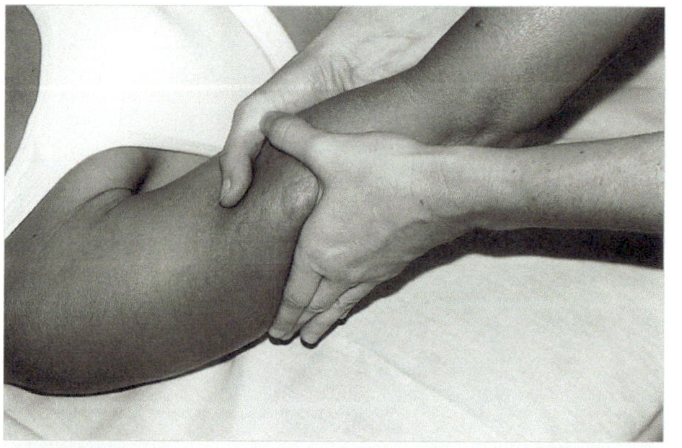

Fig. 6.6 Edema technique (superficial) on the upper arm.

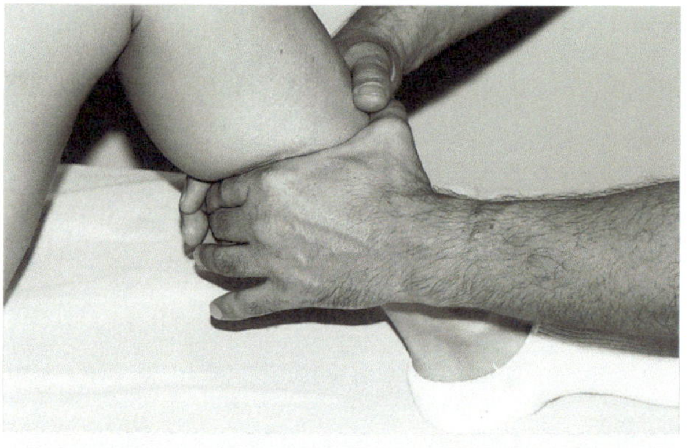

Fig. 6.7 Edema technique (deep) on the lower leg.

Edema Technique

This technique should be applied only after the drainage area located proximal to the application has been previously cleared with basic MLD strokes, the ipsilateral trunk quadrant is free of edema, and the extremity has at least begun to decongest.

The goal of edema strokes is to mobilize the free protein-rich and sluggish edema fluid in the extremities in direction of the drainage area, which necessitates increased pressure and prolonged duration (5–8 s) in the working phase. The hands move dynamically from distal to proximal between strokes to cover a certain portion of a limb.

Edema techniques may be applied with more or less intensity; the less intensive technique consists of bimanual pump techniques, which are applied simultaneously on opposing sides of the extremity. This technique can be used on the entire limb (▶ Fig. 6.6).

The deeper and more effective variation is administered circumferentially with the radial surface of both hands. The hands move simultaneously into the subcutaneous tissue and proceed to move the lymphatic fluid toward proximal. This technique is applied on the lower leg and foot and the hand and forearm (▶ Fig. 6.7).

Edema technique cannot be used if it causes pain, in painful lipedema or lipedema with accompanying lymphedema, in patients with hemophilia, in patients on anticoagulants, and in patients with varicose veins or deep venous thrombosis. Other contraindications listed later in this chapter must be observed as well.

Fibrosis Technique

The goal of this modality is to soften and break up lymphostatic fibrosis often associated with lymphedema. Fibrosis techniques should be used only if the extremity has begun to decongest and are applied directly in the area of lymphostatic fibrosis with more intensity and prolonged duration than the basic techniques of MLD; these techniques may cause local vasodilation. To optimize the softening effect on lymphostatic fibrosis, compression bandages (preferably in combination with special foam applications) should be applied directly following this modality.

Variations of the fibrosis technique include the "kneading" and the "thumb" technique. In the kneading technique, the fibrotic tissue is lifted softly from the underlying tissue with the flat finger pads. The skin fold is then softly and slowly moved using an S-shaped

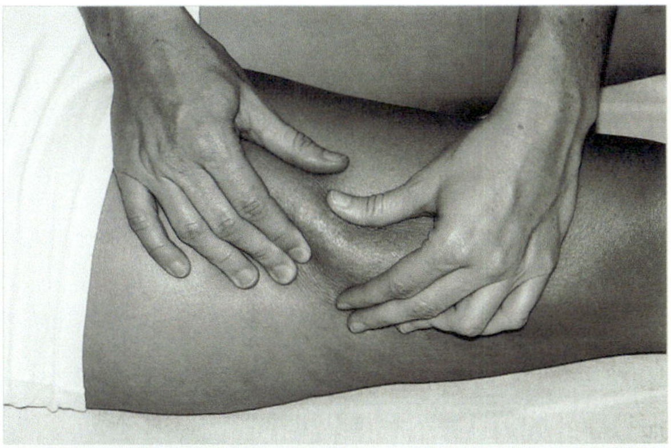

Fig. 6.8 Fibrosis technique ("kneading" technique) on the thigh.

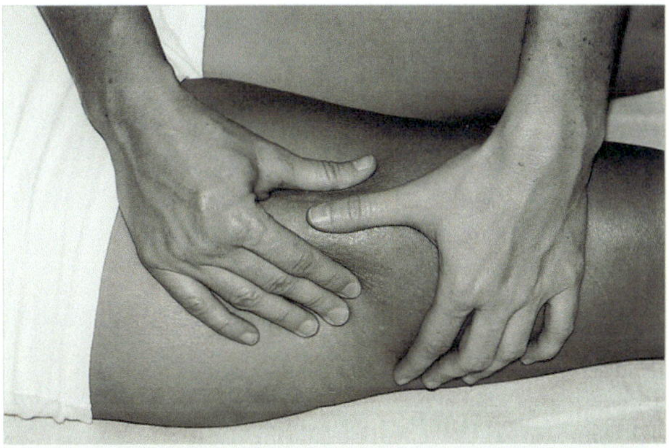

Fig. 6.9 Fibrosis technique ("thumb" technique) on the thigh.

manipulation between the thumb of one hand and the fingers of the other hand (▶ Fig. 6.8).

In the other, more intense technique, the fibrotic tissue fold is lifted softly with the flat fingers of one hand. The flat thumb of the other hand manipulates the skin fold by pressing down on it (▶ Fig. 6.9).

Contraindications include radiation fibrosis and those discussed for the edema technique.

Vasa Vasorum Technique

The vasa vasorum is a network of small blood vessels that supply the walls of large blood vessels and lymphatic vessels that drain these areas. This technique uses and optimizes the drainage pathways of the plexus-like lymphatic vessels, which can serve as auxiliary drainage pathways in the treatment of lymphedema (▶ Fig. 6.10).

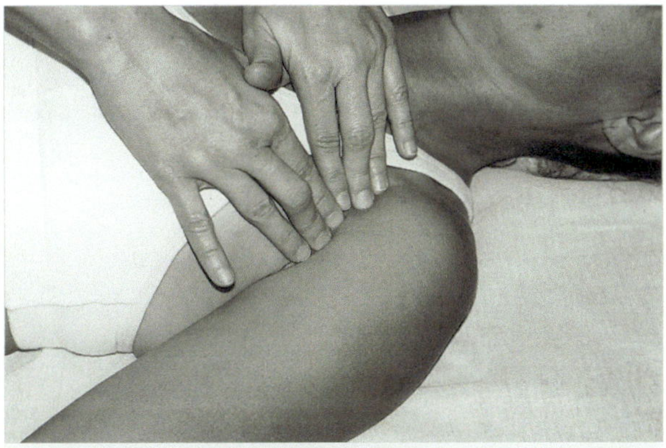

Fig. 6.10 Vasa vasorum technique (cephalic vein).

Contraindications for Manual Lymph Drainage

General and local contraindications for MLD should be critically evaluated by the lymph therapist and by the surgeon in the multiprofessional team for the indication of surgery for lymphedema (▶ Table 6.1 and ▶ Table 6.2), which may require pre- and postoperative MLD. In addition, on the one hand, contraindications for MLD may also be per se contraindications for certain microsurgical treatment options, as it is progressive chronic venous insufficiency for lymphovenous anastomosis (LVA) after a deep vein thrombosis. On the other hand, contraindications for MLD may be an exclusive indication for selected lymphoreconstructive procedures of modern surgical management in order to improve the patient's outcome even without MLD.

Compression Therapy

The primary goal of compression therapy as part of the lymphedema treatment regimen is to maintain the decongestive effect achieved during the MLD application and to prevent re-accumulation of fluid in the tissues. Correctly applied compression bandages and garments have several effects that address the lymphedematous extremity (▶ Table 6.3). Without the benefits provided by compression therapy, successful and lasting treatment of lymphedema would be nearly impossible.

The elastic fibers of the cutaneous tissues are damaged in lymphedema. This is true for lymphedema in its primary and secondary forms, as well as in those cases when lymphedema is combined with other pathologies. Although lymphedema may be reduced to a normal or near-normal size utilizing proper treatment techniques, the lymphatic vascular system is never normal again after lymphedema has been present, and the skin elasticity may never be regained completely. The affected body part is consequently at permanent risk of fluid re-accumulation. External support of the affected extremity or body part is therefore an essential component of lymphedema management.

Based on the phase of the treatment (see **Subchapter 6.3**), compression therapy is applied either by specific bandage materials, especially at the beginning of a therapeutic

Table 6.1 General contraindications for MLD

General contraindications for MLD include:

- *Cardiac edema*: MLD/CDT does not provide therapeutic benefit in edema caused by decompensated cardiac insufficiency. If cardiac edema is combined with lymphedema, MLD may be indicated, but cardiac and pulmonary functions need to be closely monitored by the referring physician.
- *Renal failure.*
- *Acute infections*: MLD may exacerbate the symptoms.
- *Acute bronchitis*: The parasympathetic stimulation associated with MLD may exacerbate the symptoms in the acute phase by producing contractions of the smooth bronchial musculature.
- *Acute deep vein thrombosis*: MLD/CDT is contraindicated on the affected extremity and the abdominal area.
- *Malignancies*: MLD/CDT may be indicated as palliative treatment; however, close cooperation between the treating therapist and the referring physician is necessary. To date, there is no scientific evidence that the application of MLD (or other manual treatment techniques) could accelerate the spread of malignant cells to other parts of the body or contribute to the growth of malignant tumors (see also the section on Limitations of CDT in Lymphedema Management later in this chapter).
- *Bronchial asthma*: The parasympathetic stimulation associated with MLD may cause the onset of an asthma attack. If bronchial asthma is associated with lymphedema, MLD generally can be applied safely if the treatment time is incrementally increased. Sessions may start at about 20 minutes of initial treatment time and if no negative reactions are noted during or after the therapy, the treatment time may be increased by 5 to 10 minutes until normal treatment time is reached.
- *Hypertension*: MLD/CDT may be applied if cardiac functions are monitored.

Abbreviations: CDT, complete decongestive therapy; MLD, manual lymph drainage.

episode, known as short-stretch bandages, by compression garments, or a combination of both modalities. In select cases, alternate compression devices, such as elastic and nonelastic padding sleeves, may have to be considered.

Nevertheless, contraindications for compression therapy remain and have to be considered individually at the beginning and during therapy (▶ Table 6.4).

Principles of Compression

The pressure applied on a body part by use of external compression is generally measured in millimeters of mercury (mmHg). To achieve the desired effects, a compression gradient from distal to proximal is imperative; correctly applied bandages and compression garments achieve this effect. Complications are common if the measurements or the chosen compression class of compression garments are faulty or if short-stretch bandages are applied incorrectly.

Table 6.2 Local contraindications of manual lymph drainage

Local contraindications are as follows:

- On the neck:
  - *Carotid sinus syndrome*: The application of MLD may cause cardiac arrhythmia in cases of hypersensitive pressure receptors on the carotid bifurcation.
  - *Thyroid dysfunction*: Manipulation on the neck may accelerate the release of thyroid hormones and/or medications into the blood.
  - *Age*: An increased risk of atherosclerosis in the cervical arteries may be associated with patients over 60 years of age.
- In the abdominal area:
  - *Unexplained pain.*
  - *Recent abdominal surgery.*
  - *Inflammatory conditions* of the small and large intestines, such as Crohn's disease, ulcerative colitis, and diverticulitis.
  - *Pregnancy.*
  - *Dysmenorrhea.*
  - *Ileus.*
  - *Diverticulosis.*
  - *Aortic aneurysm.*
  - *Deep vein thrombosis.*
  - *Radiation fibrosis, radiation cystitis, radiation colitis.*

Abbreviation: MLD, manual lymph drainage.

Table 6.3 Effects of compression therapy

Correctly applied compression bandages and garments have the following effects:

- Increase in tissue pressure, and increased pressure to the blood and lymphatic vessels contained within these tissues; the tissue pressure plays an essential role in the exchange of fluids between the blood capillaries and the tissues.
- Improved venous and lymphatic return. External compression directs these fluids in the proximal direction and improves the function of the valves contained within these vessels.
- Reduced fluid filtration in the area of the blood capillaries results in lower workload of the lymphatic system.
- Improved effectiveness of the muscle and joint pumps during activity. The activity of skeletal musculature is an important factor in the return of fluids within the venous and lymphatic systems. Together with other supporting mechanisms, the muscle and joint pump activity propels these fluids back to the heart ensuring an uninterrupted circulation. External compression provides a sufficient counter-force to the working musculature, thus improving its efficiency.
- Prevention of reaccumulation of evacuated lymphatic fluid, subsequently conserving and improving the results achieved during MLD.
- Compensation for elastic insufficiency of the affected tissue in lymphedema and support for those tissues that have lost elasticity.
- Softening of connective tissue deposits and scar tissue, which is beneficial in the treatment of lymphostatic fibrosis; this effect can be increased by the use of special foam materials in combination with compression therapy.

Table 6.4 Absolute and relative contraindications for compression therapy

Part of the evaluation process is to scan for potential contraindications and/or precautions for compression therapy to avoid adverse outcomes.
The application of compression on an extremity is absolutely contraindicated in the following cases:

- *Cardiac edema.*
- *Peripheral arterial diseases*: Compression therapy is contraindicated with an ankle/brachial index (ABI) of less than 0.8. Normal ABI values range from 0.95 to 1.3; in mild to moderate arterial disease, the values range from 0.5 to 0.8. ABI values of less than 0.5 are interpreted as severe arterial insufficiencies.
  ABI compares the systolic blood pressure of the ankle to that of the arm. These measurements are useful in the assessment, follow-up, and treatment of patients with peripheral vascular disease.
- *Acute infections* (cellulitis, erysipelas).

Relative contraindications:

- *Hypertension.*
- *Cardiac arrhythmia.*
- *Decreased or absent sensation in the extremity.*
- *Partial or complete paralysis, flaccid limbs.*
- *Age.*
- *Congestive heart failure.*
- *Mild to moderate arterial occlusive disease (ABI values 0.8–1.0).*
- *Diabetes.*
- *Malignant lymphedema.*

A normal extremity can be compared to a cylinder. If compression therapy is applied on a leg using the same tension on the distal and the proximal ends of the extremity, the pressure in the ankle area (smaller radius) would be greater than the pressure on the calf (greater radius), and the pressure on the thigh would be lower than the pressure on the calf.[4]

This principle can be applied in a true cylindrical or cone-shaped extremity. In the area of bony prominences (ankles, wrists, or the medial and lateral circumferences of the hand and foot), the pressure is higher due to the smaller radius and the greater tension of the compression material used, whereas in concave areas (behind the ankles), the applied pressure is lower.

These issues and the fact that swollen extremities generally lose their cone shape make it necessary to use foam materials for padding in combination with compression bandages to construct a more cylindrical shape.

During the manufacturing process of compression garments a compression gradient is already built into the garments, generally eliminating the need of additional padding.

Compression Bandages

Correctly applied compression bandages are safe and effective and represent an indispensable part of CDT. Only trained therapists or patients and their caregivers who have received instruction in the application of short-stretch bandages from a trained individual should apply compression bandages in the treatment of lymphedema.

The application of bandage materials can be bulky and are used primarily during the initial phase, also known as the decongestive phase of CDT. Various types of elastic bandages are available; the preferred types of bandage material used in lymphedema management are short-stretch compression bandages. The braided cotton fibers used in the production process are woven in a way to achieve a certain degree of textile-elasticity. This interwoven pattern allows for about 30% to 60% extensibility of the bandage's original length. To understand the effects of various bandage materials on the tissues and the vascular systems embedded within the tissues, it is important to discuss the difference between short-stretch and long-stretch compression bandages.

Two different qualities of sub-bandage pressure can be distinguished in compression therapy: the *working pressure* and the *resting pressure*. Relevant in the determination of these pressure qualities are the type of bandage (long-stretch or short-stretch) used, the tension employed during the application of the bandage, the number of layers, and the condition of the material (age); bandages lose some of their elasticity over time and with repetitive use and cleaning.

Working pressure: The resistance the bandage provides against the working musculature determines the working pressure. This pressure is temporary and only active during muscle expansion, and its value depends on the extent of muscle contraction. The active working pressure results in an increase of the tissue pressure in the area where the bandages are applied; in addition, the venous and lymphatic vessels in the superficial and in the deep systems are compressed, thus improving the return of fluids within these vessel systems.

The lower the elasticity of a compression bandage, the higher the working pressure. Short-stretch bandages exert a high working pressure on the tissues and form a strong support during muscle contraction.

Long-stretch bandages contain elastic fibers and retain a low working pressure. Newly manufactured long-stretch bandages allow for an extensibility of more than 140% to 300% of the bandage's original length. This relatively high elasticity exerts a low resistance against the working musculature, and the decongestive effect on the venous and lymphatic system is minimal, especially in the deep systems.

Resting pressure: This is the sub-bandage pressure exerted on the tissues at rest, i.e., without muscle contraction. The resting pressure is a permanent pressure, and its value depends on the amount of tension used during the application of the bandage. The higher the tension (or stretch), the higher the pressure the bandage exerts on the tissues. A bandage with a high extensibility will therefore result in increased pressure on the tissues during rest.

Long-stretch vs short-stretch bandages in the treatment of lymphedema

Long-stretch bandages exert a relatively high resting pressure during which the venous and lymphatic vessels in the skin are compressed. This permanent compression may cause a tourniquet effect on the bandaged extremity. Long-stretch bandages may constrict veins and lymphatic vessels at rest and provide minimal support of the tissues during muscle contraction.

Short-stretch bandages employ a very low resting pressure on the tissues and the vascular systems. The risk of a tourniquet effect is therefore relatively low if a specially trained individual applies the compression bandages correctly.

Note: Long-stretch bandages are therefore not suitable for the treatment of lymphedema.

The high working and low resting pressure qualities of short-stretch bandages make them the preferred choice in the management of lymphedema and swellings of other geneses.

If significant short-term changes of the limb volume after lymphoreconstructive surgery are expected, e.g., after lymphovenous anastomosis (LVA), the characteristics of short-stretch bandages in the postsurgical "new" decongestive phase are preferable. After achieving a "new" steady state after successful LVA treatment, compression garments are recommended again, but in general require re-sizing and replacing garments.

How to apply a short-stretch bandage correctly?

To avoid constriction of venous and lymphatic vessels and to achieve a compression gradient in the treatment of lymphedema, it is necessary to apply compression bandages in layers. Following the application of a suitable moisturizer on the skin (see the section on Skin and Nail Care later in this chapter), a cotton stockinette is applied to absorb sweat and to protect the skin from the padding materials. The goal in the use of padding is to protect bony prominences and to create a cylindrical shape around the extremity. Special soft foam materials or synthetic cotton bandages are used for this purpose. For the padding of concave areas (behind the malleoli, palm) or to increase the pressure over lymphostatic fibrosis or wounds, a denser foam material is suitable. Short-stretch bandages of various widths are then applied in layers on the extremity. Tape should be used to affix the bandage material; sharp bandaging clips or pins are to be avoided as these materials may cut into the patient's skin and cause infection.

Most patients adjust to and tolerate the compression bandage well after a few applications. Patients should maintain their normal activity level and perform the decongestive exercise program while wearing the bandages (see the section on Exercises later in this chapter).

Compression Garments

The primary role of compression garments in lymphedema management is to preserve the success achieved with treatment during the decongestion of the edematous body part. In patients with lymphedema bandages are replaced with elastic compression garments once the limb is decongested (see the section on Two-Phase Approach of CDT later in this chapter).

Note:

Compression garments by themselves do not reduce swelling and should not be worn on untreated swollen extremities or body parts.

To ensure maximum long-term benefits of compression garments, it is imperative that only trained individuals with a full understanding of the pathology of lymphedema and its related conditions take the required measurements for the garment and, together with the patient, decide on the compression class, style, and length of the garment. Ill-fitting and ineffective compression garments not only produce poor results but also can be dangerous to the patient. A number of potential limitations and specific needs of the individual patient must be addressed and resolved to arrive at a comfortable yet supportive garment. Compression garments become a part of the patient's life, much like hearing aids or eyeglasses; they must be worn on a daily basis and applied first thing in the morning.

Compression garments are available as compression gauntlets, sleeves, and stockings and are made for specific body parts (e.g., brassieres or vests). They are manufactured in several sizes, variations (circular knit, flat knit), styles, compression classes, and materials, and are available in standard sizes or be custom-made.

Note:

Compression garments should be replaced every 6 months or sooner if the garments have lost their elasticity.

Donning and doffing of compression garments may be a challenge for patients who have mobility issues, whose hands are weak, or who have pain because of osteoarthritis;

this is most challenging for patients living alone. Some patients, despite their best efforts, may not be able to reach their feet adequately in order to don elastic garments or may have limited assistance at home. Education and practice are crucial to helping patients and/or caregivers achieve independence in this skill.

Donning aids can be useful to assist in the application of compression garments. Rubber gloves, slip-on/off aids, and nonslip mats are examples of donning systems, which also help to protect the garment from damage (▶ Fig. 6.11).

Rubber gloves are an important tool for all patients as they allow for "massaging" of the garment into place and avoid pinching and pulling of the garment and damage from fingernails or jewelry.

Elastic garments, which offer effective daytime compression, are not appropriate for nighttime use because they can restrict adequate blood flow while the limb is elevated and may bunch up when worn in bed.

Circular-Knit and Flat-Knit Garments

Compression garments are produced using two main knitting methods—seamed flat-knit (▶ Fig. 6.12) and seamless circular-knit. Both types are knitted by using threads made of some form of rubber (elastomer). Cotton or a synthetic material generally covers the elastomeric thread, providing the garment with additional qualities. Covered compression threads are more durable in that they limit or regulate stretch of the elastic fiber and protect it from sweat and skin ointments (▶ Fig. 6.13). The covered fibers make the garments softer, more breathable, and easier to apply. The manufacturing process provides compression garments with a two-way elasticity (▶ Fig. 6.14); the more two-way stretch a compression garment provides, the more comfortable it is to wear.

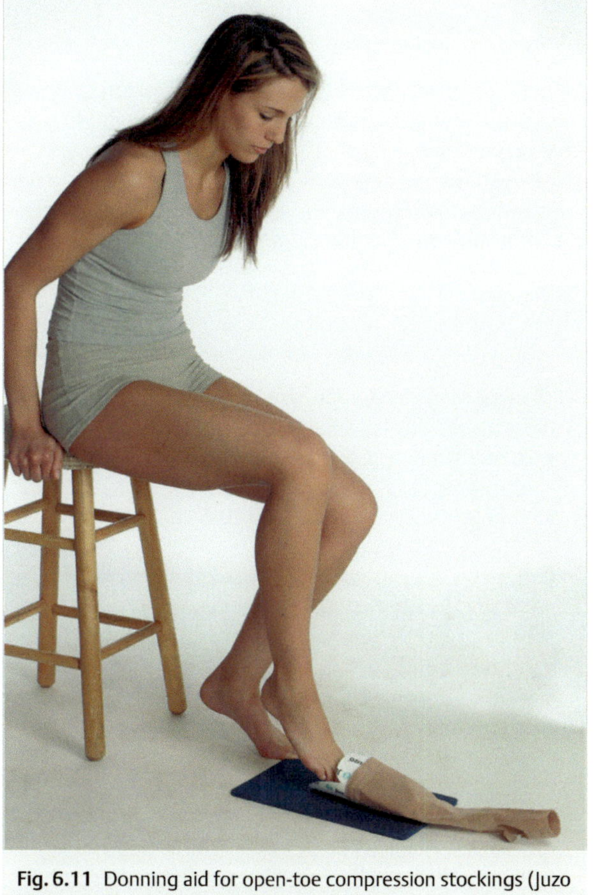

Fig. 6.11 Donning aid for open-toe compression stockings (Juzo Slippie; with permission from Juzo USA, Inc.).

Flat- or circular-knit compression garments?

The choice between flat- or circular-knit compression garments involves various considerations. Circular-knitted materials are less expensive and cosmetically more attractive than flat-knit garments because they have no seam and are produced using finer and sheerer materials. Based on the manufacturing process of flat-knit garments, these items are usually denser and more costly to produce. However, they produce a more tailored fit since the number of meshes is determined by the patient's circumferential measurements, which may be a determining factor for patients with excessively deformed extremities.

Aesthetic considerations are an important aspect in choosing the right garment. Compression garments are effective only if they are worn consistently; if the patient is unhappy with the garment and does not want to wear it, the therapeutic benefit is lost. Lower extremity stockings can be disguised by wearing a sheer (preferably dark) nylon stocking on top of them.

Styles of Compression Garments

Compression garments are manufactured in different styles and lengths and are available with a variety of fastening systems and integrated pressure pads (▶ Fig. 6.15a,b).

Fastening systems are designed to prevent the garments from sliding, which may create a tourniquet effect that may cause additional swelling and make the compression garment uncomfortable to wear for the individual. Fastening systems consist of garter belts, hip attachments (▶ Fig. 6.16), or fasteners that attach to shoulder straps. Other systems include synthetic polymers (usually silicone dots or stripes) on the inside of the proximal end of the garments (▶ Fig. 6.17). Special adhesive lotions that are available from most garment manufacturers can be used as well to prevent the garment from slipping.

Built-in pressure pads constructed of dense foam materials ensure an even distribution of pressure in concave areas, such as behind the malleoli or the palmar surface of the hand.

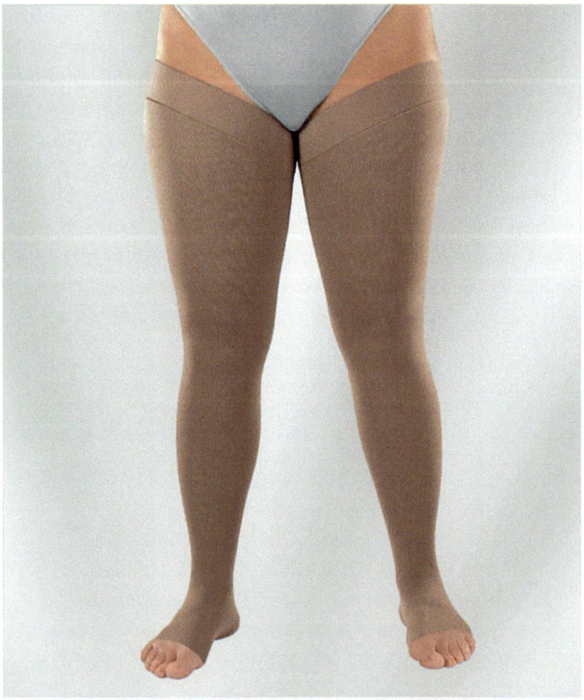

Fig. 6.12 Flat-knit thigh-high compression garment (with permission from Juzo USA, Inc.).

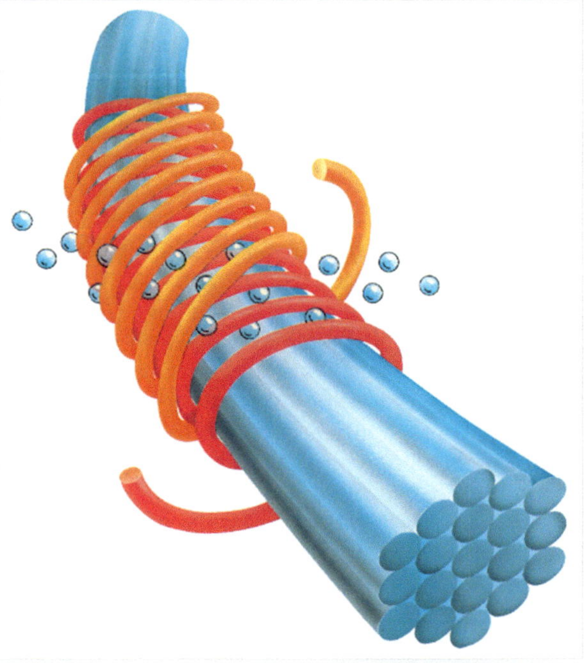

Fig. 6.13 Covered compression threads used in compression garments (Juzo USA Fibersoft) (with permission from Juzo USA, Inc.).

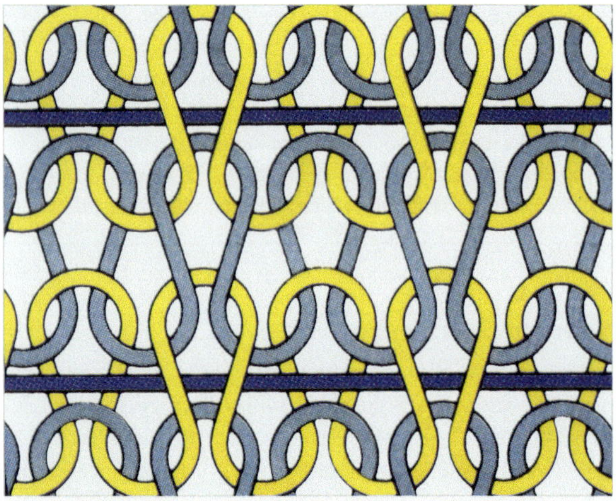

Fig. 6.14 Two-way elasticity in compression garments (with permission from Juzo USA, Inc.).

Compression Classes

Graduated compression garments are available in four main compression classes, which establish the compression value the garment produces on the skin surface and are calculated in millimeters of mercury (mmHg). The pressure values within the different classes of compression garments are measured on the distal circumference of the extremity (wrist, ankle), where the pressure is highest. To ensure the benefits of compression and promote sufficient circulation, a gradient from distal to proximal is necessary.

For seamless circular-knit garments there is no current international consensus for compression values within the different compression classes.

Compression levels for lymphedema treatment

The following values represent the compression ranges most manufacturers adhere to (▶ Fig. 6.18):

- 20 to 30 mmHg (Compression class I)
- 30 to 40 mmHg (Compression class II)
- 40 to 50 mmHg (Compression class III)

Compression levels for seamed flat-knit garments lean more toward international standards:

- 18 to 21 mmHg (Compression class I)
- 23 to 32 mmHg (Compression class II)
- 34 to 46 mmHg (Compression class III)
- Over 50 mmHg (Compression class IV)

Pressure values below 20 mmHg are generally not suitable for the management of lymphedema and are used only if a higher compression cannot be tolerated or is contraindicated.

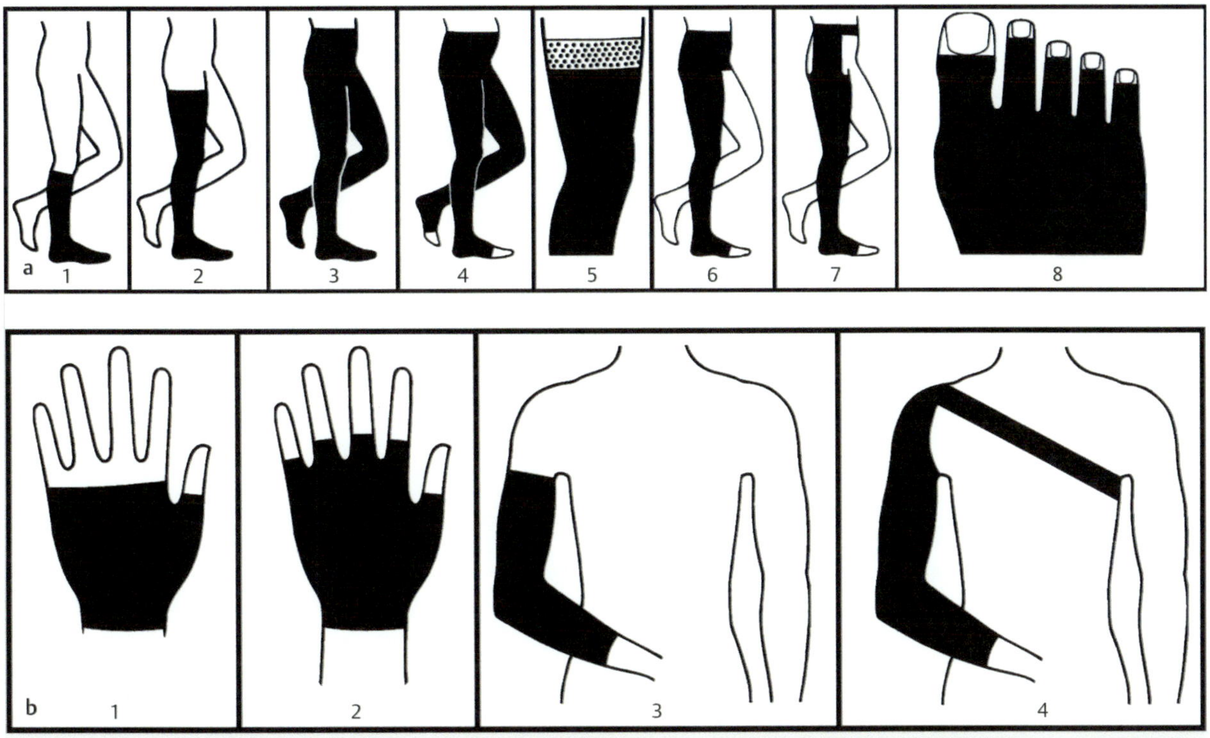

Fig. 6.15 **(a)** Compression styles for the lower extremity: 1, Knee-high stocking; 2, thigh-high stocking; 3, pantyhose; 4, pantyhose with highly elastic body part; 5, thigh-high stocking with fastening border (silicone dots); 6, thigh-high stocking with hip attachment; 7, thigh-high stocking with garter belt; 8, toe caps. **(b)** Compression styles for the upper extremity: 1, Compression gauntlet; 2, compression gauntlet with finger stubs; 3, arm sleeve; 4, arm sleeve with shoulder cover and strap (with permission from Juzo USA, Inc.).

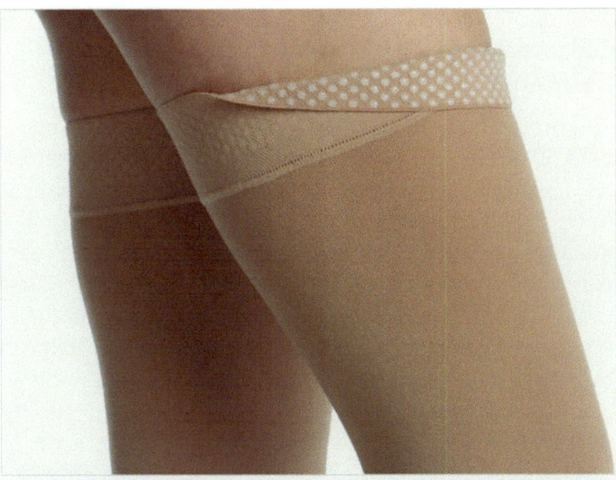

Fig. 6.16 Thigh-high compression stocking with fastening border made of silicone dots (with permission from Juzo USA, Inc.).

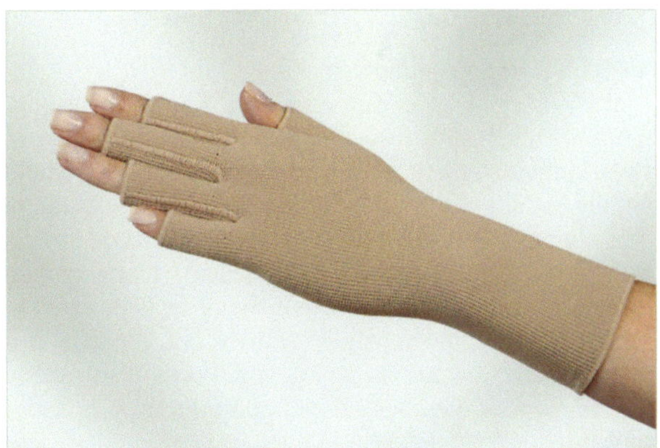

Fig. 6.17 Compression glove with finger stubs (with permission from Juzo USA, Inc.).

Many factors, such as age, activity level, skin integrity, mobility issues, congestive heart failure, partial or complete paralysis, diabetes, and wound care factors, must be considered to determine the correct compression class for a patient.

In some cases of lower extremity lymphedema, a compression of more than that available in compression class IV may have to be used. In these cases, a compression level II or III knee-high stocking may be worn in addition to a compression level III thigh-high stocking (or pantyhose). It is important to understand that the individual compression values of garments worn on top of each

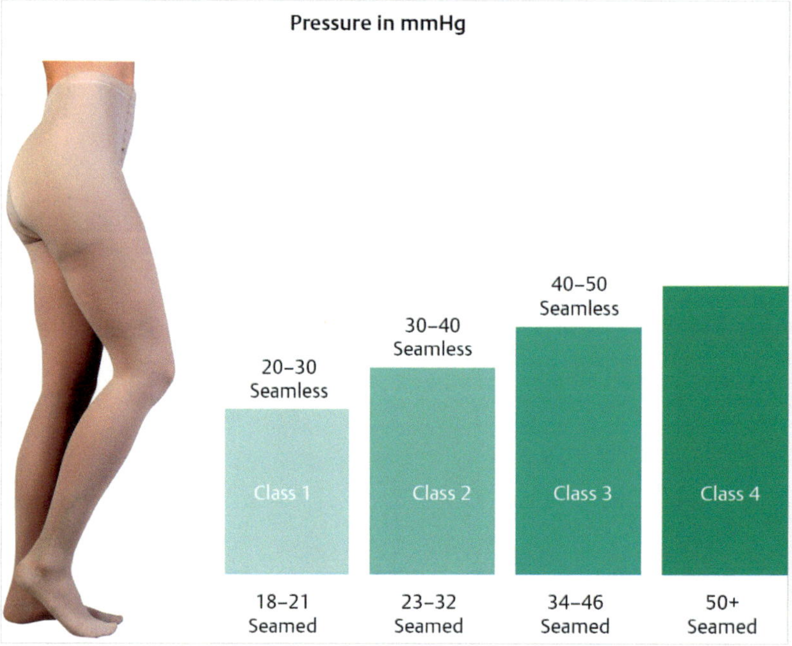

Fig. 6.18 Compression levels (with permission from Juzo USA, Inc.).

other do not double the values. Two level III stockings, for example, do not add up to a level VI; the resulting pressure would be somewhere between compression classes IV and V.

Physical limitations of the patient could be a rationale for a decision to combine two stockings. For example, an arthritic patient who requires a lower extremity garment of a higher compression level may have less difficulty donning a compression class III thigh-high with a compression class II knee-high stocking.

In most cases of upper extremity lymphedema, patients are adequately served by a compression class II arm sleeve, provided there are no contraindications that would require the use of a lower compression class, such as in the case of a partially or completely paralyzed, or flaccid limb. A patient with upper extremity lymphedema may require a compression class III arm sleeve if she or he is involved in a high-intensity and repetitive activity. For example, if a patient wishes to return to playing golf, a class III arm sleeve can be used on the involved extremity during play and a class II arm sleeve for daily activities.

Patients with lower extremity involvement usually require a compression class III garment; however, contraindications may be present that may necessitate the use of a lower level, and certain situations may require a higher level of compression.

If the patient has tolerated compression well during the decongestive phase, she or he may easily fit into the standard compression levels for the upper and lower extremities. It is important to consider the physical ability of the patient, as well as the patient's home support system when choosing a compression garment. A 70-year-old patient with lower extremity lymphedema may not be physically able to don a class III garment; thus, a class II garment may serve the patient's needs better.

The reduction of compression class is a relevant therapeutic aim to be discussed during patient education in the modern surgical management of lymphedema, as it will help to define potential phases to pause wearing compression garments without harming the overall results.

Custom-Made and Standard Compression Garments

Compression garments with a compression level of more than 50 mmHg are available only in custom-made materials. The high degree of compression requires the garment to be manufactured to the patient's exact circumferential measurements. As discussed earlier, custom-made garments may also be a better choice for those individuals with extremely deformed extremities. Some manufacturers provide custom garments with zippers, which can be a choice for patients who may be physically unable to don a closed compression garment.

Standard or ready-made garments are available in compression classes I–III; these garments can be obtained from most manufacturers in many predetermined sizes and styles that can accommodate a vast majority of extremities.

Custom-made garments are expensive, and the production time for these garments is longer. Although some lymphedema patients benefit from custom-made garments, they are certainly not requisite for all patients. The availability of a large variety of standard garments helps to reduce the cost and allows patients to wear cosmetically more attractive compression garments.

Alternative Compression Materials

Multilayered short-stretch compression bandaging remains the most adaptable compression modality for lymphedema. The application of short-stretch bandage materials in combination with appropriate padding allows customization of the compression in virtually unlimited variations. However, some patients are either unable or unwilling to apply bandages for nighttime compression, in which case alternative materials may provide the solution to counter a lack of adherence to the self-care and self-bandaging regimen.

Several adjustable elastic and nonelastic compression devices are available for patients with lymphedema and venous disorders. These devices provide gradient compression by use of adjustable bands. Some of these devices use foam pads underneath the nonelastic material to provide additional padding, others may be combined with traditional compression garments (▶ Fig. 6.19).

There is a broad consensus between clinicians that these devices should not be used to decongest a swollen limb (▶ Table 6.4). Nonelastic, adjustable compression may be used as an alternative to nighttime bandaging to balance daytime compression supplied by elastic compression garments when the extremity has decongested to a normal or near-normal size.

Alternative devices can also be utilized as a supplement to elastic garments in the daytime when elastic compression is insufficient to control edema in a limb with flaccid skin due to massive reduction or very aggressive forms of edema.

Exercises

Well-tailored regular exercise programs can have a positive impact on a healthy lifestyle, improve general well-being, increase energy level, and contribute to stress and weight management. Additional benefits of exercises for those individuals at risk of, or have, lymphedema include improved limb flexibility and range of movement, and most importantly increased lymphatic and venous return from the swollen areas, which can result in reduction of limb size and subjective limb symptoms.

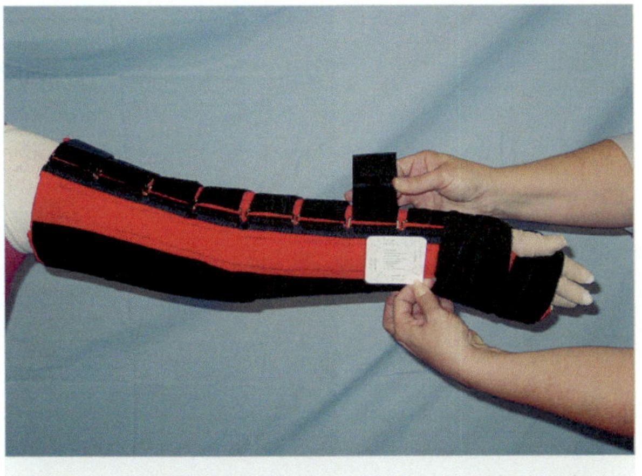

Fig. 6.19 Padded gradient compression with nonelastic adjustable bands (CircAid Measure-Up; with permission from CircAid Medical Products, Inc.).

Research indicates that the transport of lymphatic fluid and proteins from swollen areas increases during and after exercises. Studies show that lymph flow increased fivefold in the first 15 minutes and two- to threefold during the remaining time of a 2-hour exercise protocol.[5] In addition to the benefits to the lymphatic system, it is known that muscle activity and diaphragmatic breathing also have a considerable impact on venous blood returning from the extremities back to the heart, which in turn also positively affects fluid management within the interstitial spaces; increased venous return is of particular importance for those individuals affected by lower extremity lymphedema.

Decongestive Exercises

The goal of the exercise program during the intensive phase of CDT is to improve lymphatic circulation and to maximize functional ability. Exercises are performed at least twice a day for 10 to 15 minutes wearing the compression bandages. To promote patient's compliance, it is important to create an exercise protocol that is easy to learn and to perform. The therapist should monitor the exercise program regularly and the patient should assume the primary responsibility for the exercise as early as possible in the treatment program. A balanced program of recreational activities supports general well-being, improves lymphatic drainage, and controls weight. High-risk activities that could trigger a further decrease in lymphatic transport capacity should be avoided or kept at a minimum. High-risk activities for lymphedema include running, tennis and other racquet sports, soccer, wrestling, kickboxing, step aerobics, weight lifting with the affected extremity, or intense horse riding.

Abdominal Breathing Exercises

Diaphragmatic breathing exercises are a valuable tool in stimulating deep lymphatic structures, such as the cisterna chyli, the abdominal part of the thoracic duct, lumbar trunks and lumbar lymph nodes, pelvic lymph nodes, and certain organ systems.

Stimulation of these deep lymphatic structures, in particular the thoracic duct, accelerates the transport of lymphatic fluid toward the venous angles through which the lymphatic fluid is returned into the blood circulatory system.

The considerable decongestive effects on the lymphatic and venous systems also make abdominal breathing exercises a valuable tool for the treatment of upper extremity lymphedema.

Resistive Exercises

Resistive or strength exercises increase the strength in ligaments, tendons, and bones, improve muscular power, and positively contribute to weight control. Strength exercises are typically performed in a repetitive fashion against an opposing load. Improved strength assists in the prevention of overuse syndrome and restores intramuscular balance and normal biomechanics in the involved limb and surrounding joints. Resistive exercises using weights may present possible problems in regard to injury or overuse; however, with appropriate precautions resistive exercises using weights can be beneficial for patients affected by lymphedema. Negative effects in terms of accumulation of fluid in the affected limb (or the limb at risk) are unlikely if exercises are performed with compression in place on the involved extremity.[6] More research is needed to determine whether weight-training and other forms of exercise help reduce the risk of lymphedema.

Lifting heavy weights is not the best way to start a lymphedema exercise regimen; an exercise program should start gradually to avoid sprains and injury to muscles and should be followed by a warm down after active exercises. Studies have shown that a 10 to 15 minutes warming down period assists the lymphatic system in the removal of excess fluid and metabolites, which have accumulated in the interstitial space.

Aerobic Exercises

Aerobic exercises are generally performed in a repetitive fashion using large muscle groups. Some long-term benefits include decrease in resting heart rate, improved muscular strength, weight control, and increased return of venous and lymphatic fluids.

It is important to understand that certain aerobic exercises and recreational activities could trigger an increase in swelling or have higher risks of injury. Ideally, such high-risk activities (listed earlier under the section Decongestive Exercises) should be avoided or modified for patients affected by lymphedema.

Beneficial activities for upper and lower extremities

Beneficial activities for upper and lower extremity lymphedema include (but are not limited to):

Swimming or water aerobics: With the body weight reduced by approximately 90% in chest-deep water, exercises improve mobility, make movement more comfortable, and enhance strength and muscle tone. In addition, the hydrostatic pressure acts like a "full-body" compression garment and helps to reduce edema by contributing to lymphatic and venous return. Hot water (temperatures above 35 °C [94 °F]), usually found in hot tubs and Jacuzzis, must be avoided; high water temperature has a negative impact on lymphedema. Patients should be cautious with hot tubs and lakes during the summer (in warmer climates any time of the year) as they present an increased risk for various types of infections caused by bacteria. Range of motion and flexibility are increased when in a warm water pool and the cardiovascular system is working more effectively, so aerobic workout is possible.

Walking: A 20-minute walk outdoors or on a treadmill (10–15 minutes, slow walking speed), while wearing the compression garment, will stimulate the circulatory system and contribute to the individual's general well-being.

Easy biking: Easy biking for 20 to 25 minutes either outdoors or at the gym, using a comfortable and wide saddle. Legs are placed in a higher position on recumbent bikes, which makes them a better choice for individuals affected by lower extremity lymphedema.

Yoga: Several studies[7,8] indicate that yoga can have positive effects for those affected by lymphedema. Yoga can be easily adapted to the individual's particular health status, abilities, and limitations, and therefore may be preferable to more strenuous forms of exercise for some patients. In addition to increasing flexibility, muscle strength, and range of motion, yoga beneficially impacts breathing and increases venous and lymphatic circulation, both important aspects in the management of lymphedema. Some forms of yoga are fast-paced and intense, others are gentle and relaxing; techniques like "Hatha" and "Iyengar" yoga are gentle and slow, "Bikram," "Hot," and "Power" yoga are faster. The gentler forms of yoga combined with breathing exercises are preferable; challenging techniques should be avoided by those affected by lymphedema. More advanced poses, and most of the inverted poses, should be avoided as well—including headstand (too much weight on the arms and neck), shoulder stand (too much weight and pressure on the neck and shoulders), and downward facing dog (too much weight on the arms). Many cancer centers and support groups provide contacts for yoga classes specifically tailored to cancer survivors and lymphedema patients.

Lebed Method: This exercise and movement program is designed for people with lymphedema and cancer survivors. The program incorporates music and dance to focus on overall wellness, range of motion, balance, strength, and endurance.

There is no real consensus on the type of exercise regimen that can be incorporated into the patient's self-management regimen. Research suggests that a program of progressive exercises, i.e., starting with gentle exercises and increasing intensity moderately over time, tailored to each patient's needs and abilities, is not likely to increase the risk of lymphedema.

Although research has shown that strenuous exercises can be undertaken by those individuals at risk of, or already having, lymphedema without negative effects, it is advisable to start the exercise regimen slowly, which avoids the risk of increased swelling, strains, and injury to muscles, and allows the individual to observe how the edematous extremity responds to exercise.

In some cases, it is not an easy task to draft a list of exercises that should be avoided in individuals with lymphedema. Many patients find it important to continue their prelymphedema activities, even if these activities are considered high-risk for lymphedema. However, for many individuals engaging in these activities, the exercise plays such a vital role in their daily routine, and is so ingrained in their personality, that giving up these high-risk activities could have a serious impact on their well-being.

Nobody knows better than the lymphedema patient what is good for her or his body and spirit. As long as the patients are careful and under the care of a trained lymphedema therapist or health care professional with experience in lymphedema, wear their compression garment during physical activities, and the exercise regimen does not cause discomfort or pain, continuing with these activities should not have any negative impact. However, if the affected limb hurts, feels strained, or increases in volume during and after the activity, the patient should adjust as necessary and consult with the treating lymphedema therapist or physician. The key here is caution and moderation; gradual progression is imperative while trying to accomplish an improved return of lymphatic fluid without adding further stress to an impaired lymphatic system.

Skin and Nail Care

Before compression bandages are applied, appropriate moisturizers or lotions are used to cover the affected body part. During the intensive phase of CDT, patients are continuously instructed by the therapist on proper cleansing and moisturizing techniques to maintain the health and integrity of the skin and to prevent infections. This educational process includes how to inspect the skin for any wounds or signs of infection or inflammation. Patients affected by lymphedema are susceptible to infections of the skin and nails. Meticulous care of these areas is essential to the success of CDT. Skin is usually impermeable to bacteria and other pathogens, but any defect in the skin, whether from trauma, heat, or other causes, can present an entry site for pathogens or infectious agents. Lymphedematous skin can also become thickened and scaly, increasing the risk of skin cracks and fissures.

The basic consideration in skin and nail care is therefore prevention and control of infection.

Suitable ointments or lotions formulated for sensitive skin, radiation dermatitis, and lymphedema should be applied prior to lymphedema bandaging while the patient is in the decongestive phase of CDT. After the limb is decongested and the patient wears compression garments, moisturizing ointments should be applied twice daily. Ointments, as well as soaps or other skin cleansers used in lymphedema management, should have good moisturizing qualities, contain no fragrances, be hypoallergenic, and be formulated to be in either the neutral or acidic range of the pH scale (around pH 5.0).

Tight-fitting compression sleeves or stockings, as well as materials used in compression bandaging, may cause skin irritation.

In mosquito-infested areas, it is necessary to apply insect repellents to the affected extremity (some moisturizers contain natural repellents) to avoid bites, which could cause infections.

6.3 The Two-Phase Approach in Lymphedema Management

The vast majority of lymphedema patients benefit from CDT, which is performed in two phases; in phase *1*, also known as the intensive or decongestive phase, CDT is administered on a daily basis until the limb is decongested. Once the end of phase one is reached, the patient progresses seamlessly into phase *2* of CDT, also known as the self-management or improvement phase, in which the patient assumes responsibility for managing, improving, and maintaining the results achieved in phase one.

6.3.1 Intensive Phase

It is imperative for the success of the therapy that treatments are given daily and that the patient is thoroughly informed about all components of CDT before treatment is initiated. Patient's adherence to the treatment program and compliance are indispensable components to ensure treatment success.

The severity of the condition is a determining factor for the duration of the intensive phase, which averages 2 to 3 weeks for patients with upper extremity lymphedema and 2 to 4 weeks for patients with lymphedema of the leg. In extreme cases the decongestive phase may last up to 6 to 8 weeks and may have to be repeated several times. Depending on the stage of lymphedema, the involved extremity or body part may have reached a normal size at the end of the intensive phase, or there may still be a circumferential difference between the involved and the uninvolved limb. If treatment is initiated in the early stage of lymphedema, which is characterized by a soft tissue consistency without any fibrotic alterations, limb reduction can be expected to a normal size (compared with the uninvolved limb). If intervention starts in the later stages of lymphedema, in which lymphostatic fibrosis in the subcutaneous tissues has developed, the edematous fluid will recede, and fibrotic areas may soften. However, in most cases the indurated tissue will not completely regress during the intensive phase of CDT. Reduction in fibrotic tissue is a slow process, which can take several months or longer, and is achieved mainly in the second phase of CDT.

MLD in the first phase of therapy is applied at least once a day, 5 days a week. The MLD portion of the treatment generally requires 30 to 60 minutes; the duration of individual treatments is contingent on the number of involved limbs and body parts, as well as on the severity of the symptoms.

The most important aspect of MLD in the intensive phase is to identify drainage areas with sufficient and healthy lymphatics. Lymphatic pathways (lymphatic capillaries, precollectors, and collectors) as well as lymph nodes are then used to reroute the accumulated protein-rich lymphatic fluid around blocked or damaged areas from the swollen extremity or body part to areas with sufficient lymphatic drainage, and then back to the venous system.

How to practically treat an extremity with lymphedema

The basic procedural pattern of treatment in the example of a unilateral, secondary, upper extremity lymphedema.

Swelling in upper extremity lymphedema in many cases involves the ipsilateral truncal quadrant. Healthy lymphatics are generally found in adjacent truncal lymphatic territories (e.g., the contralateral upper quadrant and the ipsilateral lower quadrant) as well as in the lymphatic vessels and lymph nodes in the supraclavicular area of the same side. To maximize the therapeutic effect of MLD, the method of procedure can be broken down into the following steps:

Manipulation of lymph nodes and collectors located in the healthy adjacent quadrants as well as in the supraclavicular area on the ipsilateral side will increase lymphangiomotoricity and result in a "suction effect" on the protein-rich lymphatic fluid in the congested area. Following this initial preparation, the congested body quadrant is included in the treatment. The protein-rich lymphatic fluid located in this area is carefully moved toward the previously manipulated adjacent truncal quadrants, using primarily superficial lymphatic capillaries (initial lymphatic vessel plexus) and lymphatic collectors, which connect adjacent truncal quadrants (lymphatic anastomoses). Even though MLD is not directly applied to the swollen extremity during this period of the treatment, a volume reduction occurs, which can be noted in a decrease of circumferential measurements in the affected extremity. This volume reduction is generally observed following a series of two to four treatments.

When the extremity starts to decongest, the initial preparation is reduced to the relevant lymph nodes (in this case, axillary lymph nodes on the contralateral side and inguinal lymph nodes on the ipsilateral side) and anastomoses. The treatment area is now expanded to include the affected extremity on a step-by-step basis. To avoid overload of the healthy lymphatics in the drainage areas, it is suggested to initially include only the upper arm in the treatment protocol. In severe cases of lymphedema, it may be necessary to treat only parts of the upper arm. In the following treatments, the forearm then the hand and fingers are carefully included.

Patients should be instructed early in the course of treatment how to perform simple self-MLD techniques, which are used to stimulate lymphatic drainage during the weekends in the intensive phase as well as in the self-management phase.

Compression therapy during the intensive phase of the treatment is provided using short-stretch bandages in combination with appropriate padding materials as described earlier in this chapter.

Depending on the number of bandages and padding materials used, it may take experienced lymphedema therapists 10 to 20 minutes (in extreme cases, even longer) to apply a compression bandage.

An important aspect in this stage of the treatment is to instruct the patient, and preferably a family member or care giver, in self-bandaging techniques. This requires a lot of practice, which makes it necessary to initiate the patient instruction early in the intensive phase.

The end of the first phase of treatment is determined by the results of circumferential or volumetric measurements of the affected extremity. When the measurements approach a plateau, the end of the intensive phase is reached, and the patient progresses seamlessly into phase two of CDT.

6.3.2 Self-Management Phase

Self-management is an essential part of lymphedema treatment and specially defined in the self-management phase. Adherence to the self-care regimen designed for each individual patient is crucial to maintaining treatment results and preventing the progression of lymphedema. It is important to understand that the symptoms associated with lymphedema may have a negative psychological and psychosocial impact on some patients affected by this condition, which may create barriers to the compliance in the self-management phase of lymphedema treatment.

Many patients report that changes in body weight and climate can cause their symptoms to fluctuate. Female patients commonly report that the swelling tends to increase during the menstrual cycle. Usually, these situations can be remedied by following the self-management protocol more closely.

For those patients unable to maintain decongestion, or who experience an increase in swelling during the second phase of CDT, it is necessary to follow up with additional treatment sessions in the clinic.

The components in the self-management phase are similar to those in the intensive phase.

MLD: Simple and easy-to-perform MLD techniques are an integral part of the self-management program. In this stage, the patient has completed the intensive phase, practiced self-MLD techniques with the lymphedema therapist, and is familiar with the pressures and techniques used in MLD (see also the section on Patient Education in the following).

Compression therapy in this phase of the treatment is administered by compression garments, which are worn during the daytime hours. Measurements for compression garments are taken at the end of the intensive phase when the maximum level of decongestion is achieved. The condition of the compression garment is evaluated during regular check-ups (at least every 6 months), and the patient's measurements are taken again to ensure proper fit. Compression garments should be replaced every 6 months or sooner if the material is damaged or has lost its elasticity. Patients should have at least two sets of compression garments, one to wear and one to wash. The severity and chronicity of the symptoms determine whether a lymphedema patient should continue to apply compression bandages during the night in this phase.

In order to maintain adequate compression, bandages may be applied on top of the compression garment during times of increased swelling or activities that may trigger the onset of swelling (airplane travel, standing for long periods of time, high-risk activities).

6.3.3 Patient Education

The early involvement of the patient and family, or a professional caregiver, is of greatest importance and should begin on the first visit.

Providing patients with appropriate information and education facilitates long-term success of lymphedema management. Sufficient knowledge of the patient regarding his or her condition is the key to compliance. Patients need to know what caused the onset of their lymphedema to fully understand why self-management is a necessary component of CDT. Patients should be informed about the possible consequences if self-care for lymphedema is neglected. Knowledge about the risks involved in certain activities (air travel, extremes in temperature, etc.) helps to avoid the recurrence of symptoms.

At the end of the intensive phase, the patient should have the necessary skills to perform self-bandaging and self-MLD techniques safely and effectively and to execute a customized program of decongestive exercises.

Elements of patient education should include skin care, *self-MLD, self-bandaging, exercises, and precautions regarding extreme temperature, clothing and jewelry, exercises, and travel.*

6.4 Limitations of Complete Decongestive Therapy in Lymphedema Management

Unsatisfactory results, delayed progress during the intensive phase, or re-accumulation of fluid in the self-management phase of the treatment may be caused by insufficient patient compliance or improper treatment techniques. Nevertheless, even when CDT lymphedema management is optimal, unsatisfactory results or progress cannot be excluded and should be an indication to multiprofessional evaluation for modern surgical management of lymphedema.

Treatment is prone to failure if CDT is applied only in part (MLD as the only form of intervention, no MLD, or improper bandaging), intermittent pneumatic compression (IPC) devices are used inappropriately, or the therapist is poorly trained. The severity of the symptoms, such as progressive lymphostatic fibrosis, scarring, or infections, may also have an impact on the treatment progress; the results in these cases are generally less dramatic and take a longer time to establish.

Certain forms of lymphedema or associated pathologies may slow treatment progress as well; some examples are as follows:

- *Malignant lymphedema*: Malignant lymphedema by definition involves proximal tumor masses which physically obstruct the outflow of lymph and venous blood, affect arterial inflow, and compromise nerve structures, eliciting intense pain, numbness, or limb paralysis.
  Another complication that may present in long-standing lymphedema is the development of a vascular tumor (lymphangiosarcoma). These tumors most commonly occur in individuals who have developed chronic lymphedema following mastectomy (Stewart-Treves

syndrome)[21]; however, tumors have also been reported in individuals with chronic lymphedema of unknown etiology. These tumors are most commonly fatal. Breast cancer is one of the most common malignancies that spread to the skin. Skin metastases most often occur near the breast area, on the trunk or near the line of surgical incision, and commonly present as hardened or rubbery, light pink-red nodules with a surrounding lighter area accompanied by patchy erythema. These nodules may have the appearance of a pimple initially and are usually the size of a grain of rice; these lesions often progress to ulcers and may become infected and painful. Depending upon the disease, an adapted CDT approach will eventually follow a palliative care model. However, if energy is still high, and pain levels are managed, activities of daily living may be greatly enriching to the patient. As such, a minimal adjustment in the treatment approach may be very productive for some time, generating great relief from discomfort. It should be noted that MLD employed as a pain management modality is quite beneficial and has proven very productive as a complementary tool with no adverse effects. Even when the general health condition becomes grave, patients remain highly receptive to MLD above all other therapies. For this reason, MLD should be offered frequently for as long as possible and will be prized by the patient and family as a valuable extension of compassion during hospice care.

- *Pediatric lymphedema:* Whether pediatric cases have primary (Meige's disease, Milroy's disease, distichiasis syndrome) or secondary causes, the conventional approach to treatment must be considerably modified for the pediatric patient. Early education of the parent regarding the condition itself and child- or age-appropriate treatment adaptations are essential components in this process. The parents or caregivers play a crucial role in the therapy and become a direct extension of the therapist, and ideally continue to perform treatment elements at home. Special pediatric precautions and modifications in terms of duration of individual treatment sessions, and intensity of MLD techniques and compression therapy must be observed and conveyed to the parents so that CDT can commence at a low level of intensity yet provide valuable therapeutic benefits.
  The main limitations of CDT in the pediatric patient are the restrictions in intensity of the therapy and therefore less tangible treatment results initially. Compression is a very powerful tool that produces immediately measurable and visually apparent results. Although parents may be asked to refrain from compression until the child can tolerate this modality safely, they should know that more tools will become available when the child is 1 year old in most cases. It is therefore important for therapists to convey the plan of care as continually developing.
- *Lipo-lymphedema:* Lipedema is characterized by symmetric enlargement of the limbs, generally affecting the lower extremities, extending from the hips to the ankles secondary to the deposition of fat; upper extremities are affected in 30% of the cases. Lipedema is not rare and not caused by a disorder of the lymphatic system, but is commonly misdiagnosed as bilateral lymphedema, extreme cellulitis, or morbid obesity. This condition almost exclusively affects women. According to an epidemiologic study,[9] lipedema affects 11% of the female population, and literature suggests that lipedema is associated with extensive hormonal disorders or liver dysfunctions if present in males. Lipedema is a painful fat disorder and if left untreated can cause multiple secondary health problems, including mobility issues and lymphedema.
  The excessive amount of fatty tissue present in lipedema compresses the lymphatic collectors of the superficial lymphatic system, which are embedded in the fatty subcutaneous tissue. Lymphangiographic imaging shows that the lymphatic collectors within the proliferated fatty tissue have a coiled or corkscrew-like appearance rather than passing fairly straight toward the lymph nodes as is the case in healthy tissue. This can result in a reduced transport capacity of the lymphatic system in the affected area. If the capacity of the lymphatic system is reduced to such an extent that it becomes unable to perform one of its basic functions, which is the removal of water from the tissues, fluid will accumulate and edema develops in addition to lipedema.
  In the initial stages, the swelling may recede with elevation and rest, but over time and without adequate treatment (compression, elevation, and exercise), the constant strain on the lymphatic system may cause damage to the lymphatic vessels, leading to further reduction of its transport capacity, and swelling may be constantly present.
  As a result of prolonged overstrain of the lymphatic system, lymphedema may develop secondary to lipedema (lipo-lymphedema), thereby increasing the complexity of treatment.
  If lipo-lymphedema is associated with obesity, nutritional guidance must be provided to reduce the weight and avoid further weight gain.
  After the decongestion of the lymphedematous component in lipo-lymphedema during the intensive phase of CDT, the patient should be fitted with a compression garment, which in the majority of cases needs to be custom-made. The preferred garment is a pantyhose type of a higher compression class.
  CDT shows good long-term results in lipo-lymphedema; however, affected individuals need to understand that although the lymphedematous component responds well and generally relatively fast to CDT, the lipedema itself, i.e., the reduction of fatty tissue, responds more slowly, and sometimes not at all. Nevertheless, the

domain of successfully treating lipedema with long-lasting stable results is lipectomy, which is the main armamentarium in the modern treatment of lipedema.[25]

- *Obesity:* Excessive weight and obesity may contribute to the onset of primary and secondary lymphedema, worsen existing symptoms associated with lymphedema, and add to the complexity of CDT applications.
  Excessive weight, especially morbid obesity, can have a negative impact on the return of lymphatic fluid from the legs; additional fluid volumes associated with obesity may overwhelm an already impaired lymphatic system. Direct pressure on lymphatic vessels by excess fatty tissue, impaired diaphragmatic breathing, and decreased mobility and muscular function can also be factors contributing to the manifestation of lymphedema and impairing treatment results. Progressive venous insufficiency is commonly caused by obesity and can result in combined insufficiency characterized by phlebo-lymphedema.[10] Treatment progress in existing lymphedema may be seriously hampered in patients with a high body mass index (BMI). In patients with obesity it is often difficult to apply bandages, especially in cases of lymphedema affecting the lower extremities. Furthermore, the compressive materials (bandages, garments) applied to the affected extremities tend to slide in cases of obesity. Excessive fatty lobules may be present resulting in very irregular limb shapes, which creates a challenge to the creation of a sufficient pressure gradient when applying compression bandages. Other treatment challenges may be caused by deep skin folds, which are frequently present in the obese population. Skin folds can harbor anaerobic and/or fungal infections, which necessitates an increased focus on appropriate skin care. Compression garments may have to be custom-made, creating an additional financial burden to the patient.
- *Limb paralysis:* Lymphedema patients with extensive underlying trauma due to accidental injury, cancer therapy, or other disease processes may present with functionless, insensate, and dependent edematous limbs. Although these patients are suitable candidates for CDT, it is necessary to adjust compression therapy protocols according to the individuals' limitations. The mechanical nature of compression therapy will place them at considerable risk of additional injury if not employed with a high degree of care and skill.

Tissue atrophy, increased skin fragility, and lack of sensory feedback are risk factors that may be a causal factor for compression-related wounds. Ample padding around bony prominences and lower bandaging pressures are imperative to avoid injury (▶ Fig. 6.20 and ▶ Fig. 6.21). The skin should be inspected thoroughly on a daily basis to identify erythema caused by excessive pressure and possible skin lesions. The impact of compression bandages on limb weight and the patient's mobility should be carefully assessed. Compression garments in the self-management phase should be of a low compression class.

6.5 Additional Treatment Modalities

CDT is the therapy of choice for the vast majority of patients affected by primary and secondary lymphedemas. In addition to CDT, there are a number of treatment approaches that may be used to supplement CDT.

6.5.1 Sequential Intermittent Pneumatic Compression

The use of IPC devices in the treatment of lymphedema continues to be a topic of discussion, and their use is neither accepted as a replacement nor as a component of CDT under the accepted international gold standard of lymphedema treatment. However, recent studies suggest that there is a potential place for newer generation IPCs that may be used as a beneficial adjunct treatment to effectively control lymphedema. Following discharge from

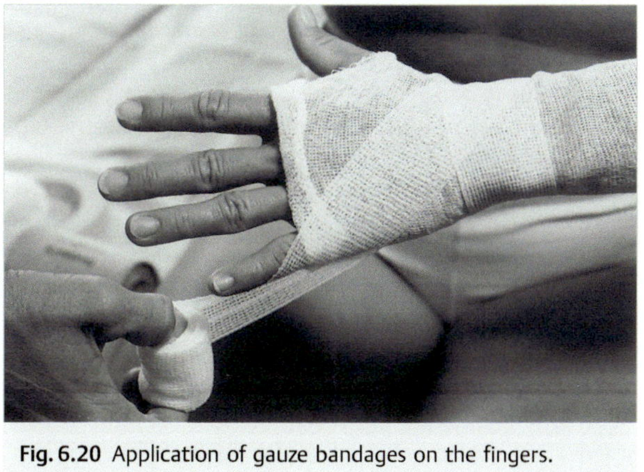

Fig. 6.20 Application of gauze bandages on the fingers.

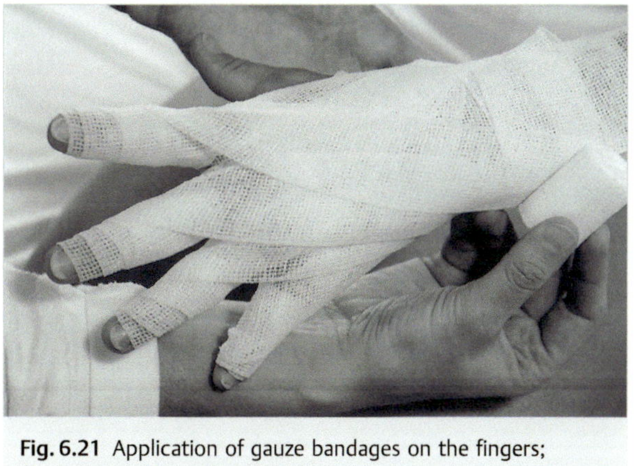

Fig. 6.21 Application of gauze bandages on the fingers; fingertips remain unbandaged.

the intensive phase of CDT, patients are instructed by the therapist to maintain the results with compression bandages and garments, self-MLD, and decongestive exercise protocols; these conservative therapy modalities are effective for most, but may not be sufficient for some individuals. An appropriate pneumatic compression device may offer an effective option to control this condition on a more ideal level for this group of patients.

An IPC device is composed of an inflatable garment consisting of multiple pressure compartments that wrap around the arm or leg and an electrical pneumatic pump, which fills the garment with compressed air. The garment is intermittently inflated and deflated in cycles whose times and pressures vary between devices.

Multichambered, segmented IPCs represent the newer generation compression devices and are equipped with multiple outflow ports on the pneumatic pump leading to distinct segments of the garment that inflate sequentially from the distal to the proximal part of the extremity until all segments are inflated. Following this phase, all compartments deflate at the same time (▶ Fig. 6.22). To maintain control of the swelling, it is necessary that compression garments and/or short-stretch compression bandages are worn between treatments with sequential pneumatic compression devices.

Two groups of multichambered IPCs can be distinguished—those without or with limited manual control and noncalibrated pressure, and devices equipped with programmable options and calibrated pressure.

Consensus on the proper pressure level and treatment frequency of IPCs for the treatment of lymphedema is nonexistent. As a general rule, the pressure level should be adjusted to the patient's level of tolerance and response to treatment. Careful instruction of the patient in the use of IPCs and surveillance by a practitioner trained to a specialist level in these devices are required. A review of the literature suggests that peak inflation pressure of 25 to 60 mmHg may be sufficient for most patients.[11] Depending on the individual situation, treatment duration of 30 minutes to 2 hours (1 hour twice a day) is generally recommended. Careful guidance by a practitioner with knowledge in lymphedema treatment is mandatory to determine optimal treatment frequency.

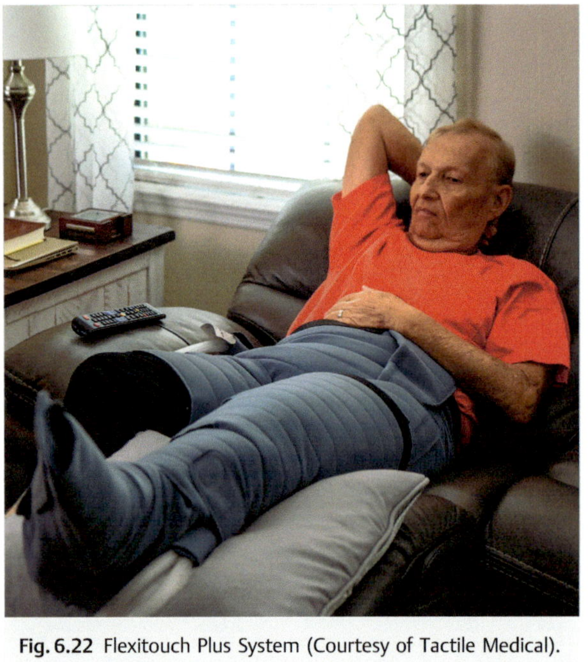

Fig. 6.22 Flexitouch Plus System (Courtesy of Tactile Medical).

Contraindications for Intermittent Pneumatic Compressions

The use of IPC devices is not advisable in the presence of the following conditions[12]: Nonpitting chronic lymphedema; known or suspected deep vein thrombosis; pulmonary embolism; pulmonary edema; thrombophlebitis; acute inflammation of the skin (erysipelas, cellulitis); uncontrolled/severe cardiac failure; ischemic vascular disease; active metastatic diseases affecting the edematous region; edema at the root of the extremity or trunkal edema; severe peripheral neuropathy.

6.5.2 Elastic Taping

Elastic taping is mostly known as a form of treatment for pain management and disabilities resulting from athletic injuries and other physical disorders. In recent years, this form of therapy also gained popularity as an emerging adjunct treatment modality for lymphedema. Although evidence of the efficacy of taping in lymphedema is currently lacking, the evolution of special taping techniques in the recent past has demonstrated positive anecdotal clinical outcomes of this modality in the treatment of lymphedema.

Based on the original technique, which was developed in the 1970s, a number of other taping variations have evolved, and different taping products were developed by various manufacturers. The tape is held in place by a hypo-allergenic and latex-free medical-grade acrylic adhesive, which is heat activated. Perforated with numerous holes the tape allows air to circulate, and while the tape's cotton fabric will absorb water, the acrylic adhesive next to the skin is waterproof, which enables the patient to shower and swim with the material in place. Elastic tape is available in rolls of various widths or pre-cut shapes; the length and pattern of the application depend on the individual pathology and drainage pathways and take into consideration additional barriers such as scars and other defects on the skin.

Present-day opinion among researchers and practitioners supports the utilization of elastic taping as an adjunct to CDT whenever possible to enhance current treatment standards; however, the use of taping as a stand-alone treatment or as replacement for any component of CDT is not advocated.

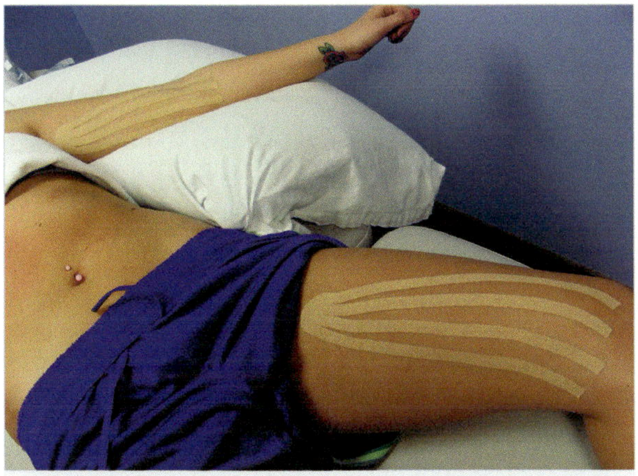

Fig. 6.23 General application of elastic taping for upper and lower extremity bundles Taping toward the involved lymph nodes may be utilized in general edema techniques or primary lymphedema. Taping toward involved lymph nodes would be avoided and a rerouting technique utilized in treatment planning for secondary lymphedema. (Courtesy of Nicolle Samuels.)

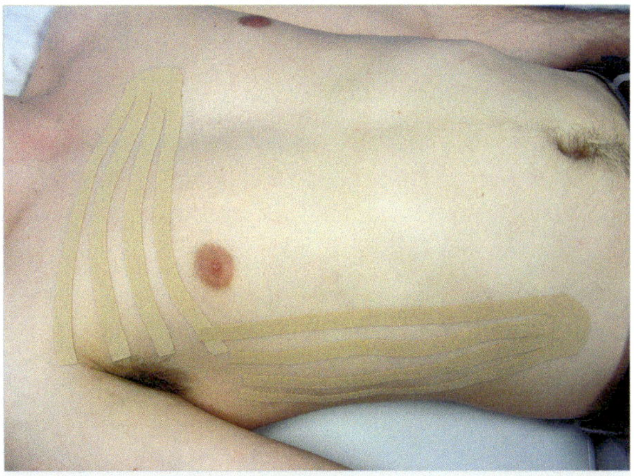

Fig. 6.24 Anastomosis technique: Taping of interterritorial anastomoses is applied with the base of the tape in the healthy quadrant crossing the watershed along the appropriate anastomoses The tails of the tape follow in the congested quadrant with resultant flow across the anastomosis into an area of normal lymphatics. (Courtesy of Nicolle Samuels.)

In the presence of contraindications or complications to MLD, elastic taping can be utilized as a viable alternative.[13] The method is particularly useful in areas affected by lymphedema where bandaging is difficult, or not possible, such as lymphedema affecting the head and neck.

The application of elastic taping in the management of lymphedema is primarily used to support uptake of tissue fluid into the lymphatic capillaries and to improve, and if necessary redirect, the flow of lymphatic fluid.

The tape generates a gentle lift on the skin, which allows the lymphatic vessels underneath to absorb and drain lymphatic fluid from the edematous area into an area with sufficient lymphatic drainage, thus reducing the volume of the edematous area.

The tape is applied to the skin with slight stretch (just to the tension required to remove the backing) and with the patient's skin in a stretched position. Once the skin returns to the resting position, the tape rebounds, and if applied correctly, rippling convolutions in the tape will become visible. This desired effect deforms the skin and slightly lifts it from the fascia below in order to create a pull force on the filaments anchoring the small lymphatic capillary vessels within the tissues. The pull force of the tape creates openings in the wall of these vessels, which allows more fluid to enter the lymphatic system and subsequently increase lymphatic flow away from the swollen area. By positioning the tape correctly, it is possible to facilitate and channel the lymphatic fluid in the desired direction without restricting muscle and joint movements.

Additional stimulation of the lymphatic system is achieved as the patient performs movements in daily activities, or performs decongestive exercises as instructed by the clinician. The tape can be worn for several days as long as there are no negative reactions on the skin.

Local contraindications, such as adverse reactions to the tape, radiation fibrosis, wounds, lymphatic cysts, and fistulas, as well as the risk of damaging the fragile skin of lymphedema patients are concerns to be considered when using elastic taping. Elastic taping should not be applied on fresh scars and incision sites.

Elastic taping in the management of lymphedema can be applied either in a way that closely follows the lymphatic anatomy, in which the tape is applied in the uncongested drainage area with the end of the tape trailing and covering the congested treatment area (▶ Fig. 6.23), or in a spiraling/crisscrossing method. The goal of the second method is to cover large areas of skin surface to maximize activation of the initial lymphatic plexus (▶ Fig. 6.24). When utilizing the initial lymph plexus, the tape may be placed in any direction toward the uncongested drainage area.

The therapist instructs the patient to properly remove the tape after several days. The adhesive bond of the tape is best broken by holding up an edge of the tape and gently pushing down the skin to dislodge it from the adhesive. The use of oil helps to neutralize the adhesive, and removal of the tape in the direction of the body hair minimizes the risk of skin irritation.

6.6 Documentation and Screening Modalities for Conservative Lymphedema Management

Researchers and clinicians have used multiple methods of screening for lymphedema and evaluation of limb volume,[14] and opinions vary regarding the most effective and accurate measurement technique (see **Subchapter 4.4**).

For both conservative treatment and modern surgical management of lymphedema, it is necessary to include diagnostic tools and scores to screen patients and evaluate subjective and functional limitations including the quality of life at the beginning of a treatment episode and during every consultation.

6.7 Role of Weight Management, Nutrition, and Supplements

There is a common misconception among patients that lymphedema may be positively affected by limiting protein intake. Although lymphedema is defined as an accumulation of water and protein in the tissues, it is essential to clarify and convey to the patient that lymphedema cannot be reduced by the limitation of protein ingestion.

A special diet for lymphedema does not exist; an accepted nutritional approach in the management of lymphedema is to follow a nutrition-balanced and portion-appropriate diet, which in addition to physical activity and exercises positively contributes to weight management. Patients should trust their own judgment regarding selection of a proper diet and make an effort to achieve and maintain a reasonable weight to reduce the risk factors associated with obesity, or they should consult with a certified nutritionist. If no other medical conditions are present, such as diabetes or heart disease, a healthy, balanced, and portion-appropriate diet should be the goal, which contributes to reducing the risk factors associated with lymphedema. A balanced healthy diet including whole grains, fish, fruits, and vegetables and avoiding fatty foods will greatly assist in achieving and maintaining a healthy weight without restricting the intake of important nutrients and vitamins. Crash diets or diets which restrict certain food groups and nutrients are not advisable. Studies[16,17] indicate that obesity and overweight negatively impact lymphatic fluid level and extremity volume.

It is also important not to limit fluid intake in an attempt to reduce the swelling. Good hydration is essential for basic cell function and is especially important before and after lymphedema treatment to assist the body in eliminating waste products.

There are no vitamins, food supplements, or herbs that have been proven to be effective in the reduction of lymphedema. In most countries there is no requirement to review dietary supplements for consistency among manufacturers, and specific standards for dosage or purity do not exist, possibly resulting in considerable variation within the products marketed as dietary supplements. However, lymphedema patients are often in need of additional vitamins and supplements, especially if they battle recurrent episodes of infections. To determine which supplements and vitamins are beneficial, individuals with lymphedema should consult with their physicians and/or nutritional specialist.

6.8 Outpatient versus Inpatient Treatment

Ideally, advanced cases of lymphedema (stages II and III) and malignant lymphedema should be treated as inpatient treatment and in rehabilitation centers specialized in the care of lymphedema for the first phase of lymphedema management[18]; inpatient treatment should also be considered for cases when previous outpatient treatments have failed.

Crucial clinical determinants for inpatient therapy should not be limited to classification of lymphedema on the basis of etiology and staging, but should also include the presence of wounds, recurrent episodes of infections, and certain comorbidities, which aggravate lymphedema, or add to the complexity of treatment. Crucial comorbidities include decompensated cardiac insufficiency, severe cardiac arrhythmia, chronic hypertension, diabetes, peripheral neuropathy, kidney and liver insufficiencies, and severe mobility impairments.

Inpatient treatment centers that are specialized in the care of lymphedema are currently limited to countries such as Australia, Germany, and Austria. Inpatient treatment centers are uniquely qualified to provide essential diagnostic procedures and tailored CDT treatment components (often provided twice daily), which may be necessary for patients with severe conditions and mobility impairments.

Lymphedema management in the United States and other countries is primarily administered in clinical outpatient settings. Early stage and uncomplicated cases of lymphedema can be successfully treated in the outpatient setting. Advanced cases that ideally require inpatient treatment can be treated if outpatient clinical settings and treatment programs are able to provide the intensity of therapy appropriate and necessary for the stage and severity of a patient's lymphedema, comorbidities, and functional limitations.[19,20]

6.9 Wound Management in Lymphedema Patients

Individuals affected by chronic lymphedema often present with a variety of skin changes, such as lymphatic cysts (▶ Fig. 6.25) and/or fistulas, fungal infections, or even open wounds and skin ulcers.

6.9.1 Types of Lymphedema-Related Wounds

Lymphatic cysts occur due to congestion and distension of lymphatic vessels, which are most commonly caused

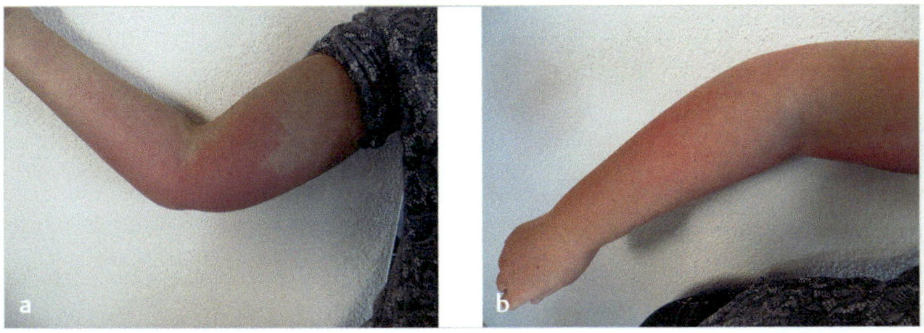

Fig. 6.25 Typical clinical manifestation of cellulitis ("erysipelas") of an upper extremity with secondary breast-cancer associated lymphedema: **(a)** medial view, **(b)** dorsal view. (Courtesy of Yves Harder.)

by congenital malformation; however, a local surgical interruption of lymphatic flow can also create sufficient collector hypertension and reflux to cause cyst formation. This is more commonly evident in areas where the skin is thin and extensible such as in the axillary and genital regions, or in the geriatric population. Depending upon the tissue structure related to the cyst (collector, capillary) a distinction can be made as to the level of congestion of surrounding tissues and the origin of the problem. If caused by primary malformation, cysts may be less correctable by decongestive therapy since the underlying cause may involve valvular insufficiency or hyperplasia of the deep lymphatic system. White cysts rather than clear cysts indicate chylous reflux from deep intestinal lymphatics or the thoracic duct itself. If chylous reflux is present, imaging studies should be considered to determine if a surgical solution is required. In some cases, clear or chylous fluid is seen weeping from the skin. Cysts are very fragile and likely to rupture when exposed to any mechanical stressors (bandages, garment, MLD, exercise). MLD techniques should not be applied in the area of lymphatic cysts (and fistulas), and a sterile, highly absorbent dressing should be applied over cysts prior to compression bandage application. Most cysts shrink or disappear once the involved region is thoroughly decongested.

The presence of lymphatic **fistulas** requires physician-directed infection prevention in addition to appropriate exudate dressing and compression. In patients with lymphedema, fistulas may be present in a variety of anatomical places, such as the genital and rectal regions, within irradiated tissue, and between arteries and veins as in complex vascular syndromes or in some cases of primary lymphedema. In cases where fistulas occur between lymphatic vessels and the skin surface, leakage of body fluids directly from these openings can create strong malodorous and infectious complications. If surgical repair can be performed, fistulas may be corrected or closed. However, when active disease such as cancer is causal, fistulas can remain persistent and untreatable. Activated charcoal pads as a palliative treatment perform well in controlling odor in these situations.

Fungal infections are commonly present in lymphedema. Although fungal infections may be acute, they are usually not regarded as strict contraindications to therapy unless the tissues are fragile or open. A normal plan of care would dictate that fungal infections be arrested prior to commencement of therapy to reduce the avoidable complication of spread to other skin regions. However, should CDT begin during an active fungal infection of lesser severity, the therapist should administer MLD proximal to the involved area, apply topical antifungal preparations (as prescribed by the treating physician), stockinette, and toe bandages with hands gloved, and discard all materials that are in contact with skin to avoid recontamination.

Open wounds associated with lymphedema may be caused by a dysfunctional vascular system or may be related to other comorbidities. They can result from trauma, allergies, surgery, or radiotherapy. These changes range from simple excoriations to complex wounds with multiple etiologies. Most common wound types associated with lymphedema include ulcerations caused by vascular dysfunction of the venous, arterial, or lymphatic system, or a combination thereof. Vascular ulcerations are most observed in the lower extremities and are associated with long-term vascular compromise. Research indicates that over 70% of these ulcerations have a venous etiology[22]; the incidence of venous ulcerations is higher in women (62%).

In comparison, skin lesions due to arterial insufficiency account for 10% to 30% of lower extremity ulcers, with as many as 15% of these lesions having both an arterial and venous component. Lesions solely caused by lymphedema are poorly discussed in the literature. Other less commonly diagnosed vascular ulcers include those with an underlying genetic or inflammatory etiology.

The key to successful treatment of wounds that result from the chronic accumulation of interstitial fluids, such as that observed with venous insufficiency or lymphedema, is reduction or clearance of the swollen tissues. MLD, along with the application of short-stretch bandaging for initial reduction of chronic fluid accumulation, followed by maintenance therapy with a compression garment, is necessary for clinical success. However, vascular status should be determined prior to any addition of compression therapy, so that ischemic limbs are not treated inadvertently. Enzymatic preparations may also assist with necrotic tissue reduction and improve wound healing. Newer antiseptic technologies that use slow-release iodine or silver preparations will help control the wound bioburden, thus reducing malodor and enhancing wound closure. Charcoal-based dressings may also be applied over a primary dressing to assist with odor control. Exercises that stimulate the calf muscle pump also accelerate the reduction of tissue edema and enhance wound healing.

6.9.2 Modification of Lymphedema Bandaging in the Presence of Wounds

There is a common consensus among wound care clinicians that the successful management of the swelling is crucial to healing, particularly in the case of lymphedema. Wounds and edema are routinely treated separately among providers in the health care industry. However, there are a number of benefits to treating both conditions simultaneously, and a dedicated multidisciplinary approach to wound care and lymphedema will greatly support successful outcomes and provide economical delivery of care for these patients and medical facilities providing their care. A simultaneous treatment approach can lead to better treatment outcomes and eliminate the need for patients to spend hours in the wound clinic for weeks or months only to be referred to a lymphedema specialist to spend additional time managing the swelling. Wound care clinicians are aware of adequate compression for edema, but typically are not trained in the application of specific compression bandages that effectively manage the swelling associated with lymphedema; on the other hand, a lymphedema therapist generally has little experience in wound dressing or the application of compression over wounds.

With CDT as part of the wound treatment regimen, all components should be included. MLD applied proximal to the wound does not require modification; MLD is not applied directly to the wound, and techniques on the wound perimeter are adapted.

Following proper wound dressing and exudate management, the lymphedema bandage is applied directly over the completed wound dressing as part of the second phase of wound treatment. However, a common challenge arising with many wound patients is that the shape of the limb may not allow for an effective and safe compression gradient when using the basic lymphedema bandage due to the frequent presence of pathologies in addition to lymphedema. This issue can be addressed with the application of strategically placed foam padding to artificially change the shape of the extremity and thereby achieving a cone shape. As the shape of the limb is changes over the course of treatment by appropriately applied short-stretch compression, it is likely the limb will become gradually more cone-shaped and the clinician will need to change the bandage approach so that it is more in line with the standard lymphedema bandage.[23]

References

[1] Granzow JW, Soderberg JM, Kaji AH, Dauphine C. An effective system of surgical treatment of lymphedema. Ann Surg Oncol. 2014; 21(4): 1189–1194

[2] Granzow JW, Soderberg JM, Dauphine C. A novel two-stage surgical approach to treat chronic lymphedema. Breast J. 2014; 20(4):420–422

[3] Zuther JE, Norton S. Lymphedema Management: The Comprehensive Guide for Practitioners. 4th ed. Thieme Publishers Germany; 2017

[4] Thomas S. The production and measurement of sub-bandage pressure: Laplace's Law revisited. J Wound Care. 2014; 23(5):234–236, 238–241, 244 passim

[5] Lane K, Worsley D, McKenzie D. Exercise and the lymphatic system: implications for breast-cancer survivors. Sports Med. 2005; 35(6): 461–471

[6] Cheema BS, Kilbreath SL, Fahey PP, Delaney GP, Atlantis E. Safety and efficacy of progressive resistance training in breast cancer: a systematic review and meta-analysis. Breast Cancer Res Treat. 2014; 148(2):249–268

[7] Moadel AB, Shah C, Wylie-Rosett J, et al. Randomized controlled trial of yoga among a multiethnic sample of breast cancer patients: effects on quality of life. J Clin Oncol. 2007; 25(28):4387–4395

[8] Bower JE, Woolery A, Sternlieb B, Garet D. Yoga for cancer patients and survivors. Cancer Contr. 2005; 12(3):165–171

[9] Földi E, Földi M. Lipedema. In: Földi M, Földi E, eds. Földi's Textbook of Lymphology. Munich, Germany: Elsevier GmbH; 2006:417–427

[10] Davies HO, Popplewell M, Singhal R, Smith N, Bradbury AW. Obesity and lower limb venous disease—the epidemic of phlebesity. Phlebology. 2017; 32(4):227–233

[11] Feldman JL, Stout NL, Wanchai A, Stewart BR, Cormier JN, Armer JM. Intermittent pneumatic compression therapy: a systematic review. Lymphology. 2012; 45(1):13–25

[12] International Best Practice Guideline for Lymphedema. Available at http://www.woundsinternational.com/media/issues/210/files/content_175.pdf (page 35)

[13] Bosman J. Lymphtaping for lymphoedema: an overview of the treatment and its uses. Br J Community Nurs. 2014 Suppl:S12–, S14, S16–S18

[14] Yahathugoda C, Weiler MJ, Rao R, et al. Use of a novel portable three-dimensional imaging system to measure limb volume and circumference in patients with filarial lymphedema. Am J Trop Med Hyg. 2017; 97(6):1836–1842

[15] Stout NL, Pfalzer LA, Springer B, et al. Breast cancer-related lymphedema: comparing direct costs of a prospective surveillance model and a traditional model of care. Phys Ther. 2012; 92(1):152–163

[16] Fu MR, Axelrod D, Guth AA, et al. Patterns of obesity and lymph fluid level during the first year of breast cancer treatment: a prospective study. J Pers Med. 2015; 5(3):326–340

[17] Helyer LK, Varnic M, Le LW, Leong W, McCready D. Obesity is a risk factor for developing postoperative lymphedema in breast cancer patients. Breast J. 2010; 16(1):48–54

[18] Földi M, Földi E, eds. Textbook of Lymphology: For Physicians and Lymphedema Therapists. Urban and Fischer; 2006

[19] Leard T, Barrett C. Successful management of severe unilateral lower extremity lymphedema in an outpatient setting. Phys Ther. 2015; 95 (9):1295–1306

[20] Pereira de Godoy JM, Azoubel LM, de Fátima Guerreiro de Godoy M. Intensive treatment of leg lymphedema. Indian J Dermatol. 2010; 55 (2):144–147

[21] Berebichez-Fridman R, Deutsch YE, Joyal TM, et al. Stewart-Treves syndrome: a case report and review of the literature. Case Rep Oncol. 2016; 9(1):205–211

[22] Spentzouris G, Labropoulos N. The evaluation of lower-extremity ulcers. Semin Intervent Radiol. 2009; 26(4):286–295

[23] European Wound Management Association (EWMA). Focus Document: Lymphedema Bandaging in Practice. London: MEP Ltd; 2005

Section V

Surgical Treatment and Techniques

Edited by Yves Harder

V

7 Basic Principles of Surgical Treatment and Accompanying Complete Decongestive Therapy

Summary

The surgical treatment of lymphedema is a constantly evolving field. Detailed patient history and clinical examination are important to assess the clinical stage of lymphedema, but imaging diagnostic techniques play an essential role in assessing the structural and functional characteristics of the lymphatic system and oedematous tissue for planning the most effective therapeutic approach. To date, there is no standardized international consensus on surgical management of lymphedema; however, the basic principles for planning the most adequate surgical strategy are based on the presence of functioning lymphatic vessels and the degree of adipose hypertrophy and fibrosis of the subcutaneous tissue. Currently, the three most common procedures for surgical treatment of lymphedema are: lymphovenous anastomosis, vascularized lymph node transfer, and suction-assisted lipectomy. In general, the surgical strategy must always be personalized, adapted for each patient based on the degree of the lymphatic system insufficiency and medical situation, and may involve a combination of techniques. The most recent trend is preventive lymphedema surgery in patients undergoing breast cancer treatment by immediate restitution of lymphatic drainage after sentinel lymph node biopsy or axillary lymph node dissection.

Keywords: autologous lymph vessel transfer (ALVT), Complete decongestive therapy (CDT), dermolipectomy, lymphovenous anastomosis (LVA), manual lymph drainage (MLD), nodevenal shunt, reconstructive procedures, reductive procedures, suction-assisted lipectomy, vascularized lymph node transfer (VLNT)

7.1 Lymphatic Surgery

Jaume Masia and Cristhian D. Pomata

7.1.1 Introduction

Lymphedema treatment is a complex and constantly evolving field that involves a wide variety of therapeutical approaches. Conservative therapy is usually the first approach and one of the pillars of lymphedema treatment (see **Chapter 6** and **Subchapter 7.3**). Complete decongestive therapy (CDT) aims to reduce the fluid component of lymphedema by increasing the lymphatic drainage through (re)absorption of proteins and fluid from the interstitial space, redirection of lymph and, eventually maintaining and optimizing the activity of the remaining functional lymphatic channels to prevent lymphedema progression, and reduce the risk of infection.[1] Nevertheless, efficacy of the CDT alone is limited, considering the existence of structural or functional damage to the lymphatic system which will continue to hinder adequate lymphatic drainage.

In the last five decades, advances in the imaging techniques have allowed a greater understanding of the anatomy and pathophysiology of the lymphatic system. Similarly, development of microscopes with higher magnification, supermicrosurgical instruments, as well as robotic assistance and suction-assisted lipectomy devices have led to the introduction of different techniques for surgical treatment of early and advanced stages of lymphedema.[2,3] Based on clinical practice and scientific evidence, this chapter introduces the basic principles of surgical management of lymphedema. At this point, it needs to be stated that successful and personalized treatment is based on specific imaging techniques to assess the lymphatic system (see **Chapter 4**) and adequate preoperative CDT to best prepare the patient for surgery (see **Chapter 6,** and **Subchapter 7.3**). More technical aspects of each surgical technique—be it reconstructive or reductive—will be presented in detail in the following chapters (see **Chapters 8–14**).

7.1.2 Pathophysiological Aspects and Clinical Considerations

Accurate patient history and physical examination are essential for diagnosis of lymphedema and proper staging according to the International Lymphedema Society (see **Chapter 4**).[4] During physical examination, the most important clinical sign to be recognized is the presence of pitting or nonpitting edema. The early clinical manifestation of lymphedema is characterized by swelling of the affected body part with a soft and pitting edema that is consequence of the interruption in the lymphatic drainage that results in accumulation of protein-rich fluid in the interstitial space (see **Chapter 2**).[5] The mechanism behind it, at cellular level, is the disbalance between (too much) free fluid bubbles that can no longer bind to the chains of glycosaminoglycans in the interstitial space, which are strongly hydrophile (polyanions) and bind to H20. Therefore, the bubbles flow freely in the interstitial space and you can push them away with the pitting test, but the 'pit' will be filled with free fluid bubbles immediately when releasing the pressure of your fingers. Subsequently, as the impaired lymphatic drainage persists over time, the lymphatic stasis within the interstitial space will generate a chronic inflammatory response inducing proliferation of adipose and connective subcutaneous tissue and progressive fibrotic degeneration of the functioning lymphatic vessels.[5,6] Accordingly, the advanced lymphedema stage is characterized by permanent swelling with rather hardened nonpitting edema that is frequently accompanied by trophic skin changes. Understanding these pathophysiological processes and clinical manifestations are essential to best offer a stage-associated and personalized surgical treatment for the patient.

7.1.3 Diagnostic Imaging Techniques

Imaging techniques play an essential role in assessing the morphological and functional characteristics of the lymphatic system in order to define the most appropriate patient-oriented surgical approach. Nowadays, the most commonly used imaging methods include lymphoscintigraphy (LS), ICG lymphangiography, and increasingly, MRL (see **Chapter 4**).

Lymphoscintigraphy

Lymphoscintigraphy has been the gold standard imaging technique for many years and is used to confirm the clinical suspicion of lymphedema. This standardized imaging technique allows for qualitative assessment of the deep lymphatic system functionality. The main parameters evaluated are the quality of uptake of the tracer that consists of a protein marked with radioactive technetium. Further, this imaging technique allows for visualization of the major lymphatic collectors and the presence of the lymph node basins, as well as the time the tracer takes to reach a region of interest and calculate the transport index (see **Subchapter 4.6**).[7]

Indocyanine Green Lymphangiography

This minimally invasive imaging technique consists of a fluorescent dye injection (ICG) that allows real-time visualization of the superficial lymphatic channels without any exposure to radiation. Currently, ICG lymphangiography is the most often used diagnostic imaging technique and the most decisive for surgical decision-making as it helps to identify the presence or absence of functioning superficial lymphatic channels up to 2-cm deep and determines the severity of lymphedema according to the type of dermal back flow (see **Subchapter 4.7**).[8]

Magnetic Resonance Lymphangiography

Essentially, surgical planning can be performed using LS and ICG lymphangiography. More recently, MRL has been introduced to overcome certain limitations of the two previous imaging techniques. MRL allows for a three-dimensional reconstruction of the entire anatomical region of interest and distribution of the adipose tissue. Further, it provides rather precise information of the morphology and functionality of both the superficial and the deep lymphatic system. Eventually, this allows for more accurate surgical planning for the reconstruction of the damaged lymphatic system (see **Subchapters 4.8** and **4.9**).[9]

7.1.4 Surgical Procedures

Since the early 20th century, various surgical procedures have been developed for lymphedema treatment. Over time, the different techniques have undergone permanent modification and enhancement in order to become more efficient and effective. Conceptually, surgical procedures for lymphedema treatment are classified into two main groups: reconstructive techniques which aim to redirect lymphatic drainage and lymphoablative techniques which aim to reduce the volume of the hypertrophied subcutaneous tissue.[2,3]

Reconstructive Techniques

There are four surgical techniques which redirect accumulated lymph into healthy lymphatic collectors and veins, respectively:

- Autologous lymph vessel transfer;
- Lymphaticolymphatic anastomoses (LLAs);
- Lymphovenous anastomosis (LVA),[10,11,12] a surgical technique which increases lymph flow through the development of new extra-nodal lympho-lymphatic and lympho-venous connections;
- Vascularized lymph node transfer (VLNT)[13,14,15,16]

In rare cases, these nodo-venal shunts are performed, particularly in filariasis-associated lymphedema.[17] Currently, the two main reconstructive techniques that are most commonly performed and have shown the greatest efficacy in reducing lymphedema-related symptoms are LVA and VLNT.

The first line in the surgical treatment of lymphedema is LVA (see **Chapter 8**). This technique is indicated when active lymphatic channels are still present, usually in the early stage of lymphedema, and consists of redirecting lymphatic drainage into the venous circulation.[18] The use of ICG lymphangiography in combination with MRL will provide the precise information to preoperatively select the most suitable lymphatic channels for anastomosis.[19]

The second line in the surgical treatment of lymphedema is VLNT and can be offered in early or advanced stage lymphedema (see **Chapter 10**). This technique consists of placing healthy lymphatic tissue, harvested from another region of the body, in areas with damaged or absent lymphatic channels and/or lymph nodes. The exact mechanism of action is not yet fully understood, but there are two theories. One proposes that the transferred lymphatic tissue may induce lymphangiogenesis and spontaneous development of lymphatic pathways at the recipient site.

The other hypothesizes that the transferred lymphatic tissue acts as a sponge to absorb lymphatic fluid from the surrounding interstitial tissue and finally redirects it into the venous circulation of the flap.[2] VLNT can be used for the treatment of lymphedema regardless the etiology; however, it is more frequently performed in patients with lymphedema secondary to cancer treatment or trauma with extensive soft tissue loss. In general, ICG lymphangiography and LS are necessary to determine if the patient is a candidate for VLNT. Moreover, when VLNT surgery is planned, an additional imaging technique is requested, the computed tomography angiography (CTA), which will provide information about the location of the superficial lymph nodes of the donor site and vascular pedicle of the flap (see **Chapters 4** and **10**). In selective cases, LVA and VLNT can be performed simultaneously during the same intervention. In the case of breast cancer-related lymphedema with postmastectomy amastia, LVA and VLNT can even be combined with autologous breast reconstruction, which is called total breast anatomy restoration (T-BAR) approach (see **Chapter 11**).[20]

It is well known that the success rate of reconstructive surgery for lymphedema treatment is most effective if performed rather soon after the clinical onset of lymphedema. Accordingly, recent trend consists of reducing the risk of developing lymphedema secondary to surgical treatment and/or radiotherapy for cancer.[21] This approach is based on intraoperative evaluation of the lymphatic system in patients undergoing sentinel lymph node biopsy and lymph node dissection, and immediate derivation of the sectioned lymphatic vessels into the neighboring veins by LVA technique.

Reductive and Lymphoreductive Techniques

Despite the revolutionary concept of surgically restoring the functionality of the impaired lymphatic system, in most cases, none of these reconstructive approaches will provide complete reduction of the swelling in advanced stages of lymphedema. Since the excess volume in very advanced stage of lymphedema are mainly related to fat hypertrophy and fibrosis, excisional or lymphoablative techniques may be needed to reduce the subcutaneous tissue (see **Chapters 14** and **15**).

In the early 1900s, treatment of advanced stage of lymphedema consisted in circumferential debulking of skin and subcutaneous tissue followed by defect coverage with skin grafts. In the following decades, many modifications of the Charles technique[22] were described with the aim of reducing excessive skin grafting after the removal of skin and subcutaneous tissue. To cover the full-thickness skin defect after excision of skin and subcutaneous tissues affected by lymphedema, newer techniques were developed based on skin flaps (1936: Homans-Miller procedure),[23] or the advancement and transposition of deepithelialized dermal flaps (1970: Thompson procedure)[24] into the underlying fascia and muscle to somehow connect the superficial lymphatic drainage system to the deep one rather[25] than skin grafts. Unfortunately, all these procedures are associated with a rather high rate of pain, wound healing complications, infection, and/or lymph fistulas. Furthermore, they are often aesthetically disfiguring. Therefore, this type of surgery is nowadays used only occasionally in industrialized countries in cases of very severe and advanced stage of lymphedema, i.e., in instances where extremities are very voluminous.

In the 1970s, the technique of removing excess fatty tissue through blunt cannulas connected to a suction machine was introduced for aesthetic purpose.[26,27,28] At the end of the 1980s, it began to be applied for the treatment of advanced stage lymphedema, becoming the preferred lymphoablative technique due to its rather low rate of complications and good aesthetic results compared to excisional techniques (see **Chapter 14**).[29] Therefore, suction-assisted lipectomy has become the third line in the surgical treatment of lymphedema. Vibration-assisted suction devices are preferred for removal of adipose and fibrosed tissues from the affected body part that must be performed circumferentially using a technique that does not damage the vascular components and the remaining functioning lymphatic channels.

7.1.5 Conclusions

The treatment of lymphedema is complex and often requires a multistage surgical approach that combines different reconstructive and lymphoablative techniques.[30,31,32] The surgical strategy should always be individualized for each patient based on the structural and functional involvement of the lymphatic system of the affected body part. Early diagnosis and prompt surgical treatment are the key to successful management of lymphedema when conservative treatment fails.

7.2 Complete Decongestive Therapy in the Pre- and Postoperative Setting

Nele Adriaenssens, Ellen Vandyck, and Sarah Harnie

7.2.1 Introduction

CDT has an added value both during the pre- and postoperative phases when using microsurgical reconstructive techniques to treat lymphedema, including LVA and VLNT.

Preoperatively, CDT drains excessive extracellular lymphatic fluid to clear the surgical field, making lymphatic and vascular structures visible and surgically accessible, while preparing the lymphatic system for the newly formed surgical structures.

Manual lymphatic drainage, combined with compression therapy, induces contractions of the lymphangions during the postoperative phase, redirecting lymphatic flow toward and through the surgically created channels that are able to drain after LVA or VLNT and later on through the spontaneously developed drainage networks following VLNT. Postoperative CDT aims at obtaining the results of surgery and preventing worsening of symptoms, in particular volume increase and infection. Skin and wound care as well as lifelong physical activity and exercise should be standard of care in management of lymphedema.

However, scientific evidence on how to optimally standardize CDT protocols for daily clinical practice before and after reconstructive microsurgery of the lymphatics is lacking. Therefore, an international survey was conducted to elaborate consensual recommendations on how to offer best practice. Interprofessional referral and management are key to success in lymphedema treatment.

7.2.2 Background

CDT (see **Chapter 6**) treats lymphedema-induced symptoms in most cases, whereas reconstructive microsurgery of the lymphatic system may result in a causative treatment. Accordingly, this type of surgery has recently shown growing interest to treat impaired and dysfunctional lymphatic systems. It is important to acknowledge that reconstructive microsurgery of the lymphatic system and CDT go hand-in-hand, i.e., CDT may optimally condition and maintain the surgically induced results, whereas lymphatic microsurgery may improve the efficacy of CDT.[33,34,35,36,37,38,39]

To understand the added value of CDT in the perioperative phases of lymphedema treatment, the aims of the different CDT modalities are briefly discussed below.

- Manual lymphatic drainage (MLD): In MLD, extracellular fluid and proteins are gathered (recalled) and reabsorbed from the interstitial space and contractions of the lymphangions are activated and intensified to transport the lymphatic fluid toward the lymph nodes and finally into the blood stream.[40] A lymphangion is defined as the functional unit of a lymphatic vessel (collector) between two consecutive valves (▶ Fig. 7.1), innervated by the autonomic nervous system (▶ Fig. 7.2 and ▶ Fig. 7.3).[40] Besides the physiologically active lymphatic vessel network, inactive anastomosis (e.g., interaxillary; ▶ Fig. 7.4 and ▶ Fig. 7.5) can also be addressed through MLD (in pathophysiological conditions such as cancer-related lymphedema) in order to redirect lymphatic fluid to healthy and intact lymphatic structures in neighboring body parts.[41] This may also apply for newly formed collateral pathways and, therefore, for newly formed lymphatic (or lymphovenous) anastomosis and transplanted lymphatic tissues (vessels and/or nodes).[42]

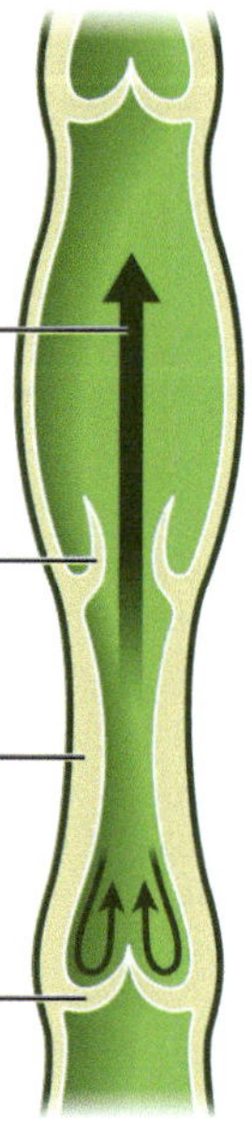

Fig. 7.1 The interaction of valves and musculature of the vessel wall during contraction of a lymphangion, i.e., the segment of a lymph vessel in between two valves.

- Compression therapy: Preoperatively, compression therapy with short-stretch multilayer bandages (preferred over a compression sleeve or stocking) wrings out the edematous tissue to clear the surgical field, reduce filtration into the interstitial space, and, therefore, make it as dry as possible. Bandages are applied when volume changes over time. Postoperatively, these multilayer short-stretch bandages or, if possible, custom-made pressure garments (preferably dressed on the patient in the operating room postoperatively) are generally indicated for additional pumping function and thus improvement of lymphatic flow, regulation in homeostasis (Starling's law), and prevention of skin damage. Custom-made garments are applied when the volume is stable over time.[36,43]
- Wound and skin care: Necessary throughout the patient's postoperative care to avoid infections, prevent surgical complications, and prepare the skin (elasticity) to a smaller volume.[36]
- Physical exercise (and a healthy lifestyle, e.g., decrease of body mass index since being overweight is an important risk factor for cancer-related lymphedema):
  - Exercise-lymphology is a relatively new but interesting field. Four important physiological mechanisms of aerobic (walking, cycling, swimming, etc.) and strengthening (to enforce the muscles with

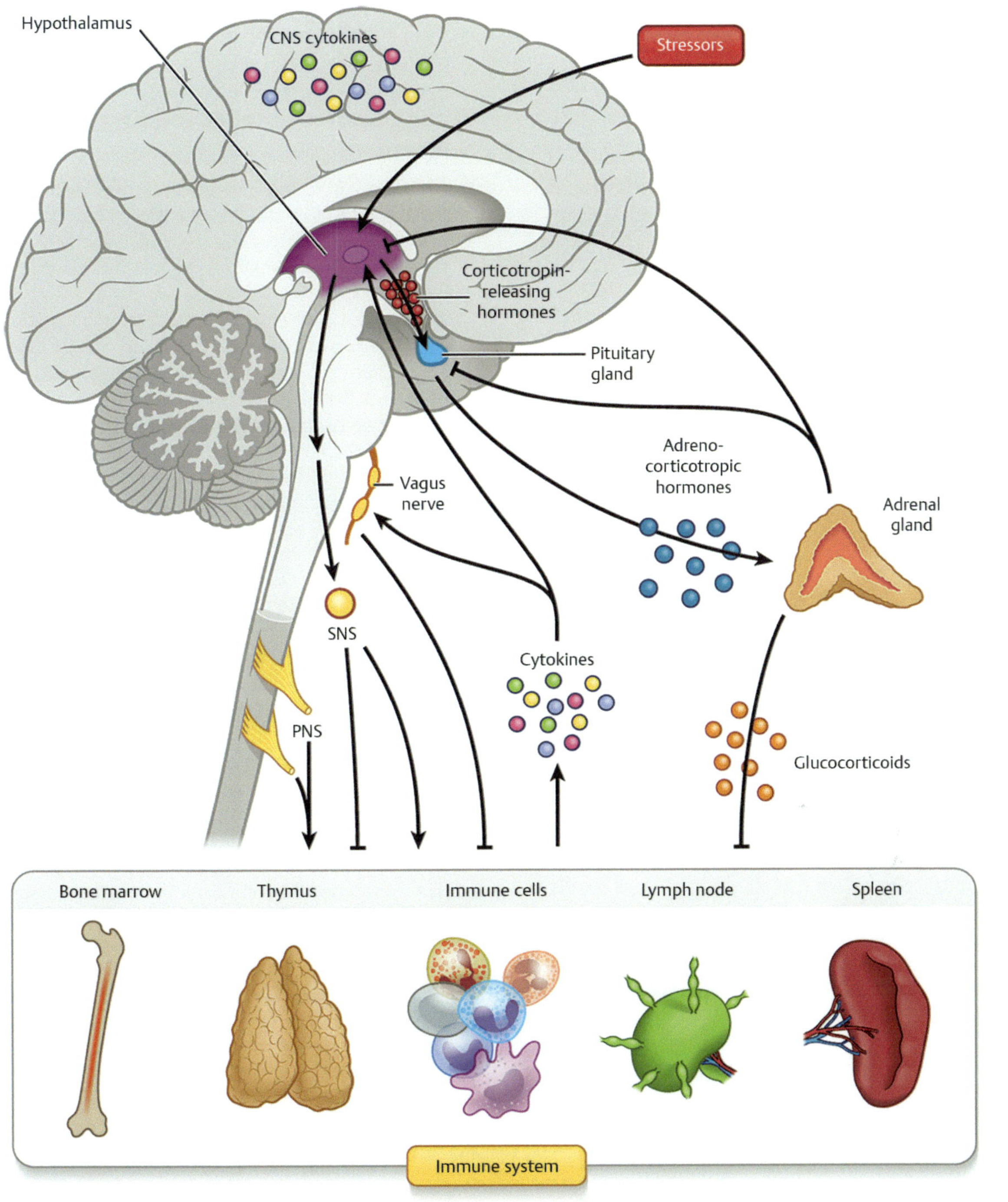

Fig. 7.2 Interplay between the immune system and the autonomic nervous system. CNS, central nervous system; PNS, parasympathetic nervous system; SNS, sympathetic nervous system.

elastic bands, weights, etc.) exercise may influence the lymphatic system.[44,45]

- Exercise therapy increases interstitial pressure and strains on the extracellular matrix because of an increase in capillary pressure and thus capillary filtration. This results in the opening of microvalves of lymphatic capillaries and draining of extracellular fluid.

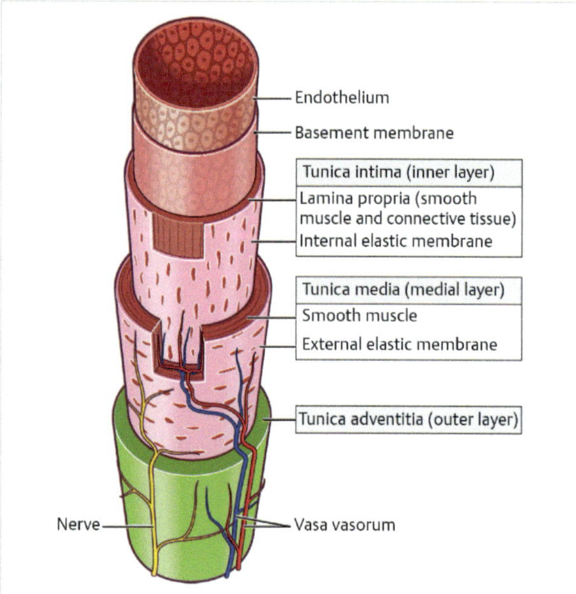

Fig. 7.3 Innervation of lymphatic collectors to induce contraction of lymphangions.

  - Muscle contractions close the microvalves and transport lymphatic fluid from the interstitial space into the lymphatic capillaries to be transported unidirectionally.
  - When systematic resistance training is applied, a decrease in mean blood pressure could lead to less filtration into the interstitial space and thus less load on the lymphatic system.
  - The wall of the lymphatic vessels (collectors) consists of a smooth muscle layer whose contraction rate is regulated by pacemaker cells and influenced by the autonomic nervous system. Exercise therapy activates the sympathetic nervous system, increasing the contraction rate by which lymphatic fluid is transported and hence drained more efficiently.

Therefore, the aim of CDT in the perioperative phases of lymphedema treatment is threefold:

- CDT is important in the *preoperative phase* to drain excessive extracellular lymphatic fluid and thereby clear the surgical field to make lymphatic and vascular structures visible and accessible. It is important that the surgery can be performed in the most optimal conditions, increasing the success rates.
- CDT, in general, and MLD, in particular, activate contractions of the lymphangions in the *postoperative phase*, redirecting lymphatic fluid progressively toward and through the newly formed lymphatic (or lymphovenous) or lympho-lymphatic anastomosis or the lymph nodes in the transplanted flap.
- CDT in the *postoperative phase* aims at maintaining the results obtained by surgery and preventing worsening of symptoms, in particular volume increase and infection.

Timing and Teamwork are Key to Success

In order to offer the best possible treatment, timing when to refer patients to surgery is of great importance. When the lymphatic vessels are continuously drenched in fluid, they slowly dissolve, becoming unsuitable for LVA and VLNT.

Accordingly, physical therapists play an important role in this interdisciplinary and often complex clinical decision-making. Thorough interprofessional communication and integrated patient care between surgeon, lymphologist, physical therapist, and patient is essential.[46,47,48]

Currently, there is no clear recommendation about the appropriate timing when to offer reconstructive microsurgery of the lymphatic system, i.e., LVA and/or VLNT. Most commonly, 1 year of CDT after lymphedema onset is sufficient to evaluate whether or not conservative treatment is effective. Damaged or insufficient lymphatic vessels can regenerate spontaneously or neoformation of lymphatic collaterals occurs to bypass the nonfunctional area. If the patient is nonresponsive to CDT for at least 6 months to 1 year, this process of spontaneous regeneration and vascular neoformation can be considered terminated.[34,38]

If CDT fails and reconstructive microsurgery is not initiated within 2 years after onset of lymphedema, the risk of irreversible changes to subcutaneous and cutaneous tissues, such as fat hypertrophy and tissue fibrosis, increases.[34,39] The International Society of Lymphology (ISL) states that: "If intensive conservative, non-operative treatment offered in a specialized center that takes care of lymphedema and is managed by an experienced lymphologist has been unsuccessful, CDT has to be considered as failed."[36] Although clear indications to surgery are not well defined, Maclellan and Greene recommend reconstructive microsurgery in instances when conservative measures fail and/or when significant complications occur, including recurrent infections, impaired function of the affected body part, as well as decreased quality of life and/or psychosocial distress due to the aesthetic aspect of the affected body part.[35]

7.2.3 Evidence-Based Practice for Perioperative Complete Decongestive Therapy

Microsurgical procedures and CDT including MLD, compression therapy, skin care, and physical exercise vary considerably with regard to frequency, intensity, and techniques, and the patient population suffering from lymphedema is very heterogeneous. Literature about

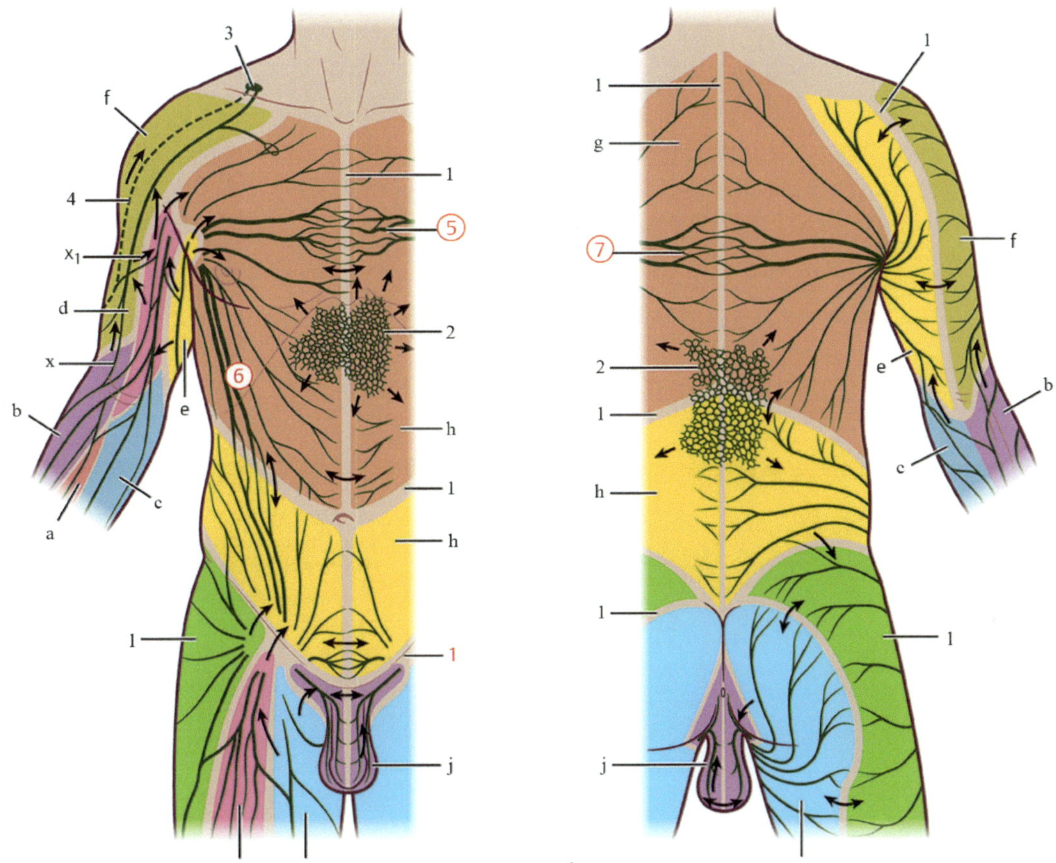

a b

1 Lymphatic watershed (divide) at the borders of the lymphatic territories
2 Cutaneous lymph vessel network
3 Supraclavicular lymph nodes
4 Lateral bundle of the upper arm (long type: continuous line, short type: dotted line)
5 Ventral interaxillary anastomoses
6 Axillo-inguinal anastomoses
7 Dorsal interaxillary anastomoses
a Middle territory of the forearm
b Radial territory of the forearm
c Ulnar territory of the forearm
d Middle territory of the upper arm
e Dorsomedial territory of the upper arm
f Dorsolateral territory of the upper arm with deltoid bundle
g Upper territory of the trunk
h Lower territory of the trunk
i Dorsomedial territory of the thigh
j Territory of the outer genitalia and the perineal region
k Territory of the ventromedial bundle
l Dorsolateral territory of the thigh
x, x_1 Anastomotic branches

Fig. 7.4 Ventral **(a)** and dorsal **(b)** cutaneous territories of the trunk and the adjacent territories of the extremities (arrows mark the possible drainage pathways after lymphadenectomy). Numbers 5, 6, and 7 show the transpectoral, the ipsilateral axillo-inguinal, and the transdorsal anastomoses, respectively, allowing transport of lymph between different territories of the body following, for example, breast cancer surgery.

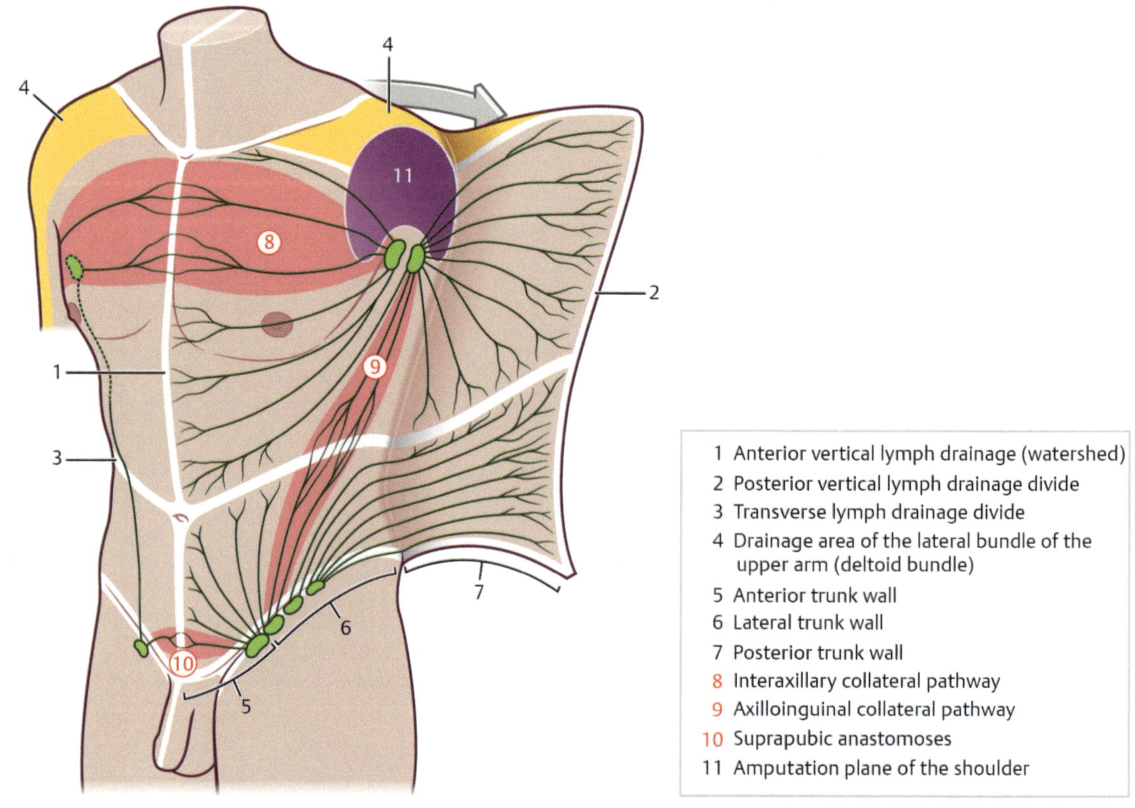

Fig. 7.5 Schematic diagram of the lymphatic drainage of the trunk (skin of the back retracted sideways). Numbers 8, 9, and 10 show the transpectoral, ipsilateral axillo-inguinal, and transpubic anastomoses, respectively, allowing transport of lymph between different territories of the body.

specific protocols or recommendations on perioperative CDT accompanying reconstructive microsurgery in lymphedema patients is scarce. Hence, currently it is impossible to define a gold standard for perioperative CDT protocols, in particular in the absence of consensus-based recommendations and randomized clinical trials comparing different perioperative CDT protocols.

Therefore, this chapter highlights available protocols by November 2021 on pre- and postoperative CDT to be applied after *LVA and/or LNT* for lymphedema treatment of the *extremities*. Note that the published protocols of specialized and skilled professionals in literature are institution-dependent.

Manual Lymphatic Drainage

The majority of the patients suffering from lymphedema get MLD since the onset of lymphedema, while the minority initiates MLD only 2 weeks *prior to surgery*. The frequency of preoperative MLD sessions per week lies between three and seven.[34,37,39,49,50,51]

Currently, no clear recommendations are available regarding MLD after reconstructive microsurgery *during hospitalization stay*.[35,39,52] Every center seems to apply in-house protocols that are often based upon personal experience and best adapted to the available infrastructure and personnel.

A majority of the surgically treated patients get MLD *following surgery* for a time period of 4 to 12 months. The frequency of postoperative MLD sessions initially varies between three and seven times a week to be gradually decreased to one session a week or every 2 weeks in most cases.[34,37,49,50,51,53]

Compression Therapy

Scientific evidence regarding perioperative compression therapy is sparse. Some reviews recommend initiation of local compression between 1 and 6 weeks *prior to surgery* for at least 5 days a week. Thereby, the grade of compression should amount to class II and class III for the upper and lower extremities, respectively.[33,35,37]

Note:

Over 50% of the studies reviewed in the meta-analysis of Basta et al. propose initiation of compression therapy *immediately after surgery* if possible or at latest within 1 month as an alternative. Most often, custom-made garments are tailored to the patient in the operating room.[54]

According to Winters et al.,[43] approximately one-third of the patients used low pressure elastic bandaging in the *postoperative phase*, while other authors mention the use of custom-made, low-pressure garments. Low pressure usually corresponds to 20 to 30 mmHg (class II) or higher (class III) for the lower extremity, depending on the supplier and country (▶ Table 7.1).[55,56]

ISL recommends wearing a short-stretch elastic stocking or sleeve.[33,36] Penha et al. recommend indefinite continuation of compression therapy following LVA surgery, whereas after VLNT surgery, only 33% were wearing compression garments for approximately 6 months. After 2 years, patients who had undergone VLNT completely ceased wearing compression therapy.[53]

Currently, the literature states inconsistently that compression bandage is worn between 1[57] and 4 weeks[58] and between 4 and 10 weeks[37] following surgery. Some recommend daily replacement of the bandage, whereas others do not.[37] Interestingly, the grade of applied pressure differs a lot among studies and the ideal pressure to be applied is unknown.[57,58,59]

Exercise Programs

Evidence on detailed exercise programs *prior to surgery* is very scarce. McKey and Alappattu recommend a moderate-intensity, home-based program with exercises five times a week.[37]

Table 7.1 Different classes and respective pressures generated by compression garments for patients with peripheral lymphedema (adapted from Todd[55])

Class	British (mmHg)	French (mmHg)	German (mmHg)
I	14–17	10–15	18–21
II	18–24	15–20	23–32
III	25–35	20–36	34–46
IV	n/a	> 36	> 49

Almost in all known cases, patients are allowed to mobilize themselves and walk freely *immediately* or at least 1 day *following surgery*.[39,58,60,61]

After hospital discharge, most approved protocols recommend exercise.[37,39,58,60,61]

Skin Care

Skin care and personal hygiene (e.g., manicure/pedicure, prevention of bacterial or fungal infection) are essential during all phases of lymphedema treatment because they play an important role in preventing infections (erysipelas), eventually reducing the risk of onset of new lymphedema formation and worsening of preexisting lymphedema. If the infection is local, accurate treatment (intravenous antibiotics) should be initiated immediately to best prevent the potential loss of benefit on lymphedema due to surgery.[33,34]

7.2.4 Best Practices—the Expert's Opinion

To define best clinical practices of perioperative CDT with reconstructive microsurgery, a survey has been organized worldwide, including experts in the field. A total of 12 surgeons participated from all over the world: Australia, Belgium, France, India, Italy, Japan, Peru, Spain, Taiwan, and United States of America.

Results of the survey were presented at the 44th Congress of the European Society of Lymphology, September 20–22, 2018, Prague, Czech Republic, by the authors and published in the proceedings of *The European Journal of Lymphology and Related Problems*. In ▶ Table 7.2, the most relevant results are presented.

Results for LVA and VLNT are quite similar with the following exceptions:

- MLD
  - MLD for VLNT can be initiated from day 1 after surgery, while for LVA at least 1 week post operation is requested to start MLD. About 70% of VLNT patients undergo MLD compared to only 58% following LVA.
- Compression
  - Preoperatively to LVA always use multilayer bandages (not single layer).
  - Bandages are worn in the majority of LVA patients (70%), mostly (63%) immediately following surgery, while only one out of three patients wears compression bandages following VLNT. Half of all VLNT patients start wearing compression bandages at least 1 day following surgery, whereas the other half usually start wearing compression bandages 3 to 4 weeks postoperatively.
  - A compression sleeve is worn by 75% of all LVA patients immediately following surgery, whereas 25% wait between 1 week and 3 months after surgery. About 75% of all VLNT patients initiate a

compression sleeve between 1 and 4 weeks following surgery.
- Mobilization and physical exercise
  - Hospital stay varies between 0 and 7 days for VLNT, and between 1 and 6 days for VLNT.
  - About 25% of LVA patients are totally immobilized during hospital stay and 75% partially, while for VLNT only 33% are immobilized completely and 100% partially.
  - Physical exercise is performed twice a week following VLNT in the majority of the patients, while after LVA, frequency of exercise is performed three or more times a week.

7.2.5 Discussion

The aim of MLD prior to LVA is (1) to clear the surgical field as much as possible (2) in order to ideally turn a pitting edema into a nonpitting edema and eventually (3) to activate and intensify drainage within preexisting lymphatic vessels, especially distal to the planned LVA site.

MLD prior to VLNT is meant to activate and stimulate drainage within afferent lymphatic vessels toward the recipient site and is much more patient dependent than prior to LVA, which may be explained by the variety of donor and recipient sites, as well as the differences in surgical techniques.

MLD protocols for LVA and VLNT **following reconstructive surgery** are far more specific than the preoperative protocols:
- Despite the frailty of the new structures following reconstructive microsurgery, only one out of three patients are partially immobilized following surgery and MLD can be initiated from day 1 (for VLNT) and week 1 (for LVA) following surgery.
- Intensity and frequency of MLD needs to be scaled up progressively following microsurgery (from two to five times a week in the first 3 months).
- After 3 months, decreasing the frequency from five back to two or three times a week seems to have beneficial effects as per our clinical experience.
- Furthermore, 6 to 12 months after surgery and depending on the evolution of the surgical outcome that is patient dependent, MLD can be further reduced to once a week or even once every 2 weeks.

Similar to MLD, the aim of **preoperative compression** is to reduce filtration and hence to best clear the extremity in general and the surgical field in particular in order to maintain the state of decongestion, stimulating the pumping function of the lymphatic vessels. Therefore, compression therapy can also be applied **postoperatively** to prevent from new volume increase in the extremity (preferably following MLD), thereby perpetuating the effect of MLD in the long run.

Basically, elastic bandages have a higher rest pressure and a lower working pressure than nonelastic bandages. Working pressure corresponds to the external pressure caused by the bandage when a patient is physically active and therefore uses the muscles in the concerned area. In contrast, rest pressure is the pressure a bandage is inducing on the body part when the patient is not using the diseased or affected body part. Therefore, elastic bandages are more often used in sedentary or immobilized patients, whereas nonelastic (short stretch) bandages support the pumping pressure, especially during physical activity.

After surgery, more patients who underwent VLNT wear a compression sleeve or stocking rather than a bandage when compared to patients that underwent LVA surgery. Since the volume of the body part will decrease progressively particularly in the early postoperative phase, wearing bandages is indicated during the acute postoperative phase until volume starts to stabilize in order to change to a custom-made compression garment for the phase of maintenance. It is also recommended to use customized garments made of flat knitted elastic tissue rather than garments made of circular knitted elastic tissue because the latter has the tendency to tighten at the narrowest areas and apply overpressure in bulky areas.

The expert group did not consent on any duration of postoperative compression treatment, but clinical experience shows that the first 12 months after surgery are crucial to determine the success of surgery. Basically, compression can be recommended lifelong, and patients should be aware of this prior to surgery because the request for help, i.e., the desire of patients to undergo reconstructive microsurgery, can be based on banishing compression treatment in particular and CDT in general. Currently, scientific evidence is lacking on how to progressively reduce and downgrade compression treatment following surgery although there are cases reported with beneficial effects following several years without compression. Comparable to MLD, intensity of bandaging should be increased until a compression sleeve can be fitted on a stabilized volume of the body part. Classes of sleeves that should be used largely follow the ISL guidelines of the consensus document where for lymphedema stages I–II class II for the upper and class III for the lower extremity are recommended.[36]

Preoperative exercises may increase the pumping effect that is inherent to the lymphatic vessels, i.e., the active contractions of the lymphangions. Most often home-based exercise programs are recommended. For many surgical interventions, starting exercise therapy as early as possible is recommended to prepare the body (physical fitness called prehabilitation) and more specifically the lymphatic system for the scheduled microsurgical procedure.[62,63]

Table 7.2 Summary of the results of an international survey showing current best clinical practice of perioperative CDT in combination with reconstructive microsurgery to treat lymphedema

	MLD	Compression	Exercise	Skin Care
Preoperative phase	• Executed by 86% of patients • ≥3×/week (50% of patients) or 1–2×/week (50% of patients)	• Pneumatic compression (40–90 mmHg) executed by 33% of patients • Bandages indicated 1–4 weeks prior to surgery executed by 60%–75% of patients	• Executed by 81% of patients • Usually 3×/week and usually home-based • Initiation at latest 1–2 weeks prior to surgery executed by 33% of patients	• 91% of the patients receive advice on skin care, primarily to avoid infection
Comments on preoperative phase	• Sessions of 30–60'	• Bandages: Mostly multilayer and inelastic (short-stretch) and the majority wears them day and night • Sometimes sleeves instead of bandages (alternating), but usually only during the day	• Sessions of 30–60' • Most commonly aerobic exercise	
Postoperative phase	• Remarkable differences for LVA and VLNT • ≥2×/week	• Bandages and compression sleeves: Remarkable differences between LVA and VLNT • Compression sleeves: 75% of patients wear them	• Initiation 3–4 weeks postoperatively (61%) • Usually home-based • Limit session to 30' in the beginning	• 86% receives advice on skin care, primarily to avoid infection
Comments on postoperative phase	• Sessions of 30–60'	• Pneumatic compression is rare (since pressure cannot be controlled manually at distinct locations, which is necessary in the postoperative phase) • Most commonly worn day and night, never only during the night		• Advice is similar to preoperative information

Abbreviations: CDT, complete decongestive therapy; MLD, manual lymphatic drainage; LVA, lymphovenous anastomosis; VLNT, lymph node transfer.

Exercise needs to be built up progressively in intensity and frequency **following microsurgery**. The first sessions intend to intensify lymphatic circulation through progressive pumping function (lymphangion contractions) and eventually increase lymphatic flow through the newly created lymphovenous or lympho-lymphatic structures. It is essential to combine aerobic exercise with strengthening training aiming at reinforcing the muscles in a supervised environment.[64] The effect of additional and specific respiratory exercises that induce a repeated and alternate over- and under-pressure in the chest to eventually induce a suction effect from the extremities toward the center of the body (thoracic duct) is currently not sufficiently studied.[65] Anyhow, as in almost all patients with chronic disease, exercise therapy and healthy lifestyle (through behavioral changes and continuous patient education) should be undertaken lifelong, particularly in lymphedema patients.

Skin care is an essential part of conservative lymphedema treatment to prevent infection. Every single infection of the affected extremity constitutes an additional risk to further destroy compromised or nonfunctional lymphatic structure. Accordingly, an episode of infection can induce lymphedema formation or deteriorate preexisting lymphedema state. Therefore, patients have to be repeatedly informed and instructed whenever possible by every single member of the interprofessional lymphedema care team.

Recently, combination therapy (CDT and surgery) was proposed for lymphedema in a clinical trial. Good results were obtained in the diseased body parts, including volume reduction and prevention of cellulitis.[66]

Take-home messages

- Preoperatively, follow the standard ISL guidelines[4] of CDT (especially **MLD** and **compression**) for early lymphedema in the acute (reduction) phase.[36]
- The first postoperative year is crucial to benefit best from lympho-reconstructive surgery. Personalized CDT, adapted to the needs of every single patient (especially **MLD** and **compression**), is a must in the interprofessional care of lymphedema patients who underwent lympho-reconstructive microsurgery.
- Postoperatively, it is strongly recommended to use short-stretch multilayer **bandages** until the volume reaches a stable state, followed by wearing a custom-made flat knitted **compression garment**.
- Correctly dosed **exercise** (mixed aerobic and resistance exercise associated with a healthy active lifestyle) may have an additional benefit on lymphatic function and eventually lymphedema state prior to and especially following surgery.
- Educate and strongly encourage patients about meticulous **skin care** during every phase, before and after surgery.

7.2.6 Conclusions

CDT is an essential and integral part of lymphedema care, as well as prior to and following microsurgical interventions. Accordingly, CDT and reconstructive microsurgery have to be considered complementary to achieve best possible surgical outcomes for the patients.

Neither CDT nor reconstructive surgery of the lymphatic system can cure chronic lymphedema, yet in many cases complete restoration can be achieved, particularly in a well-organized and coordinated interprofessional setting. Although best clinical practices are promising, current literature is too heterogeneous and the level of evidence is insufficient to define an internationally recognized consensus on perioperative CDT.

References

[1] Lasinski BB, McKillip Thrift K, Squire D, et al. A systematic review of the evidence for complete decongestive therapy in the treatment of lymphedema from 2004 to 2011. PM R. 2012; 4(8): 580–601

[2] Chang DW, Masia J, Garza R, III, Skoracki R, Neligan PC. Lymphedema: surgical and medical therapy. Plast Reconstr Surg. 2016; 138(3) Suppl:209S–218S

[3] Kung TA, Champaneria MC, Maki JH, Neligan PC. Current concepts in the surgical management of lymphedema. Plast Reconstr Surg. 2017; 139(4):1003e–1013e

[4] International Society of Lymphology. The diagnosis and treatment of peripheral lymphedema: 2013 Consensus Document of the International Society of Lymphology. Lymphology. 2013; 46(1):1–11

[5] Scallan JP, Zawieja SD, Castorena-Gonzalez JA, Davis MJ. Lymphatic pumping: mechanics, mechanisms and malfunction. J Physiol. 2016; 594(20):5749–5768

[6] Koshima I, Kawada S, Moriguchi T, Kajiwara Y. Ultrastructural observations of lymphatic vessels in lymphedema in human extremities. Plast Reconstr Surg. 1996; 97(2):397–405, discussion 406–407

[7] Yoshida RY, Kariya S, Ha-Kawa S, Tanigawa N. Lymphoscintigraphy for imaging of the lymphatic flow disorders. Tech Vasc Interv Radiol. 2016; 19(4):273–276

[8] Yamamoto T, Yamamoto N, Doi K, et al. Indocyanine green-enhanced lymphography for upper extremity lymphedema: a novel severity staging system using dermal backflow patterns. Plast Reconstr Surg. 2011; 128(4):941–947

[9] Neligan PC, Kung TA, Maki JH. MR lymphangiography in the treatment of lymphedema. J Surg Oncol. 2017; 115(1):18–22

[10] O'Brien BM, Shafiroff BB. Microlymphaticovenous and resectional surgery in obstructive lymphedema. World J Surg. 1979; 3(1):3–15, 121–123

[11] Koshima I, Inagawa K, Urushibara K, Moriguchi T. Supermicrosurgical lymphaticovenular anastomosis for the treatment of lymphedema in the upper extremities. J Reconstr Microsurg. 2000; 16(6):437–442

[12] Gilbert A, O'Brien BM, Vorrath JW, Sykes PJ. Lymphaticovenous anastomosis by microvascular technique. Br J Plast Surg. 1976; 29(4): 355–360

[13] Becker C, Hidden G. [Transfer of free lymphatic flaps. Microsurgery and anatomical study]. J Mal Vasc. 1988; 13(2):119–122

[14] Chen HC, O'Brien BM, Rogers IW, Pribaz JJ, Eaton CJ. Lymph node transfer for the treatment of obstructive lymphoedema in the canine model. Br J Plast Surg. 1990; 43(5):578–586

[15] Becker C, Hidden G, Godart S, et al. Free lymphatic transplant. Eur J Lymphol Rel Prob.. 1991; 6:25–77

[16] Park KE, Allam O, Chandler L, et al. Surgical management of lymphedema: a review of current literature. Gland Surg. 2020; 9(2): 503–511

[17] Nielubowicz J, Olszewski W. Surgical lymphaticovenous shunts in patients with secondary lymphoedema. Br J Surg. 1968; 55(6):440–442

[18] Chang DW, Suami H, Skoracki R. A prospective analysis of 100 consecutive lymphovenous bypass cases for treatment of extremity lymphedema. Plast Reconstr Surg. 2013; 132(5):1305–1314

[19] Pons G, Clavero JA, Alomar X, Rodríguez-Bauza E, Tom LK, Masia J. Preoperative planning of lymphaticovenous anastomosis: the use of magnetic resonance lymphangiography as a complement to indocyanine green lymphography. J Plast Reconstr Aesthet Surg. 2019; 72(6):884–891

[20] Masià J, Pons G, Rodríguez-Bauzà E. Barcelona lymphedema algorithm for surgical treatment in breast cancer-related lymphedema. J Reconstr Microsurg. 2016; 32(5):329–335

[21] Boccardo F, Casabona F, De Cian F, et al. Lymphatic microsurgical preventing healing approach (LYMPHA) for primary surgical prevention of breast cancer-related lymphedema: over 4 years follow-up. Microsurgery. 2014; 34(6):421–424

[22] Charles RH: The surgical treatment of elephantiasis. Ind Med Gaz 1901; 36: 84–99.

[23] Homans J. The treatment of elephantiasis of the legs. A preliminary report. N Engl J Med. 1936; 215:1099–1104

[24] Thompson N. Buried dermal flap operation for chronic lymphedema of the extremities. Ten-year survey of results in 79 cases. Plast Reconstr Surg. 1970; 45(6):541–548

[25] Sistrunk WE. Contribution to plastic surgery: removal of scars by stages; an open operation for extensive laceration of the anal sphincter; the Kondoleon operation for elephantiasis. Ann Surg. 1927; 85(2):185–193

[26] Fischer A, Fischer G. First surgical treatment for molding body's cellulite with three 5 mm incisions. Bull Int Acad Cosmet Surg. 1976; 3:35
[27] Schrudde J. [Lipectomy and lipexhaeresia in the area of the lower extremities (author's translation)]. Langenbecks Arch Chir. 1977; 345:127–131
[28] Illouz YG. Surgical remodeling of the silhouette by aspiration lipolysis or selective lipectomy. Aesthetic Plast Surg. 1985; 9(1):7–21
[29] Brorson H, Svensson H. Complete reduction of lymphoedema of the arm by liposuction after breast cancer. Scand J Plast Reconstr Surg Hand Surg. 1997; 31(2):137–143
[30] Granzow JW, Soderberg JM, Kaji AH, Dauphine C. Review of current surgical treatments for lymphedema. Ann Surg Oncol. 2014; 21(4): 1195–1201
[31] Granzow JW, Soderberg JM, Kaji AH, Dauphine C. Review of current surgical treatments for lymphedema. Ann Surg Oncol. 2014; 21(4): 1195–1201. Epub 2014 Feb 21
[32] Granzow JW. Lymphedema surgery: the current state of the art. Clin Exp Metastasis. 2018; 35(5-6):553–558. Epub 2018 Jul 6
[33] Szuba A, Rockson SG. Lymphedema: classification, diagnosis and therapy. Vasc Med. 1998; 3(2):145–156
[34] Lee BB, Laredo J, Neville R. Reconstructive surgery for chronic lymphedema: a viable option, but. Vascular. 2011; 19(4):195–205
[35] Maclellan RA, Greene AK. Lymphedema. Semin Pediatr Surg. 2014; 23(4):191–197
[36] Executive Committee of the International Society of Lymphology. The diagnosis and treatment of peripheral lymphedema: 2020 Consensus Document of the International Society of Lymphology. Lymphology. 2020; 53(1):3–19
[37] McKey KP, Alappattu MJ. Physical therapy intervention to augment outcomes of lymph node transfer surgery for a breast cancer survivor with secondary upper extremity lymphedema: a case report. Int J Stud Scholarsh Phys Ther. 2015; 1:30–44
[38] Boccardo F, Campisi CC, Molinari L, Dessalvi S, Santi PL, Campisi C. Lymphatic complications in surgery: possibility of prevention and therapeutic options. Updates Surg. 2012; 64(3):211–216
[39] Demirtas Y, Ozturk N, Yapici O, Topalan M. Comparison of primary and secondary lower-extremity lymphedema treated with supermicrosurgical lymphaticovenous anastomosis and lymphaticovenous implantation. J Reconstr Microsurg. 2010; 26 (2):137–143
[40] Földi M, Földi E. Földi's Textbook of Lymphology for Physicians and Lymphedema Therapists. 2nd ed. Munich, Germany: Mosby Elsevier GmbH; 2006:115–117
[41] Leduc O. Drainage lymphatique manuel selon la « méthode Leduc ». EMC - Kinésithérapie-Médecine Physique-Réadaptation 2013. Doi: 10.1016/S1283-0887(13)56651-5
[42] Medina-Rodríguez ME, de-la-Casa-Almeida M, Martel-Almeida E, Ojeda-Cárdenes A, Medrano-Sánchez EM. Visualization of accessory lymphatic pathways, before and after manual drainage, in secondary upper limb lymphedema using indocyanine green lymphography. J Clin Med. 2019; 8(11):1917
[43] Winters H, Tielemans HJP, Sprangers PN, Ulrich DJO. Peri-operative care for patients undergoing lymphaticovenular anastomosis: a systematic review. J Plast Reconstr Aesthet Surg. 2017; 70(2):178–188
[44] Lane K, Worsley D, McKenzie D. Exercise and the lymphatic system: implications for breast-cancer survivors. Sports Med. 2005; 35(6): 461–471
[45] Carlson DJ, Dieberg G, Hess NC, Millar PJ, Smart NA. Isometric exercise training for blood pressure management: a systematic review and meta-analysis. Mayo Clin Proc. 2014; 89(3):327–334
[46] Chang D, Dayan J, Fried P, et al. Establishing standards for centers of excellence for the diagnosis and treatment of lymphatic disease. Lymphat Res Biol. 2021; 19(1):4–10
[47] Lentz R, Shin C, Bloom Z, et al. From bench to bedside: the role of a multidisciplinary approach to treating patients with lymphedema. Lymphat Res Biol. 2021; 19(1):11–16
[48] Marchica P, D'Arpa S, Magno S, et al. Integrated treatment of breast cancer-related lymphedema: a descriptive review of the state of the art. Anticancer Res. 2021; 41(7):3233–3246
[49] Maegawa J, Yabuki Y, Tomoeda H, Hosono M, Yasumura K. Outcomes of lymphaticovenous side-to-end anastomosis in peripheral lymphedema. J Vasc Surg. 2012; 55(3):753–760
[50] Wong MM-K, Liu H-L. Treatment of physiotherapy-refractory secondary upper limb lymphedema with vascularized lymph node transfer: a case report with clinical and bioimpedance analysis correlation. Breast Dis. 2015; 35(4):263–266
[51] Yamamoto T, Yamamoto N, Hayashi A, Koshima I. Supermicrosurgical deep lymphatic vessel-to-venous anastomosis for a breast cancer-related arm lymphedema with severe sclerosis of superficial lymphatic vessels. Microsurgery. 2017; 37(2):156–159
[52] Salgado CJ, Sassu P, Gharb BB, Spanio di Spilimbergo S, Mardini S, Chen H-C. Radical reduction of upper extremity lymphedema with preservation of perforators. Ann Plast Surg. 2009; 63(3):302–306
[53] Penha TR, Ijsbrandy C, Hendrix NA, et al. Microsurgical techniques for the treatment of breast cancer-related lymphedema: a systematic review. J Reconstr Microsurg. 2013; 29(2):99–106
[54] Basta MN, Gao LL, Wu LC. Operative treatment of peripheral lymphedema: a systematic meta-analysis of the efficacy and safety of lymphovenous microsurgery and tissue transplantation. Plast Reconstr Surg. 2014; 133(4):905–913
[55] Todd M. Selecting compression hosiery. Br J Nurs. 2015; 24(4): 210–212
[56] A Brown. Flat knit hosiery and compression wraps: managing lower limb lymphoedema. Journal of Prescribing Practice. 2019; 1(Sup11): S8--S14
[57] Winters H, Tielemans HJP, Hameeteman M, et al. The efficacy of lymphaticovenular anastomosis in breast cancer-related lymphedema. Breast Cancer Res Treat. 2017; 165(2):321–327
[58] Demirtas Y, Ozturk N, Yapici O, Topalan M. Supermicrosurgical lymphaticovenular anastomosis and lymphaticovenous implantation for treatment of unilateral lower extremity lymphedema. Microsurgery. 2009; 29(8):609–618
[59] Koshima I, Narushima M, Yamamoto Y, Mihara M, Iida T. Recent advancement on surgical treatments for lymphedema. Ann Vasc Dis. 2012; 5(4):409–415
[60] Belcaro G, Errichi BM, Cesarone MR, et al. Lymphatic tissue transplant in lymphedema—a minimally invasive, outpatient, surgical method: a 10-year follow-up pilot study. Angiology. 2008; 59(1):77–83
[61] Koshima I, Nanba Y, Tsutsui T, Takahashi Y, Itoh S, Fujitsu M. Minimal invasive lymphaticovenular anastomosis under local anesthesia for leg lymphedema: is it effective for stage III and IV? Ann Plast Surg. 2004; 53(3):261–266
[62] Brahmbhatt P, Sabiston CM, Lopez C, et al. Feasibility of prehabilitation prior to breast cancer surgery: a mixed-methods study. Front Oncol. 2020; 10:571091
[63] Freire de Oliveira MM, Costa Gurgel MS, Pace do Amaral MT, et al. Manual lymphatic drainage and active exercise effects on lymphatic function do not translate into morbidities in women who underwent breast cancer surgery. Arch Phys Med Rehabil. 2017; 98(2):256–263
[64] Johnstone PA, Hawkins K, Hood S. Role of patient adherence in maintenance of results after manipulative therapy for lymphedema. J Soc Integr Oncol. 2006; 4(3):125–129
[65] Shields JW. Central lymph propulsion. Lymphology. 1980; 13(1):9–17
[66] Onoda S, Nishimon K. The utility of surgical and conservative combination therapy for advanced stage lymphedema. J Vasc Surg Venous Lymphat Disord. 2021; 9(1):234–241

Section VI

Lymphoreconstructive Procedures

Edited by Yves Harder, Christoph Hirche, Katrin Seidenstücker, and Moustapha Hamdi

VI

8 Lymphovenous Anastomosis

Johnson Chia-Shen Yang and Christoph Hirche

Summary

Supermicrosurgical lymphovenous anastomosis has become one of the workhorses for lymphedema treatment and is a targeted procedure with limited invasiveness, which of all reconstructive surgical procedures does the least harm to the patient. It is a bypass procedure that is characterized by anastomosis of distal lymphatic vessels to a recipient vein in the lymphedematous limb. The concept entails several patent lymphovenous anastomoses per extremity. The technique requires veins without major backflow and functional and detectable lymphatic collectors, ideally adjacent to the veins which are localized with the help of blue dye, indocyanine green, magnetic resonance lymphangiography, or simply surgical exploration. Although most surgeons have defined lymphovenous anastomosis as most indicated for early to mid-lymphedema stages, some surgeons have shown successful exploration and lymphovenous anastomosis with comparable outcomes to vascularized lymph node transfer even in advanced stages in which the dermal backflow makes the navigation to functional collectors more difficult. Primary lymphedema may not be a good candidate for lymphovenous anastomosis due to a high probability of lymphatic vessel hypo- or even aplasia. Several configurations of anastomosing the lymphatic collector(s) to the vein, including intravascular stenting superfine instruments constitute the microsurgeon's armamentarium to consistently and successfully perform lymphovenous anastomoses using 0.3- to 0.8-mm vessel.

Keywords: end-to-end anastomosis, end-to-side anastomosis, functional lymphatic vessels, lambda shape, lymphedema, lymphovenous anastomosis (LVA), minimally invasive, octopus technique, supermicrosurgery

8.1 Introduction

8.1.1 Definition

Lymphovenous anastomosis (LVA) is a bypass procedure which works quite straightforwardly through anastomosing the lymphatic vessels to the recipient vein (or venule) in the lymphedematous limb, and new routes are created for draining the accumulated lymph into the peripheral venous system distal to the injured zone.

LVAs are generally performed in regions where lymphatic vessels are least affected by previous surgery or irradiation. A small incision and relatively shallow dissection are required for LVAs, making it a minimally invasive procedure that is the least harmful to the patient as compared to other surgical interventions for lymphedema treatment (▶ Fig. 8.1).

Multiple LVAs in several regions of the lymphedematous limb including functional lymphatic collectors of various draining areas together represent the LVA concept to treat an affected limb. The number of LVAs required to treat an affected extremity successfully varies significantly and has not been finally determined, and patients have been treated with LVAs ranging between 1 and 18 and more incisions sites and anastomosis.

After the introduction of supermicrosurgical LVA by Professor Isao Koshima in 2000,[1] LVA has become a workhorse for lymphedema treatment. When LVA was first introduced in the 1960s, concerns among microsurgeons as to whether proper anastomosis could be achieved in such small lymphatic vessel–which is usually about 0.3 to 0.8 mm in diameter–were not uncommon. With advancements of supermicrosurgical instruments and high-power microscopes in the past decades, lymphatic surgery has been made relatively easier. Nevertheless, LVA remained a technically demanding procedure requiring advanced microsurgical skills, super-thin instruments, and special equipment. Thus, solid basic microsurgical training and proper microsurgical concepts are key for performing a proper LVA. "True" LVA as a supermicrosurgical anastomosis with high magnification, super-thin instruments and special suture of United States Pharmacopeia (USP) size 11–0 to 12–0 restricts its application by surgeon/equipment-related factors, and its effectiveness is further limited by technical constraints. The lymphovenous implantation or "octopus" LVA technique is an alternative "anastomosis" in which several distal lymphatic vessels are placed and sleeved in the lumen of a vein, addressing the above problems (also see **Subchapter 8.5**).

Supermicrosurgery

Supermicrosurgery is a new technique and concept based on further development of microsurgery that allows very small vessels (e.g., arteries, veins/venules, and lymphatic vessels) with a diameter of less than 1 mm (usually 0.3–0.8 mm) to be dissected and sewed for new surgical options. Preconditions, which enabled supermicrosurgery, are particularly fine surgical instruments and microscopes with up to 40 × magnification and high depth of shield and resolution. Extremely thin sutures are used which, according to the USP classification, have a thickness of 11–0 to 12–0, i.e., less than 0.1 mm.

The method has expanded the surgical possibilities to close soft tissue defects after accidents with flaps with reduced donor sites, fingertip replantation, and successful implementation of LVA or lymphaticolymphatic and lymphaticonodule anastomosis to treat lymphedema.

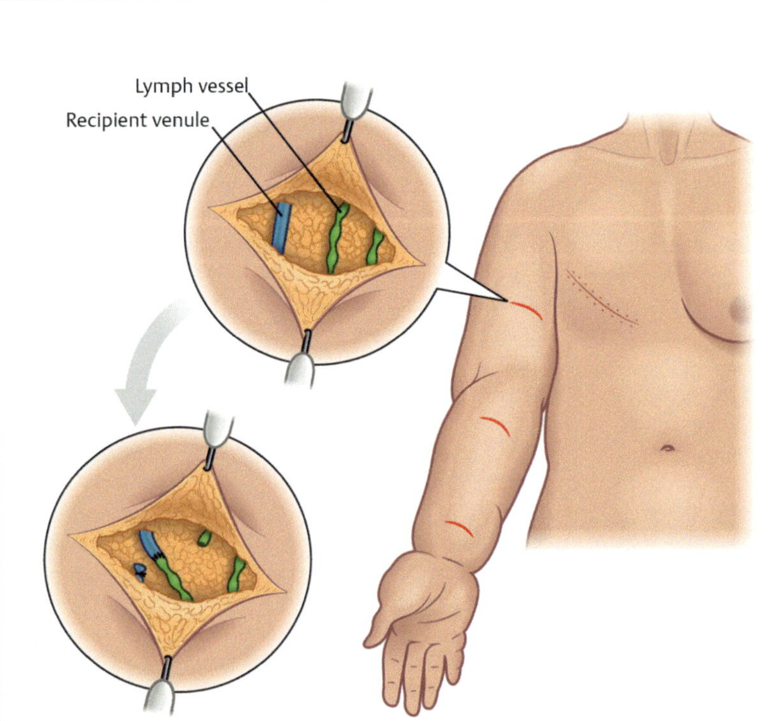

Fig. 8.1 Lymphovenous anastomosis are performed through small skin incisions, followed by gentle dissection of the superficial fat of the edematous extremity. In instances of the identification of functional lymphatic vessels and a sufficient recipient vein/venole, a bypass procedure by anastomosing a distal lymphatic vessel (green) to a proximal recipient vein (or venule) is performed. Different configurations of connecting lymphatic vessels to veins or venules are possible (end-to-end in the present figure, with ligature/clip to distal vein and the proximal lymphatic vessel) in order to drain the accumulated lymph into the peripheral venous system distal to the injured zone.

The masking effects of dermal backflow in indocyanine green lymphangiography

For patients with advanced lymphedema, indocyanine green (ICG) is disseminated in the superficial/dermal layer of the integument due to partially or completely obstructed lymphatic flow. The skin literally "lights up" under a near-infrared camera. The intensity of ICG enhancement from the dermal backflow (DB) can be much brighter than the fluorescent lymphatic vessels underneath. A masking effect from the DB is created, despite having functional lymphatic vessels below. Under such circumstances, it is commonly believed that no functional lymphatic vessels exist in these regions, rendering LVA unsuitable. However, more deeply located functional lymphatic vessels may be present and still be found with meticulous dissection. They are simply "masked" by the superficial DB. As an additional tool to provide further "insights" and three-dimensional resolution, magnetic resonance lymphangiography (MRL) is a useful modality to "demask" functional lymphatic vessels under a DB pattern.

8.1.2 Key Concepts of Supermicrosurgical Lymphovenous Anastomosis

Surgical Considerations for Lymphovenous Anastomosis

Three key components of LVA, as indicated in the title, are the lymphatic vessels/collectors, the recipient vein/venules, and the anastomosis. Ideally, to obtain optimal results from LVA, functional lymphatic vessels, which are uninjured and without morphological changes and (fully) capable of transporting lymph, a reflux-free recipient vein, and an impeccable anastomotic technique are required.

Preparation

When it comes to supermicrosurgical LVA, it is no surprise that everyone focuses mainly on the anastomotic skills. However, the lymphatic vessel and the recipient vein must be well-prepared before any anastomosis can be performed. Successful anastomoses rely on proper preparation of the desirable vessels, as in any type of microsurgery. The key to success is "preparation." The anastomosis part comes later.

Soft Tissue Manipulation

Lymphatic Vessels

To dissect and skeletonize lymphatic vessels smaller than 1 mm is not an easy task. To have a sense of feeling during soft tissue manipulation takes years of training. To isolate the lymphatic vessel when they are buried in the surrounding adipose tissue takes attentiveness. With the help of a microscope-integrated NIR source for lymphangiography, the identification of ICG-enhanced lymphatic vessels is made easier intraoperatively. Alternatively, a blue dye with lymph vessel affinity (e.g., Toluidine Blue, Patent Blue V) can be injected as a second tracer just a few centimeters distal to the LVA incisional site to visualize the uptake to the lymphatic vessel without NIR of the microscope (▶ Fig. 8.2).

> **Note:**
>
> Be mindful of injection pressure and distance, as "blue contamination" may occur throughout the entire LVA situs.

Recipient Vein

A general consideration prior to the choice of recipient vein and its individual function is to exclude severe venous insufficiency of the affected extremity, as it is a lymphedema aggravating disease and will improve the reflux in a way that the LVA becomes afunctional.

The dissection for the recipient vein per se is relatively easier as compared to lymphatic vessels. The recipient veins are somewhat larger with thicker walls. However, the recipient veins are not as abundant as one would think, especially in the thigh area. Therefore, preserving all the veins in the operative field is advised, unless it obstructs further dissection of the lymphatic vessels. When dissecting the recipient vein, as in regular microsurgery, all the branches on the recipient vein should be ligated properly with nylon 11–0 to prevent vessel spasm and hematoma. A great deal of patience is required for vessel preparation. It will eventually pay off. Ideally, avoiding the use of a recipient vein with reflux is the key, although it is not up to microsurgeons to decide most of the time.

The Concept of a Functional Lymphatic Vessel

Pathological changes to lymphatic vessels can occur due to factors such as genetics, aging, infection, trauma, and irradiation. Prolong lymphedema and subsequent cellulitis can further lead to lymphatic vessels deterioration, ultimately causing total occlusion of lymphatic vessels such as sclerosis. As stated earlier, one of the key components for a successful LVA is the identification of functional lymphatic vessels before LVA is performed. Without proper identification, many potentially functional lymphatic vessels can be overlooked and decrease the chance for lymphedema reduction.

Definition of Functional Lymphatic Vessels

What really defines a "functional" LVA should be its ability to directedly transport lymph. ICG lymphangiography has become a popular tool for identifying lymphatic vessels with linear pattern. Logically, ICG-enhanced lymphatic vessels are considered "functional" for its capability to uptake and transport contrast-containing lymph.[3] In contrast, lymphatic vessels not enhanced by ICG are mistakenly regarded as "nonfunctional" and are often abandoned for LVA nowadays. However, many factors can influence whether a lymphatic vessel has an ICG uptake, such as injection site etc.

> **The concept of lymphosome**
>
> The concept of lymphosome was first introduced by Suami et al.[4] A lymphosome is defined as a specific anatomical region where the interstitial fluid is drained by a specific lymphatic vessel. Therefore, whether a lymphatic vessel can be enhanced or not is influenced by the location, the depth, and the amount of ICG injected intradermally. A functional lymphatic vessel will remain nonenhanced due to no contrast in the region it is designated to drain once it stops receiving dye injection. Based on a previous study,[3] we recommend supermicrosurgeons doing LVA to endorse this novel concept of what really defines functional lymphatic vessels. An ICG-nonenhanced, but flow-positive lymphatic vessel should be considered as functional. With this concept in mind, the number of functional lymphatic vessels used for LVA can be increased significantly, and therefore a better outcome can be achieved.

The Concept of Using a Reflux-Free Recipient Vein

A successful LVA relies on two key components: (1) being able to identify "functional" lymphatic vessels, which are still capable of transporting lymph, as stated above; and (2) a nearby recipient vein that is, ideally, reflux-free. As venous pressure is usually higher than the pressure in the lymphatic vessel, a recipient vein with reflux can backflow into lymphatic vessels after anastomosis. This, supposedly, can lead to a lower long-term LVA patency rate, as stated by Yamamoto et al.[2]

Vein Finders/Visualizers

The localization of a recipient vein for LVA can be done using a vein visualizer. A commercially available, noninvasive

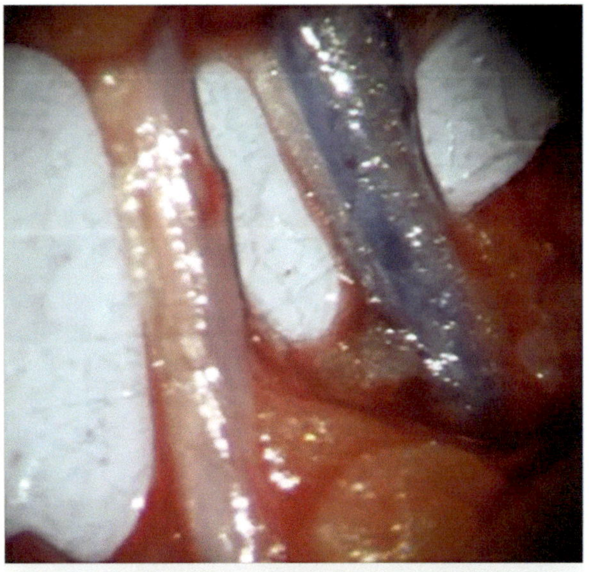

Fig. 8.2 A blue dye with lymph vessel affinity (Patent Blue V) has been injected as a second tracer just a few cm distal to the lymphovenous anastomosis incisional site to visualize the uptake to the lymphatic vessel (stained blue, right vessel) without near-infrared of the microscope.

"vein visualizer" can be used not only for recipient vein localization, but also for selecting a reflux-free vein simultaneously, as stated in our previous publication.[5] The instantaneous, live image from the vein visualizer enables the use of the milking test to identify an ideal reflux-free vein. The advantages of having the locations of both functional lymphatic veins and reflux-free recipient veins preoperatively are as follows: (1) preoperative planning of the incision site, allowing for a smaller incision; (2) predetermination of the orientation of LVA (e.g., end-to-end, end-to-side, side-to-end, or side-to-side); (3) reduction in the operative time because of less time needed for exploration; (4) improvement of surgical outcome mainly because of better long-term LVA patency rate; and (5) reducing the need for valvuloplasty (▶ Fig. 8.2).

The vicinity of reflux-free veins and functional lymphatic vessels can be localized and marked for targeted incisions by combining the of use of vein finders/visualizers and ICG lymphangiography and by MRL in combination with intradermally and intravenously injected contrast agent with three-dimensional marking of veins/venules and lymphatic vessels.

Limitations do exist for finding reflux-free veins with the use of vein visualizer. With limitation in the depth of detection, only superficial veins can be detected. It is reserved for anatomical locations such as dorsal hand/foot, wrist, and elbow for mild lymphedema cases. In proper candidates, the use of a vein visualizer is easy, is associated with a short learning curve, and offers an ideal solution for identifying a reflux-free vein.

8.2 Indications and Contraindications for Lymphovenous Anastomosis

8.2.1 Current Consensus Regarding Surgical Treatment for Lymphedema with Lymphovenous Anastomosis

The algorithm and current concept for the surgical treatment of lymphedema is based on the severity/stage of the lymphedema and the remaining regional function of the lymphatic system of the affected extremity. The International Society of Lymphology (ISL) staging system based on the clinical phenotype is the most commonly used system for evaluating the severity of lymphedema. An additional staging system especially for the indication of microsurgical treatment involves ICG lymphangiography first described by Ogata et al.[6] and the transcutaneous detection of directed or nondirected flow of the affected lymphedematous extremity resulting in the stages (normal, splash, stardust, diffuse (see **Subchapter 4.7**).

For ISL stages 0–I, near-normal to mild lymphedema, the perceptions among some microsurgeons and the advocates for free vascularized lymph node transfer (VLNT) nowadays supported the idea that LVA should be reserved only for mild lymphedema cases, where lymphatic vessel with linear pattern is evident after intradermal ICG injection. ICG-enhanced lymphatic vessels with a linear pattern are considered functional collectors, with the capability to uptake ICG from the interstitial fluid and transport ICG within the lymphatic channels. LVA is therefore recommended when linear lymphatic vessel is not recognized by ICG.

For ISL stages II–III, moderate to severe lymphedema, with a more prominent swelling or severely deformed lymphedematous limbs, a "dermal backflow" either with splash, star dust, or diffuse pattern becomes evident. Lymphatic vessels generally cannot be observed after ICG injection.

Indocyanine Green Lymphangiography Visualizing Dermal Backflow

For mild lymphedema patients, ICG-enhanced lymphatic vessels with linear patterns can be observed with the use of NIR camera. This enables microsurgeons to pinpoint the lymphatic vessel preoperatively, which can reduce the need for blind dissection and thus shorten operative time. Other than linear pattern which represents functional lymphatic vessels, a phenomenon called "dermal backflow" can be observed, signifying total or partial obstruction of lymphatic system. Dermal Backflow (DB) is a result of the inability of lymphatic vessels to absorb and transport the ICG proximally, leaving the epidermis and dermal layer "flooded" with the static or slow migrating ICG. The disseminated contrast will light up the integument under NIR camera. The severity of lymphedema can be correlated to the different patterns of DB such as splash, star dust, and diffuse.[2]

8.2.2 Indications

Based on the current guidelines for the surgical treatment of lymphedema by Kung et al.,[7] LVA is reserved only for mild lymphedema patients where lymphatic vessels can be identified either with MRL or ICG lymphangiography. VLNT or dermolipectomies are recommended for moderate to severe lymphedema patients. The main reason for abandoning LVA is based on the concept that lymphatic vessels are considered nonfunctional when they cannot be detected either by MRL or ICG lymphangiography.

Note:

Functional lymphatic vessels can be visualized with the ICG lymphangiography in early stages but can be masked in progressed stages II and III, where remaining functional vessels can be principally approached for LVA. In early stages, it is more likely to find several lymphatic vessels successfully for LVA than in progressed stages, but LVA should not be reserved only for mild lymphedema cases.

The anastomosis is performed within the adipose tissue, with minimal damage to the soft tissue. Therefore, LVA is the least harmful among all the procedures for surgical lymphedema treatment. The major limitation for LVA is the quality of lymphatic vessels. The pathological changes of the lymphatic vessels such as sclerosis will render lymphatic vessels functionless and minimize the capability of lymphatic vessels to transport lymph, as mentioned by Mihara et al.[8] The sclerotic changes are usually irreversible once they have occurred.

Due to its minimally invasive character, LVA should be considered as the first line of treatment for lymphedema and even for much more severe cases, such as lymphorrhea with infection. Even though DB has obscured lymphatic vessels, it does not signify nonexistence or nonfunctional lymphatic vessels. Although successful exploration and finish of LVA can be expected in early-stage lymphedema I and II, more decisive and exhausting dissection may be expected in progressed stages II and III. In addition, patients require informed consent that in progressed stages LVA may not be successful to significantly resolve lymphedema, and failed exploration may occur, requiring VLNT, suction-assisted lipectomy, or surgical excision by dermolipectomy.

8.2.3 Contraindications

Primary lymphedema, such as Milroy's disease, may not be a good candidate for LVA because of the high probability of missing lymphatic vessel due to lymphatic system aplasia. As for the severely deformed lymphedematous limb, performing LVA alone is not enough. Although LVA is able to provide a route to relief lymphostasis, excisional therapy is needed to correct the excessively distorted soft tissue. Central lymphatic obstruction such as partial or total obstruction of thoracic duct should be ruled out for patient without any prior history. For those with central venous partial obstruction such as iliac vein compression or kinking, interventions such as stenting should be done before receiving LVA.

For peripheral venous insufficiency, such as varicose veins, it is considered as a contraindication for LVA, as peripheral venous insufficiency must be regarded as lymphedema aggravating disease with increased peripheral pressures which do not enable acceptable pressure gradients for functional LVA. Due to valvular insufficiency, part of the venous blood becomes static, resulting in engorged vein. However, varicose veins might not be evident in moderate to severe lymphedema patients since it can be masked by the swollen, tense integument. Such cases can still benefit from LVA, where varicose veins have become more prominent after lymphedema reduction, even when anastomoses were carried out on recipient veins with dysfunctional valve. The transportation of lymph into the recipient vein after LVA can be aided by both the internal and external pump.

8.3 Preoperative Evaluation and Planning

Preoperative evaluation regarding the general condition of the patient, the severity of lymphedema, and in particular the LVA-related criteria such as the location of lymphatic vessels and recipient vein using imaging modalities can help the surgeons to obtain information to plan ahead as to where to perform the anastomoses before the operation (see **Chapter 4**).

8.3.1 Medical History

As emphasized in almost every medical textbook, a detailed history of present illness is essential, including previous surgical operation received for cancer treatment, the extent of lymphadenectomy, the implementation of adjuvant chemotherapy/radiotherapy, the timing of lymphedema onset, the frequency of cellulitis episode, prior treatment received for lymphedema (i.e., complete decongestive therapy, free lymph node transfer, lipectomy, stenting [for venous obstruction]), and medications such as diuretics, anticoagulants, and steroids.

Note:

Peripheral venous diseases such as deep vein thrombosis and varicose veins, venous insufficiency, and relevant preceding surgeries to the venous system are particularly relevant for LVA surgery.

8.3.2 Preoperative Evaluation for Lymphovenous Anastomosis

A successful LVA relies on two key components: (1) being able to identify "functional" lymphatic vessels, which are still capable of transporting lymph; and (2) a nearby recipient vein that is, ideally, reflux-free. The advantages of locating functional lymphatic collecting vessels and reflux-free recipient veins preoperatively are as follows:

- Preoperatively planned incision sites can allow smaller incisions (targeted incision).
- Based on the number, the proximity, and the orientation of target lymphatic vessels, the type of LVA can be often predetermined (e.g., end-to-end, end-to-side, side-to-end, or side-to-side anastomosis).
- Reduced operative time.
- No damage of target lymphatic vessels due to blind exploration.
- Improved surgical outcome by utilizing functional lymphatic vessels and reflux-free recipient vein.
- Use of reflux-free recipient veins can reduce the need for additional manipulations such as valvuloplasty.
- Informed patient consent for second-line treatment as VLNT in instances of lack of functional lymphatic vessels and frustrated exploration in the same operation.

8.3.3 Identifying Functional Lymphatic Vessels

For the staging of lymphedema severity,[2] ICG lymphangiography is the basis to indicate LVA with its particular ICG severity pattern including DB patterns and is regarded to be superior to lymphoscintigraphy.[15]

For mild lymphedema patients, localization of functional lymphatic vessel is possible with ICG lymphangiography, but the penetration depth is limited to 1 to 2 cm and it is most useful for the distal parts of the extremities.

The portability of the system allows detection of "functional" lymphatic vessels in the ward, outpatient clinic, and operation theater.

It provides much-needed information for the surgery and is more sensitive than lymphoscintigraphy.

It is a useful tool for planning the site and length of incisions, when combined with vein finder for location of recipient veins, allowing shorter operative time.

8.3.4 Timing for the Indocyanine Green Injection for the Identification of Functional Lymphatic Vessels

The timing for locating lymphatic vessel requires some experience and should take the following issues into consideration:

Linear pattern with good visibility of lymphatic vessels can sometimes be observed immediately after ICG injection in mild to moderate patients. However, due to lymphatic flow obstruction, ICG will eventually become saturated in the dermal layer, causing the phenomenon of DB, and make the linear pattern of lymphatic vessel shortly invisible. The more severe the lymphedema, the faster the DB will appear. A window of opportunity does exist for locating linear lymphatic vessels right after ICG injection in some moderate lymphedema patients, requiring early action for marking on the skin before the DB takes over.

The speed with which ICG travels proximally is equal to the lymphatic velocity, which is dependent on the severity of lymphedema. The more severe the lymphedema, the slower the ICG will travel proximally. Oftentimes, the ICG remains static distally, even with manual massage to force the ICG proximally. Lymphatic vessels cannot be identified in such a scenario; however, for mild to moderate cases, with partial lymphatic flow obstruction, some lymphatic vessels are visible immediately after ICG is injected intradermally. The best time for ICG injection is in the operating room (OR) after general anesthesia and locating linear lymphatic vessel whenever possible.

Based on the authors' experience, the dorsal foot, ankle, and dorsal hands regions have higher possibilities to local "functional" lymphatic vessels with ICG lymphangiography.

With this concept in mind, one should realize that when patients present with DB, such as splash, stardust, and diffuse pattern, it does not signify that there are no lymphatic vessels, nor that they are nonfunctional underneath. DB is only a phenomenon of ICG spreading across dermal layer due to obstructed lymphatic flow, masking lymphatic vessels underneath. In fact, most of the lymphatic vessels uncovered underneath DB remain functional, and they are capable of reducing lymphedema when anastomosed properly to a recipient vein.

8.3.5 Identifying Reflux-Free Veins with a Vein Finder (Vein Viewer)

Venous pressure is usually higher than lymphatic collecting vessel pressure, thus a recipient vein with reflux can flood back into the lymphatic collecting vessel after LVA (backflow test). This can lead to a lower long-term LVA patency rate.

A commercially available, noninvasive "vein visualizer" can be used not only for recipient vein localization, but

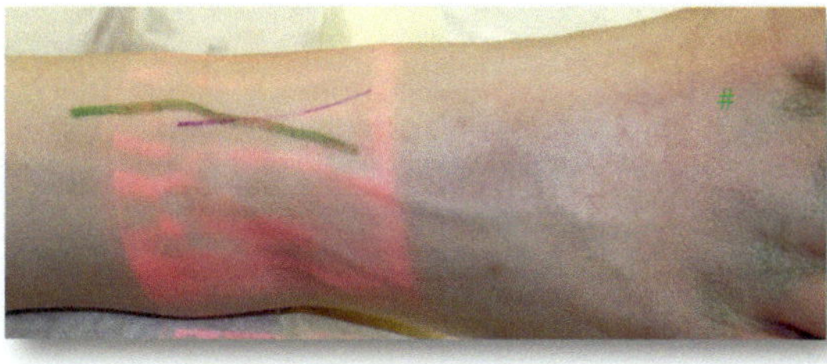

Fig. 8.3 The use of a vein finder with near-infrared technique is shown, identifying dorsal foot veins, which are marked in green on the skin for further surgery. A milking technique enables the identification of functional, nonreflux veins.

also for selecting a reflux-free vein simultaneously. The instantaneous, live image from the vein visualizer enables the use of the milking test to identify an ideal reflux-free vein (▶ Fig. 8.3).

However, there are limitations to finding a reflux-free vein with a vein visualizer. Because of its limitation as to the depth of superficial vein it can detect, it can be used only for mild to moderate lymphedema cases and reserved for anatomical locations such as dorsal hand/foot, wrist, and elbow. Despite this limitation, the use of a vein visualizer is easy, is associated with a short learning curve, and offers an ideal solution for identifying a reflux-free vein in suitable patients.

▶ Fig. 8.3 shows the use of a vein finder with NIR technique for identifying dorsal foot veins. A milking test enables the identification of functional, nonreflux veins. The injection site of ICG to the folds between the toes is shown with "#" sign.

8.3.6 Other Imaging Studies for Preoperative Evaluation and Planning of Lymphovenous Anastomosis

Lymphoscintigraphy was considered to be the golden standard for lymphedema diagnosis; however, other diagnostic modalities are emerging (see **Chapter 3**). It can be used as a prognostic factor to predict patient's response to complete decongestive therapy,[9] or as a surgical indicator for performing LVA.[10] Nevertheless, some limitations for LVA remain:

- The images from lymphoscintigraphy are too coarse which provide limited information regarding lymphatic vessel orientation to be used for LVA.
- It is a painful and long-lasting procedure requiring special, huge equipment and thus is not suitable as a screening technique in outpatient clinic and for intraoperative navigation.
- Accessibility is limited, and not every hospital is equipped with nuclear medicine and radiocolloid. Advanced appointments needed for examination due to radiocolloid availability.

MRL has shown higher sensitivity in lymphedema detection as compared to lymphoscintigraphy.[11] MRL is suitable for identification of both lymphatic vessel and vein for LVA with several technical and software-based solutions to render ideal LVA points.[12]

It has the advantage of combining MRL, resolution of fat content, and limb volumetry for accurate measurement of the volume of lymphedematous limb. The soft tissue composition can be distinguished with MR images.

Nevertheless, claustrophobia is an issue for patients, and most patients have complained about MRI being too noisy, even with ear plugs. It is time-consuming as a scan takes 40 to 60 minutes on average, and patients need to lie down flat and maintain their position, which can be stressful for the elderly. The technique is not useful as a screening tool for LVA or intraoperative navigation.

Ultrasound has been well-demonstrated by Hayashi et al.,[14] and has the chance to overcome the shortcoming of ICG lymphangiography, where LVs are masked by DB. The identification of deeper lymphatics is made possible with ultrasound. It is portable for use at the ward, at the outpatient clinic, and for intraoperative navigation for LVA. The main advantage of using ultrasonography is to be able to identify the lymphatic vessels and the recipient veins simultaneously. It further provides information about the relative depth of lymphatic vessels. It can be regarded as a supplement to ICG lymphangiography.

There are several, noteworthy limitations: Ultrasound and its use for LVA evaluation has a steep learning curve, and it is not as intuitive as compared to ICG lymphangiography. It is an operator-dependent modality. Lymphatic vessels < 0.3 mm may be mistaken as nerve fascicle. A high-definition ultrasound machine is needed, including probes with 45 to 70 MHz.

8.4 Surgical Setting and Technique

8.4.1 Anesthesia: Local, Regional, or General

Whether supermicrosurgery using LVA should be performed under general or local anesthesia really depends on the hospital resources/policy, the patient's individual considerations and wishes, and the surgeon's choice. Local anesthesia for LVA carries minimal risk as illustrated by Chan et al.,[17] but patient's compliance needs to be taken into consideration since they will be conscious and have to lie down for a minimum of 4 to 5 hours, with minimal allowance for movements during supermicrosurgery; it is no easy task, especially for the elderly patient. Local anesthesia is best suited for patients who are at high risk with general anesthesia. However, to achieve this task in such a short time, multiple microscopes and supermicrosurgeons are needed. This can be problematic for a smaller facility.

Supermicrosurgery performed under general anesthesia, on the other hand, allows for longer operating hours, as the patient's compliance is no longer a factor, and the surgery does not need to be rushed. The use of general anesthesia is also best suited for the entry-level supermicrosurgeons who need time to think and adjust intraoperatively. The disadvantage, however, is that long-lasting elective surgeries conducted on single patients mean that fewer patients can be treated in a given timeframe. The economic pressure faced by certain health-care systems has therefore resulted in the avoidance of long-lasting surgeries performed under general anesthesia in order to make better use of OR-capacity and to treat more patients who might also need surgery. Another factor worth considering is that, despite recent advancements in general anesthesia, it still carries a higher risk for the patient as compared with local anesthesia.

Regional anesthesia with spinal anesthesia for the lower extremity and plexus anesthesia for the upper extremity can be a good compromise for reducing movements to the treated extremity without the risks of general anesthesia. Nevertheless, some drawbacks from local anesthesia remain for the patient.

Note:

The use of virtual reality (VR) glasses and headphones can render long-lasting LVA surgery performed under local or regional anesthesia much more comfortable for the patient.

8.4.2 Intraoperative Position

Posture

The most important thing about microsurgery, especially supermicrosurgery, is the ability to find the most comfortable intraoperative posture for the surgeon. To endure such a long operation, for at least 4 to 5 hours, a supermicrosurgeon must have a relaxed, aligned back, sitting on an adjustable, properly cushioned operative chair. Knowing how to find and fine-tune the optimal posture while gazing into the microscope is no less important than the supermicrosurgery itself. Without proper posture, one can get tired easily; once that happens, hand tremor becomes obvious, which can be problematic when trying to complete an anastomosis at the level of supermicrosurgery.

Three-dimensional LVA with 3D glasses and screens for both the surgeon and the surgeon's assistant has recently been reported to improve comfortable intraoperative posture for the surgeon and ergonomics for supermicrosurgery (▶ Fig. 8.4a,b).[16]

Proper Cushioning

Even with an optimal upright posture, hand tremors can still be obvious without proper cushioning. When performing an extremely delicate surgery such as LVA, proper support of the wrist and hypothenar area is essential before the shoulder, elbow, and wrist can be relaxed properly. This can minimize any unwanted tremors originating from the larger joints from the upper limb, allowing only intrinsic muscles in the hands to maneuver the needle holder and microforceps. An added cushion can be prepared with the use of rolled-up surgical draping.

Note:

An optimal patient positioning in combination with the abovementioned recommendation is the basis for optimal posture and proper cushioning for supermicrosurgeons.

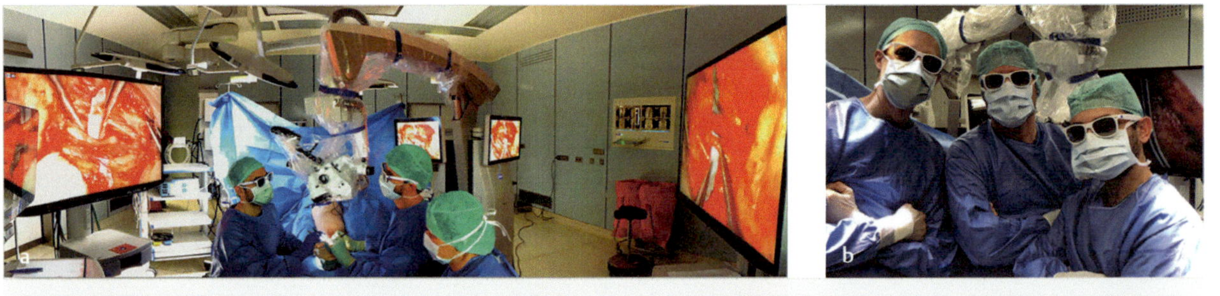

Fig. 8.4 Hybrid visualization microscopy involves the combined use of optics and digital displays. **(a)** This setup allows a comfortable ergonomic posture, providing the surgeon with more freedom of movement. Furthermore, it also allows better communication with the rest of the team, who can also follow the surgeon's movement on the screens and can include several observers. The surgical microscope (Zeiss Kinevo 900, Germany) is positioned over the patient in a conventional way. A magnified image of the operative field is projected on two opposite large high-resolution screens, which in combination with 3D glasses **(b)** can provide an immersive three-dimensional experience.

8.4.3 Technique of Supermicrosurgical Lymphovenous Anastomosis

Lymphatic Vessels—the Donor

Multisite Anastomosis

Since LVA is a bypass surgery, it is therefore sensible to perform as many LVAs as possible in order to create more routes and diversions for lymphatic drainage, as stated by Mihara et al.[18] Nevertheless, the impact of the number of LVAs in relation to the effect on relief of lymphedema has not been evaluated on a standardized LVAs as possible in order to create more routes and diversions for lymphatic drainage level, so surgeons around the world still have different approaches to applying multisite LVA, and 1 to 18 LVAs per extremity have been reported.

As there is an occlusion rate of approximately 50% after 2 years detected in smaller series, a minimum of three LVAs should be applied, keeping in mind that more LVAs create more routes and diversions for lymphatic drainage.

Intravascular Stenting

It was first mentioned by Narushima et al.[19] in 2010 and is one of the most useful technical steps applied for LVA. It can be used on nearly transparent lymphatic vessels, such as the ectatic type. The lumen of an ectatic lymphatic vessel will tend to collapse and becomes flattened after it is transected. With the placement of a stent within the lumen, it makes the anastomosis much more feasible. It can also be applied to lymphatic vessels with constriction type, where they are small in diameter and is difficult to be visualized under the microscope. The stent is commercially available, but due to health ministry regulation in different countries, it is not always certified. For a do-it-yourself stent, use a segment of a blue nylon 5–0, about 1 mm in length. The stenting method is not limited to lymphatic vessels only. It can also be applied to the recipient vein in the same fashion.

Note:

A lymphatic vessel that requires a stent smaller than nylon 5–0 is considered too small for LVA. There is no need to spend time on such a small lymphatic vessel, unless there is no other choice.

Double Barrel Lymphatic Vessels

Occasionally, two lymphatic vessels can be found aligned to each other closely, which grossly resemble a "double barrel shotgun." These small lymphatic vessels are usually in the range of around 0.3 to 0.4 mm, which might be too small for a direct anastomosis to a larger vein. These double barrel vessels can be fused together to obtain a larger caliber for anastomosis to the recipient vein, either with fusion lymphoplasty or monocanalization as mentioned by Yamamoto et al.[20]

Veins and Venules—the Recipients

With increasing experience in LVA, one will realize that locating a suitable recipient vein is not an easier task than finding functional, sizable lymphatic vessels. The truth is that the recipient veins are not as abundant as we once thought. The density of recipient vessels is inverse proportional to the proximity in the limbs. The recipient veins are abundant in the dorsal foot/ankle, or in the dorsal hand/wrist, but scarce in the thigh and upper arm. Oftentimes incisions need to be extended to locate the recipient veins. But with the help of vein visualizer and Doppler echo, the incidence of not finding a recipient vein can be decreased. Several vein grafting methods were described by Yamamoto et al.[21] with *in situ* vein grafting and t-shaped vein graft by Visconti et al.[22] To reduce the possible venous reflux, Yamamoto and Koshima implemented the idea of neo-valvuloplasty.[23]

Microvascular Lymphovenous Implantation—"Octopus Lymphovenous Anastomosis"

"True" LVA has been shown to have a higher patency rate as compared to lymphovenous implantation in a rat model, although no significant difference in the clinical effect is noted.[25] However, sizable lymphatic vessels are not always available, even after much time and effort spent. There are times where only lymphatic vessels smaller than 0.2 mm can be found. For such small lymphatic vessels, direct anastomosis is technically difficult and time-consuming. The efforts put into such small lymphatic vessels can be disproportional to post-LVA improvement. This is where lymphovenous implantation by Campisi et al.,[25] or the "octopus" method by Chen et al.,[26] comes into play. Multiple small caliber lymphatic vessels can be implanted into a larger vein with a few anchoring sutures. It can be done in a relatively short period of time as compared to supermicrosurgical LVA. However, anastomotic site leakage is not uncommon among lymphovenous implantation since a watertight seal cannot be obtained simply by anchoring sutures. The leakage is usually due to venous reflux for recipient veins larger than 0.8 mm. A recipient vein with reflux is regarded to have a lower long-term patency rate. Hematoma as well as iatrogenic lymphatic fistula can also result from anastomotic leakage after lymphovenous implantation or "octopus," which can also result from leakage after "true" LVA.

Originally, the technique had been described for more proximally located "octopus" anastomosis, often as a single anastomosis site, to a major vein in vicinity to the hiatus saphenous, directly to the injured groin in lower extremity lymphedema or the axillary vein directly after axillary lymph node dissection, which is referred to as a prophylactic approach.

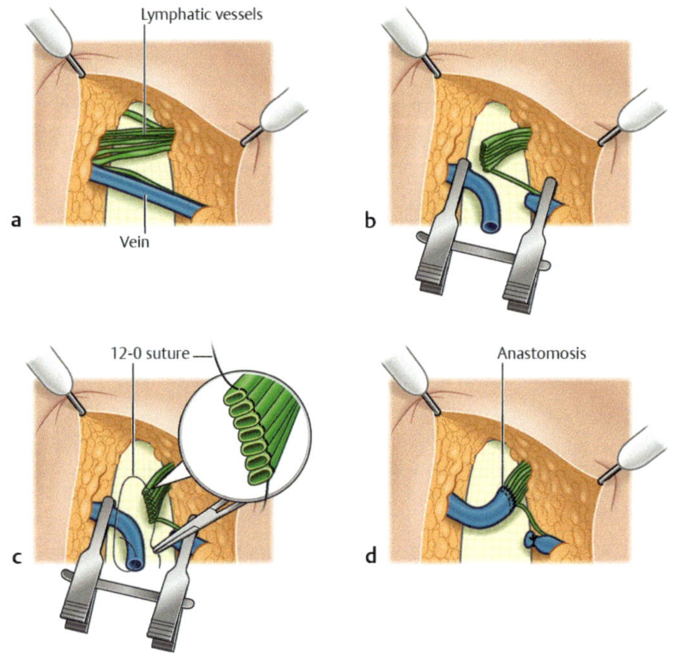

Fig. 8.5 The "octopus" technique is an alternative way to anastomose lymphatic vessels to a vein or venule, by connecting several very small distal adjacent lymphatic vessels into a proximal vein or venule in the presence of a relevant size mismatch **(a,b)**. The lymphatic vessels are ligated/clipped proximally and sleeved into the vein, then fixed using adventitial stitched to somehow "intubate" the vein that is further restricted to match the lymphatic's diameter. The vein is further distally ligated/clipped. After skeletonizing and aligning the lymphatic vessels **(a)**, a supermicrosurgical suture (e.g., 12–0) is first placed through the vein (outside inside), then continued by piercing stepwise the adventitia of each lymphatic vessels that are placed in a parallel row **(b)**. The suture's loop is then completed by placing the stitch back through the vein (inside outside) **(c)**. The lymphatic vessels intussuscept into the vein's lumen. Eventually, additional stitches are placed between the adventitia of the vein and the lymphatic vessels to tighten up the anastomosis **(d)**. (Adapted with permission from Chen et al.[27] and Boccardo F, Casabona F, De Cian F, et al. Lymphedema microsurgical preventive healing approach: a new technique for primary prevention of arm lymphedema after mastectomy. Ann Surg Oncol 2009;16(3):703–708.)

Patients are reported to have a prompt relief of lymphedema symptoms with stable long-term results analogous to the "true," segmental anastomosis. Overall, the technique is found to be easier compared to the standard supermicrosurgical LVA and could be performed using a standard surgical microscope.

It remains an alternative to the standard LVA technique and has the potential of simplifying this technically challenging procedure. Until today, a direct comparison to the "true" LVA is missing, and from some microsurgeons' perspective the placement without a proper anastomosis with less magnifying equipment does not allow sufficient standardization.

Nevertheless, the "octopus" technique, that is the sleeving in of lymphatic vessels into a greater vein with a mismatch of size, can definitely be regarded as a drawback option in cases with very low diameter lymphatic vessels even for segmental LVA (▶ Fig. 8.5).

8.4.4 Which Suture Technique is Best Suited for Supermicrosurgery?

General factors that influence the type of suturing technique used for supermicrosurgery are:
- adhesive forces;
- hydrophilic property of nylon 11–0;
- hypocoagulative state of lymphatic fluid.

In most lymphedema patients, the raw surface is usually filled with interstitial fluid or the precursor as lymph. In some severe cases, a constant flux of lymph out of the incision wound is not uncommon. Keeping the operative field near to dry is almost an impossible task. The combination of adhesive force from the lymph and the unique hydrophilic property of nylon makes nylon particularly "sticky" when it comes in contact with the lymphatic fluid. The hypocoagulative state of lymph, mainly due to the lack of coagulation factor and platelet, although not as strong as blood, can still coagulate but at a slower speed. This sticky situation makes it difficult to manage and tie the nylon, especially the loops from continuous-interrupted sutures before the stitches are tied individually. An extremely tiny suture such as nylon 11–0 definitely makes it even more difficult.

The authors' recommendations include:
- Using interrupted sutures to complete most of the stitches, and continuous-interrupted sutures for the last three to four stitches to exclude iatrogenic occlusion due to stitches to the back wall.

- Continuous suture is difficult to be adjusted properly due to distortion to the anastomosis site after tightening the sutures to prevent leakage.
- Hydrophobic suturing material such as Prolene (Polypropylene) may be considered. Prolene is also stiffer than nylon which can help to maintain its shape as loops, which should make tying the stitches easier.

LVA anastomosis in "magnified" steps

Anterior wall-first approach: This is the most commonly adopted method used by microsurgeons. It can only be used when the vessels can be flipped over. It has a high possibility to catch the posterior wall.

Posterior wall-first approach: It is very useful when the lymphatic vessel and the recipient vein cannot be flipped over to do anastomosis for microsurgery. This method minimizes the chance of unnoticed catching of the posterior wall. However, high magnification with the operative field almost flooded with interstitial fluid can make this approach much more difficult. Regardless, it is a much-needed skill when performing supermicrosurgery. One should master anterior approach first before attempting posterior wall approach.

8.4.5 Documentation

The authors recommend keeping standardized and accurate records of all intraoperative surgical interventions as well as the relevant parameters that are significant for the OR protocol and evaluation of the procedure, ideally also using a drawing nearby the planned LVA, as summarized in ▶ Fig. 8.6.

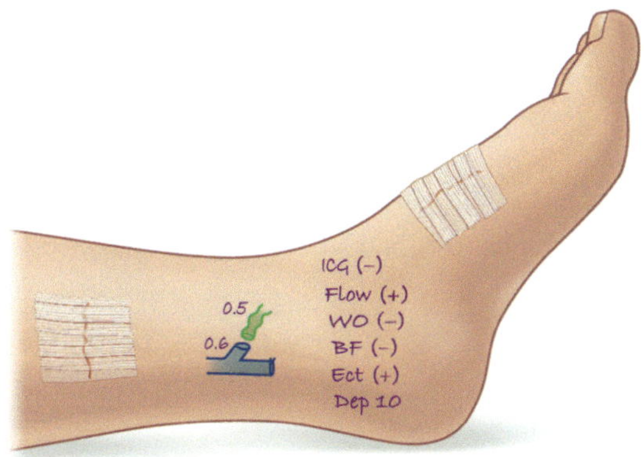

- Lymph vessel diameter (mm)
- Vein diameter (mm)
- ICG enhancement (++/+/–)
- Flow of lymph fluid from collector (++/+/–)
- Washout (of vein after LVA) (++/+/–)
- Backflow (of vein prior to LVA) (++/+/–)
- Morphological changes: Reg(ular)/Ect(asia)/Scl(erosis)
- Depth of lymph collector (mm)

Fig. 8.6 Intraoperative documentation of a lymphovenous anastomosis on the patient's extremity with lymphovenous anastomosis specific characteristics using ++ full, + moderate, - absent for the level of expression. The worm-like vessel (green) represents the lymph collector, the straight wall vessel (blue) the vein. The markings on the foot summarize the individual results, based on the general, specific characteristics in the table.

8.4.6 Dressing

As LVA is a minimally invasive procedure, the dressing including sterile strips and water-resistant dressing should enable early discharge and less limitations in daily routine. A transparent dressing allows incisional site follow-ups to exclude infection (▶ Fig. 8.7).

Note:

LVA should not be a first-line consideration for young microsurgeons, simply owning to indetectable anastomotic failure—the LVA will not immediately turn blue or white in instances of anastomotic insufficiency. The limited-invasive LVA involves a high responsibility as patients' expectations due to the burden of lymphedema are irrevocably high.

8.5 Type and Configuration of Lymphovenous Anastomosis

8.5.1 Key Factors for a Successful Lymphovenous Anastomosis

Sound microsurgical skills are indispensable. Supermicrosurgery is not as simple as microsurgery made smaller. In the world of supermicrosurgery, the commonly encountered difficulties during regular microsurgery are amplified. LVA should be avoided until solid microsurgical skill is obtained to achieve patent supermicrosurgical anastomosis.

Starting from skin incision to the dissection and skeletonization of the lymphatic vessels and recipient vein, and finally the anastomosis, are the key technical aspects of LVA. The type of anastomosis which is most suitable to perform is influenced by the size, the number, the configuration, the proximity, and the relative orientation between the lymphatic vessel and the recipient vein within the same incision. The objective is to maximize the number of LVAs to channel the accumulated lymph

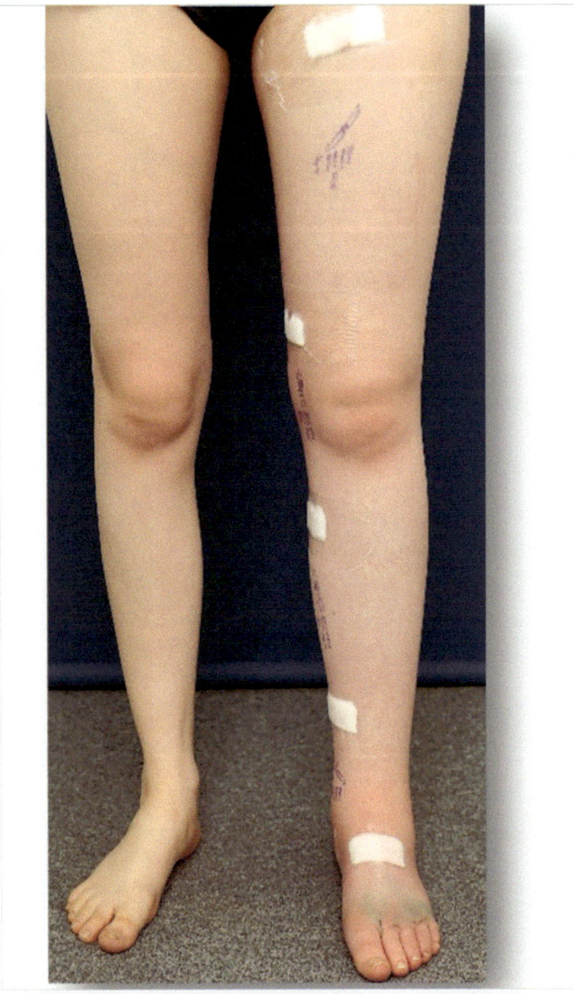

Fig. 8.7 Dressing and state after lymphovenous anastomosis.

into the recipient vein(s) and reduce the lymph load arriving to the injured zone. Both technical aspect and decision-making are essential for a successful LVA.

8.5.2 End-to-End Lymphovenous Anastomosis

End-to-end lymphovenous anastomosis (LVEEA) is perhaps the most commonly used anastomosis for LVA (▶ Fig. 8.8 and ▶ Fig. 8.13).

- Prerequisite: Size discrepancy and the distance between lymphatic vessels and recipient vein can be tolerated to certain extent.
- Advantages: May be the only method to anastomose lymphatic vessels and recipient vein which are some distance apart in the same incision. Dissection of lymphatic vessels proximally and recipient vein most distally is needed to obtain adequate length to bridge the distance between them before anastomoses.
- Disadvantages: Size discrepancy between lymphatic vessels and recipient vein is not uncommon. The recipient vein is usually significantly larger than lymphatic vessels, making LVEEA difficult and prone to leakage. It only allows one anastomosis for each recipient vein, and it can only drain the accumulated lymph distal to the site of LVA.

8.5.3 End-to-Side Lymphovenous Anastomosis

End-to-side lymphovenous anastomosis (LVESA) is performed e.g., in instances of size mismatch between the lymphatic vessel and vein/venule (▶ Fig. 8.13).

- Prerequisite: Lymphatic vessels and recipient vein within certain proximity; relatively larger recipient vein.

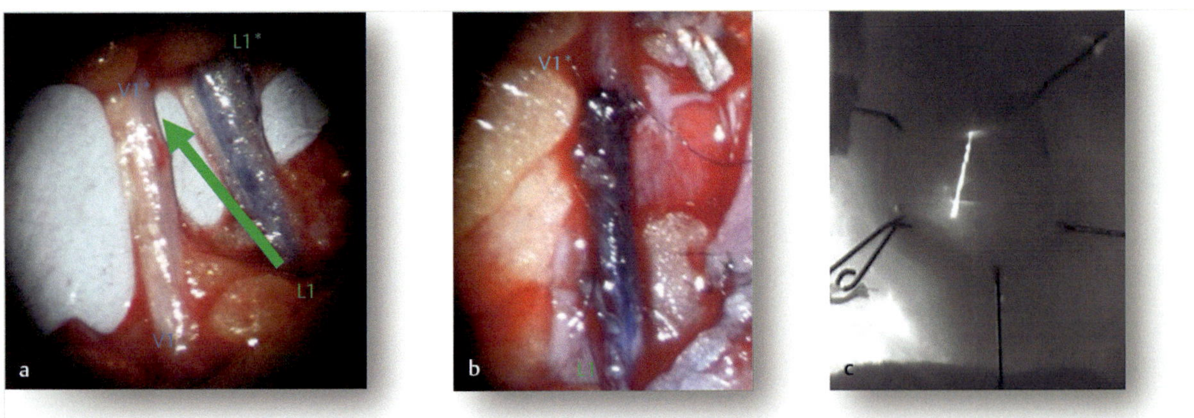

Fig. 8.8 Pre–lymphovenous anastomosis **(a)**, post–lymphovenous anastomosis **(b)**, and post–lymphovenous anastomosis ICG lymphangiography **(c)**: End-to-end lymphovenous anastomosis can be assumed as the most commonly used anastomosis for lymphovenous anastomosis. The concept and anastomotic steps of end-to-end lymphovenous anastomosis are summarized **(a, b)** with ICG confirmation of the patency and washout with ICG near-infrared imaging after the end-to-end lymphovenous anastomosis **(c)**. The lymphatic vessel has taken up blue dye injected distal to the incision site in this case for navigation. L, lymphatic vessel; V, venule.

- Advantages: Multiple lymphatic vessels can be anastomosed to one single recipient vein to increase lymphatic drainage. Ante/retrograde anastomoses of the lymphatic vessels can be done to drain both the proximal/distal of the incision. Ideal windows can be created to overcome size discrepancy between lymphatic vessels and the recipient vein.
- Disadvantages: Technically more demanding as compared to LVEEA.
- Relatively stable recipient vein. LVESA is easier to perform as compared to LVEEA, as during LVEEA, both ends of the lymphatic vessel and the recipient vein become loose after they are severed, making them more difficult to manipulate. In LVESA, the recipient usually remains intact, with the distal part of the recipient vein ligated with nylon 9–0 to prevent antegrade influx of venous blood. It is much easier to perform anastomosis by dealing with one loose end.
  - Some microsurgeons consider LVESA is more technically more demanding as compared to LVEEA. But with practice, LVESA can be quite handy to deal with complex anastomosis (▶ Fig. 8.9 and ▶ Fig. 8.13).

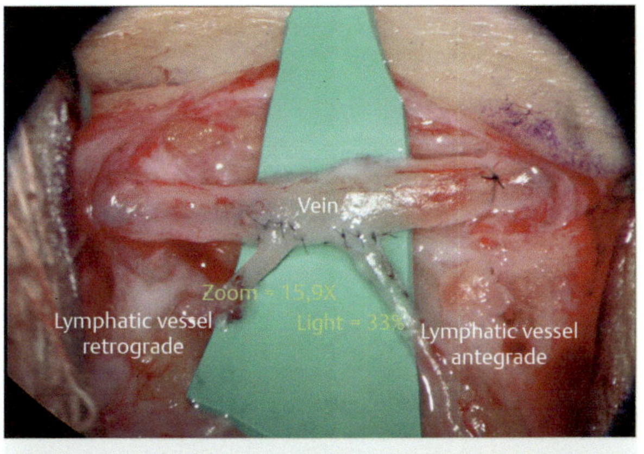

Fig. 8.9 The concept and anastomotic steps of end-to-side lymphovenous anastomosis is summarized, using two lymphatic vessel anastomoses of both the retrograde (proximal) and antegrade (distal) lymphatic vessel to drain the extremity from both areas due to the pathophysiology of lymphedema.

8.5.4 Side-to-End Lymphovenous Anastomosis

Side-to-end lymphovenous Anastomosis (LVSEA) allows to maintain the integrity of the lymphatic collector axis (▶ Fig. 8.10).

- Prerequisite: Lymphatic vessels and recipient vein within certain proximity; relatively larger lymphatic vessel.
- Advantages: It enables ante/retrograde lymphatic drainage with one anastomosis. In healthy people, retrograde lymphatic flow does not occur because valves in the lymphatic vessel are working to support antegrade flow. In secondary lymphedema with increased lymph load, lymph retention and lymphatic hypertension occur and valvular dysfunction induces retrograde lymphatic flow, which can be successfully addressed by double LVSEA including the retrograde LVA to be more efficient in drainage and relief.
- Disadvantages: It is technically more demanding as compared to LVEEA. Posterior-wall approach is usually the only technique to start the anastomosis since it is difficult to flip the vessels to approach the posterior side.

8.5.5 End-to-End Lymphovenous Anastomosis in Conjunction with End-to-Side Lymphovenous Anastomosis: The Lambda-Shaped Lymphovenous Anastomosis

The Lambda (λ)-shaped LVA enables ante/retrograde lymphatic drainage with one anastomosis (▶ Fig. 8.11 and ▶ Fig. 8.13).

- Prerequisite: Lambda-shaped LVA with one LVEEA and one LVESA, lymphatic vessels and recipient vein within certain proximity.
- Advantages: It enables ante/retrograde lymphatic drainage with one anastomosis; technically less demanding as compared to two LVESA.

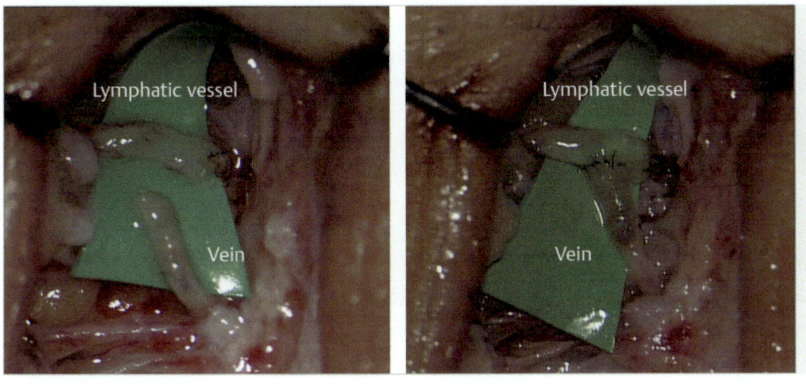

Fig. 8.10 The concept and anastomotic steps of side-to-end lymphovenous anastomosis is displayed; to maintain the integrity of the lymphatic collector axis, the side-to-end lymphovenous anastomosis is performed with residual physiological drainage and/or retrograde drainage and augmented site drainage to the venule due to the pathophysiology of lymphedema.

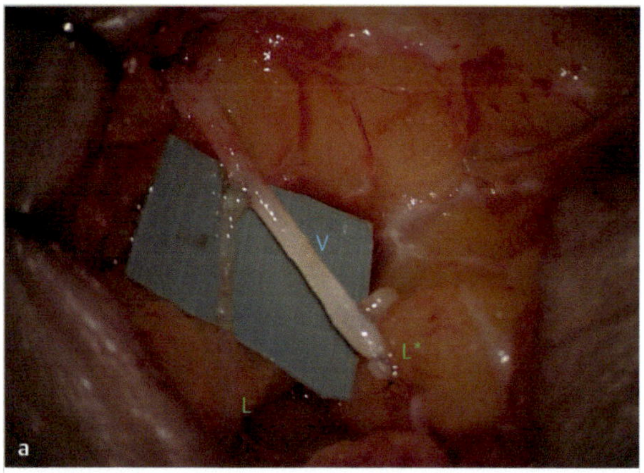

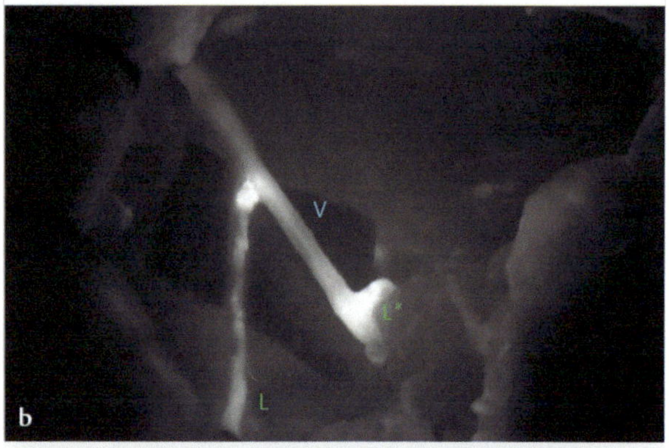

Fig. 8.11 The concept and anastomotic steps of the lambda-shaped lymphovenous anastomosis configuration with two lymphovenous anastomoses, one end-to-end lymphovenous anastomosis and one side-to-end lymphovenous anastomosis, are summarized after anastomosis **(a)** and with the use of intraoperative ICG near-infrared imaging **(b)** to prove the washout of the anastomoses. V: vein, L lymph collector and L* second collector

8.5.6 Side-to-Side Lymphovenous Anastomosis

Side-to-side lymphovenous anastomosis (LVSSA) maintains the integrity of both the lymphatic collector and vein/venule axis and enables ante/retrograde lymphatic drainage (▸ Fig. 8.12 and ▸ Fig. 8.13).

- Prerequisite: Lymphatic vessels and the recipient vein need to be in close proximity. A relatively same diameter between the lymphatic vessel and recipient vein will be more suitable, best for normal to ectatic lymphatic vessels.
- Advantages: It enables ante/retrograde lymphatic drainage with one anastomosis, which is similar to SEA.
- Disadvantages: It is technically more demanding as compared to EEA. Posterior-wall approach is usually the only technique to start the anastomosis since it is difficult to flip the vessels to approach the posterior side.

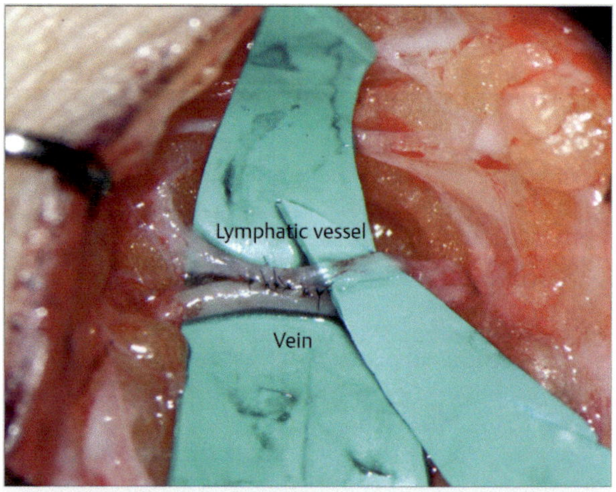

Fig. 8.12 The concept and anastomotic steps of side-to-side lymphovenous anastomosis is summarized with both retrograde (proximal) and antegrade (distal) lymphatic vessel to drain the extremity from both areas due to the pathophysiology of lymphedema.

8.5.7 End-to-Side Lympholymphatic Anastomosis

End-to-side lympholymphatic anastomosis (LLESA) is a helpful step to bridge lymphatic vessels for a recipient vein (▸ Fig. 8.13).

- Prerequisite: Lymphatic vessels are within certain proximity; when the recipient vein is too far away or no more space for the recipient vein to perform LVESA.
- Advantages: One or more lymphatic vessels are used to bridge other lymphatic vessels to the recipient vein to enhance lymphatic drainage.
- Disadvantages: Usually the distal lymph is drained; technically more demanding; difficult to perform for lymphatic vessels with constriction or sclerotic change.

8.5.8 Comparison among Different Lymphovenous Anastomosis Types

The different types and configurations of lymphovenous anastomoses and lympholymphatic anastomoses addressing variable matches and mismatches between the lymphatic vessel's and venule's/vein's size requiring different physiological consideration for anastomosis are outlined in ▸ Table 8.1.

The several types and configuration addressing various matches and mismatches between the LV and Venule/vein size and different physiological consideration of LVA anastomosis are summarized in ▸ Fig. 8.13, and it is useful to have most of them in the toolbox to address individual differences of the vein and LV anatomy.

Table 8.1 The different types of lymphovenous anastomoses and lympholymphatic anastomoses

Type	Prerequisite	Advantages	Disadvantages
LVEEA	Minimal size discrepancy	May be the only method to anastomose lymphatic vessels and recipient vein which are some distance apart	Size discrepancy One anastomosis for each recipient vein Only for distal drainage
LVESA	Certain proximity Relatively larger recipient vein	Allow multiple LVAs onto one single recipient vein Allow ante/retrograde anastomoses for proximal/distal drainage Less size discrepancy	Technically more demanding as compared to EEA
LVSEA	Certain proximity Relatively larger lymphatic vessel	Enables ante/retrograde lymphatic drainage with one anastomosis	Technically more demanding as compared to EEA
LVSSA	Lymphatic vessels and the recipient vein need to be in close proximity	Enables ante/retrograde lymphatic drainage with one anastomosis, which is similar to SEA	Technically more demanding as compared to EEA
LLESA	Certain proximity	Multiple lymphatic vessel anastomoses to enhance drainage to a single recipient vein	Draining only distal lymphedema; technically more demanding; difficult to perform with constriction/sclerotic lymphatic vessels

Abbreviations: LVEEA, end-to-end lymphovenous anastomosis; LVESA, end-to-side lymphovenous anastomosis; LVSEA, side-to-end lymphovenous Anastomosis; LVSSA, side-to-side lymphovenous anastomosis; LLESA, end-to-side lympholymphatic anastomosis.

- A reflux-free recipient vein is preferred for all LVAs.
- Distal vein ligation is recommended to prevent venous reflux from the distal vein in all configuration types.
- After mastering the basic anastomosis for LVA, combination of different types of anastomoses can be improvised to maximize the effect of LVA.
- Combination of LVEEA and LVESA with the lambda (λ) shape.

8.5.9 Lymphovenous Anastomosis for Single Recipient Vein and Multiple Lymphatic Vessels

Occasionally, multiple lymphatic vessels with one single recipient vein can be identified within the same incision. Since LVA is a bypass procedure, having more channels to bypass the accumulated lymph into the venous system will definitely aid in the reduction of lymphedema. It is imperative to anastomose as many lymphatic vessels as possible.

- The utilization of LVESA, LVSEA, and LVSSA can help to achieve this goal.
- Yamamoto et al.[27,28] mentioned the use of ladder-shaped SSA and triple-SSA for lymphatic vessels and EEA for recipient vein.
- Since there is only one recipient vein, the stakes are high if improper anastomoses were made and increase the risk of venous/lymph thrombosis.

8.5.10 Lymphovenous Implantation or "Octopus" Anastomosis

- Prerequisite: Only lymphatic vessels with a diameter of < 0.3 mm are found making "true" LVA technically impossible alternative to the standard LVA technique with the potential of simplifying this technically challenging procedure.
- Advantages: Several small caliber lymphatic vessels are used to be place and fix into a larger vein to enhance lymphatic drainage with anchoring sutures (see ▶ Fig. 8.5).
- Disadvantages: Anastomotic site leakage (hematoma, lymph fistula).

8.6 Surgical Equipment

8.6.1 Surgical Microscopes (Selection)

- Zeiss Pentero 900 or Kinevo 900 surgical microscope with 25 × magnification and additional 50% magnification by magnification extender on the eyepiece. Kinevo 900 also allows three-dimensional usage with special glasses for comfortable ergonomic posture, providing the surgeon with more freedom of movement and a special supermicrosurgical experience (see **Subchapter 8.5.2** and ▶ **Fig. 8.4**).
- Mitaka MM51 surgical microscope with up to 42 × magnification, which is very useful for showing

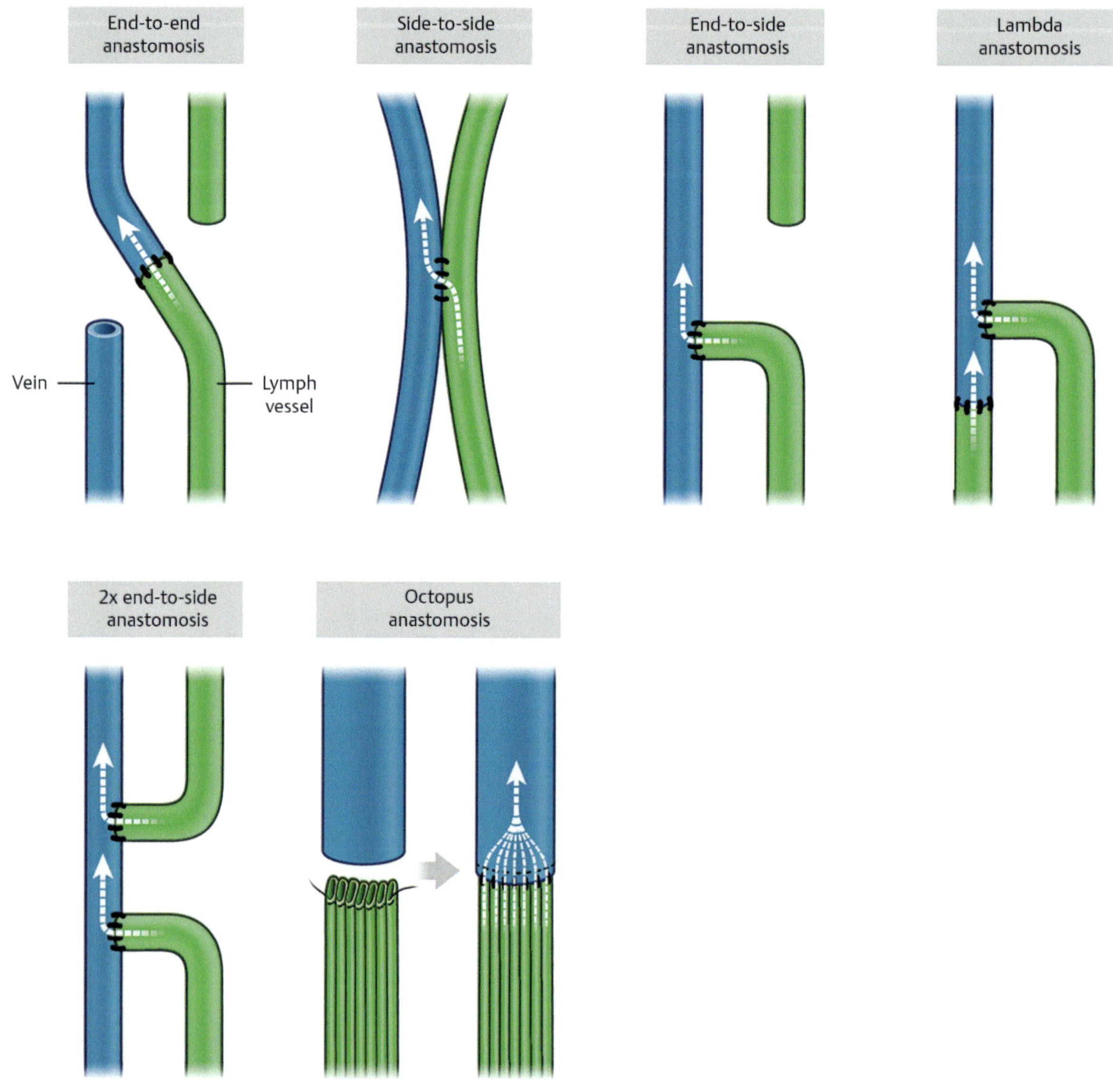

Fig. 8.13 Different commonly used configurations of lymphvenous anastomosis.

great details in anastomosing lymphatic vessel < 0.3 mm.

- Both microscopes can be equipped with NIR system for ICG lymphangiography which is very useful intraoperatively for identifying ICG-enhanced lymphatic vessels and for anastomosis patency authentication.

8.6.2 Mobile Indocyanine Green Near-Infrared Systems (Selection)

Several systems with high resolution and Laser class 1 and 2 are available nowadays. Technical features with individual preference include handheld probe versus fixed suspensions, special software solutions as panoramic view, photo, and video management as well as connection to picture archiving and communication system (PACS). A comprehensive testing to evaluate individual needs for the setting, which allow outpatient clinic screening as well as intraoperative navigation, is recommended prior to the purchase of the system.

- Fluobeam 800 or LX, Fluoptics, Grenoble, France, is a system with handheld probe and several software solutions, both for outpatient clinic and operation theater.

- EleVision IR Plattform, Medtronic, Freiburg, Germany, is rather a suspension system with potential handheld use with high-definition resolution and several software solutions, both for outpatient clinic and operation theater.
- Spy System, Stryker, USA, is a complex solution with several features with a high resolution and a suspended imaging system, rather for the operation theater.

8.6.3 Supermicrosurgical Instruments (Selection)

Super-fine instruments are necessary for handling the tissue and the sutures. Careful handling by the nurse, the surgeon, and the sterilization team is necessary to extend the usage time.

- EMI microsurgery instruments are nice to have, especially for someone who is just starting supermicrosurgery. The ability to use a locking needle holder can help to decrease hand tremor, and it definitely helps to attack difficult-to-reach areas. The fingers do not need to exert forces onto the needle holder to hold the needle in place. The tremor will become quite obvious under 20 × magnification.
- Two supermicro forceps. The anastomosis can also be done with two supermicro forceps. Personal advice is to use a wider forceps as needle holder for 11–0 or 12–0. With the wide tip and increased contact surface area between the forceps and needle, there will be much less rotational force from the needle which it is used to penetrate the lumen of lymphatic vessels or the recipient vein.
- The titanium-made instruments are very nice to have, but great care is needed since they are more delicate than the stainless-steel instruments. Most mishaps happen during cleansing and preparation for sterilization after operation.
- Smooth mosquito and micro pickup are very useful for dull soft tissue dissection.
- Supermicrosurgical scissor is a must-have.
- Suture lines: Nylon 11–0 for suture and 12–0 for LVA, nylon 9–0 for opening a perfect window for end-to-side, side-to-end, or side-to side anastomoses.
- Wound retraction: Fishhooks with rubber band. Comes in different sizes. Avoid skin compression by placing gauze underneath as cushion.
- Stents. More suitable for normal or ectatic lymphatic vessels. Be careful about performing SEA to severe ectatic lymphatic vessel due to extremely thin, almost transparent, lymphatic wall. It is prone to tear and leakage during anastomosis. Lymphatic lumen will become indistinguishable due to thin, transparent lymphatic wall. Intraluminal stenting technique with a commercially available stent (Crownjun, Japan) or a fragment of nylon 5–0 (1–2 mm) can aid to overcome this problem.

8.7 Additional Intraoperative Tools

8.7.1 Indocyanine Green Lymphangiography

ICG lymphangiography can be provided by external devices (see **Chapter 4** and **Subchapter 8.7.2**) which are portable and can be used in the outpatient clinic for screening and intraoperatively for navigation and microscope-integrated solutions. Magnification and resolution of the portable machine are not detailed enough for seeing lymphatic vessels in the operative field. Microscope-integrated NIR microscope is able to zoom in on the lymphatic vessels based on the magnification of the microscope, offering a close-up view of the lymphatic vessels. However, the field of view also becomes smaller as the magnification increases. The penetration depth of NIR in the microscope is also shallower as compared to handheld devices.

8.7.2 Blue Dye

Visual aids such as Patent Blue V dye can also be helpful in identifying lymphatic vessels intraoperatively (see **Chapter 4** and **Subchapter 8.7**). Blue dye in the recipient vein is also indicated to observe LVA patency. However, Patent Blue V can stain surgical field blue during dissection, which can obscure lymphatic vessel and make LVA patency incomprehensible. In comparison, the directly green staining effect of ICG is much less since visualization of ICG is mainly based on fluorescence.

8.8 Patient Education

8.8.1 Before Lymphovenous Anastomosis

The degree of lymphedema reduction after LVA is dependent on the size and quality of the lymphatic vessels found and used for LVA.

8.8.2 After Lymphovenous Anastomosis

- Light compression with bandage after LVA; start compression garment 1 week after LVA. The compression garment should be replaced every 6 months or when it losses elasticity. Custom-made compression garment is preferred (see **Subchapter 8.5**).
- The next day after LVA: indoor ambulation.
- First week after LVA: light activity.
- Second week after LVA: resume normal activity.
- Prophylactic antibiotic therapy in patients at risk as lymphedema per se involves a local immunoincompetence.
- After 1 month of LVA: resume the use of pneumatic compression garment and regular exercise. The intensity

of exercise should be adjusted according to the status of lymphedema improvement and one's general condition.
- Avoid insect bites or open wounds, for example, mosquito bites, to prevent cellulitis.

8.9 Robotic Lymphovenous Anastomosis Microsurgery

The use of robotic arms to assist microsurgical reconstruction has yet to gain popularity since most reconstructions are performed on the surface. However, recent publications[34,35] have discussed the opportunities of robotic-assisted microsurgical reconstruction, including learning curves, reduction of tremor, and a microsurgeon's longer professional longevity, even for LVA surgery (see **Subchapter 10.11**).

8.10 How to Advance Your Supermicrosurgical Skills for Lymphovenous Anastomosis[29]

- Dry lab
  - Needle manipulation: The training usually starts with dry lab where basic manipulation starting with nylon 9–0 and gradually advance to nylon 11–0 and 12–0, with increased magnification.
  - Suture on synthetic material: This anastomosis practice aims to enhance needle manipulation. Supermicrosurgical simulation is performed by placing sutures onto synthetic vessel (hydrogel), silicon tubes, or prosthetic lymphatic channels.[30]
- Soft tissue simulation
  - Chicken thigh[31]
  - Rat thigh lymphatic vessels by Yamamoto et al.[32] and femoral vessels[33]

8.11 Perspective

LVA is still a very microsurgeon-dependent procedure, and the type, manner, and quality of the anastomosis, the configuration of the LVA, and the number of LVAs per patient vary significantly for lack of profound data. Mixed opinions do exist among supermicrosurgeons and other lymphatic surgeons due to mixed outcomes for LVA. It should be our quest as the supermicrosurgeons to deliver the much-needed scientific merits to accredit the role of supermicrosurgery in treating lymphedema, and possibly, for the standardization of treatment protocol.

8.12 Clinical Cases

The efficiency of LVA can be observed shortly after the LVA procedure (in contrast to long-masked results after VLNT) and improves in weeks to months depending on the degree of damage to the tissue of lymphedema. Slight relief of swelling with recurrent wrinkles to the distal extremity are an early sign of functioning of the bypasses after LVA.

For patient education, successful results after LVA are important to be discussed along with unsuccessful surgery.

Case 1

The results after successful treatment with LVA to the lower extremity after lymphorrhea with dermal alterations (▶ Fig. 8.14).

Case 2

The results after successful treatment with LVA to the upper extremity after breast cancer (▶ Fig. 8.15).

8.13 Pearls and Pitfalls

- LVA is a supermicrosurgical, minimally invasive, and targeted procedure, which does the least harm to the patient.
- The lymphedema will not get worse even if LVA does not work.
- The patient can benefit greatly from this procedure when LVAs are performed with functional lymphatic vessels and reflux-free recipient veins and supermicrosurgical skills.
- Fast postoperative recovery due to small incisions.

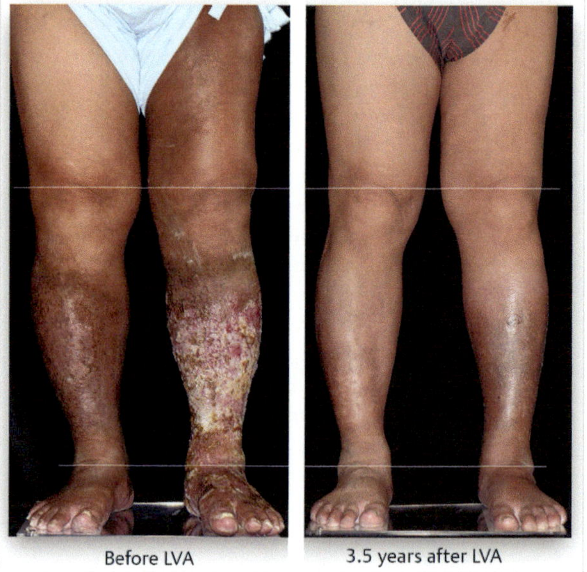

Fig. 8.14 The results following the successful treatment of the lower extremity with LVA after lymphorrhea with dermal alterations before and after a period of 3.5 years.

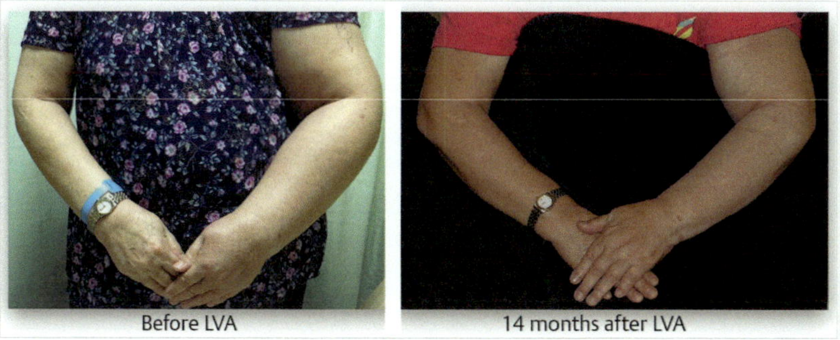

Fig. 8.15 The result following the successful treatment of the upper extremity with LVA after breast cancer before and after a period of 14 months.

- Surgery to be optionally performed in local or regional anesthesia.
- LVA has the least complications as compared with other procedures.
- Supermicrosurgical LVA is a very technically dependent procedure. Years of training are required to obtain the solid microsurgical skills for LVA.
- A whole procedure of several LVAs is a long operation with a lot of patience required.
- The degree of pathological changes among the lymphatic vessels is irreversible; the microsurgeon needs to work with what is given.
- DB in moderate to severe lymphedema hinders preoperative functional lymphatic vessel identification.
- Several variables, especially configurations and types of LVA anastomosis as well as a large number of LVAs per patients, make it remarkably difficult to compare the results and efficiency.
- The anastomotic patency after LVA remains uncertain. The only way to confirm the patency is by the progress of lymphedema reduction. Technically, ultrasound and ICG lymphangiography are able to visualize the patency in most patients.
- Compression garment is needed after LVA. The duration of compression required is patient dependent and not evaluated yet.
- No answers are yet available as to how many LVAs should be performed to yield result.

References

[1] Koshima I, Inagawa K, Urushibara K, Moriguchi T. Supermicrosurgical lymphaticovenular anastomosis for the treatment of lymphedema in the upper extremities. J Reconstr Microsurg. 2000; 16(6):437–442

[2] Yamamoto T, Yamamoto N, Doi K, et al. Indocyanine green-enhanced lymphography for upper extremity lymphedema: a novel severity staging system using dermal backflow patterns. Plast Reconstr Surg. 2011; 128(4):941–947

[3] Yang JC, Wu SC, Chiang MH, Lin WC, Hsieh CH. Intraoperative identification and definition of “functional” lymphatic collecting vessels for supermicrosurgical lymphatico-venous anastomosis in treating lymphedema patients. J Surg Oncol. 2018; 117(5):994–1000

[4] Suami H, Yamashita S, Soto-Miranda MA, Chang DW. Lymphatic territories (lymphosomes) in a canine: an animal model for investigation of postoperative lymphatic alterations. PLoS One. 2013; 8 (7):e69222

[5] Yang JC, Wu SC, Chiang MH, Lin WC. Targeting reflux-free veins with a vein visualizer to identify the ideal recipient vein preoperatively for optimal lymphaticovenous anastomosis in treating lymphedema. Plast Reconstr Surg. 2018; 141(3):793–797

[6] Ogata F, Azuma R, Kikuchi M, Koshima I, Morimoto Y. Novel lymphography using indocyanine green dye for near-infrared fluorescence labeling. Ann Plast Surg. 2007; 58(6):652–655

[7] Kung TA, Champaneria MC, Maki JH, Neligan PC. Current concepts in the surgical management of lymphedema. Plast Reconstr Surg. 2017; 139(4):1003e–1013e

[8] Mihara M, Hara H, Hayashi Y, et al. Pathological steps of cancer-related lymphedema: histological changes in the collecting lymphatic vessels after lymphadenectomy. PLoS One. 2012; 7(7):e41126

[9] Yoo J, Choi JY, Hwang JH, et al. Prognostic value of lymphoscintigraphy in patients with gynecological cancer-related lymphedema. J Surg Oncol. 2014; 109(8):760–763

[10] Mikami T, Hosono M, Yabuki Y, et al. Classification of lymphoscintigraphy and relevance to surgical indication for lymphaticovenous anastomosis in upper limb lymphedema. Lymphology. 2011; 44(4):155–167

[11] Bae JS, Yoo RE, Choi SH, et al. Evaluation of lymphedema in upper extremities by MR lymphangiography: comparison with lymphoscintigraphy. Magn Reson Imaging. 2018; 49(49):63–70

[12] Zeltzer AA, Brussaard C, Koning M, et al. MR lymphography in patients with upper limb lymphedema: the GPS for feasibility and surgical planning for lympho-venous bypass. J Surg Oncol. 2018; 118(3):407–415

[13] Akita S, Ogata F, Manabe I, et al. Noninvasive screening test for detecting early stage lymphedema using follow-up computed tomography imaging after cancer treatment and results of treatment with lymphaticovenular anastomosis. Microsurgery. 2017; 37(8):910–916

[14] Hayashi A, Yamamoto T, Yoshimatsu H, et al. Ultrasound visualization of the lymphatic vessels in the lower leg. Microsurgery. 2016; 36(5): 397–401

[15] Mihara M, Hara H, Narushima M, et al. Indocyanine green lymphography is superior to lymphoscintigraphy in imaging diagnosis of secondary lymphedema of the lower limbs. J Vasc Surg Venous Lymphat Disord. 2013; 1(2):194–201

[16] Will PA, Hirche C, Berner JE, Kneser U, Gazyakan E. Lymphovenous anastomoses with three-dimensional digital hybrid visualization: improving ergonomics for supermicrosurgery in lymphedema. Arch Plast Surg. 2021; 48(4):427–432

[17] Chan VS, Narushima M, Hara H, et al. Local anesthesia for lymphaticovenular anastomosis. Ann Plast Surg. 2014; 72(2):180–183

[18] Mihara M, Hara H, Tange S, et al. Multisite lymphaticovenular bypass using supermicrosurgery technique for lymphedema management in lower lymphedema cases. Plast Reconstr Surg. 2016; 138(1):262–272

[19] Narushima M, Mihara M, Yamamoto Y, Iida T, Koshima I, Mundinger GS. The intravascular stenting method for treatment of extremity lymphedema with multiconfiguration lymphaticovenous anastomoses. Plast Reconstr Surg. 2010; 125(3):935–943

[20] Yamamoto T, Yamamoto N, Ishiura R. Fusion lymphoplasty for diameter approximation in lymphatic supermicrosurgery using two

lymphatic vessels for a larger recipient vein. J Plast Reconstr Aesthet Surg. 2016; 69(9):1306–1308

[21] Yamamoto T, Yoshimatsu H, Yamamoto N, Yokoyama A, Numahata T, Koshima I. Multisite lymphaticovenular anastomosis using vein graft for uterine cancer-related lymphedema after pelvic lymphadenectomy. Vasc Endovascular Surg. 2015; 49(7):195–200

[22] Visconti G, Hayashi A, Salgarello M, Narushima M, Koshima I, Yamamoto T. Supermicrosurgical T-shaped lymphaticovenular anastomosis for the treatment of peripheral lymphedema: bypassing lymph fluid maximizing lymphatic collector continuity. Microsurgery. 2016; 36(8):714–715

[23] Yamamoto T, Koshima I. Neo-valvuloplasty for lymphatic supermicrosurgery. J Plast Reconstr Aesthet Surg. 2014; 67(4):587–588

[24] Visconti G, Salgarello M. Venule valve graft in lymphatic supermicrosurgery: a novel strategy for managing blood backflow. Microsurgery. 2017; 37(8):958–959

[25] Campisi C, Davini D, Bellini C, et al. Lymphatic microsurgery for the treatment of lymphedema. Microsurgery. 2006; 26(1):65–69

[26] Chen WF, Yamamoto T, Fisher M, Liao J, Carr J. The "octopus" lymphaticovenular anastomosis: evolving beyond the standard supermicrosurgical technique. J Reconstr Microsurg. 2015; 31(6):450–457

[27] Yamamoto T, Kikuchi K, Yoshimatsu H, Koshima I. Ladder-shaped lymphaticovenular anastomosis using multiple side-to-side lymphatic anastomoses for a leg lymphedema patient. Microsurgery. 2014; 34(5): 404–408

[28] Yamamoto T, Furuya M, Harima M, Hayashi A, Koshima I. Triple supermicrosurgical side-to-side lymphaticolymphatic anastomoses on a lymphatic vessel end-to-end anastomosed to a vein. Microsurgery. 2015; 35(3):249–250

[29] Pafitanis G, Narushima M, Yamamoto T, et al. Evolution of an evidence-based supermicrosurgery simulation training curriculum: a systematic review. J Plast Reconstr Aesthet Surg. 2018; 71(7):976–988

[30] Tsunashima C, Kannan R, Koshima I. Supermicrosurgery simulation using prosthetic lymphatic channels. J Plast Reconstr Aesthet Surg. 2016; 69(7):1013–1014

[31] Chen WF, Eid A, Yamamoto T, Keith J, Nimmons GL, Lawrence WT. A novel supermicrosurgery training model: the chicken thigh. J Plast Reconstr Aesthet Surg. 2014; 67(7):973–978

[32] Yamamoto T, Yamamoto N, Yamashita M, et al. Establishment of supermicrosurgical lymphaticovenular anastomosis model in rat. Microsurgery. 2017; 37(1):57–60

[33] Liu HL. Microvascular anastomosis of submillimeter vessels—a training model in rats. J Hand Microsurg. 2013; 5(1):14–17

[34] Ibrahim AE, Sarhane KA, Selber JC. New frontiers in robotic-assisted microsurgical reconstruction. Clin Plast Surg. 2017; 44(2): 415–423

[35] Struk S, Qassemyar Q, Leymarie N, et al. The ongoing emergence of robotics in plastic and reconstructive surgery. Ann Chir Plast Esthet. 2018; 63(2):105–112

9 Autologous Lymph Vessel Transfer

Ruediger Baumeister, Andreas Frick, and Christiane G. Stäuble

Summary

Autologous lymph vessel transfer is indicated for patients with lymphedema caused by a localized interruption of the lymphatic system. The anatomical regions at risk are the lymph node basins in the axilla, the groin, and the pelvic region. This is the case in most patients suffering from secondary lymphedema in Europe, usually cancer related, with a potential indication for autologous lymph vessel transfer. Compared to other reconstructive techniques, autologous lymph vessel transfer is performed within the lymphatic system itself. Lymph vessels are harvested as grafts. Thus, the medial side of the thigh is a common donor site area. Preoperative scintigraphy is indicated to document lymph flow at the graft harvesting site.

Keywords: autologous lymph vessel transfer (ALVT), bypass, interposition, lymphatic graft, lymphatic vessel (LV), lymphedema

9.1 Indications and Contraindications

Transfer of lymphatic vessels is, in principle, a vascular surgical bypass procedure of lymphatic vessels to treat lymphedema. Autologous lymph vessel transfer (ALVT) technique is favored for patients with lymphedema caused mainly by a localized impairment of the lymphatic transporting system in the axillary, groin or pelvic region. The medial side of the knee region may be also affected, after orthopedic interventions, as well as distal areas of extremities, after peripheral interventions and trauma.

Note:

Compared with other techniques that aim to restore lymphatic flow (see **Chapters 8, 10,** and **12**), ALVT is performed within the preexisting vascular network of the lymphatic system that demonstrates a virtually normal lymph flow.

This means that the reconstruction respects the intrinsic lymphatic pressure gradient. Furthermore, the reconstruction within the lymphatic vascular system takes advantage of the low coagulation behavior of lymph compared to blood. The wall of the lymphatic vessel can be solely nourished by the lymphatic fluid. The lymphatic collectors are used due to their active transport mechanism, which has been shown in experimental studies even outside of the body after immersion in an organ bath.[1,2] This is important as chronic lymphedema leads to fibrosis of the lymphatic collectors and the surrounding tissue. Consequently, the collectors lose their innate elasticity, and the active transport capacity of the lymph diminishes. Since lymphatic grafts are independent of an active inflow, they act as pumps and enable lymph flow with a negative pressure gradient. In advanced fibrosis of lymphatic collectors, the lumen usually remains partly patent and not completely occluded. This has been demonstrated in histological studies.[3] In his lymphographic studies, Kinmonth described one type of primary lymphedema with localized atresia in one groin or pelvis region. This specific type may also be treated using an ALVT.[4] Nowadays, MRL allows for the selection of these special types of primary lymphedema that are suitable to ALVT.

9.2 Preoperative Considerations

Prior to the surgical procedure, the patient should undergo conservative treatment (see **Chapter 6** and **Subchapter 7.3**). The cause of lymphedema should be elucidated. Only lymphedemas with a localized, impaired lymphatic transport are suitable for this method. The donor site requires diagnostic workup to determine whether the harvesting of lymphatic collectors is possible. This requires lymphangiography of the deep system to exclude any damage, which is possible with either lymphatic scintigraphy or MRI-based techniques (see **Chapter 4**). For the donor site, presence of edema, damage to lymphatic vessels or persistent malignancies has to be exlcluded.

9.3 Operative Technique

Final evaluation for suitable lymphatic collectors to be harvested is made at the beginning of surgery during dissection and is based upon stained lymphatic collectors.

Accordingly, and after induction of general anesthesia, a dye with affinity to the lymphatic drainage system (e.g., 2 ml Patent Blue V) is injected intra- and subdermally into the first and second web spaces of the foot respectively. The leg is actively moved in order to enhance lymphatic flow. The lymphatic collectors will be stained after about 15 minutes. After skin incision, lymphatic collectors can be harvested as grafts only if several stained lymphatic collectors are present. If these requirements are not fulfilled, lymphatic grafting should not be performed in order to avoid donor site lymphedema.

There are two anatomical regions in the lower extremity where the lymphatic vascular network is particularly at risk when manipulating surgically, i.e., the groin, including the inguinal lymph nodes and the medial side of the knee where the lymphatic collectors of the lower leg course. Therefore, these two regions have to be avoided during surgical preparation and the suitable lymphatic collectors must be harvested distal to the groin respectively proximal to the knee. ALVT is performed within subcutaneous tissue and therefore represents a surgical risk comparable to surgery on superficial veins.

The grafts always run within the subcutaneous tissue. In order to minimize any friction, tubes with a greater diameter like Redon tubes or urinary catheters with a length corresponding to the length of the distance are inserted first. Before that, a polyfil thread (2–0) is inserted and fixed outside on both openings in order to pull the lymphatic grafts later on. The tubes are moistened; the tiny suture of the graft is connected to the thicker thread within the tube. Now, within the moistened tube, the graft is pulled without friction to the opposite side. The tube is removed and the graft lies within the subcutaneous tissue without tension.

Experimental work has shown that the lymphoid wall is resistant to longitudinal stress, but not to oblique tension.[6] Therefore, the so-called tension-free technique is applied. This means that in contrast to the common microsurgical techniques in arteries and veins, a lymphatic vessel should not be turned on corner sutures.[9] The low pressure within the vessels needs only three to four stitches. We prefer absorbable suture material.

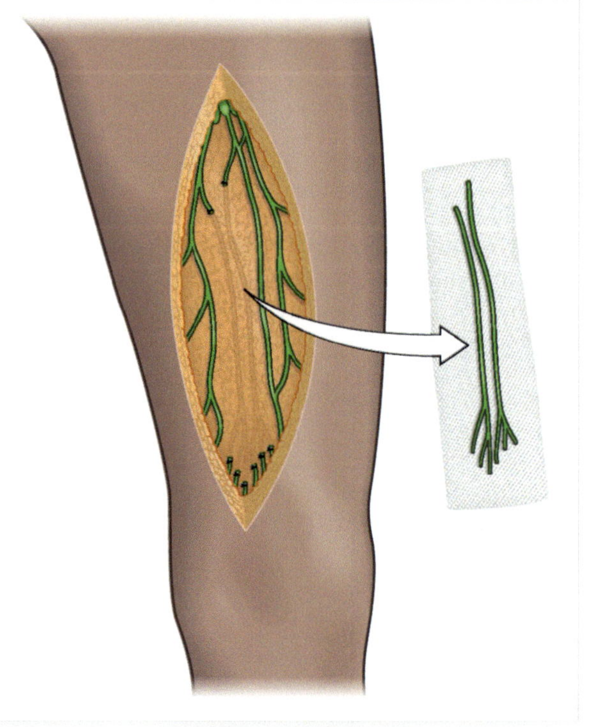

Fig. 9.1 Harvesting of lymphatic collectors from the anteromedial aspect of the patient's healthy thigh for subsequent autologous lymphatic interpositional grafts.

9.3.1 Harvesting the Lymphatic Graft

For all types of VLNT surgeries, the patient is in a supine position. For harvesting lymphatic collectors at the lower extremity, the leg is usually rotated outwards and flexed at the hip and knee region respectively, in order to facilitate the access to the medial thigh region (in a frog-leg position).

A short, longitudinal superficial skin incision is made medial to the femoral artery, After the blunt dissection, stained lymphatic vessels are sought out, right down to the fascia, since the bigger collectors are found just above this structure. The lymphatic collectors are stained greenish blue. The incision is lengthened according to the course of the stained lymphatic collectors. Staining indicates a collector is functional. Within the knee region, the collectors are very close together, whereas above this area lymphatic collectors are spreading and building a network. Therefore, the harvesting should be stopped above the knee region. Oftentimes, at the peripheral part of the grafts, small branches can be seen and dissected. Using these branches allows for a greater number of anastomoses compared to the number of chosen bigger collectors. One to three collectors of the ventromedial bundle, consisting of about 16 ones, are normally taken resulting in four to six possible peripheral anastomoses. Centrally, the main collectors are also often divided and about three to four anastomoses can be performed at the central endings of the grafts, if the lymphatic collectors are harvested as free grafts (▶ Fig. 9.1).

If the lymphatic collectors are used as a transpositional graft from one lower extremity to the other, the lymphatic collectors remain attached to the inguinal lymph nodes of the healthy leg.

For a free graft, the collector is fixed with a long thread. Distally, the remaining lymphatic vessel is sealed. The peripheral ending of the graft remains open.

The grafts always run within the subcutaneous tissue. In order to minimize any friction, tubes with a greater diameter like Redon tubes or urinary catheters with a length corresponding to the length of the distance are inserted first. Before that, a polyfil fixed with a long thread (2–0) is inserted in order to pull the lymphatic grafts later on. The tubes are moistened; the suture of the graft, with its 3-0 pulling thread, is connected to the thicker suture within the tube. Now, within the moistened tube, the graft is pulled without friction to the opposite side. The tube is removed and the graft lies within the subcutaneous tissue without tension.

9.3.2 Autologous Lymph Vessel Transfer to the Axilla Region

To treat an arm lymphedema, the arm is placed on an arm-table and the head rotated to the opposite side to access the neck region. An oblique superficial incision is made at the inner aspect of the upper arm, distal to the axilla and superficial to the brachial artery (▶ Fig. 9.2). With blunt dissection, the tissue is evaluated for structures running in a longitudinal direction. Small nerves, thickened fibers, small veins and arteries, and lymphatic vessels are found. Since the dye is not correctly transported within extremities with lymphedema, no staining is performed. Under the operating microscope, lymphatic collectors have a grey-like appearance, whereas nerves look white and have oblique stripes; thickened fibers dissolve under pincers, and arteries and veins contain blood. Finally, transection of the functional lymphatic collectors should reveal clear fluid and a lumen. The bigger lymphatic collectors are found just superficial to the fascia and used preferably. Proximal to the axilla, the next healthy lymphatic structures are found at the neck. Here, lymphatic collectors run from the head toward the venous angulation. They are found beneath the sternocleidomastoid muscle, lateral to the internal jugular vein. These collectors are mostly thin-walled and vulnerable. End-to-side or end-to-end anastomoses with the grafts are performed. Anastomoses between the grafts and lymph nodes is often easier. Their capsule is carefully opened to gain direct access to the nodal sinuses. The lymphatic graft is sutured to the capsule with about four single stitches. Experimental studies have shown that this direct suturing results in an inflow into the lymph nodes.[5]

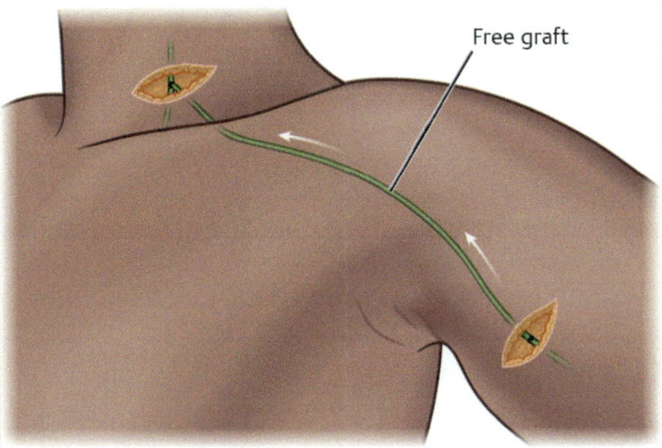

Fig. 9.2 Interpositional free grafts of one lymphatic collector to bypass the affected axilla. After harvesting of the lymphatic collector, a subcutaneous tunnel is prepared to insert the graft and connect it using two lympho-lymphatic anastomoses both the at the neck and at the upper arm proximally to re-establish directed lymph flow (white arrow).

9.3.3 Autologous Lymph Vessel Transfer in the Groin Region

To treat unilateral lymphedema of the lower extremities or scrotal lymphedema the vessel grafts remain attached to the inguinal lymph nodes and are transpose to the opposite groin or the lateral penile and scrotal region. ▶ Fig. 9.3 illustrates the treatment of contralateral leg edema.

Treating lymphedema of the contralateral leg the lymphatic vessel grafts remain attached to the inguinal lymph nodes at the harvest region. The peripheral ends of the grafts are pulled to the edematose leg ore area using the tubing technique. Finally, the grafts are anastomosed to ascending lymph collectors within the lymphedema.

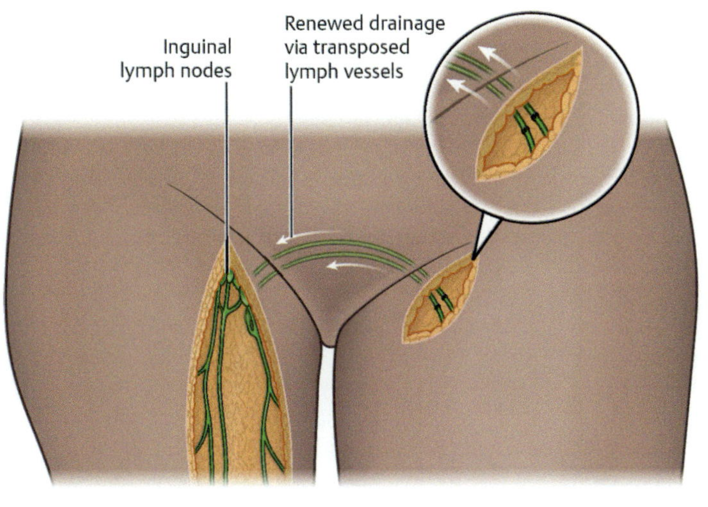

Fig. 9.3 Autologous lymph vessel transfer from the healthy thigh on the right to the groin of the affected extremity; identification and dissection of lymphatic collectors within the subcutaneous tissue of the healthy thigh. Distal transection of the healthy, uncongested collectors, subcutaneous transposition of these collectors that remain connected to the efferent lymphatic system proximally. Lympho-lymphatic anastomoses of healthy collectors to congested collectors of the affected side to reestablish directed lymph flow (white arrows).

Penal and scrotal edema are treated in a similar way (▶ Fig. 9.3).

9.4 Type of Vessel Transfer

Lymphatic collectors are specialized in transporting lymph. Since the motility is autonomic, it can be preserved, even if used as non-vascularized grafts. This is of major importance in cases where lymphatic collectors within the lymphedematous tissue are no longer able to transport lymph through their own active motion.

The grafts are harvested from the antero-medial region of the healthy thigh to serve as a nonvascularized lymphatic graft (▶ Fig. 9.1). Most of the time, they can be harvested in a length of about 20 to 30 cm depending on the length of the thigh. Usually, this length is always sufficient to bridge defects in the axilla and the groin.

9.5 Interpositional Graft

In order to bridge lymphatic gaps (also in peripheral parts of the extremities, after trauma, surgical intervention or for treating lymphoceles), free grafts are necessary and is referred to as an interposition. The central endings, peripheral to the inguinal nodes, are fixed by long threads and separated from the nodes. At the peripheral endings, the grafts remain open after the peripheral transection. Adjacent bigger particles of fat are removed in order to facilitate the passage within the tubes.

These tubes are temporarily inserted to bridge the gap at the recipient site. With the help of a thread within the tube, the grafts can be pulled through the tube. In order to minimize the friction, it is important to moisten the grafts as well as the tubes. Sometimes, the course must be curved in order to have the grafts placed within an adequate subcutaneous tissue.

9.6 Number of Used Lymphatic Collectors

In the literature, there has been a discussion as to why certain patients do not develop lymphedema despite extensive damage to the axilla. The anatomical situation provides an explanation. There is a long lymphatic upper arm bundle connecting the arm and the lymphatic vessels behind the clavicle. If this long bundle is present, it bypasses the axilla, and the patient does not develop lymphedema. This long lymphatic bundle consists of one to two lymphatic collectors. The number of collectors are also used for lymph vessel transplantation. Scintigraphic measurements show that regaining normal lymphatic transport is possible using lymphatic collectors for transplantation.[10]

Normally, two collectors are harvested for grafting, which has been shown not to affect the lower extremity drainage, which is based on approximately 16 collectors.

9.7 Surgical Equipment

For the anastomosing process, the operating microscope with the highest possible magnification and the finest available instruments are used, after a long intensive micro-surgical and lymphological training. Magnification up to 40-fold should be achieved.

9.8 Postoperative Management

After surgery, the affected extremity and the donor site leg are treated with bandages and kept in an elevated position. Bed rest is advised for 3 days, and active decongestive movements are performed by the patient after surgery. No specific postoperative manual decompression therapy (MDT) is recommended.

Patients are advised to wear custom-made elastic stockings for 6 months on the extremity with lymphedema in order to improve the influx from the peripheral lymphatic vessels into the grafts.

9.9 Pearls and Pitfalls

Even though the authors describe a positive impact on quality of life following ALVT and report that these patients no longer require further treatment[7] because the affected extremity is equal in size compared to the healthy extremity, some pitfalls of the procedure should be mentioned. One major risk of ALVT concerns the possible donor site morbidity that may occur, in the worst case, in a surgery-associated lymphedema at the graft donor site. Moreover, a rather large longitudinal scar at the donor site after harvesting of the lymphatic collector cannot be prevented. The procedure of ALVT has not established itself internationally over the years as improvements in imaging (see **Chapter 4**) and the further development of the lymphovenous anastomosis (LVA) technique offer a less minimally invasive and probably equally effective alternative to ALVT. Furthermore, LVAs aim at redirecting the excess lymphatic fluid directly into the venous system as opposed to the lymphatic circulation in ALVT.

However, there is still merit in seeking to improve this type of lymphatic surgery. The ALVT is a milestone in the history of lymphedema surgery based on the plastic surgery principle of replacing like with like. The senior author is the pioneer of reconstructive lymphedema surgery in Germany.

Please also note that the foregoing pearls relate to patients where no further treatment became necessary, where the extremity had the same size as the unaffected arm and the postoperative, nuclear-medical measurement of the lymphatic flow was normal.

The pitfall is given when. despite the normal scintigraphic lymphatic flow at the harvesting site at the beginning of the surgery, only single lymphatic collectors are stained and lymphatic grafting seems therefore not advisable.

9.10 Clinical Cases

Case 1

Free lymphatic grafts were used to reconstruct the interruption of the lymphatic pathway in the axillary region (▶ Fig. 9.4).

Case 2

The transpositioning of lymphatic vessels from a non-affected leg. Vessel grafts from a healthy lower extremity may remain attached to the inguinal lymph nodes while being transposed to the affected groin for the anastomosis (▶ Fig. 9.5)

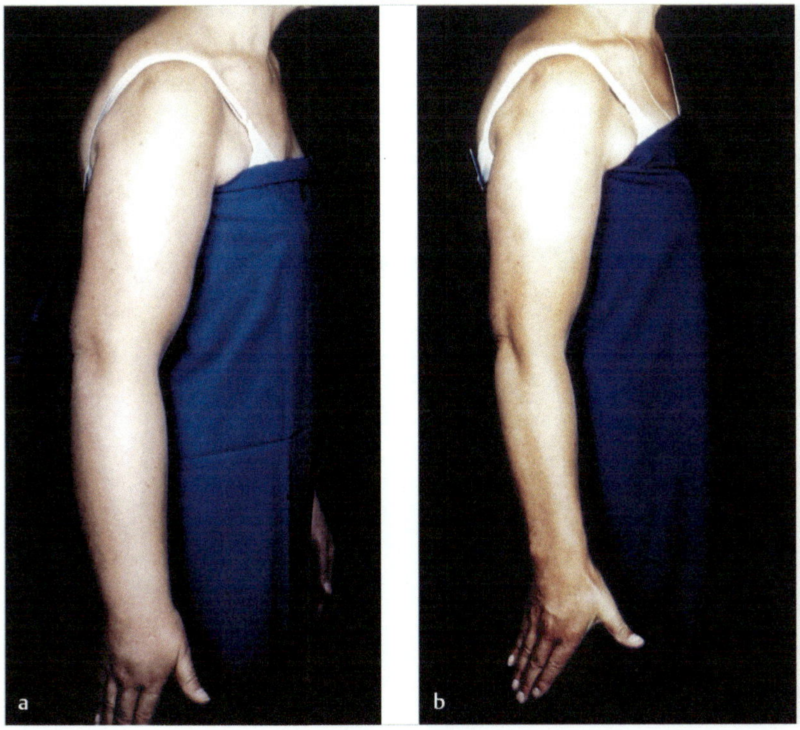

Fig. 9.4 A 50-year-old woman after axillary dissection. **(a)** Preoperative and **(b)** 5 months after autologous lymph vessel transfer.

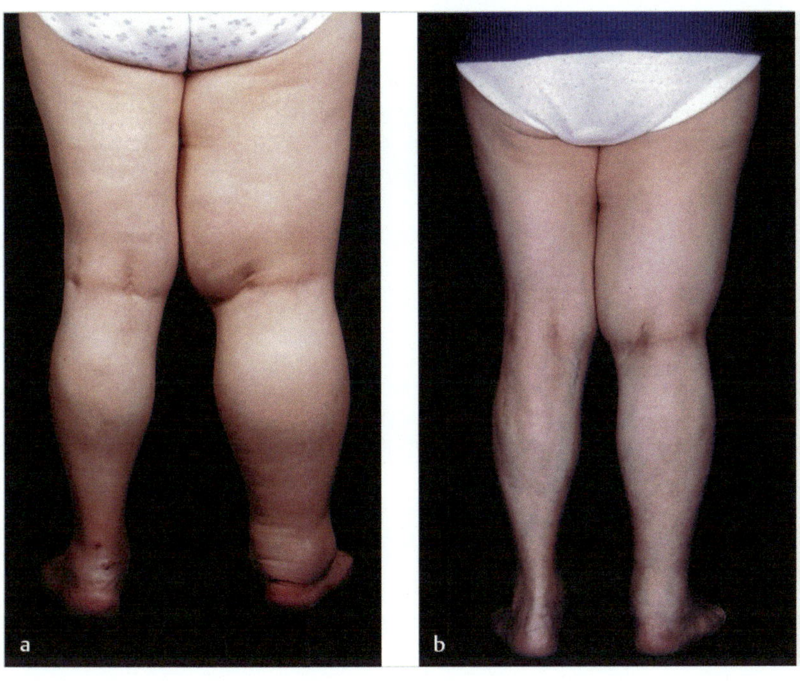

Fig. 9.5 **(a)** A 70-year-old patient with unilateral secondary lymphedema on the right leg. **(b)** Twelve years after transpositioning lymphatic vessels from the nonaffected leg.

References

[1] McHale NG, Roddie IC. The effect of transmural pressure on pumping activity in isolated bovine lymphatic vessels. J Physiol. 1976; 261(2): 255–269

[2] McHale NG. The lymphatic circulation. Ir J Med Sci. 1992; 161(8): 483–486

[3] Frick A, Wiebecke B, Baumeister RGH. Histologische Befunde von Lymphgefäßen, gewonnen bei Lymphgefäßtransplantationen. In: Baumeister RGH, ed. Lymphologica Jahresband 1990. München: Medikon Verlag; 1990

[4] Kinmonth JB. The Lymphatics. London: Edward Arnold; 1982

[5] Wallmichrath J, Baumeister RGH, Herrler T, et al. Experimental study on the microsurgical or spontaneous formation of lympho-lymphonodular anastomoses in the rat model. J Plast Reconstr Aesthet Surg. 2012; 65(4):494–500

[6] Baumeister RGH, Seifert J, Wiebecke B. Transplantation of lymph vessels on rats as well as a first therapeutic application on the experimental lymphedema of the dog. Eur Surg Res. 1980; 12 Suppl2:7–8

[7] Springer S, Koller M, Baumeister RGH, Frick A. Changes in quality of life of patients with lymphedema after lymphatic vessel transplantation. Lymphology. 2011; 44(2):65–71

[8] Baumeister RG, Seifert J, Wiebecke B, Hahn D. Experimental basis and first application of clinical lymph vessel transplantation of secondary lymphedema. World J Surg. 1981; 5(3):401–407

[9] Baumeister RG, Siuda S. Treatment of lymphedemas by microsurgical lymphatic grafting: what is proved? Plast Reconstr Surg. 1990; 85(1): 64–74, discussion 75–76

[10] Weiss M, Baumeister RGH, Frick A, Wallmichrath J, Bartenstein P, Rominger A. Lymphedema of the upper limb: evaluation of the functional outcome by dynamic imaging of lymph kinetics after autologous lymph vessel transplantation. Clin Nucl Med. 2015 Feb;40(2):e117–23

[11] Weiss MF, Baumeister RG, Zacherl MJ, Frick A, Bartenstein P, Rominger A. [Microsurgical autologous lymph vessel transplantation: does harvesting lymphatic vessel grafts induce lymphatic transport disturbances in the donor limb? Handchir Mikrochir Plast Chir 2015;47:359-64.

[12] Wallmichrath, J, Schoepfer D, Frick A. Investigations on the donor limb after harvest of lymphatic vessels for lymphedema surgery. J Vasc Surg Venous Lymphat Disord. 2022

10 Vascularized Lymph Node Transfer

Summary
Lymphedema is a pathologic condition that involves the accumulation of lymphatic fluid leading to tissue swelling. Options for surgical treatment of lymphedema can be categorized into two groups: excisional and physiological methods. The goal of physiological treatment is to restore the lymphatic drainage. The vascularized lymph node transfer is a free tissue transfer with lymph nodes has been practiced in lymphatic surgery for two decades. It is unclear whether the transferred lymph nodes act as a sponge to absorb lymphatic fluids into the venous system, or if they really induce lymphangiogenesis. The groin has been considered as the first choice for many years. However, other donor sites have been lately described as alternative options, with less risk of potential iatrogenic lymphedema at the donor site. Indocyanine green images and reverse lymphatic mapping technology are mandatory when vascularized lymph node transfer is planned. This chapter will describe the different available donor sites, indications, surgical techniques, and outcomes.

Keywords: gastroepiploic lymph node transfer (GELNT), jejunal mesenteric lymph node transfer (JMLT), lateral thoracic/thoracodorsal lymph node transfer (LTLNT), lymph nodes, omental lymph node transfer (OLNT), robotic, submental lymph node transfer (SMLNT), superficial inguinal lymph node transfer (SILNT), supraclavicular lymph node transfer (SCLNT), transplantation, vascularized, vascularized lymph node transfer (VLNT)

10.1 Donor Sites: Anatomical Basics and Clinical Reality

Moustapha Hamdi, Chieh-Han Tzou, and Julia Roka-Palkovitz

10.1.1 Inguinal Lymph Node Transfer

The anatomy of the groin area for harvesting superficial inguinal node transplants (hereafter referred to as superficial inguinal lymph node transfer [SILNT]) is complex[8], and an understanding of this anatomy is crucial for safe flap harvesting without creating donor site lymphedema.

The primary anatomic landmarks in the groin are the pubic tubercle (PT), inguinal ligament, anterior superior iliac spine (ASIS), femoral artery and veins, femoral nerve, and sartorius muscle. The femoral artery lies lateral to the femoral vein and branches to form the superficial circumflex iliac artery (SCIA), deep circumflex iliac artery (DCIA), superficial inferior epigastric artery (SIEA), and deep inferior epigastric artery (DIEA) (▶ Fig. 10.1). The SCIA divides further into a direct superficial (and more medial) branch and a deeper (and more lateral) branch, which runs below the deep fascia, piercing the sartorius, before traveling more superficially.

Lymph nodes of the groin are located medially/laterally and deep/superficially to the femoral vessels. Based on several studies, a mean number of lymph nodes of 6.5 per groin are present.[2,3,4] In the area where SILNT is safely performed, a mean of 3.1 lymph nodes is counted. In some rare cases, no lymph nodes are found.

Describing the territories of the superficial lymphatic system and their corresponding lymph nodes is possible with the concept of "lymphosomes," presented by Scaglioni and Suami in 2015. The superficial lymph nodes in the inguinal region are divided into three subgroups based on the connecting lymphatic vessels: the abdominal group, the lateral thigh group, and the medial thigh group (▶ Fig. 10.2).

The abdominal lymph node group can be targeted for SILNT, whereas the medial thigh lymph node group must be preserved. The lymph nodes responsible for abdominal lymphatic drainage are located along the lower edge of the inguinal ligament and supplied by the SCIA or SIEA and anonymous branches from the common femoral artery. In addition, lymph drainage from the leg via the sentinel lymph nodes and their efferent lymphatic vessels should be respected.

In a similar concept, Zeltzer et al.[4] divided the superficial groin into three zones regarding their lymph node drainage patterns: Zone I is the area medial to the superficial inferior epigastric vein (SIEV), draining the lower extremity, whereas Zone II drains the lower abdomen, lower back, and upper gluteal region and is between the SIEV and the superficial circumflex iliac vein (SCIV). Within this zone, the most medial and caudal nodes could also pour the lower extremity. Zone III is lateral and caudal to the SCIV and drains the lower extremity.

The authors described a "golden triangle" within Zone II, where superficial inguinal lymph nodes can be found and harvested safely (▶ Fig. 10.2).

It was found to be 48 mm from the PT when projected on a line from the PT to the ASIS, 16 mm caudal to this line, and 20 mm above the groin crease. It was 41 mm lateral to the SCIV–SIEV confluence (▶ Fig. 10.3).

In summary, the SILNT design should include a functional group of lymph nodes out of Zone II. Lymph nodes that drain the lower extremity should be excluded. Lymph nodes medial to the femoral artery drain the lower extremity. Staying lateral to the artery during flap

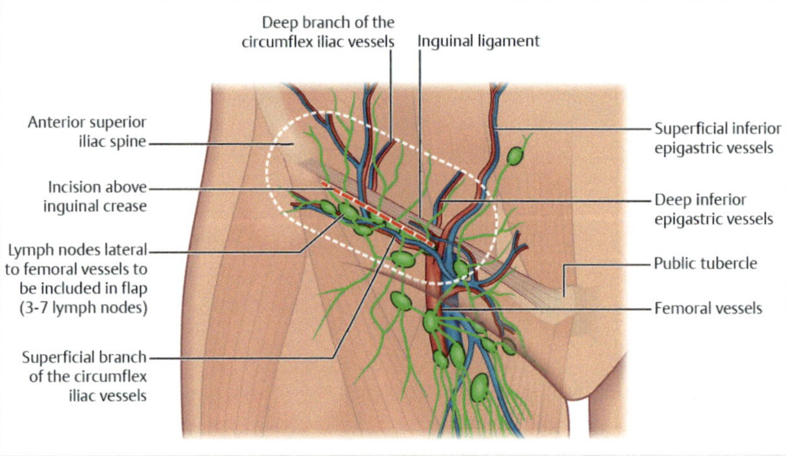

Fig. 10.1 Anatomy of the inguinal region: Different lymph node groups adjacent to the femoral vessels and superficial branch of the circumflex iliac vessels. Marking of the inguinal vascularized lymph node flap (dotted line).

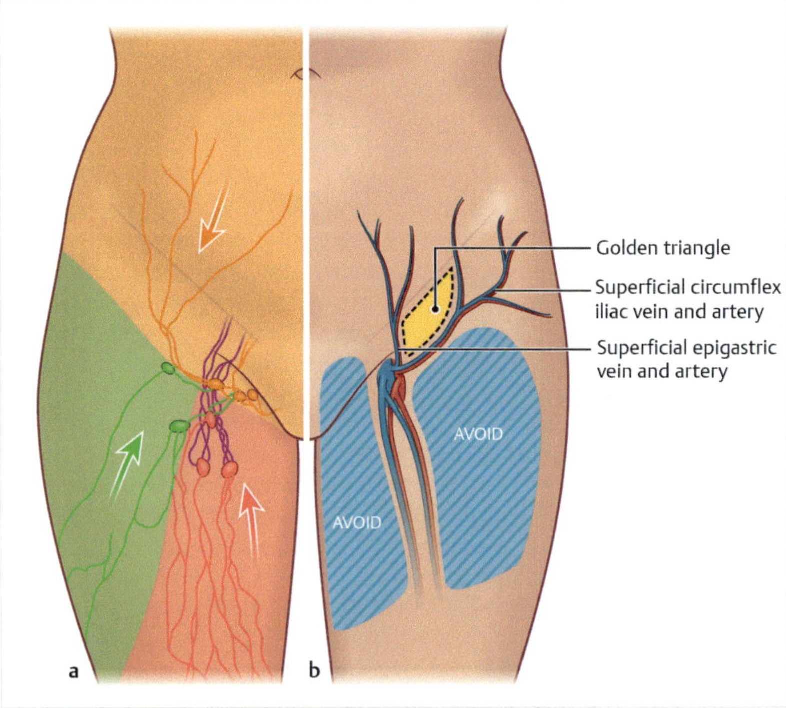

Fig. 10.2 Anatomy of the inguinal region: The different groups of superficial inguinal lymph nodes with their corresponding drainage zones (lymphosomes) of the right abdominal region and thigh: abdominal in yellow, lateral thigh in green, and medial thigh in red (a). The lymph nodes that drain the medial zone of the thigh (red) and which are usually found medially to the femoral vessels have to be preserved. Anatomic boundaries of the "Golden Triangle" (yellow). The zones marked in blue often contain lymphatic tissue and therefore should not be included in the LN flap (a).

harvest is not sufficient in terms of safety. Secondary lower extremity lymphatic impairment can still occur after SILNT. A study by Dayan et al.[7] describing the anatomy of the flap was completed using magnetic resonance angiography imaging. The study suggested that there was a cluster of lymph nodes at the confluence of the SCIA/SCIV and the SIEV, which could be included in the flap harvest. However, a cadaveric study suggests that lymph nodes at the confluence, along the SIEV and caudal to the SCIV, can contribute to lymphatic drainage of the lower extremity. Including these lymph nodes with the flap harvest may increase the risk of lower extremity lymphedema.

10.1.2 Supraclavicular Lymph Node Transfer

The supraclavicular chain of lymph nodes, also known as the "transverse" chain, is located along the transverse cervical artery (TCA). It receives afferent vessels from the anterolateral neck skin, chest wall, mammary gland, and occasionally from the upper extremity and the infraclavicular lymph nodes. Anterior tributaries connecting the superficial anterior cervical lymph nodes are located in the anterior jugular pathway, draining lymph from skin and muscles of the infrahyoid region, the isthmus of the thyroid gland, and the infraglottic part of the larynx.

Tributaries arise laterally from the accessory lymphatic chain, and channels from the superficial external jugular lymph nodes.

The majority of the lymphatic pathways from the breast toward the supraclavicular apical lymph nodes, typically terminating in the scalene lymph nodes posterior to the sternocleidomastoid and the clavicle, may drain to the supraclavicular lymph nodes. An "axillary bypass" directly into these lymph nodes may be present in 5% to 17% of cases.

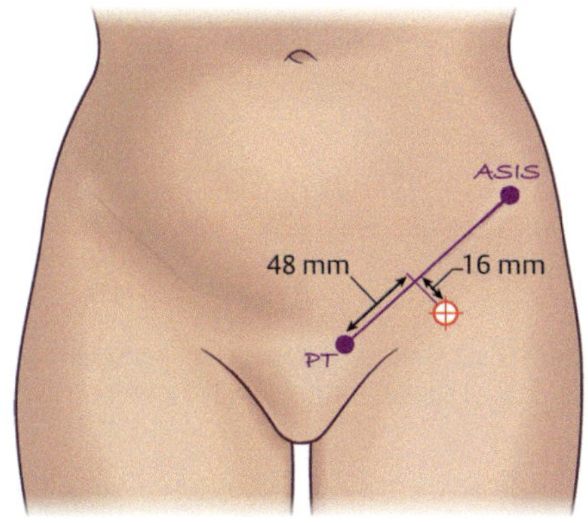

Fig. 10.3 Anatomical landmarks to plan the vascularized lymph node flap of the groin: A line is marked between the pubic tubercle and the anterior superior iliac spine. In this case, the lymph nodes to be harvested are located adjacent to a perforating vessel identified 48 mm lateral to the pubic tubercle and 16 mm caudal to the marked line.

Efferent lymphatics (typically two to three) form the supraclavicular trunk, which enters the subclavian venous angle either directly, or via the thoracic duct (or the right lymphatic duct).

In the left neck, the last lymph node intercalated within the thoracic duct, after its ascendance in the chest, is referred to as Virchow's node. It is located at or near the jugulo-subclavian venous junction (referred to as the venous angle).

There is significant anatomic variability of the arterial and venous supplies of the supraclavicular region.

The blood supply of the skin component of this flap is based on the supraclavicular artery (SCA) (1.0–1.5 mm) and vein (1.0–1.5 mm). Cadaver dissections have shown that the SCA arises 3 to 4 cm from the origin of the TCA, which is found in the triangle between the dorsal edge of the sternocleidomastoid muscle (SCM), the external jugular vein (EJV), and the medial part of the clavicle. Moreover, the SCA runs along with two accompanying veins; one or two veins may drain into the transverse cervical vein, and the other may drain into the EJV (▶ Fig. 10.4).

When the lymph nodes are harvested without a skin paddle, blood supply comes from various branches of the transverse cervical artery and vein as they course through these lymph nodes (▶ Fig. 10.5). However, one must be aware that the vascular anatomy in this area can vary significantly both in terms of the location and size of the vessels. Major important nerves present in this area are the phrenic nerve and the vagus nerve (lateral and medial to internal jugular vein [IJV], respectively).

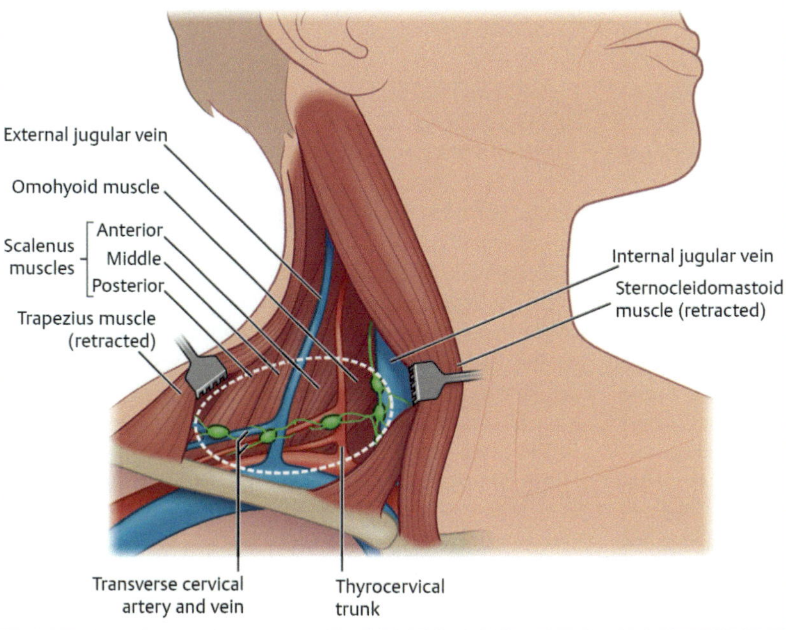

Fig. 10.4 Anatomy of the supraclavicular region: Anatomical relationship between the transverse cervical vessels originating from the thyro-cervical trunk and the adjacent lymph nodes. Marking of the supra-clavicular vascularized lymph node flap (dotted line).

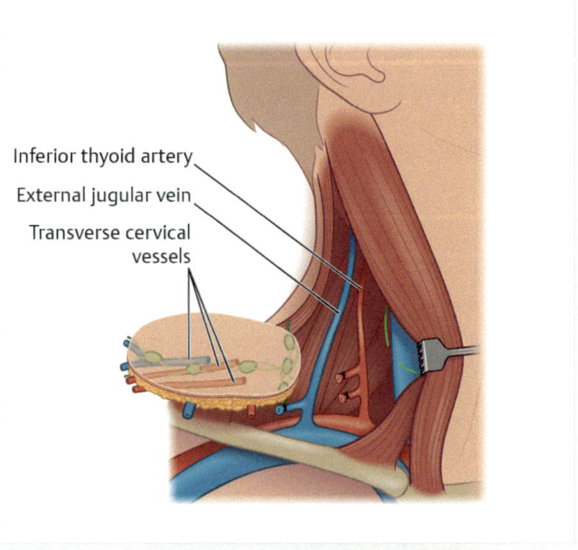

Fig. 10.5 Anatomy of the supraclavicular region: Multiple vascular perforators originate from the transverse cervical artery and perforate the platysma muscle towards the skin in order to perfuse the corresponding skin island. The actual lymph node flap includes the transverse cervical artery, its side branches and concomitant veins being the flap's pedicle. The lymph nodes of the supraclavicular regions are in part located adjacent to these blood vessels. When dissection this flap, the external jugular vein is usually included into the skin island of the flap to become the dominant subcutaneous vein for additional venous drainage.

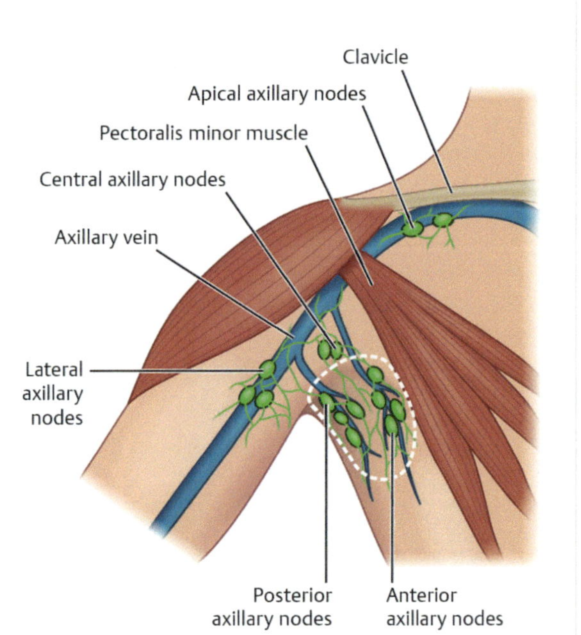

Fig. 10.6 Anatomy of the axillar region: The three axillary lymph node groups, i.e., lateral, posterior and anterior. Marking of the axillary vascularized lymph node flap of the lateral thoracic region (dotted line).

10.1.3 Lateral Thoracic/Thoracodorsal Lymph Node Transfer

The lateral thoracic lymph node flap involves the transfer of lymph nodes from the lower part of the axilla between the anterior and posterior axillary lines. Anatomical studies of the lymphatic drainage of the axilla have demonstrated discrete organization of the sentinel lymph node drainage of the thorax and upper extremity, and this forms the basis of lymph node transfer from this region.

Branches of the lateral thoracic vessels are identified as well. Lymph node harvest is limited to level 1 (inferior to lateral border of pectoralis minor) lymph nodes to avoid damaging the draining lymphatics of the arm. A freestyle flap is designed, and the lateral thoracic vessels are usually chosen as their branches tend to preferentially supply the lymph nodes.

The axilla may be conceptualized as containing five groups of lymph nodes: lateral, central, posterior, anterior, and apical. Beginning distally along the axillary vein, the lateral group drains the arm and continues into a central group that receives drainage from the back via posterior group based on the thoracodorsal axis and from the chest via an anterior group based on the lateral thoracic axis. The central group then drains into the apical group of lymph nodes located proximally along the axillary vein. These lymph nodes drain superiorly into supraclavicular lymph nodes. In practice, these groups are not clearly defined and there is cross-over drainage between groups that makes identification of drainage patterns based on anatomy alone unreliable. It is worth mentioning that there is a separate drainage pathway, named after Mascagni, which runs along the cephalic vein in the deltopectoral groove. Some lymphatics from this pathway may cross over the clavicle and drain directly into deep cervical lymph nodes, thus bypassing the axillary nodal groups.

The anterior and posterior groups of lymph nodes are targeted for harvest in axillary VLNT (▶ Fig. 10.6). The blood supply to these lymph nodes is not consistent due to variations in the vascular anatomy in the axilla. The lateral thoracic artery may arise from the thoracodorsal or subscapular artery in 29% of cases. The lateral thoracic vein typically arises as a separate branch from the axillary vein. The artery is 1.3 mm, and the vein is 2.6 mm.

The lateral thoracic artery, which is the classic pedicle to the lateral thoracic lymph nodes, originates from the axillary artery, but anatomic variations can exist, with variable origin or complete absence of the lateral thoracic artery altogether.

An alternative pedicle is the thoracodorsal artery, which can also supply the lateral thoracic lymph nodes. However, if the thoracodorsal vessels are utilized for a lateral thoracic lymph node transfer, this sacrifices the latissimus dorsi and precludes the use of a workhorse flap in breast reconstruction.

An anatomical study revealed on average 13.40 ± 3.13 lymph nodes within the flap. Perforators to the overlying skin were present in 87.5% of anatomical dissections, allowing for transfer of a skin paddle.

10.1.4 Submental Lymph Node Transfer

In the subplatysmal space, key structures can be found within the various layers of the investing layer of the cervical fascia. The main arterial sources to neck structures include branches of the external carotid system. The arterial supply to the submental vascularized lymph node (VLN) flap is based on the submental artery, which is a consistent branch of the facial artery. The facial artery can be found approximately 2.0 to 2.5 cm anterior to the mandibular angle at the level of the lower mandibular border. Approximately 0.5 cm below this point and 6.5 cm from the origin of this artery, the submental artery can be found originating as an anterior branch from the facial artery. The average arterial diameter at the origin is approximately 1.5 to 2.0 mm. The key anatomic structures of the submental region are shown in ▶ Fig. 10.7.

The emergence of the submental artery is in close relation to the submandibular gland. In a majority of cases, the submental artery can be found between the lower border of the mandible and the submandibular gland.[12] Occurring less frequently, the artery runs on the superficial surface of the gland or running between the lobes of the gland. Following the course past the gland, the artery travels on the superficial surface of the mylohyoid muscle, which separates the neck structures from the oral cavity. During the arterial course, the submental artery supplies various skin perforators through the platysma muscle. The distal aspect of the artery can have a variable course in relation to the anterior belly of the digastric muscle. In approximately 70% of patients, the distal submental artery travels deep to the digastric muscle, while the remaining travels superficial to the muscle.[13] It terminates in the submental region, where it anastomoses with the contralateral submental artery. During its course, it gives rise to several septocutaneous perforating branches, also supplying the adipose tissue containing submental (Ia) and submandibular (Ib) lymph nodes.

Venous return is ensured by the submental vein draining into the facial vein, according to a satellite course of the artery. The facial vein drains inconsistently into the thyrolinguofacial venous trunk and then into the internal jugular vein, via a more superficial course than that of the facial artery, generally above the posterior belly of the digastric muscle.

Special consideration is warranted for the location of the marginal mandibular branch of the facial nerve (MMN). If not, an otherwise successful lymphedema-related surgical result will be overshadowed by the morbidity of injury to this important structure. Injury to the MMN manifests as weakness and/or inability to move the ipsilateral lower lip downward and laterally. Muscles responsible for this action are the depressor anguli oris (DAO) and depressor labii inferioris (DLI). Injury is apparent on animation of the face and from asymmetry during smiling.

Harvested vascularized lymph nodes included in the submental VLN flap are based on the level I lymph nodes in the Ia and submandibular Ib regions. Ib sublevel is drawing attention as a lymph node hotspot. These lymph nodes are located in the subplatysmal plane atop the deep cervical musculature and perfused by the submental artery. The hyoid bone, the mandible, and the anterior belly of the digastric muscle form the submental triangle. The anatomic landmarks of the submandibular group of lymph nodes are posterior to the submental region and continue from the digastric muscle posteriorly to the posterior aspect of the submandibular gland. Altogether, both groups comprise the level I lymph nodes and are in close proximity to the submental/facial artery system (▶ Fig. 10.7).

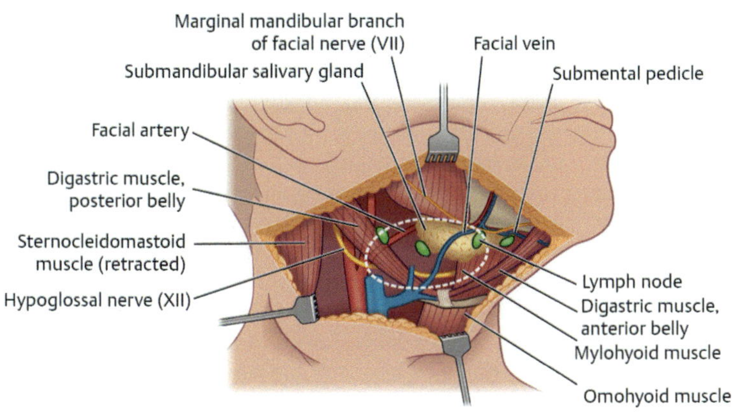

Fig. 10.7 Anatomy of submandibular region: Relationship between lymph nodes, facial artery and vein, submental pedicle of the flap, and marginal branch of the facial nerve and hypoglossal nerve. Marking of the submandibular vascularized lymph node flap (dotted line).

10.1.5 Omental Lymph Node Transfer

The omental flap comprises two dominant pedicles, the right and left gastroepiploic vessels. The right gastroepiploic artery (RGEA) is preferred because it is larger, has more epiploic branches, and is easily accessible through a laparoscopic approach. The omentum consists of a vast network of lymphoreticular bodies that drain into the lymphatic collecting system along the right gastroepiploic pedicle and should be preserved during dissection.

10.1.6 Gastroepiploic Lymph Node Transfer

The gastroepiploic flap is a modification of the free omental flap, such that the omental tissue is harvested laparoscopically and is limited to the area adjacent to the gastroepiploic vascular arcade, since the lymph nodes are located around these vessels. This allows for the creation of relatively small lymph node flap (mean: 3 cm × 7 cm) that allows placement in the distal extremity with minimal impact on cosmetics (▶ Fig. 10.8). The flap is harvested using the right gastroepiploic artery (RGEA) due to greater accessibility compared with the left side.

The lymph nodes within the RGEA distribution can be reliably found within 3 cm surrounding the artery within the first 9 cm of the RGEA from its origin. Most patients have at least three lymph nodes within this basin, which is comparable to other lymph node basins prepared for VLNT. These findings are consistent and reliable: 75% of individuals in this study population had identifiable lymph nodes in the RGEA perfusion area. This lymphosome confers the additional advantage of being located within the abdomen, in an area without a known risk of causing iatrogenic lymphedema. Of note, 25% of individuals included in this study did not have identifiable lymph nodes in the RGEA lymphosome. Whether these individuals truly do not have lymph nodes in the RGEA distribution or whether they were perhaps missed on imaging remains to be determined. Certainly, this difference supports the use of CT angiography before harvesting RGEA lymph nodes to verify that there are lymph nodes in the RGEA basin before beginning surgery (▶ Fig. 10.8).

Recent studies have characterized the anatomy of the vessel and associated lymph nodes with preference for the RGEA.[14] The right gastroepiploic lymph node basin for VLNT has become popular due to minimal donor site morbidity. Although anatomy varies from person to person, CT angiography may help to plan VLNT. The diameter of RGEA is between 1.5 and 3 mm, and the lymph nodes are within 3 cm. Although the right gastroduodenal artery (GDA) is typically 4 cm away from the RGEA takeoff, that distance can be much less, so one must identify it before dissection. With these principles, the plastic surgeon can safely take the RGEA and surrounding 3 cm of tissue to include three lymph nodes when planning for a right gastroepiploic VLNT.

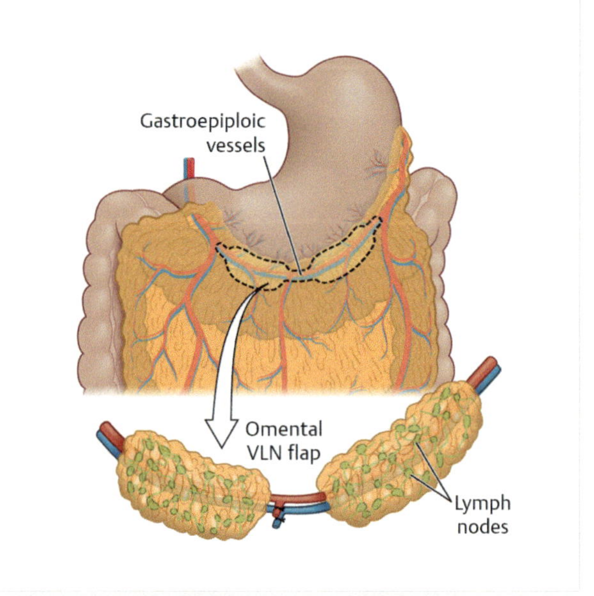

Fig. 10.8 Anatomy of gastroepiploic region: Omental vascularized lymph node flap based on the gastroepiploic vessels. Marking of the omental vascularized lymph node flap (dotted lines) including several lymph nodes adjacent to the gastroepiploic vessels along the greater curvature of the stomach.

10.1.7 Jejunal Mesenteric Lymph Node Transfer

The jejunum is the middle segment of the small intestine and functions primarily in the digestion and absorption of enteric contents. It comprises approximately two-fifths of the total length of the small intestine and itself measures roughly 2.5 m in length. The mesentery, which is a double fold of the peritoneum, suspends the small and large intestines from the posterior abdominal wall and houses their vascular, lymphatic, and nervous supply.

The jejunum receives its blood supply from the superior mesenteric artery (SMA), which originates from the aorta anterior to L1 and approximately 1 cm inferior to the takeoff of the celiac artery. From there, the SMA proceeds inferiorly, passing behind the neck of the pancreas and the splenic vein, before giving rise to several jejunal arteries, which run in parallel to each other within the layers of the mesentery. As these vessels travel toward the small intestine, the jejunal arteries further divide into branches that have numerous anastomoses with adjacent branches to form a series of arterial arcades. The collateral flow conferred by these anastomoses serves as the basis for the ability to selectively divide mesenteric branches without causing ischemia. The venous drainage of the small intestine occurs through the superior mesenteric vein, which ultimately joins the splenic vein to empty into the portal system.[18]

Cadaveric investigation has found that the greatest number of lymph nodes exist within the proximal third of the jejunum, where there is an average of 19.2 total lymph nodes, a significantly greater number than in the middle and distal thirds. The lymph nodes can be divided into those located in the periphery of the mesentery closer to the bowel and the more plentiful lymph nodes located centrally and closer to the larger vessels at the root of the mesentery. The lymph nodes present in the periphery are usually supplied by vessels that measure approximately 1.5 to 3 mm in diameter (with the vein measuring approximately 0.5 mm larger than the associated artery) and have a more robust capillary network around the lymph nodes, making them an ideal target for a standard end-to-end or end-to-side anastomosis at the recipient site. The arterial inflow and venous outflow should be well balanced in these flaps as they represent more of an “end organ” to the pedicle, not unlike other fasciocutaneous flaps that we routinely use, such as the anterolateral thigh flap. However, these peripherally located lymph node flaps may include the anastomotic loops and straight arteries to the jejunum and thus may potentially devascularize a segment of the bowel and should be carefully chosen by transillumination. Use of these relatively smaller vessels for microsurgical transfer, compared to those in proximity to the root of the mesentery, achieves a better size match with the flap itself, which typically measures approximately 3 cm.

The lymph nodes located toward the root of the mesentery can be harvested with less concern about related bowel ischemia due to the tremendous arborization and redundant vascular connections through anastomotic loops toward the periphery of the mesentery. However, the larger vessels at the mesenteric root (the artery and vein typically measure approximately 3 mm and 4-6 mm, respectively) carry a tremendous amount of blood to and from the jejunum, which largely bypasses the small capillary perforators to the lymph nodes in this area. Therefore, a standard end-to-end vascular connection of the flap pedicle to donor vessels at the recipient site may result in a significant vascular inflow and outflow imbalance and even flap loss, unless a more physiologic connection, such as a flow-through design of the flap artery and vein or an arteriovenous loop at the distal end of the flap pedicle, is included.

10.2 Indications and Contraindications

Holger Engel

Indications for autologous lymph node transfer have developed dramatically in the last 10 years and knowledge of lymphatic surgery has increased. Initially, lymph node transfer was indicated for certain lymphedema staging/classification levels (e.g., International Society of Lymphology [ISL] stage II/III) or after a fixed period of conservative treatment, not infrequently for up to 2 years, without any improvement or worsening conditions. Currently, the indication and the time point of intervention for autologous lymph node transfer are determined based on a specific patient-centered assessment and in an embedded multimodal therapy setting. This approach is supported by recently published data demonstrating that patient-reported outcomes might be more critical in predicting long-term health-related quality of life than clinician-measured results.

A sequential approach in a multimodal setting is described in detail in the algorithm in **Chapter 18**. In brief, lymph node transfer is indicated when options for conservative treatment and lymphovenous anastomosis (LVA) have already been used and reached their limits. This is the case when, for example, total occlusion of lymphatics or partial occlusion on lymphoscintigraphy combined with increasing episodes of cellulitis is present. This could already be the case in lymphedema severity stage I on the ISL scale and in “stardust” or “diffuse” formation described by Yamamoto et al.[16] The controversy between one stage versus sequential use of combined surgical procedures is discussed in **Subchapter 15.5**. Patients with ISL stage III or IV should undergo adjunctive lipectomy or debulking procedures before lymph node transfer.

Contraindications are dependent on patients' health status and expected donor site morbidities. In general, the patient should be healthy enough to survive the operation and should also be able to follow a dedicated aftercare schedule postoperatively. One should act with extreme caution with patients suffering from tumor, e.g., local recurrences and distant metastasis. Additionally, undetected metastasis, or a local tumor disease, within the lymph node transplant could be brought to the recipient site, making oncologic therapy difficult or impossible. Depending on the tumor type, prognosis, and expected treatment, in select cases there could be an indication if there is a high probability of increasing quality of life by decreasing lymphedema suffering.

Patients suffering from brachial plexus neuritis or chronic regional pain syndrome are also contraindicated.

Relative and absolute contraindications are present in the event of pre-existing disease, trauma, operation, or radiotherapy of the donor site. For example, a patient with multiple operations of the intestine is not an ideal candidate for jejunal mesenteric lymph node transfer due to the extensive scarring and increased donor site morbidity. Patients with lymphedema of the lower extremity develop rerouting lymphatic ducts to the other side of the groin area. Therefore, it is obsolete to harvest groin lymph nodes from that area. The same principle applies to patients suffering from head and neck lymphedema after modified unilateral neck dissection. Submental lymph nodes are obsolete in this condition.

10.3 Preoperative Evaluation and Planning

Holger Engel

Preoperative evaluation and planning are crucial for selecting the right patients for VLNT and achieving the best outcomes. The preoperative assessment contains a thorough clinical examination, ICG lymphangiography, ultrasound, and MRI. Patient selection is also based on the severity of the disease and patient-specific characteristics.

The clinical examination can be used to determine the patient's ISL stage, identify previous surgeries and scars, and inspect available donor/recipient sites. Any skin changes, cellulitis, or open wounds associated with advanced lymphedema stages will affect the selection of VLNT recipient sites due to the risk of postoperative infections. Sometimes, lymphoablative surgery must be performed before or concurrently with reconstructive VLNT. Patients with severe lymphedema visible as "pitting edema" should undergo conservative treatment first with complete decongestive therapy to optimize the condition before VLNT.

Severe obesity should be treated first because of its negative influence on the whole healing process and has to be differentiated from fat depositions of the extremities caused by chronic inflammation of lymphedema. With massive fat deposits, lipectomy should also be considered.

ICG lymphangiography is one of the essential tools for evaluating lymphatic function, accurate diagnosis, and staging.[16] In patients with advanced dermal backflow called the "diffuse pattern" after Yamamoto, no functioning lymph collectors are visible, and lymph node transfer is recommended. Because ISL staging is not a reliable tool for treatment planning and tracking outcomes, Cheng's grading can be an alternative. Direct VLNT is recommended for Cheng's grade II or above.[17]

Preoperative ultrasound and MRI can help to evaluate the donor and recipient sites. The goal is to clarify anatomical details and to include as many lymph nodes as possible within the lymph node flap. The recipient vessels should be patent with adequate flow and size.

CT angiography is not mandatory unless a history of trauma or peripheral vascular disease is present. Duplex Doppler helps to clarify the patency of the venous system regarding superficial or deep venous incompetence.

10.4 Choice and Management of Donor and Recipient Sites

Holger Engel and Katrin Seidenstücker

The choice of the donor and recipient sites depends on various factors. The surgeon's preference may differ regarding the experience level, anatomical knowledge, and armamentarium that is available. Patient factors include previous surgeries, scars, and cosmetic concerns. There are anatomical differences regarding the quantity and density of donor lymph nodes, reliable and sizable pedicles, and iatrogenic lymphedema risks.

Initially, the groin area was a popular area for harvesting superficial inguinal lymph node transplants.[5,21] Unfortunately, without thoroughly performed intraoperative reversed mapping, there is a risk of iatrogenic lymphedema. This is also true for thoracodorsal lymph node transplants, where axillary reverse mapping (ARM) is mandatory. Therefore, preferences have shifted from the groin area and thoracodorsal lymph nodes to submental, supraclavicular, and abdominal donor sites for VLNT. They are utilized only when there is a contraindication for the other VLNT, due to patients' preference, for cosmetic reasons, or due to an inadequate number or size of lymph nodes.

Submental, supraclavicular, and jejunal mesenteric donor sites could demonstrate a high quantity and density of lymph nodes with minimal risks of iatrogenic lymphedema as well as reliable pedicles.[21] In contrast, gastroepiploic and omental donor sites have revealed a lower number of lymph nodes per transplant. A drawback of jejunal mesenteric lymph node transplants is often the short and small pedicle, making the dissection and anastomosis tedious.

An advantage of submental and jejunal mesenteric VLNT is that multiple flaps (submental two/jejunal mesenteric up to three) can be harvested from one donor site at the same time.[22] These flaps can be transplanted to different recipient sites in a one-stage operation.

The recipient site's choice depends on previous surgery scars, cosmetic concerns of the patient, availability of the recipient's vessels, and different severity of lymphedema at various levels of the extremity. Whether the surgeon believes in the "pump-gravity theory" or not is also essential.

10.4.1 Proximal versus Distal Recipient Area, Scar Management, and Flap Types

In general, recipient sites are divided into proximal anatomic areas such as the axilla and groin and distal "nonanatomic" sites such as the elbow, wrist, knee, and ankle.

There is still controversy regarding whether proximal or distal recipient sites are superior. Surgeons and authors who prefer the proximal recipient area emphasize the advantages of extensive scar removal along with the replacement of well-vascularized tissue in the site. Another advantage is that the scars are easily hidden and therefore provides acceptable to good cosmetic results. On the other hand, with extensive scarring, recipient vessel dissection is technically more challenging. If the dissection proceeds deep into the axilla, a

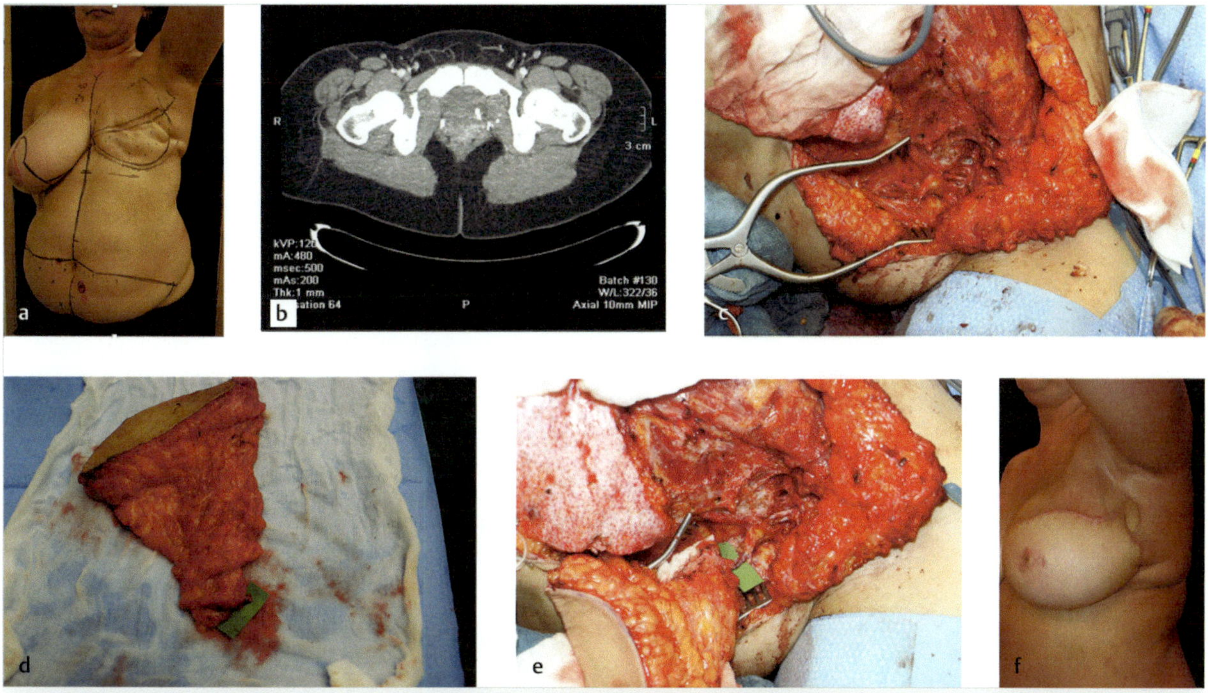

Fig. 10.9 Concomitant autologous breast reconstruction and vascularized lymph node transfer to treat breast cancer-related chronic lymphedema of the left upper extremity after mastectomy: (a) 45-year-old patient who developed left upper extremity lymphedema after mastectomy with axillary lymph dissection followed by radiotherapy 3 years ago. The patient was scheduled for deep inferior epigastric artery perforator flap breast reconstruction with simultaneous groin vascularized lymph node transfer to the axilla. (b) Computed tomography angiography scan was done to map the deep inferior epigastric artery perforator and also to identify the localization of lymph node. The left lymph nodes were selected for transfer. (c) The axilla was released from scar tissue and branches of the thoracodorsal vessels were prepared for anastomoses. (d) The groin vascularized lymph node flap was harvested based on the superficial inferior epigastric artery/vein. (e) The groin flap was transferred to the axilla and the microsurgery was done. (f) The outcome with significant reduction of lymphedema. (Courtesy of Moustapha Hamdi.)

vein graft may be needed. Some authors have stated that with proximal recipient sites, there is a higher probability of having to wear compression garments afterward.[9] Another disadvantage is transferring lymph nodes to drain the lymph fluid from distal to proximal areas against gravity.

Surgeons who prefer distal, "nonanatomic" recipient areas believe in the "pump action" of VLNT at the level of the elbow, wrist, knee, and ankle. They recommend removing a part of the deep fibrotic tissue large enough to create an adequate pocket for flap inset to allow tension-free wound closure without compression on the flap. Additionally, removing the adventitia should be performed to remove thick and fibrotic vascular adventitia. This also applies to arteries and especially veins. Hemostasis is crucial in preventing hematoma. Change et al.[9] demonstrated a more significant circumferential reduction of the wrist, but no difference was found proximal to the elbow. A better outcome was reported using the dorsal wrist compared to the palmar wrist (▶ Fig. 10.11). At the elbow and knee level, reduced gravity effects are present to support lymph fluid drainage into the venous system. The best outcome was encountered for the wrist and ankle recipient site. If there are cosmetic concerns, the popliteal fossa or elbow level can be chosen.

The function of the skin paddle has long been considered unclear. The skin paddle is essential for flap monitoring and for achieving tension-free wound closure.

10.4.2 Inguinal Vascularized Lymph Node Transfer to Distal Recipient (Wrist)

An interesting concept was published by Hayashi's group.[26] They described a new physiological treatment strategy for lymphedema, "lymphatic system transfer," comprising the transfer of vascularized afferent lymphatic vessels along with their draining lymph nodes. This approach could give the skin paddle a new role because the afferent lymphatic vessels are transferred within; therefore, a presumably lesser degree of lymphangiogenesis is required. Even though the number of patients assessed in this study was low, the results indicate that lymph node transplants with a skin paddle have an advantage over adipolymphatic flaps.

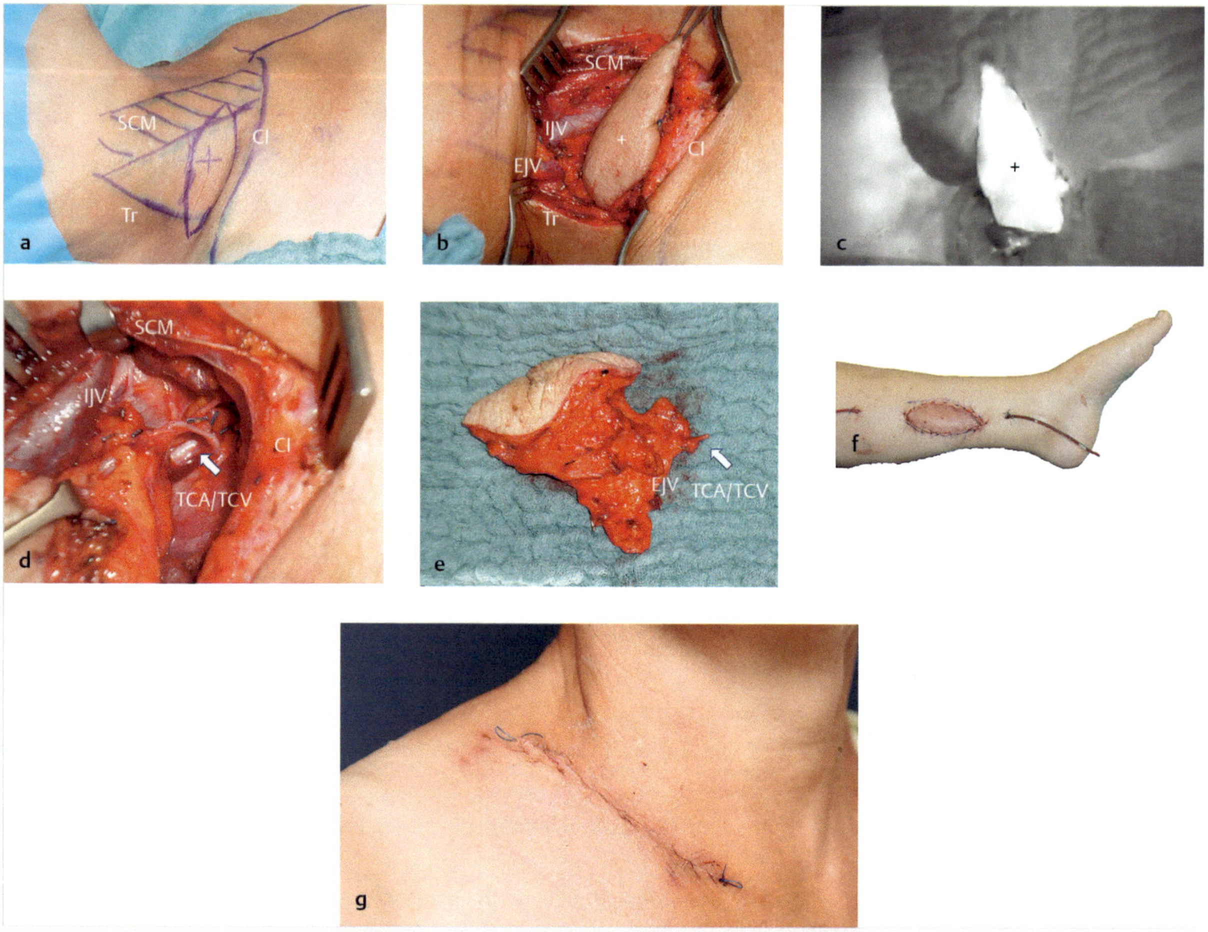

Fig. 10.10 Supraclavicular lymph node flap to treat chronic lymphedema of the left lower extremity: **(a)** Right supraclavicular region, side view, with the patient in prone position. Cl, clavicle; SCM, sternocleidomastoid muscle with lateral border; Tr, trapezius muscle; + skin island with marked perforator detected with pencil doppler probe. **(b)** Right supraclavicular region, side view, with the patient in prone position. Cl, clavicle; EJV, external jugular vein; IJV, internal jugular vein; SCM, sternocleidomastoid muscle with lateral border; Tr, trapezius muscle; + skin island after circumcision. **(c)** Right supraclavicular region, side view, with the patient in a prone position; ICG near-infrared imaging, after dissection of the pedicle + skin island of lymph node flap, abdominal linen/tissues wrapped around (dark color). **(d)** Right supraclavicular region, side view, with the patient in a prone position. Cl, clavicle; IJV, internal jugular vein; SCM, sternocleidomastoid muscle with lateral border; + skin island after circumcision; flap pedicle with transverse cervical artery/vein. (TCA/TCV). **(e)** Supraclavicular lymph node flap after harvesting; + skin island; EJV, external jugular vein as secondary vein; flap pedicle with transverse cervical artery/vein (TCA/TCV).
(f) Supraclavicular lymph node flap after inset close to the main lymphatic collectors to the distal leg and anastomosis to the dorsal tibial artery and two accessory veins (EJV and TVC); + skin island. **(g)** Donor site after 14 days. (Courtesy of Emre Gazyakan and Christoph Hirche.)

Intraoperative positioning of the patient and the physician depends on the team approach, recipient, and donor site.

Whenever possible, a two-team approach—one team for the donor and the other for the recipient site—is recommended. The units should be able to work independently without hindering each other.

Patient positioning: All of the lymph node transplants can be harvested in the supine position. The lateral thoracodorsal lymph nodes can also be harvested in the lateral position if desired. These strategies also apply to most of the recipient sites, including scar excision of the axilla. Therefore, inside the operating room, the patient should be centered in such a way that the donor and recipient sites can be approached simultaneously. If the upper extremity is the recipient site, the oblique asymmetric positioning of the patient can provide some extra space, if needed.

Equipment/Staff: Extra space should also be considered for positioning the microscope, fluorescence camera (if not included within the microscope), instrumentation table, back table, staff, and guests.

Submental and supraclavicular VLNT: The patient's head should be in slight reclination and flexible for mobilization. The intubation tube should be fixed at the teeth for intraoral anchoring and stitched to the columella for

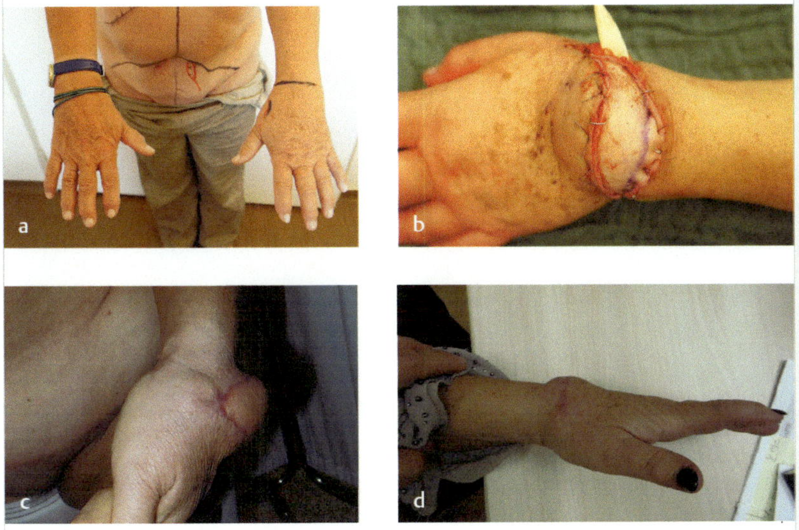

Fig. 10.11 Supraclavicular lymph node flap to treat chronic lymphedema of the left lower extremity: **(a)** A 67-year-old patient who underwent left mastectomy and axillary dissection with radiotherapy. She developed a painful and resistant hand lymphedema. The patient was scheduled for deep inferior epigastric artery flap breast reconstruction with a groin VLNT to the affected zone (left wrist). **(b)** The groin vascularized lymph node transfer was hooked to a branch of radial artery in the snuff box. **(c)** The result with wound healing. The patient no longer felt any pain, and the lymphedema was reduced significantly. However, the major concern of the patient was the aesthetic aspect. **(d)** A moderate lipectomy with skin paddle removal was done 6 months postoperatively with acceptable wrist contouring. (Courtesy of Moustapha Hamdi.)

intranasal usage. Sterile coverage should allow the surgeon to stand next to or cranial to the patient's head. Long ventilation tubes are necessary for an adequate distance of the anesthesia team.

For thoracodorsal VLNT, sterile wash should include the upper extremity for maximum mobility and the possibility to rest the extremity at the arm table.

Jejunal mesenteric, gastroepiploic, and omental VLNT allows team one to stand next to the patient at the abdominal height and team two at the recipient site upper or lower extremity.

10.5 Surgical Technique

Moustapha Hamdi, Holger Engel, and Katrin Seidenstücker

10.5.1 Vascularized Inguinal Lymph Node Transfer

Superficial inguinal lymph node transfer (SILNT) was one of the first lymph nodes to be transplanted and has gained popularity and been used by many surgeons. These lymph nodes are selectable only in lymphedema of the upper extremity. If lymphedema is present in the lower extremity on one side, lymphatic duct collaterals to the other side are present. Harvesting in that area could lead to worsening of lymphedema. To prevent donor site lymphedema, preoperative lymphoscintigraphy should be performed on every patient undergoing SILNT to identify the sentinel lymph nodes draining the leg. It is also advisable to use the intraoperative "reverse mapping technique" to exclude important sentinel lymph nodes and their efferent drainage system.

The anatomic landmarks are marked as described in **Subchapter 10.2**. The PT, antero-superior iliac spine (ASIS), inguinal ligament, and groin crease are marked. Lymph nodes within Zone II are identified as follows: On a line projected from PT to ASIS, a mark is made at 48 mm from the PT. A second mark is made 16 mm caudal to this point. This point is the center of an elliptical flap design with its axis parallel to the inguinal ligament/vascular pedicle of the SCIV/A (▶ Fig. 10.1). Care has to be taken not to include skin and subcutaneous tissue below the groin crease or medial to the SIEV/caudal to the superior circumflex iliac vein (SCIV), by staying inside the "golden triangle." A Doppler probe can help to frame the right zone through the identification of SIEV and SCIEV. The flap is first incised superiorly and laterally, and the superficial circumflex iliac pedicle and the SIEV are localized first. The flap is elevated from lateral to medial. Care is taken not to harvest any lymph nodes caudal to the circumflex pedicle and medial to the femoral artery. Dissection of the venous structures is carried out medial to the femoral artery to ensure that the veins are skeletonized of any lymphatic tissue. The venous drainage of the flap is by the SCIV. Alternatively, the SIEV can be included in the flap and used for extra drainage. The flap is harvested on the superficial branch of the SCIA, thus superficial to the deep fascia. Harvesting deep to the deep fascia, thus with the deep branch of the SCIA, can cause injury to the perisartorius superior lymph nodes, which can cause lymphedema of the donor site in some cases. (▶ Fig. 10.9).

10.5.2 Vascularized Supraclavicular Lymph Node Transfer

Harvesting the supraclavicular lymph nodes is relatively straightforward and based on three landmarks: the clavicle, SCM, and internal jugular vein.[10]

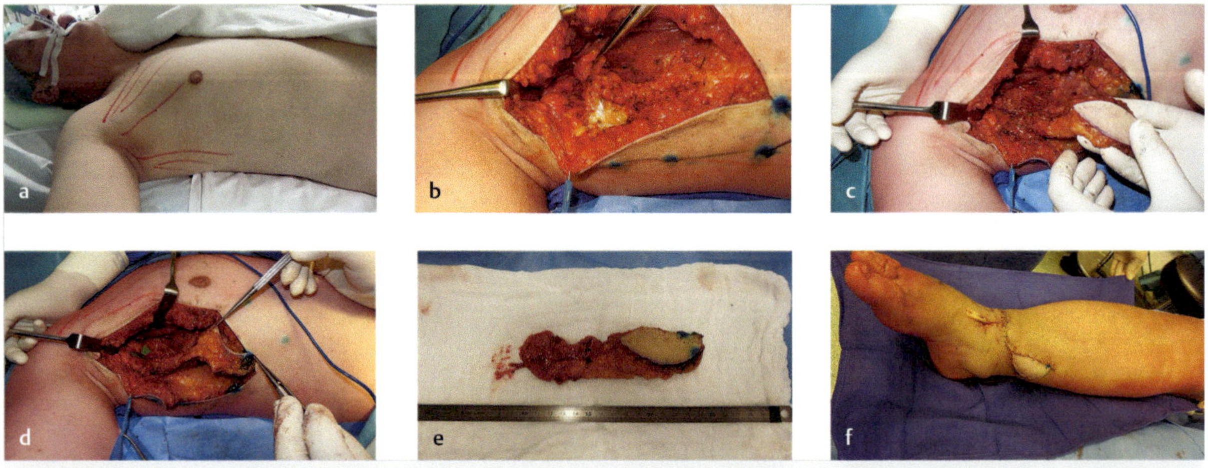

Fig. 10.12 Lateral thoracic lymph node flap to treat chronic lymphedema of the right lower extremity: 38-year-old male patient who developed bilateral lower extremity lymphedema after radiotherapy for non-Hodgkin lymphoma. A vascularized lymph node transfer was planned from the right lateral thoracic region to the right ankle. **(a)** The anatomical outlines marked between the anterior border of the latissimus dorsi muscle and the lateral border of the major pectoral muscle. **(b)** The lymph node group between the lateral thoracic pedicle and the thoracodorsal pedicle was dissected based on Patent Blue V injection. **(c)** The vascularized lymph node transfer with a skin paddle was dissected based on the lateral thoracic vessels. **(d)** The harvested flap. Note the Patent Blue V tracing from the skin to the lymph nodes. **(e)** The vascularized lymph node transfer flap was completely harvested. **(f)** The vascularized lymph node transfer flap was placed at the medial aspect of the right ankle. The microanastomoses were done to the dorsalis pedis vessels (artery end-to-side and vein end-to-end). Simultaneously, a lymphovenous anastomosis was also performed at the dorsum of the foot. (Courtesy of Assaf Zeltzer and Moustapha Hamdi.)

It is a thin, pliable flap suitable for distal extremity placement and the resulting scar can be well concealed by clothing. Injury to the supraclavicular nerve, however, may result in paresthesia of the upper anterior chest. Although the right side is typically preferred for harvesting to avoid risk of injury to the thoracic duct, it contains fewer lymph nodes than the left side.

This flap can be harvested with or without a skin flap (▶ Fig. 10.10). When a skin flap is included, it is typically designed with an elliptical skin paddle oriented horizontally just above the clavicle.

The posterior border of the clavicular insertion of SCM is usually the midpoint of the ellipse. The skin and the supraclavicular lymph nodes are harvested en bloc with the skin paddle serving as monitor.

Preserving the skin and subcutaneous tissue also obviates disruption of lymphatic channels that, in theory, may re-establish connections to recipient site lymphatics. The dimensions of the skin flap that enable tension-free primary closure are approximately 3 × 10 cm. As mentioned above the EJV runs through the flap and is typically the major outflow, and thus should be selected for the venous pedicle. Depending on the position of the arterial perforator relative to the skin paddle and required pedicle length, the TCA pedicle may be designed in an antegrade or retrograde fashion, although usually the antegrade pedicle is used.

No attempt is made to look for the perforator as this may result in injury to the small vessels encased within the fatty tissues of the flap. Several lymph nodes are reliably incorporated when harvesting the adipose tissue surrounding the pedicle. Some lymph nodes are easily visible but smaller ones may not be. Superficial sensory nerves traversing the flap toward the upper chest are sacrificed. Caution must be taken not to transect the large lymphatic ducts both on right and left sides of the neck to avoid developing a lymphocele or chyle leak. While the spinal accessory nerve lies deep to the flap and lateral to the area of dissection, the surgeon must be cognizant of its proximity and avoid injuring it.

10.5.3 Vascularized Lateral Thoracic Lymph Node Transfer

The harvesting technique varies based on the location and blood supply to the lymph nodes. The reverse lymphatic mapping allows to identify the lymph nodes that drain the chest and back area from those that drain the arm.

In short, a longitudinal line is drawn anterior to the latissimus dorsi muscle and lateral to the breast (▶ Fig. 10.12).

Branches of the lateral thoracic vessels, identified as thoracodorsal branches, are dissected back to the latissimus pedicle.

The lymph nodes may be supplied by the lateral thoracic artery or the thoracodorsal vessels. If the thoracodorsal vessels are included in the flap, the thoracodorsal nerve should be preserved. However, if any small nerve branches come between the vascular pedicle and the lymph nodes, those branches should then be sacrificed.

10.5.4 Vascularized Submental Lymph Nodes Transfer

Design of the submental VLN flap begins with palpitation and identification of the facial artery. The axis of the submental artery can be determined by the relationship of the artery and the lower border of the mandible. The submental artery is a reliable branch of the facial artery and is located at approximately 0.5 cm below the lower edge of the mandible.[13] In most cases, a skin island is needed to allow for recipient site closure. The elliptical skin paddle is oriented along the long axis of the submental artery in order to capture perforating vessels to the skin. The superior half of the ellipse is limited to approximately 1 cm below the lower border of the mandible. It leaves a scar from the angle to the symphysis. This is based on submental perforators, at the junction of the distal facial vessels. Preservation of the marginal mandibular nerve is critical, and some recommend taking the anterior digastric belly to maintain the perforators. This flap leaves a scar at the level of the mandible, and cosmetic considerations do play a role, including the patient's propensity to scar poorly. Placing a higher incision may result in inevitable visibility of the scar on donor site closure. The lower half of the ellipse is then made and is adjusted based on neck skin laxity and the possibility of donor site closure. The limits of the skin paddle can extend to the midline or further depending on the needs of the surgeon. Narrower skin islands may be designed, which allow for decreased tension along the donor site closure and potentially a smaller scar along the lower border of the mandible.

The incision is placed parallel to the inferior border of the mandible over the submental artery, and a skin paddle may be raised on perforators arising from this artery. The arterial pedicle length is short and of small caliber, and there may be anatomical variability of the facial artery and vein. Care should be taken to preserve branches of the marginal mandibular nerve. The flap is low volume, making it suitable for distal extremity placement, and there is very low risk of donor site lymphedema. The resultant scar, however, may be visible in the submandibular area.

10.5.5 Vascularized Jejunal Mesenteric Lymph Node Transfer

The jejunal mesenteric lymph node flap has been described as both a flap harvested from the periphery of the mesentery and from closer to the root of the mesentery; the latter approach avoids the risk of disruption to the vascular supply to the adjacent bowel segment and subsequent ischemic bowel complications, and a flow-through design is favored.[22] The low flap bulk makes it suitable for distal extremity placement; however, remote monitoring is typically required. Harvest is by means of a mini-laparotomy or abdominoplasty approach.

The flap is harvested through a midline supraumbilical mini-laparotomy incision that is 3 to 5 cm in length. The desired section of the jejunum, generally the proximal third, is identified and delivered from the abdomen extracorporally onto the surgical field. Lymph nodes are identified using transillumination and confirmed with palpation and inspection. Once a favorable cluster of lymph nodes with adequately sized vessels for microvascular anastomosis is identified, one side of the peritoneum is scored around the distal periphery of the flap, and distal vascular branches are ligated. An arcade immediately adjacent to the intestine is preserved to ensure vascularity to the jejunum. The flaps are then elevated from the periphery toward the root of the mesentery, preserving the other peritoneal layer. Dissection continues until vessel caliber is adequate for microvascular anastomosis while preserving all major vessels to the jejunum. The pedicle length is generally short (1–3 cm) but can be increased by dividing branches. The flap is raised en bloc with the cluster of lymph nodes and mesenteric vascular pedicle. The average size of the flap is approximately 2 to 3 cm. Bowel continuity is preserved. We avoid lymph node clusters located at the root of the mesentery to avoid sacrificing a major blood supply to the bowel and, more importantly, to optimize arterial inflow and venous outflow for the flap itself by including an adequate capillary network and avoiding excessively large inflow and outflow vessels.

10.6 Robotic-Assisted Omental Lymph Node Harvest for Lymphedema Treatment

Moustapha Hamdi, Assaf Zeltzer, and Karl Waked

Since its proper introduction in the year 2000, robotic-assisted surgery (RAS) has been implemented for all kinds of surgical procedures, mainly to limit the number of scars, decrease the postoperative pain, and reduce donor site morbidity. Recently, RAS made its entrance in lymphatic surgery as well. Not only can it help the surgeon to successfully perform lymphovenous anastomoses, but it may also be an asset in the dissection of intra-abdominal lymph node flaps for lymphedema treatment.

Despite the reported precautions described above, the search for an optimal lymph node flap donor site continues. More recently, the abdomen became a region of interest for VLNT. Given the vast majority of lymph nodes in that region, the risk of iatrogenic donor site lymphedema appears to be minimal to nonexistent. Possible donor sites include the omental lymph node flap (based on the left or right gastroepiploic artery[23]), the mesenteric lymph node flap (based on the arcuate artery of the mesojejunum), the appendicular lymph node flap (based and the appendicular artery, a branch of the ileocolic artery),

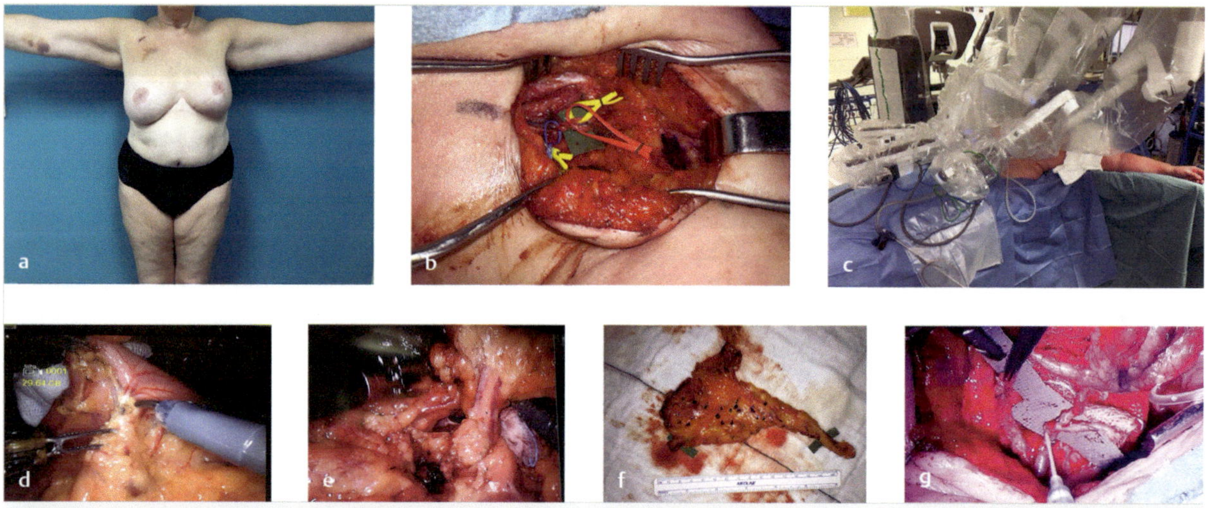

Fig. 10.13 Robotic-assisted omental lymph node flap to treat chronic lymphedema of the left upper extremity: **(a)** 61-year-old female patient with lymphedema of the left arm following breast segmentectomy and axillary clearance. **(b)** Thorough debridement of all fibrous tissue in the recipient site is necessary before flap transfer. **(c)** Setup of the Da Vinci Robotic Surgical System during mental lymph node flap harvesting. **(d)** The omentum is detached from the great curvature of the stomach, carefully ligating the cranial branches. **(e)** The flap based on the right gastroepiploic artery. **(f)** The flap with vascular pedicle. Flap dimensions can range up to 10 to 12 cm in length and 5 to 7 cm in width. **(g)** Situs during anastomosis with robotic system. (Courtesy of Assaf Zeltzer and Moustapha Hamdi.)

and the ileocecal lymph node flap (based on the ileal or colic branch of the ileocolic artery). Interestingly, the *omental lymph node flap* became quite popular in recent years thanks to its well-studied anatomy[15] and relative ease of harvesting[24] (▶ Fig. 10.13). Nourished by the gastroepiploic artery (GEA), it is located at the great curvature of the stomach and can contain up to 15 lymph nodes. Thanks to the rich intestinal vasculature, the risk of gastric ischemia is negligible (under the condition that there is no history of gastric surgery) and potential complications, mainly pancreatitis and gastric paresis, are rather seldom.

Harvesting technique: Usually, a Veress needle is used to insufflate the abdomen with CO_2 in a standard laparoscopic manner. One 12-mm incision and two 8-mm incisions are made in the abdomen for both the robotic camera and two robotic work instruments, respectively. The instrument ports are placed at both the left and right fossa, while the camera port is placed either suprapubic or supraumbilical. The right instrument port houses a grasper, while the left port is used to pass through the monopolar cautery with added scissors. Additionally, a 5-mm incision is made at the level of the left hypochonder for an assistance port. The assisting surgeon will use a classic laparoscopic grasping forceps to aid the head surgeon during lymph node flap dissection.

After insufflation of the abdomen, exploration starts at the great curvature of the stomach and the transverse colon. If needed, intraperitoneal adhesions are released in order to visualize the omentum. The right gastroepiploic vessels are identified within the omentum, after which the latter is detached from the transverse colon, as well as from the stomach, starting at the antrum until about halfway the great curvature.

Vertical gastric branches between the omental flap and the stomach are carefully ligated in order to avoid any postoperative bleeding. Flap dissection continues up until the origin of the right gastroepiploic vessels laterally and in a craniocaudal fashion medially, ligating the interconnections with the left gastroepiploic system. If the lymph node flap would be based on the left gastroepiploic system, a similar dissection is needed, but in a craniocaudal fashion, starting from the fundus and making sure to spare the splenic vessels. Before clipping the pedicle, the vascularization of the omental flap is checked using the Firefly technique, which is built in the Da Vinci surgical robot. After ensuring good vascularization, the right gastroepiploic vessels are clipped at their origin using laparoscopic hemoclips and the lymph node flap is exteriorized through a prolonged suprapubic or fossa incision. Average omental flap dimensions range from 10 to 12 cm in length and 5 to 7 cm in width.

10.7 Surgical Equipment and Intraoperative Tools

Holger Engel

Autologous lymph node transfer is best performed with a professional set of surgical instruments, microscopy,

ICG lymphangiography, and other additional tools, such as blue dye. Various companies offer this equipment. It is recommended to test different devices and companies because there are many differences in quality, on-site service, etc. Ultimately, the hardware should match perfectly to the surgeon's preferences.

It is recommended that surgical instruments are separated in microsurgery and supermicrosurgery boxes in detail. The microsurgical sieve should contain at least a straight and curved needle holder. Five forceps should be included: one of the Pierse styles, two fixation forceps with tooth, two straight forceps, and one curved forceps. One straight and one curved adventitia scissors should also be included. For vessel management, six "Acland" and six "Müller" clips, two of them straight, two curved, and two angled should be included. Additional "bulldog" clips with small, medium, and large sizes are recommended.

The supermicrosurgery instrument box should contain one dissection scissor, one curved needle holder, two straight forceps with a plateau for knot tightening, one vessel dilatator, and one mini-bipolar instrument. VLNT is generally feasible with a microsurgical sieve. If the vessels are tiny or an additional anastomosis of the efferent lymph collector is performed, the supermicrosurgery instrument box should be used.

Most standard surgical microscopes can deliver adequate magnification and high-resolution quality for microsurgery. In the context of lymphatic surgery, including LVA/supermicrosurgery techniques, a model with a fluorescence unit and a magnification above 20-fold is strongly recommended. Several options are available and should fit the surgeon's preference (e.g., Mitaka MM51, Zeiss Pentero, and Leica PROvido). In some cases, former models are upgradable in terms of adding a magnification extender or a separate fluorescence unit. However, the quality with magnification extenders is not as good as that with the new optics.

Standard sutures from 8.0 to 9.0 are usually sufficient for regular microsurgical anastomosis. Various companies offer high-quality surgical equipment, e.g., Ethicon, Braun Melsungen, Boston Scientific, Medtronic, and others. For lymphatic surgery, some surgeons might consider custom-made equipment with specific needle curvature, length, etc. Some companies are offering customized sutures 10–12.0 in size.

Intraoperative usage of ICG lymphangiography can be useful in evaluating the desired recipient site, monitoring lymph node transplant perfusion after anastomosis, discovering possible lymph leakage of the recipient site after preparation and scar excision, and detecting lymph collectors for additional LVA procedures. In addition to microscopes with fluorescence units, several separate near-infrared camera unit options are available.

Blue dyes can additionally help to stain lymphatic drainage, lymph collectors, etc., to identify efferent collectors for VLNT and to assist in reverse mapping to spare relevant lymph channels. Different dyes are on the market. Not all of them are recommended due to toxicity and affinity to stain lymphatic. Isosulfan blue (e.g., Lymphazurin) is a good option.

In some cases of lymph node dissection and LVA, it is helpful to use hemoclips instead of bipolar clips. Fine and superfine microclips can support a delicate dissection with ligation of vessels and lymphatic channels (e.g., GEM Superfine Microclips [TSG Medical, Toronto, Canada]).

A stable operative field is also helpful. Retraction hooks with different styles, sizes, lengths, etc., add value (e.g., Lone Star Elastic Stays [CooperSurgical, Trumbull, CT, USA]).

A rapidly evolving field is the usage of robotics in the operating room. Especially in the field of micro- and supermicrosurgery, we will see the establishment of these new adjuncts. The ability to stabilize and to scale down the surgeon's movements during the procedures will make submillimeter scale approaches safe and push the limits further (e.g., Microsure MUSA [EA Son, Netherlands] microsurgery robot).

10.8 Postoperative Management

Katrin Seidenstücker

Postoperative care after VLNT involves postoperative antibiotic prophylaxis, anticoagulation, a protocol for free flap monitoring, and a protocol for the use of compression and manual lymph drainage (MLD).

The information about postoperative management is rare in the literature. Antibiotics are indicated postoperatively to avoid cellulitis. Some studies specified routine postoperative antibiotic prophylaxis for 1 week in patients without a history of recurrent cellulitis and 6 months or more in patients with a history of recurrent cellulitis. In our department we just use a single-shot antibiotic like in other free flap surgery and had no problems with perioperative infections in more than 150 flaps in the last 4 years. Regarding the patient group with recurrent cellulitis, a long-term antibiotic therapy with, for example, long-lasting penicillin should be considered. The patient should be operated in an infection-free period.

Perioperative anticoagulation should be used like other microsurgical procedures.[1] For free flap transfer to the upper extremity, mobilization of the patient could be performed the day after surgery. Distal lower extremity flaps may require bed rest in the first few days after surgery followed by a postoperative dangling protocol.

For VLNT the postoperative free flap monitoring is different depending on the use of a monitor island or not. Following the Paris school of Corinne Becker, the free flap is hidden as close to the veins as possible and the monitor skin island was not required so the flap set-up was easier. This always gives rise to a discussion in the international meetings from passionate microsurgeons who always monitor their flaps for the possibility of early revision to save the flap in the event of anastomosis problems. The process of your flap monitoring could be taken over from your established free flap protocols (control of the temperature, color, capillary refill, and skin turgor and pinprick and handheld Doppler tests). There is no special recommendation for the monitoring of a VLNT flap.

The protocol for use of conservative treatment has to take into consideration the recommendations of manual decompression therapy and the placement of the flap. Use of compression stockings has been reported to be variable in the literature, from either not recommended in the immediate postoperative period or within 1 month of surgery, to on as-needed basis until 6 months indispensable.

A standardized rehabilitation program should ideally include manual lymphatic drainage toward the lymph node flap (or off the lymph node flap ["reverse flow"] in case of extra-anatomical distal flap inset), starting immediately after surgery, using the same frequency as before surgery for approximately 4 to 6 months. Furthermore, it should be recommended that class II compression garments with a compression of approximately 30mg Hg are worn, starting immediately after surgery, at least during daytime (in case of anatomical proximal flap inset to the axilla) as well as at night (in case of lymph node transfer to the groin) for arm and leg lymphedema. If the flap is placed distally, primary wound healing should be respected for at least 2 weeks after surgery until the free flap endures the compression.

Some surgeons also educate the patients to apply gentle pumping pressure onto the flap for emptying the excess fluids several times daily for the first 3 months.

10.9 Patient Education

Katrin Seidenstücker

As mentioned in the previous chapters it is important to set the patients' expectations accordingly. Lymphedema mostly needs a lifetime of conservative treatment with compression garments and MDT. Patients who have a history of recurrent cellulitis should continue with long-term prophylactic antibiotic therapy for further 6 months, along with the general advice to avoid trauma and skin injuries. MDT should be continued for at least 6 months in the same frequency the patient received it before surgery without pressure on the sore area in the first 2 weeks. A good self-management and the right reaction to worsening of the lymphedema with an increase in circumference is important. In the event of a worsening condition, the patient should increase the frequency of MDT and the compression class. Sometimes bandaging in the night or after MDT is a useful additional tool. Giving general advice is difficult because every country offers different possibilities for additive treatments, offered across different health care systems.

10.10 Pearls and Pitfalls

Katrin Seidenstücker

- VLNT is one of the physiological methods to restore the lymphatic drainage.
- VLNT acts by acting like a sponge to absorb lymphatic fluids into the venous system and by inducing lymphangiogenesis.
- VLNT is indicated when options for compression and MDT and LVA have already been used.
- Different donor sites provide safe lymph node harvesting.
- Donor site morbidity is based on extensive knowledge of anatomy, correct surgical technique, and pre- and intraoperative lymphatic mapping.
- ICG images and reverse lymphatic mapping technology are mandatory when VLNT is planned.
- Robotic-assisted lymph nodes harvesting is an additional tool to reduce donor site morbidity.
- Proximal versus distal recipient site depends on the scar tissue/lymphatic images/lymphedema stage.
- A standardized postoperative rehabilitation program should include manual lymphatic drainage toward the flap.

References

[1] Becker C, Assouad J, Riquet M, Hidden G. Postmastectomy lymphedema: long term results following microsurgical lymph node transplantation. Ann Surg. 2006; 243(3):313–315

[2] Goh TLH, Park SW, Cho JY, Choi JW, Hong JP. The search for the ideal thin skin flap: superficial circumflex iliac artery perforator flap—a review of 210 cases. Plast Reconstr Surg. 2015; 135(2):592–601

[3] Scaglioni MF, Suami H. Lymphatic anatomy of the inguinal region in aid of vascularized lymph node flap harvesting. J Plast Reconstr Aesthet Surg. 2015; 68(3):419–427

[4] Zeltzer AA, Anzarut A, Braeckmans D, et al. The vascularized groin lymph node flap (VGLN): anatomical study and flap planning using multi-detector CT scanner. The golden triangle for flap harvesting. J Surg Oncol. 2017; 116(3):378–383

[5] Poon Y, Wei CY. Vascularized groin lymph node flap transfer for postmastectomy upper limb lymphedema: flap anatomy, recipient sites, and outcomes. Plast Reconstr Surg. 2014; 133(3):428e

[6] Viitanen TP, Mäki MT, Seppänen MP, Suominen EA, Saaristo AM. Donor-site lymphatic function after microvascular lymph node transfer. Plast Reconstr Surg. 2012; 130(6):1246–1253

[7] Dayan JH, Dayan E, Kagen A, et al. The use of magnetic resonance angiography in vascularized groin lymph node transfer: an anatomic study. J Reconstr Microsurg. 2014; 30(1):41–45

[8] Tourani SS, Taylor GI, Ashton MW. Anatomy of the superficial lymphatics of the abdominal wall and the upper thigh and its implications in lymphatic microsurgery. J Plast Reconstr Aesthet Surg. 2013; 66(10):1390–1395

[9] Chang EI, Chu CK, Hanson SE, Selber JC, Hanasono MM, Schaverien MV. Comprehensive overview of available donor sites for vascularized lymph node transfer. Plast Reconstr Surg Glob Open. 2020; 8(3):e2675

[10] Ooi ASH, Chang DW. 5-step harvest of supraclavicular lymph nodes as vascularized free tissue transfer for treatment of lymphedema. J Surg Oncol. 2017; 115(1):63–67

[11] Ngo QD, Munot S, Mackie H, et al. Vascularized lymph node transfer for patients with breast cancer-related lymphedema can potentially reduce the burden of ongoing conservative management. Lymphat Res Biol. 2020; 18(4):357–364

[12] Cheng MH, Lin CY, Patel KM. A prospective clinical assessment of anatomic variability of the submental vascularized lymph node flap. J Surg Oncol. 2017; 115(1):43–47

[13] Piyaman P, Patchanee K, Oonjitti T, Ratanalekha R, Yodrabum N. Surgical anatomy of vascularized submental lymph node flap: sharing arterial supply of lymph nodes with the skin and topographic relationship with anterior belly of digastric muscle. J Surg Oncol. 2020; 121(1):144–152

[14] Howell AC, Gould DJ, Mayfield C, Samakar K, Hassani C, Patel KM. Anatomical basis of the gastroepiploic vascularized lymph node transfer: a radiographic evaluation using computed tomographic angiography. Plast Reconstr Surg. 2018; 142(4):1046–1052

[15] Cook JA, Sasor SE, Tholpady SS, Chu MW. Omental vascularized lymph node flap: a radiographic analysis. J Reconstr Microsurg. 2018; 34(7):472–477

[16] Yamamoto T, Narushima M, Doi K, et al. Characteristic indocyanine green lymphography findings in lower extremity lymphedema: the generation of a novel lymphedema severity staging system using dermal backflow patterns. Plast Reconstr Surg. 2011; 127(5): 1979–1986

[17] Cheng MH, Pappalardo M, Lin C, Kuo CF, Lin CY, Chung KC. Validity of the novel Taiwan lymphoscintigraphy staging and correlation of Cheng lymphedema grading for unilateral extremity lymphedema. Ann Surg. 2018; 268(3):513–525

[18] Demiri E, Dionyssiou D, Tsimponis A, et al. Donor-site lymphedema following lymph node transfer for breast cancer-related lymphedema: a systematic review of the literature. Lymphat Res Biol. 2018; 16 (1):2–8

[19] ScaglioniMF, Arvanitakis M, Chen YC, Giovanoli P, Chia-Shen Yang J, Chang EI. Comprehensive review of vascularized lymph node transfers for lymphedema: outcomes and complications. Microsurgery. 2018; 38 (2):222–229

[20] Cheng MH, Chen SC, Henry SL, Tan BK, Chia-Yu Lin M, Huang JJ. Vascularized groin lymph node flap transfer for postmastectomy upper limb lymphedema: flap anatomy, recipient sites, and outcomes. Plast Reconstr Surg. 2013; 131(6):1286–1298

[21] Althubaiti GA, Crosby MA, Chang DW. Vascularized supraclavicular lymph node transfer for lower extremity lymphedema treatment. Plast Reconstr Surg. 2013; 131(1):133e–135e

[22] Coriddi M, Wee C, Meyerson J, Eiferman D, Skoracki R. Vascularized jejunal mesenteric lymph node transfer: a novel surgical treatment for extremity lymphedema. J Am Coll Surg. 2017; 225(5):650–657

[23] Ciudad P, Date S, Lee MH, et al. Robotic harvest of a right gastroepiploic lymph node flap. Arch Plast Surg. 2016; 43(2):210–212

[24] Özkan Ö, Özkan Ö, Çinpolat A, Arıcı C, Bektaş G, Can Ubur M. Robotic harvesting of the omental flap: a case report and mini-review of the use of robots in reconstructive surgery. J Robot Surg. 2019; 13(4): 539–543

[25] Ciudad P, Manrique OJ, Date S, et al. A head-to-head comparison among donor site morbidity after vascularized lymph node transfer: pearls and pitfalls of a 6-year single center experience. J Surg Oncol. 2017; 115(1):37–42

[26] Yoshimatsu H, Visconti G, Karakawa R, Hayashi A. Lymphatic system transfer for lymphedema treatment: transferring the lymph nodes with their lymphatic vessels. Plast Reconstr Surg Glob Open. 2020; 8 (4):e2721

11 Autologous Breast Reconstruction in Conjunction with Lymphatic Surgery

Randy De Baerdemaeker, Assaf Zeltzer, and Moustapha Hamdi

Summary
Surgical treatment for lymphedema has undergone tremendous advancements over the years. While the earliest techniques focused on lymphoablative procedures such as lipectomy and direct excision of excess tissue, modern advancements in technology, equipment, imaging, and microscope optics enabled physiologic procedures to emerge and become the standard of care for lymphedema at high-volume institutions and centers of excellence. Lymphovenous anastomosis and vascularized lymph node transfer have both proven to be effective approaches to treat lymphedema and improve the quality of life of patients suffering from lymphedema. Mastectomy—nowadays the most often performed in a skin-sparing manner—and surgery and/or radiotherapy of the axillary lymph node basin is standard of care in the multimodal approach of breast cancer. Therefore, breast cancer-related lymphedema after mastectomy constitutes to be a particular challenge among all patients suffering from lymphedema due to the fact that these patients often desire both reconstruction of the breast and treatment of the lymphedema. Nowadays, surgical techniques allow for both the reconstruction of the breast using autologous tissue as well as the restoration of lymphatic drainage pathways. Whereas breast reconstruction using microvascular flaps has attained a very high success rate, the true efficacy of reconstructive surgery of breast cancer associated lymphedema is still somehow unclear. This chapter describes how reconstruction of breast and lymphatic drainage can be improved. Accordingly, and depending on the individual situation of the patient that considers the history of surgery and radiotherapy of the breast and the axilla as well as the presence or absence of functional lymphatics, various approaches are discussed, including simultaneous reconstruction of the breast and the lymphatic pathways, the use of lymphovenous anastomosis, and/or vascularized lymph node transfer, as well as prophylactic surgery to reduce the risk for lymphedema development.

Keywords: autologous breast reconstruction, axillary lymph node dissection (ALND), breast cancer associated lymphedema, deep inferior epigastric perforator (DIEP), prophylactic surgery, scar release, serial or simultaneous reconstruction, vascularized lymph node transfer (VLNT)

11.1 Indications and Contraindications

Breast cancer treatment is one of the major causes for developing lymphedema in high-income countries. Breast cancer has a relatively good prognosis, with a 5-year overall survival rate of 88.0% in females and 78.2% in males, and a 5-year survival rate ranging from 99.4% in stage I to 28.0% in stage IV breast cancer. The overall 5-year survival rate of breast cancer patients has been increasing by approximately 2% per year in the past decade, although breast cancer incidence remains stable. This implies that the population of breast cancer survivors is constantly growing every year and thus patients will be more frequently confronted with the long-term side effects of breast cancer treatment including secondary lymphedema.

The exact incidence of lymphedema is unknown as there are many inconsistencies in the diagnostic and measurement tools (see **Chapters 2** and **4**). Although the time of onset of lymphedema is highly variable as is its rate of progression, about 75% of lymphedema symptoms occur within a year of initial cancer treatment with an estimated 20% of the breast cancer population that will develop secondary lymphedema.[1]

Despite the poor understanding of the pathophysiology of lymphedema, many different hypotheses have been proposed, including injury to the lymph nodes and their lymphovascular network which seems to be a major contributor to developing lymphatic dysfunction and eventually lymphedema. Surgery-associated lymphedema is often worsened by adjuvant radiotherapy that may further cause fibrosis of the tissues and lymphvenous sclerosis.

The most widely used classification system of lymphedema is the clinical staging according to the International Society of Lymphology (ISL), which corresponds to the different described histological stages.[2]

Sentinel lymph node biopsy (SLNB) has been introduced in order to reduce the surgery-associated side effects of the axillary lymph node dissection (ALND) of oncologically unaffected lymph nodes.[5] The risk of developing lymphedema after ALND varies from 5% to 50%, according to literature.[6,10] A large series of over 4,000 patients have demonstrated that the overall risk of developing breast cancer-related lymphedema amounted to 27%, disregarding surgery in the axilla and/or radiotherapy.[7]

Interestingly, the incidence of lymphedema following SLNB was reported to be between 6% and 10%, identifying certain risk factors among other things high body mass index (BMI), previous infection injury to the arm, radiotherapy, chemotherapy (e.g., taxanes), a high number of positive lymph nodes, advanced age, and tumor size.[8,9,11] Accordingly, it is of utmost importance to inform the patients that the so-called minimally invasive SLNB is associated with some risk of developing secondary lymphedema.

A meta-analysis has shown that autologous breast reconstruction after mastectomy for breast cancer treatment would have a beneficial effect on lymphedema, although the underlying mechanisms are yet not fully clear.[12] Unfortunately, lymphedema impacts the quality of life in many ways and has a heavy impact on physical and psychological state of the patient.[13] Therefore, combined reconstruction of the breast and treatment of the lymphedema may be a fantastic option for these patients suffering from chronic disease impacting daily life and distortion of the body image using ideally autologous tissue from the abdomen (e.g., deep inferior epigastric perforator [DIEP] flap) and vascularized lymph node flap from the groin.[14]

11.2 Surgical Technique

11.2.1 Lymphatic Anatomy of the Recipient Site

Lymphatic Anatomy of the Upper Limb and Axillary Area

The superficial lymphatic network in the upper limb follows mainly the cephalic and basilic veins and the radial and ulnar side, respectively. However, it can be visualized over the entire surface of the forearm. The number of lymphatic vessels varies between individuals. In a nonpathologic situation, proximal to the elbow, these vessels converge and drain toward the axillary lymph nodes. The majority of the lymphatic vessels from the upper limb drain into one major "primary" lymph node in the axilla that is usually bigger in size and has interconnections with other "secondary" nodes. Some lymphatic vessels on the posterior side of the upper arm drain directly into those "secondary" smaller lymph nodes in the axilla; many anatomical variations do exist.[18]

When looking at the gross anatomy of the thorax, an important cross-over can be seen between a major lymph node draining part of the upper lateral thorax and breast and the lymphatics from the upper limb. This anatomic condition is the reason why some patients may develop lymphedema even after an axillary SLNB for breast cancer or other causes (▶ Fig. 11.1).[8]

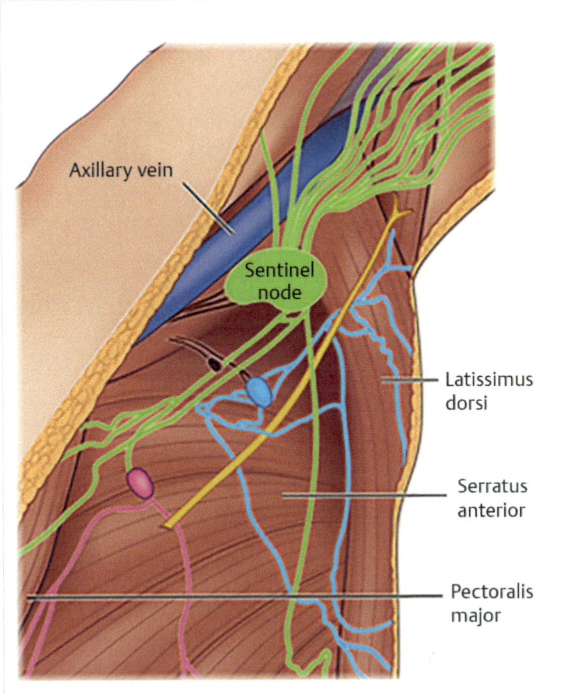

Fig. 11.1 Schematic drawing of the left axillary region. The sentinel node is connected with lymphatic vessels from both the upper limb and the upper torso.[19]

Postoperative Derivative Lymphatic Pathways

After ALND or even SLNB, lymphatic fluid can sometimes be deviated through "dormant lymphatic pathways" that are recruited to become patent and functional to counteract augmentation of pressure within the lymphatic network in the initial stages of lymphedema before swelling can be observed clinically.

The following pathways have been described:

- Extra-axillary:
  - Mascagni: Alongside the cephalic vein[20] (▶ Fig. 11.2)
  - Caplan: Posterior scapular pathway[21]
- Intra-axillary:
  - Ciucci: Radio-humeral pathway[22]

These derivative pathways are of particular importance in the initial stage of subclinical lymphedema for draining lymph by bypassing the area affected by the surgery, radiotherapy, and/or infection, to be targeted for MLD. Unfortunately, later on these pathways often increasingly fail due to a progressive fibrosis of the interstitial tissue in general and the lymphatic vessels in particular.

11.2.2 Lymphatic Anatomy of the Donor Site

Lymphatic Anatomy of the Lower Limb and Inguinal Area

The lower limb has about an equivalent network of lymphatic structures compared to the upper limb, i.e., a superficial system, a deep system, as well as interconnections and perforating vessels. Especially the superficial lymphatic vessels that are located superficial to the superficial fascia (Scarpa's fascia and equivalents) are well developed and drain to the inguinal region. The dominant vessels run alongside both the great and small saphenous veins. The lymphatic vessels following the great saphenous vein are usually constant in presence and size and

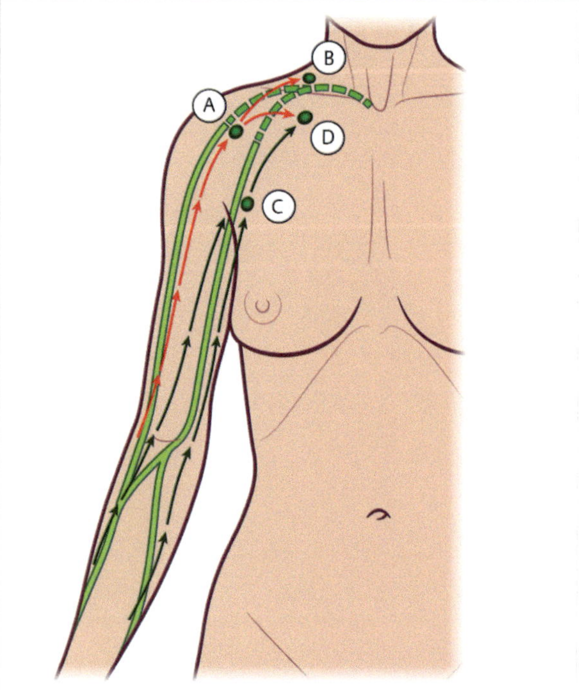

Fig. 11.2 Overview of the dominant axillary drainage pathway of the superficial lymphatic vessels passing trough C–D. Alternative extra-axillary pathway A–B defined by Mascagni et al. at the level of the delto-pectoral groove that can be recruited to become the only derivative pathway in the event of severed axillary pathway.[21]

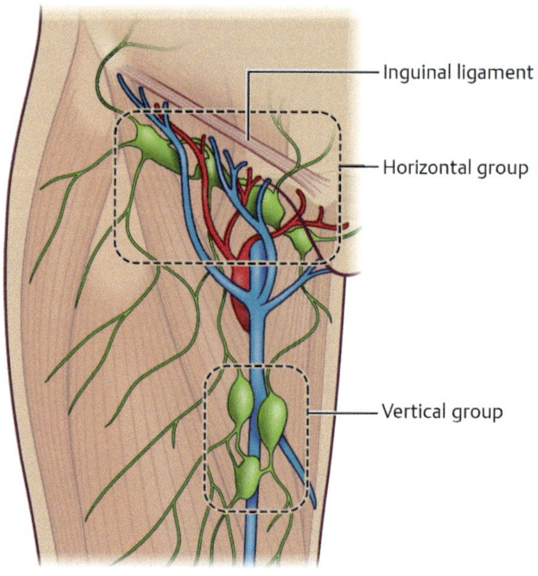

Fig. 11.3 Distribution of lymph nodes of the superficial inguinal region according to Quenu et al.[26]

drain to the superficial inguinal lymph nodes, whereas the ones following the small saphenous vein are more variable in development.[24]

The lymphatic vessels running deep to the superficial fascia are only few in number. The draining structures of the deep lymphatic system running deep to the muscle fascia are relatively small and drain toward the popliteal femoral lymph nodes to finally connect to the lymph nodes of the external iliac chain.[25]

For the superficial region of the groin, several classifications have been proposed to group the lymph nodes. However, with time, the classification proposed by Quenu has won recognition, dividing the inguinal region into four quadrants.[26] According to this classification, four to five different subgroups of lymph nodes can be observed within the groin that are distributed in a horizontal and vertical way and described according to the blood vessel they follow (▶ Fig. 11.3):

- Upper horizontal nodes (parallel to the inguinal ligament)
  - Lateral circumflex group
  - Superficial inferior epigastric group
  - Medial pudendal group
- Lower vertical nodes (parallel to the saphenous vein)
  - Medial saphenous group
  - Lateral saphenous group

The lymph nodes of the lower vertical groups and the lymph nodes of the medial pudendal group, partly drain the lower limb; thus, particular care should be taken when dissecting in this anatomical region.

11.2.3 Value and Extent of Scar Release of Axillar Recipient Site

Axillary scar tissue removal is an essential, yet critical, step for the overall reduction of arm volume since breast cancer associated lymphedema is usually caused by axillary surgery and/or radiotherapy. Wide surgical removal of scar tissue from the axilla is required to improve upper limb mobility, on the one hand. On the other hand, a wound bed of healthy, unscarred tissue is prerequisite at the recipient site in order to allow the transferred and perfused lymph node flap to integrate within its neighbouring tissues and create connection with the preexisting transected and blind ending lymph vessels. To do so, the recipient vessels for the lymph node flap must be identified within this scar tissue.

11.2.4 Breast Reconstruction in Conjunction with Vascularized Lymph Node Flap

The most common donor site for vascularized lymph node (VLN) flap is the inguinal area. The superficial inguinal lymph nodes may be harvested based on several vascular pedicles such as the superficial circumflex iliac artery or the superficial inferior epigastric artery. Alternative donor sites include the lateral thoracic lymph nodes, the submental lymph nodes, the supraclavicular lymph nodes, and the more recently described intra-abdominal lymph nodes within the greater omentum.[39]

Recipient sites include the axilla, the elbow, and the wrist. Recipient sites distally may be more efficient in draining the arm.[27] Comparative studies have not demonstrated significant functional differences between the various lymph node donor sites, except for the lymph nodes of the lateral thoracic region that are associated with a higher risk of donor site morbidity.[28]

Staged Reconstruction

Patients with breast cancer associated lymphedema may require both breast reconstruction and surgical treatment for lymphedema. These patients can be offered a chimeric flap using a combined abdominal flap for restoration of volume and shape of the breast and an inguinal lymph node flap for lymphedema treatment. This approach was first described by Saaristo et al.,[29] a concept that has been further confirmed by De Brucker et al.[13] and Nguyen et al.[30,31]

The seroma formation and wound healing complication rate in the combined group of simultaneous DIEP flap and VLNT was demonstrably higher compared with the VLNT group only (20% versus 8%), a fact that should be disclosed to patients undergoing combined procedures. This has to be balanced with the fact that simultaneous autologous breast reconstruction VLNT from the groin is associated with superior outcome compared to VLNT alone.[31] This may indicate that the transfer of vascularized tissue devoid of lymph nodes into the mastectomy site brings additional benefits. Further, it has been shown that simultaneous breast reconstruction with autologous tissue and VLNT was associated with greater improvement of lymphedema-associated symptoms compared to patients receiving LVA. Unfortunately, when analyzing the impact of breast reconstruction on lymphedema using autologous tissue, the authors did not note any benefit associated with abdominal flap-based breast reconstruction to either the LVA or the vascularized lymph node flap.[32]

Simultaneous Reconstruction

Patients planned for this procedure first undergo perforator mapping of the abdomen to visualize the vascular arborization and path of the feeding vessels of the DIEP flap, mainly using CTA scan.[34] CT scan is also able to confirm the number of functional lymph node units in the the Golden Triangle of the groin (see **Subchapter 10.2**).[33] The design of the abdominal flap should be adapted accordingly and its perforator selection should take into account the side of lymph node flap harvest to guarantee feasible and effective microsurgical anastomosis of both flap pedicles to the anteromedial thorax (i.e., internal mammary vessels) and the axilla (some branch distal to the subscapular vessels).

It is advisable to place the abdominal flap for breast reconstruction medially on the chest and the lymph node flap laterally into the axilla. To guarantee optimal shaping of the new breast and best placement of the lymph node flap onto the axillary vessels, it is preferable to use two independent flaps with two separate sets of arteriovenous anastomoses. Once integrated, it is hypothesized that the transferred, yet viable, lymph nodes will act as a "sponge" and "pump" reabsorbing lymph and interstitial fluid and pumping it into the venous vascular network through intrinsic, intranodal LVA. This concept has been confirmed using lymphoscintigraphy after VLNT, demonstrating that lymph is rerouted through the transferred lymph nodes into the recipient vein.[35] ▶ Fig. 11.5 illustrates planning of inguinal VLNT.[33]

VLNT is indicated in patients with stage I or II lymphedema, regardless of whether healthy superficial lymphatic vessels are present or not. VLNT can be used to treat patients with damaged lymphatic vessels as well as those with decreased lymph node function. Further, VLNT can be offered simultaneously not only with breast reconstruction, but also combined with LVAs or lipectomy. The major risk associated with VLNT is surgery-associated lymphedema of the lower extremity after inguinal lymph node harvest.

Taking into consideration the anatomy of the groin, this flap should ideally be harvested superficially to the deep fascia of the muscle, between the superficial inferior epigastric vein (SIEV) and superficial circumflex iliac vein (SCIV) (zone II). Lymph nodes in this region drain the lower abdomen, the lower back, and the upper gluteal region. The most medial and caudal lymph nodes in this region may drain the lower extremity. Eventually staying cranially to the inguinal crease and lateral to the femoral artery will significantly reduce the risk of secondary lymphedema.[33]

Reverse lymphatic mapping has therefore been suggested to identify the lymph nodes of the groin that drain the lower extremity. Therefore, ICG or Patent Blue V dye is injected between the toes in order to identify the injected dye in one of these lymph nodes in order to exclude them from harvesting, since they participate in draining the lower extremity (see **Subchapter 4.7**).

Surgical Technique to Harvest the Inguinal Lymph Node Flap

A two-team approach is recommended to allow for simultaneous recipient-site preparation in the axilla and flap harvesting. All axillary scar tissue must be removed surgically in order to reach healthy tissue. Of the various donor areas, the groin is the first option to be used for this type of combined reconstruction. First, the anatomic landmarks are outlined, including the pubic tubercle (PT), the anterosuperior iliac spine (ASIS), the inguinal ligament, and the groin crease. The second step is to mark the lymph node unit (LNU). A point along the inguinal ligament that is halfway minus 1 cm the way between the PT and ASIS is marked. This point marks the average distance of the LNU from the PT or the X coordinate. Thereafter, a 2 cm wide circle is drawn around this point. A distance of 2 cm corresponds to approximately two standard deviations around the X point and should include 95% of the LNUs. The LNU should be located superficial to the deep fascia within this circle. Importantly, excision of subcutaneous or lymphatic tissue medial to this circle is avoided. To ease subsequent donor site closure, the lymph node flap is designed as an ellipse with its central axis running parallel to its vascular pedicle including both superficial circumflex iliac artery (SCIA) and SCIV. Finally, the flap markings are checked based on the location of the groin crease, the SIEV and the SCIV. Skin and subcutaneous tissue caudal to the groin crease should not be included in the flap (▶ Fig. 11.4). illustrates planning, harvest and postoperative result.

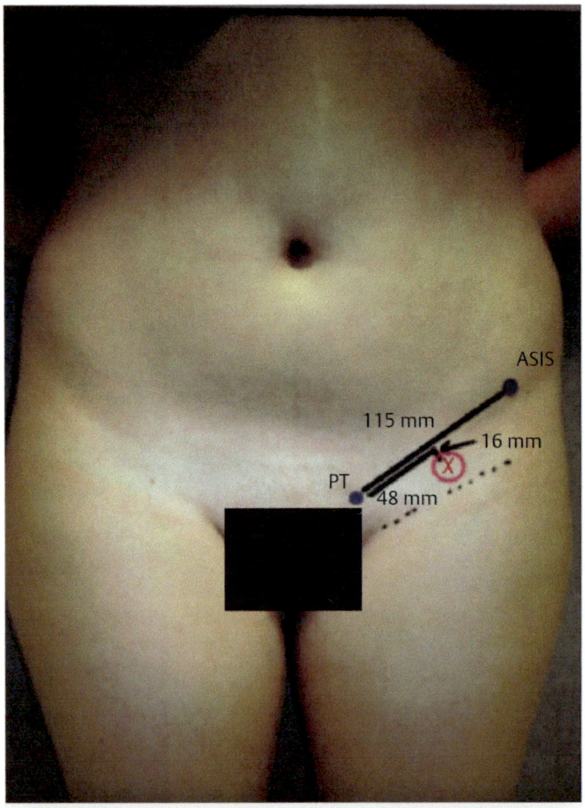

Fig. 11.4 Anatomic landmarks to plan inguinal lymph node flap in the left groin.[33] ASIS, anterosuperior iliac spine; PT, pubic tubercle.

Using handheld Doppler, the course of both the SCIV and the SIEV is marked. The space between these lines corresponds to zone II that delimits the flap, i.e., indicate “no-go” area. Based on preoperative imaging by either CTA or lymphoscintigraphy, LNUs are identified. If not, this side should be avoided for lymph node flap harvest. In the absence of LNUs bilaterally in the groin, a different donor site should be chosen for lymph node flap harvest.

About 12 hours prior to surgery as well as just before initiating surgery, 1 ml of Patent Blue V is injected into the web spaces of the toes. According to the draining pathways of the usually healthy extremity, the bue dye will reach the corresponding lymph nodes that have to be strictly avoided during flap dissection. Indeed, if the targeted nodes for the flap are stained blue, flap harvest should be ceased. Accordingly, patients should be well informed of this eventuality beforehand.

The skin of the lymph node flap will be first incised superiorly and laterally to identify the vascular pedicle of the SCIA and SCIV in the depth. The flap is then elevated from lateral to medial, making sure that blue dye cannot be seen within the flap in general and the lymph nodes in particular. The latter might be difficult since the lymph nodes are very often only identified by palpation within the flap. Essentially, during flap preparation, the lymph nodes should neither be visualized directly nor skeletonized as this may devascularize the nodes and impair their survival following transfer and eventually limit their function. Particular care is taken not to harvest any lymph nodes caudal to the circumflex femoral artery and medial to the femoral artery. Dissection of the venous structures is carried out medial to the femoral artery, making sure

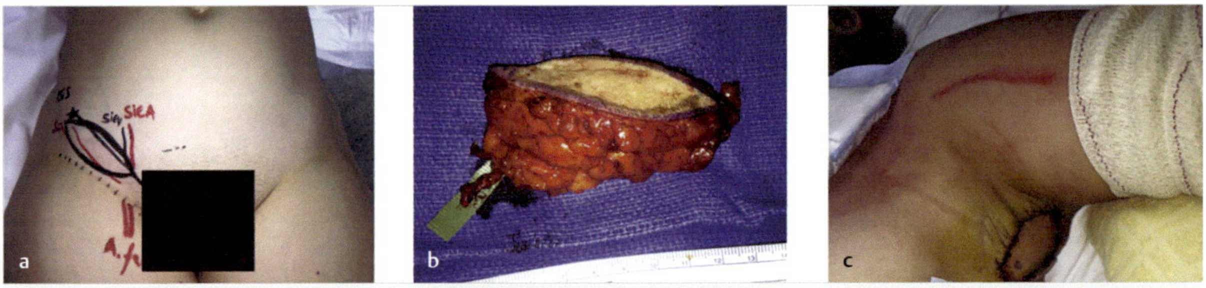

Fig. 11.5 (a) Preoperative planning of inguinal flap. (b) Flap after harvesting. (c) Final result after axillary scar release and flap inset.[4]

that the superficial veins are separated from any lymphatic tissue. The venous drainage of the flap is usually provided by the SCIV. Alternatively, the SIEV can be included into the flap or used for additional drainage. Including the vascular pedicle of the SCIA and SCIV, the flap is harvested superficial to the deep fascia of the muscles. Flap dissection deep to the deep fascia including the deep branch of the SCIA and SCIV can injure the superior lymph nodes nearby the medial border of the sartorius muscle, potentially resulting in donor site lymphedema.

After the lymph nodes have been harvested, the DIEP flap can be harvested in its usual fashion. Nevertheless, closure of the abdominal donor site can present some challenge as dissection of the inguinal lymph node flap can result in unilateral undermining, resulting in a hollow-like concavity in the region, which has propensity for seroma or lymphocele formation.

If harvested as a stand-alone flap, it should be harvested with a skin island. The skin island allows for clinical flap monitoring early on after surgery and often is needed to bring healthy and elastic skin in the retracted area due to scarring following surgery and/or radiotherapy. After microvascular anastomosis have been performed, the lymph node flap must be fixed in very close proximity to the axillary veins to best guarantee integration and formation of new lympho-venular connection.

Alternative Flaps for Breast Reconstruction

If the abdominal donor site is not suitable for adequate flap harvest, due to lack of excess tissue and/or previous surgery with abdominal scarring impeding its harvesting, alternative flaps for breast reconstruction have to be considered, including the transverse myocutaneous gracilis (TMG) flap, the profunda artery perforator (PaP) flap, the superior gluteal artery perforator (sGAP) flap, the inferior gluteal artery perforator (iGAP) flap, the fasciocutaneous infragluteal (FCI) flap, and the lumbar artery perforator (LAP) flap. Any successful harvesting of lymph nodes that are in continuity with one of these flaps has not been described. In most of the donor sites other than the abdomen, lymph nodes have to be harvested as a separate flap usually distant to the flap needed for breast reconstruction, or the risk of donor site lymphedema is far too high, as described with the TMG flap.

Fortunately, all the abovementioned flaps that are suitable for breast reconstruction can be combined with a second stand-alone lymph node flap, ideally from the inguinal area if available and suitable or from any other donor site as described earlier.

A surgical alternative that combines breast reconstruction and lymphedema using a chimeric flap may be the pedicled latissimus dorsi myocutaneous flap that contains lymph nodes from the lateral thoracic area (usually level I lymph nodes). However, this approach is only possible if breast cancer treatment has not required any type of axillary lymph node clearance since classical lymphadenectomy considers removal of level I and II lymph node basins. Sometimes, contralateral latissimus dorsi myocutaneous flap can be an option for breast reconstruction since it can—as in any other flap—be used as a free flap, including the corresponding lymph. This combined approach has proven to be efficient in treating breast cancer associated lymphedema also, similar to the breast reconstruction using the abdominal flap and inguinal lymph nodes. To date, it is not clear if one of these techniques is superior in reducing lymphedema-associated symptoms.[36,37] Accordingly, one has to also consider the surgery-associated morbidity resulting from each of these combined flap harvests.

Management of Recipient Vessels

The internal mammary vessels are the preferred recipient vessels for the free flap to be used for breast reconstruction due to its consistent anatomy, straightforward surgery, and possibility to ideally place and shape the new breast, particularly in the cleavage region. Recipient vessels for the lymph node flap usually include either the vascular branches of the serratus muscle, the circumflexa scapulae vessels, a side branch of the thoracodorsal vessels, or the thoracodorsal vessels themselves. The latter has to be avoided since it will compromise future harvesting of a pedicled latissimus dorsi flap for ipsilateral breast reconstruction, since this easily dissectable flap is somehow the “lifeboat” in case other reconstructive options of the breast fail. Furthermore, it needs to be taken into consideration that these vessels might have been injured during axillary nodal clearance and/or radiotherapy. Finally, it has to be considered that not every arterial branch with an adequate caliber for microanastomosis and flap perfusion that is arborizing distal to the subscapular artery has a corresponding vein's diameter which will match the SCIV or the SIEV.

Performing an additional anastomosis for the contralateral abdominal flap area containing the lymph nodes is an area of considerable debate if this flap is harvested in continuity with the DIEP flap. Often, ICG angiography demonstrates that one flap pedicle connected to the internal mammary (IM) vessels medially is sufficient to adequately perfuse the chimeric flap. Clinically, one should exclude arterial insufficiency and/or venous congestion, otherwise a second set of anastomoses is indicated in the axillary groove.

11.2.5 Breast Reconstruction in Conjunction with Lymphovenous Anastomosis

Breast cancer associated lymphedema treatment can include LVA to treat lymphedema, not only as a stand-alone procedure (see **Chapter 8**) but also simultaneously with breast reconstruction. To do so, patients must have intact functional lymphatic collectors that may be localized with ICG lymph angiography. Further, preoperative MRL can identify areas containing healthy lymph vessels and adjacent venules in close proximity, an ideal condition to perform LVAs. Furthermore, intraoperative ICG use or blue dye injection may help in localizing the healthy lymphatic vessels together with percutaneously marked coordinates defined by the radiologist and based upon the anatomical landmarks. These conditions are usually found in patients who present with stage 0 or stage I lymphedema.

The risks of LVA are minimal and the surgery can be performed as an outpatient procedure under local or general anesthesia. Lymphovenous shunt surgery is not helpful in the later stages of lymphedema or in patients without healthy functional superficial lymphatic vessels.

Basically, it is advised to perform LVA during breast reconstruction to treat lymphedema, if the local situation allows for it. Unlike lymphedema treatment with VLNT, scar release is not necessary when performing LVAs. LVAs consist of surgically bypassing lymph from congested lymph vessels into veins, whereas VLNT's success will depend on spontaneous development of new lympho-lymphatic and lymphovenous connections. Accordingly, LVAs are rather effective in early-stage lymphedema, whereas VLNTs are successfully used in later stage lymphedema.

Therefore, the far less invasive LVA has to be offered in early-stage lymphedema over the VLNT in order to have an adequate backup in the event of lymphedema progression despite LVA surgery. In other words, the surgery-associated morbidity of VLNT is too high to treat stage 0 and stage I lymphedema.

11.2.6 Breast Reconstruction in Conjunction with Lymph Node Flap and Lymphovenous Anastomosis ("Barcelona Cocktail" or Total Breast Anatomy Restoration)

Nowadays, a skin-sparing mastectomy is almost standard, requiring immediate breast reconstruction. Further, breast cancer treatment is currently facing escalation of adjuvant radiotherapy, despite surgical de-escalation. In the event of autologous breast reconstruction, the combination of DIEP and inguinal lymph node flaps as described above can therefore be also offered in a purely preventive approach. Accordingly, performing an additional LVA in the upper limb that is at risk for secondary lymphedema after breast cancer treatment is the third surgery that results in a synergistic effect to best prevent breast cancer associated lymphedema, i.e., autologous breast reconstruction after mastectomy, lymph node flap, and LVA. This approach is called the total breast anatomy restoration (T-BAR). Preoperative mapping of the anatomical state of the axilla along with the functional state of the lymphatic system is performed with ICG lymphangiography and MRL, which provides the necessary information to adequately plan one or more LVAs together with the combined abdominal and lymph node flap.[38]

11.3 Intraoperative Position

The patient is positioned supine with the ipsilateral arm in 90 degrees abduction to allow simultaneous access to the groin, abdomen, chest, and axillary region, as well as to the arm to simultaneously harvest the flaps and prepare the recipient sites, including axillary scar release, dissection of the recipient vessels for the flaps, and donor vessels for the LVA. Ideally this type of complex surgery is performed in a two-team approach.

Given the large surface area of the surgical wound and the considerable exposure time, the patient should ideally be placed on a heating blanket with adequate pressure point relief.

11.4 Postoperative Management

As with any breast reconstruction using microvascular flaps, there is a risk of developing complications in general and surgery-associated complications in particular. Even more so if breast reconstruction is associated with surgical lymphedema treatment. Besides postoperative flap monitoring, efforts should be made to avoid donor site lymphedema, including MLD and bandaging of the donor site extremity. Prolonged drainage of the surgical wound and repeated percutaneous aspiration of seroma or lymphocele might be necessary. Patients are usually administered thromboprophylaxis and antibiotics postoperatively. Further, they are instructed to avoid elevation of the affected arm above 90 degrees and to avoid carrying weights of more than 15 to 20 kg during approximately 6 weeks following surgery.

11.4.1 Complete Decongestive Therapy

Manual Lymphatic Drainage

MLD should avoid any incision sites of LVAs or recipient sites of VLNT in the immediate postoperative period for about 10 days. It is, however, indicated to start with MLD very early after surgery in order to stimulate the neighboring lymph node basins to activate the lymphatic pumping function.

Compression Therapy

Compression bandages should not be applied to the upper extremity until MLD is reinitiated 10 days postoperatively. Compression garment (class 1) can be applied safely once all the incision sites have healed nicely. They should be adjusted in a timely fashion. Wearing of customized compression garments should be avoided for at least 4 weeks if the heterotopic recipient site of the VLN flap is at the wrist or elbow.

11.4.2 Follow-up

Follow-up evaluation of the affected extremity can be done by different means, using both noninvasive and invasive tools. Clinical evaluation, including measurement of the circumference, is performed on a regular basis, whereas lymphoscintigraphy and ICG lymphangiography are undertaken 1 year after surgery.

Non-Apparative Evaluation

- Clinical: Pitting, nonpitting, swelling, fat hypertrophy, tissue fibrosis, skin changes such as discoloration, vesicles, lymph fistulas
- Circumference and volumetric measurements: Tape measurements, volume calculation, scan, water displacement, etc.
- Infrared opto-electric volumetry (perometer), bio-impedance
- Imaging: Ultrasound, elastometry, three-dimensional scan
- Quality of life questionnaires

Apparative Evaluation

- Lymphoscintigraphy
- SPECT-CT
- Magnetic resonance Lymphangiography (MRL)
- ICG near-infrared imaging (see **Chapter 4**)

11.5 Patient Education

Usually, lymphedema is not a life-threatening condition, yet it can have a major impact on the patient's quality of life due to its chronic nature, resulting in isolation and absenteeism. Therefore, patient education is of paramount importance and should include the understanding of the basic disease mechanisms, the clinical characteristics, and consequences as well as the mode of action of the different treatment modalities. It should also include potential behavioral changes, including dietary restriction and weight loss, if indicated.

From a surgical point of view, it is very important to set measured expectations with regard to postoperative volume reduction of the extremity, further need for compression garments, and MLD. Therefore, the patients are informed that CDT is key before surgery to best "prepare" the patient for reconstructive surgery. However, it is as important in the postoperative phase. The course will say intensity and/or frequency of the conservative treatment may be progressively reduced or eventually ceased, which requires close dialogue and collaboration with dedicated physiotherapists.

Skin care and prevention of injury to the affected limb:

- Wash with a mild soap every day to keep the skin clean.
- Use lotions to prevent skin from getting dry and cracked.
- Use electric rather than manual shaving of the hair-bearing skin.
- In general, avoid injury to the affected limb.
- Take particular care while performing manicure.
- Use sun protection to the skin.
- Wear gloves when gardening, cooking, or doing other manual work with the risk of skin injuries.
- If you suffer a small cut, a scrape, or an insect bite, clean it well with soap and water and apply an antibiotic or antiseptic cream.
- Avoid any medical procedure such as intravenous withdrawal of blood sample or measurement of blood pressure with an arm cuff.

Prevention of swelling of the treated extremity:

- Do not wear any clothes that may restricts lymph flow (e.g., tight T-shirt).
- Avoid activities that could interfere with lymph flow.
- Wear compression garments to reduce rate of filtration and eventually limit swelling.
- Execute MLD with a physical therapist on a regular basis.
- Keep weight under control. Excessive weight gain or being overweight can worsen lymphedema and may limit the effectiveness of compression garments.
- Avoid sauna and hot tub use.

11.6 Clinical Cases

Case 1

A 61-year-old active smoker, normal weight, right-handed woman with breast cancer-related lymphedema of the right upper limb.

The patient underwent skin-sparing mastectomy of the right breast and 1°-stage expander-based reconstruction and ALND for invasive ductal carcinoma of the breast followed by adjuvant chemotherapy with taxanes radiotherapy of the chestwall and axilla. Severe radiotherapy-induced fibrosis of the mastectomy skin developed resulting in expander removal 1 year later and followed by breast reconstruction with a pedicled latissimus dorsi flap. In the operation protocol of this surgery, the axilla was described to be very hostile, and the thoracodorsalis pedicle was not dissectable out of the radio-fibrotic mass. She also has radio pneumonitis of the right upper lung.

Lymphedema was graded both I and II, combining pitting and nonpitting edema. Initial CDT comprised of MLD two to three times a week and compression stocking every day. Lack of compliance to CDT measures needed to control progression of lymphedema led to a progression of lymphedema as seen in the measurement of arm circumference.

Lymphoscintigraphy of the upper limbs showed a lack of of tracer in the right axilla, both at rest and after physical activity, as well as in the early and late phase of the examination, indicating severe drainage insufficiency of the right upper limb.

Surgery comprised of extensive heterotopic VLNT from the left groin to the right elbow and LVAs.

Patent Blue V was injected the night before surgery into the web spaces I and III of both feet.

Before prepping and draping, ICG lymphangiography of the right upper extremity was performed, showing a linear pattern and a splash pattern of the fluorescent dye at the level of the lower arm and the elbow, respectively, the latter signalling dermal backflow (▶ Fig. 11.6a).

The recipient site of the VLN flap was marked (▶ Fig. 11.6b) at right elbow. The donor site for the VLN flap at the right groin was marked identifying with hand-held Doppler the femoral vessels and the flap's pedicle (SCIA and SCIV) parallel to the inguinal ligament to harvest the lymph node flap lateral to the femoral vessels and cranial to the inguinal ligament (▶ Fig. 11.6c).

Using a two-team approach, one team harvested the lymph node flap. The lymph node flap contained a skin island. While preparing the flap more deeply, all the afferent lymph vessels were clipped, and no Patent Blue V was seen during flap harvest, indicating that no lymph nodes draining the lower extremity were included in the flap (▶ Fig. 11.6d). This flap offered two veins joining each other proximally (medially SIEV and laterally SCIV) and one artery (SCIA). In this case, the artery was a direct side branch of the common femoral artery with a total pedicle length of 1.5 cm (▶ Fig. 11.6e,f).

Simultaneously, a second team performed two LVAs at the right forearm, one distally ulnodorsal and one more proximally radiodorsal (▶ Fig. 11.6g). This team also prepared the recipient site to receive the lymph node flap, creting a pocket to accommodate the often "bulky" flap and the recipient vessels to the elbow groove, allowing for vascular end-to-end anastomosis between the lymph node flap vessels and the recipient vessels, inferior ulnar collateral artery, concomitant vein of the inferior ulnar collateral artery, and a superficial vein medial (side branch of the basilic vein) in the elbow groove (▶ Fig. 11.6h).

After flap transfer from the left groin to the right elbow groove, donor site closure was performed using quilting sutures and placement of a suction drain (▶ Fig. 11.6i).

Adhering to standard postoperative recommendations, including thromboprophylaxis and antibioprophylaxis for 10 days, limited motion of the right arm and well-defined bandaging to avoid compression of the elbow region, and compression garment for the left groin for 6 weeks, the postoperative course was uneventful (▶ Fig. 11.6j-k).

MLD of the right arm was discontinued for 2 weeks until stich removal. Suction drain in the left groin remained

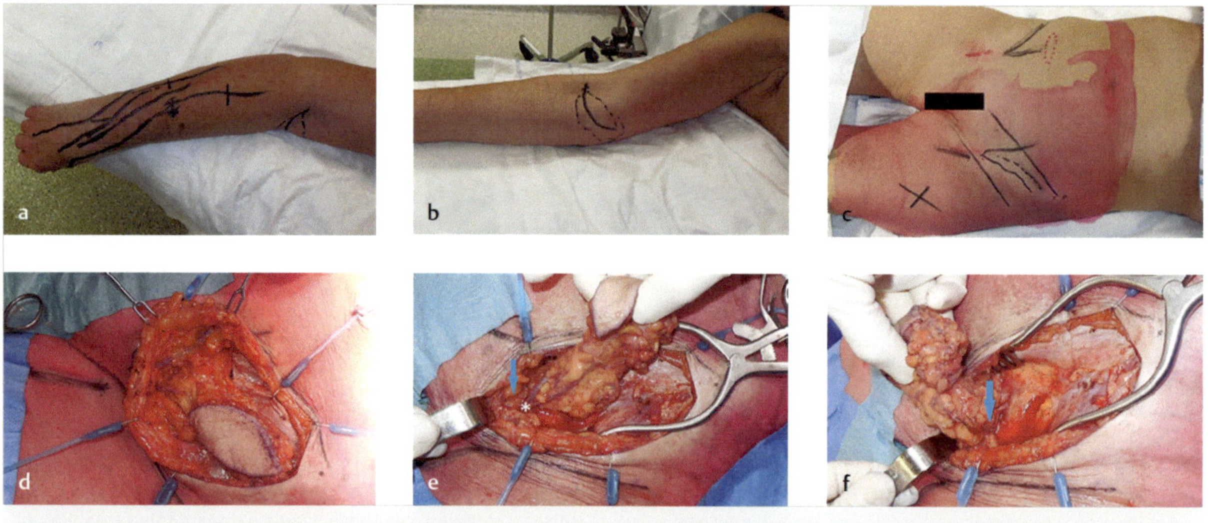

Fig. 11.6 Inguinal lymph node flap to treat breast cancer-related chronic lymphedema of the right upper extremity: **(a)** Preoperative markings of the lower arm according to linear pattern lymph drainage. **(b)** Recipient site for vascularized lymph node flap at the right elbow groove. **(c)** Preoperative markings of the flap donor site at the left inguinal region. **(d)** Clipping all afferent lymphatic vessels that are identified after incision of the flap's skin island and dissection into the depth. **(e)** Inguinal lymph node flap based on superficial inferior epigastric vein and superficial circumflex iliac vein, joining proximally (asterisk). **(f)** Inguinal lymph node flap based on superficial circumflex iliac artery with a rather short pedicle (blue arrow).

(Continued)

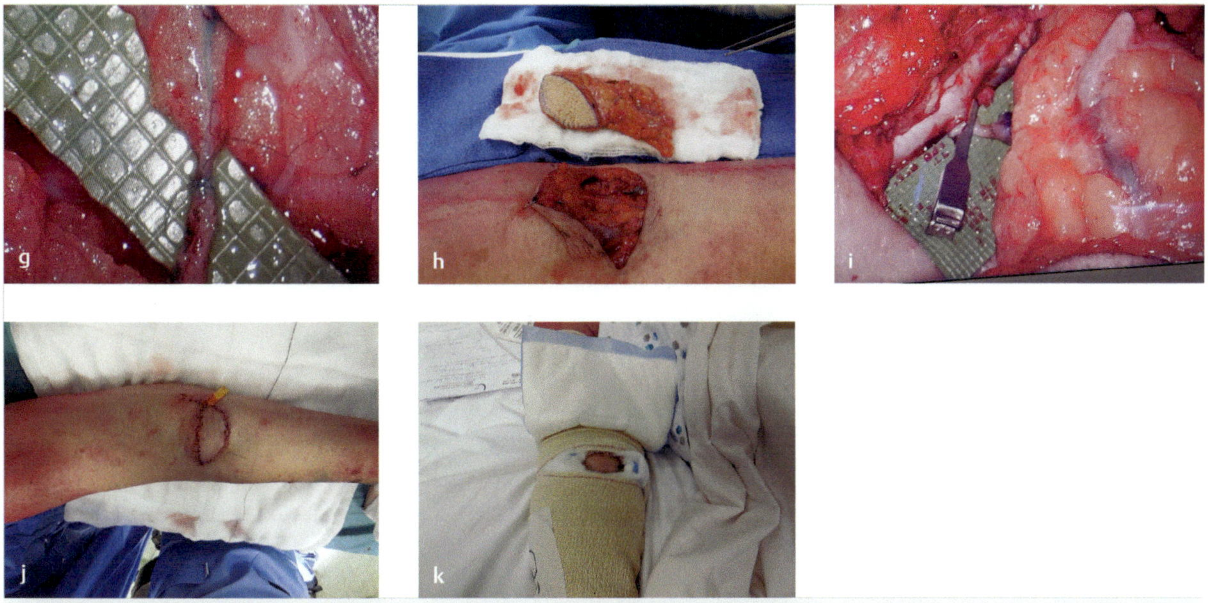

Fig. 11.6 *(Continued)* **(g)** Anterograde lymphovenous anastomosis using single sutures (11–0) for end-to-end anastomosis (asterisk = distal lymph vessel). **(h)** Lymph node flap after transfer to its recipient site at the ulnar side of the right elbow. **(i)** Arterial end-to-end anastomosis between superficial circumflex iliac artery (right) and recipient vessels at the elbow's groove (left). **(j)** After flap inset to the elbow groove and closure of the recipient site. **(k)** Postoperative circular bandage of the operated limb with "window" to monitor the flap's perfusion.

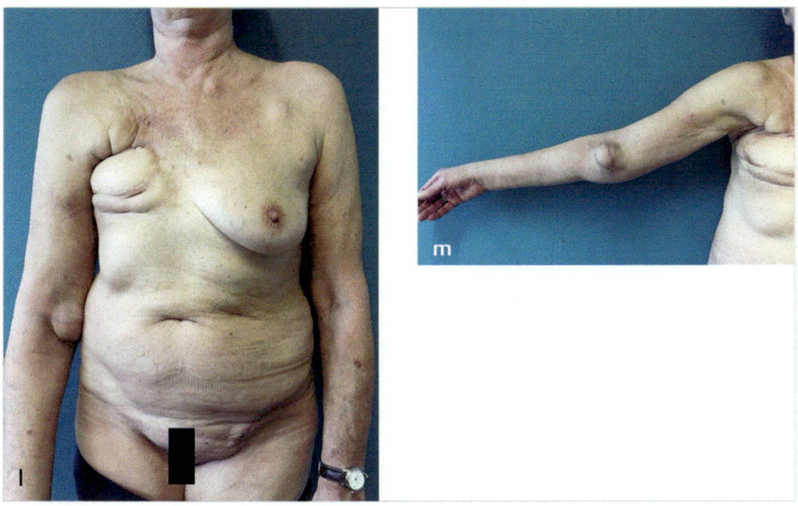

Fig. 11.6 *(Continued)* **(l, m)** One month after surgery and uneventful healing, the flap in the elbow groove is still bulky.

for 2 weeks, and donor site seroma was evacuated requiring one puncture.

At 1 month follow-up, all the wounds were healed, and CDT has been reinitiated (▸ Fig. 11.6l–m).

Case 2

58-year-old patient with chronic breast cancer-related lymphedema of the left nondominant upper extremity, suffering from recurrent infections (erysipela) 15 years after mastectomy of the left breast, SLNB, and adjuvant radiotherapy followed by mastectomy of the right breast, axillary lymph node clearance, and adjuvant radiotherapy 13 years later, now seeking bilateral breast reconstruction and surgical treatment of the arm's lymphedema (▸ Fig. 11.7a,b). Lymphedema was more pronounced on the left.

Bilateral autologous breast reconstruction was performed using a hemiabdominal DIEP flap to reconstruct each breast and was associated with bilateral VLNT from the groin region to treat lymphedema (▸ Fig. 11.7c–e).

At 16 months postoperative (▸ Fig. 11.7f,g), significant reduction of lymphedema was achieved, predominantly

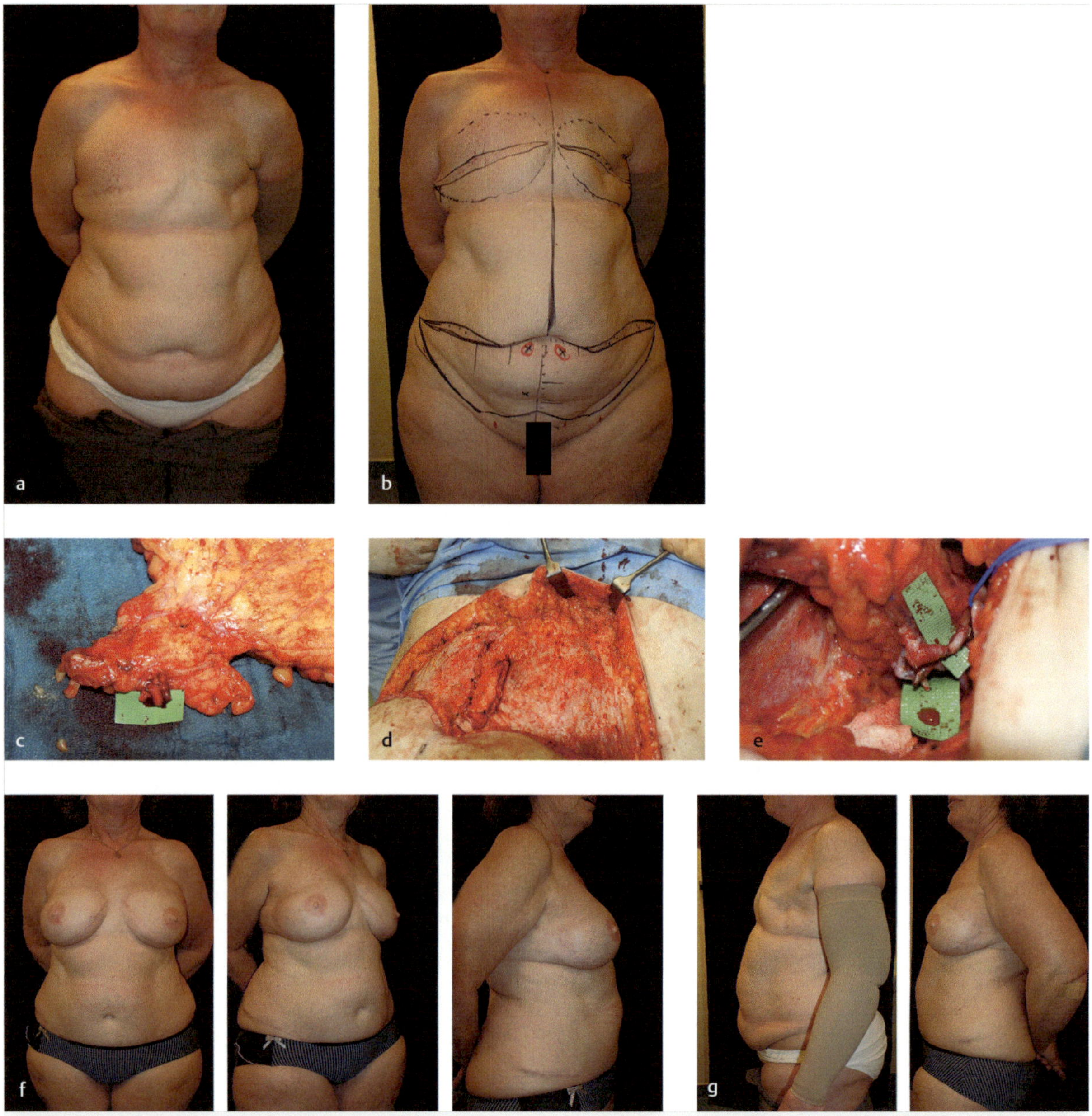

Fig. 11.7 Concomitant bilateral autologous breast reconstruction and unilateral vascularized lymph node transfer to treat breast cancer-related chronic lymphedema of the right upper extremity after bilateral mastectomy: **(a)** Frontal view after bilateral mastectomy and adjuvant radiotherapy, showing radiotherapy-induced skin changes on the right. **(b)** Frontal view with preoperative markings of the deep inferior epigastric perforator flap harvest indicating the flap's perforators in the periumbilical region after identification with handheld Doppler (red circle, black arrow). **(c)** Lymph node flap based on the superficial circumflex iliac artery and superficial circumflex iliac vein (asterisk). Note the short vascular pedicle in continuity with the deep inferior epigastric perforator flap (double asterisks) used for breast reconstruction. **(d)** Attention to the layered closure, using tissue glue and quilting sutures, of the donor sites after bilateral vascularized lymph node flap harvest is paid in order to avoid postoperative seroma formation. **(e)** Additional vascular anastomosis of the pedicle of the lymph node flap (superficial circumflex iliac artery and superficial circumflex iliac vein) to the lateral thoracic vessels. **(f)** Postoperative follow-up at 16 months with completed breast reconstruction, including the nipple-areolar complex. Note the absence of postoperative compression garment at the left arm. **(g)** Preoperative and 16 months postoperative follow-up result.

at the level of the forearms. Bilaterally, a 3-cm circumferential volume reduction was measured at both wrists and forearms, and at the upper arm a 1.5-cm reduction was achieved. The patient perceived less heaviness of the upper limbs, more softness of the tissues, and increased mobility at the shoulder joints also. After surgery, the patient did not suffer from infections anymore; further, the patient could get rid of the compression garments.

11.7 Pearls and Pitfalls

- Preoperative evaluation of functionality of the lymphatic system is key to correctly select candidates for lympho-reconstructive techniques.
- Currently available imaging techniques are key to assess both the anatomy and the function of the lymphatic system in order to accurately plan surgery.
- Axillary scar tissue removal (i.e., "scar release") is a critical step for the reduction of arm volume and improvement of shoulder mobility. An axillary recipient site devoid of scar tissue resulting from surgery and/or radiotherapy is needed for adequate integration and regeneration of new lympho-venular anastomosis after VLNT. The flap should be positioned in the apex of the axilla alongside the axillary veins to replace removed or nonfunctional lymph nodes.
- The risk of seroma formation can be reduced using quilting sutures, fibrin glue, and drains while closing the donor site of the abdominal and lymph node flap.
- The risk of iatrogenic lymphedema secondary to lymph node flap harvesting is reduced if meticulous dissection is performed within the given anatomical landmarks, namely, the femoral vessels medially and superficial circumflex iliac vessels caudally.
- Reversed lymphatic mapping during surgery is needed to distinguish lymph nodes that do not drain the extremity from the ones that drain the extremity. The latter lymph nodes should be excluded from the lymph node flap.
- Including the skin overlapping the adipose tissue containing the lymph nodes provides flap tissue that may replace skin at the recipient site (e.g., scar retraction after axillary lymph node clearance and/or radiotherapy) and allows clinical flap monitoring.
- The patient should receive accurate instructions regarding postoperative behavior, mobilization, and physical therapy according to in-house protocols.

References

[1] DiSipio T, Rye S, Newman B, Hayes S. Incidence of unilateral arm lymphoedema after breast cancer: a systematic review and meta-analysis. Lancet Oncol. 2013; 14(6):500–515

[2] International Society of Lymphology Executive Committee.. The Diagnosis and Tratment of Peripheral Lymphedema. Lymphology. 1995; 28(3):113–117

[3] Mihara M, Hara H, Hayashi Y, et al. Pathological steps of cancer-related lymphedema: histological changes in the collecting lymphatic vessels after lymphadenectomy. PLoS One. 2012; 7(7):e41126

[4] Zeltzer AA, Anzarut A, Hamdi M. A review of lymphedema for the hand and upper-extremity surgeon. J Hand Surg Am. 2018; 43(11): 1016–1025

[5] Veronesi U, Paganelli G, Viale G, et al. A randomized comparison of sentinel-node biopsy with routine axillary dissection in breast cancer. N Engl J Med. 2003; 349(6):546–553

[6] Soares EWS, Nagai HM, Bredt LC, da Cunha AD, Jr, Andrade RJ, Soares GVS. Morbidity after conventional dissection of axillary lymph nodes in breast cancer patients. World J Surg Oncol. 2014; 12:67

[7] Schünemann H, Willich N. [Secondary lymphedema of the arm following primary therapy of breast carcinoma]. Zentralbl Chir. 1992; 117(4):220–225

[8] McLaughlin SA, Wright MJ, Morris KT, et al. Prevalence of lymphedema in women with breast cancer 5 years after sentinel lymph node biopsy or axillary dissection: objective measurements. J Clin Oncol. 2008; 26(32):5213–5219

[9] Ozcinar B, Guler SA, Kocaman N, Ozkan M, Gulluoglu BM, Ozmen V. Breast cancer related lymphedema in patients with different loco-regional treatments. Breast. 2012; 21(3):361–365

[10] Shaitelman SF, Chiang YJ, Griffin KD, et al. Radiation therapy targets and the risk of breast cancer-related lymphedema: a systematic review and network meta-analysis. Breast Cancer Res Treat. 2017; 162(2):201–215

[11] Mehrara BJ, Greene AK. Lymphedema and obesity: is there a link? Plast Reconstr Surg. 2014; 134(1):154e–160e

[12] Siotos C, Sebai ME, Wan EL, et al. Breast reconstruction and risk of arm lymphedema development: a meta-analysis. J Plast Reconstr Aesthet Surg. 2018; 71(6):807–818

[13] De Brucker B, Zeltzer A, Seidenstuecker K, Hendrickx B, Adriaenssens N, Hamdi M. Breast cancer-related lymphedema: quality of life after lymph node transfer. Plast Reconstr Surg. 2016; 137(6):1673–1680

[14] Hirche C, Autologous Breast Reconstruction in Conjunction with Lymphatic Microsurgery in Breast Cancer-Related Lymphedema. Handchir Mikrochir Plast Chir. 2022;54(4):326–338

[15] Pusic AL, Cemal Y, Albornoz C, et al. Quality of life among breast cancer patients with lymphedema: a systematic review of patient-reported outcome instruments and outcomes. J Cancer Surviv. 2013; 7(1):83–92

[16] Yamamoto T, Yamamoto N, Doi K, et al. Indocyanine green-enhanced lymphography for upper extremity lymphedema: a novel severity staging system using dermal backflow patterns. Plast Reconstr Surg. 2011; 128(4):941–947

[17] Zeltzer AA, Brussaard C, Koning M, et al. MR lymphography in patients with upper limb lymphedema: the GPS for feasibility and surgical planning for lympho-venous bypass. J Surg Oncol. 2018; 118 (3):407–415

[18] Suami H, Taylor GI, Pan W-R. The lymphatic territories of the upper limb: anatomical study and clinical implications. Plast Reconstr Surg. 2007; 119(6):1813–1822

[19] Suami H, O'Neill JK, Pan W-R, Taylor GI. Superficial lymphatic system of the upper torso: preliminary radiographic results in human cadavers. Plast Reconstr Surg. 2008; 121(4):1231–1239

[20] Mascagni P. Vasorum lymphaticorum corporis humani. Historia et Ichonographia. Siena: Pazzini Carli; 1787:XIX–XXV

[21] Caplàn I. Traitement Physique de l'Ce Déme Du Bras. 1981

[22] Latorre J, Ciucci J, Rosendo A. Anatomia del sistema linfatico del miembro superior. An Cirugìa Cardìaca y Vasc. 2004; 10(3):184–198

[23] Suami H, Chang DW. Overview of surgical treatments for breast cancer-related lymphedema. Plast Reconstr Surg. 2010; 126(6):1853–1863

[24] Yamazaki S, Suami H, Imanishi N, et al. Three-dimensional demonstration of the lymphatic system in the lower extremities with multi-detector-row computed tomography: a study in a cadaver model. Clin Anat. 2013; 26(2):258–266

[25] Caplan I. El sistema linfatico ganglionar de la region polpitea [Doctoral thesis]. Buenos Aires: Tesis; 1966

[26] Quenu E, Lejars F. Etudes Sur Le Système Circulatoire. Vol. 1. Paris: Steinheil; 1894

[27] Cheng MH, Chen SC, Henry SL, Tan BK, Chia-Yu Lin M, Huang JJ. Vascularized groin lymph node flap transfer for postmastectomy upper limb lymphedema: flap anatomy, recipient sites, and outcomes. Plast Reconstr Surg. 2013; 131(6):1286–1298

[28] Scaglioni MF, Arvanitakis M, Chen YC, Giovanoli P, Chia-Shen Yang J, Chang EI. Comprehensive review of vascularized lymph node transfers for lymphedema: outcomes and complications. Microsurgery. 2018; 38 (2):222–229

[29] Saaristo AM, Niemi TS, Viitanen TP, Tervala TV, Hartiala P, Suominen EA. Microvascular breast reconstruction and lymph

node transfer for postmastectomy lymphedema patients. Ann Surg. 2012; 255(3):468–473

[30] Nguyen AT, Chang EI, Suami H, Chang DW. An algorithmic approach to simultaneous vascularized lymph node transfer with microvascular breast reconstruction. Ann Surg Oncol. 2015; 22(9):2919–2924

[31] Akita S, Tokumoto H, Yamaji Y, et al. Contribution of simultaneous breast reconstruction by deep inferior epigastric artery perforator flap to the efficacy of vascularized lymph node transfer in patients with breast cancer-related lymphedema. J Reconstr Microsurg. 2017; 33(8):571–578

[32] Engel H, Lin C, Huang J, Cheng M. Outcomes of lymphedema microsurgery for breast cancer-related lymphedema with or without microvascular breast reconstruction. Ann Surg. 2018; 268(6):1076–1083

[33] Zeltzer AA, Anzarut A, Braeckmans D, et al. The vascularized groin lymph node flap (VGLN): anatomical study and flap planning using multi-detector CT scanner. The golden triangle for flap harvesting. J Surg Oncol. 2017; 116(3):378–383

[34] Hamdi M, Van Landuyt K, Van Hedent E, Duyck P. Advances in autogenous breast reconstruction: the role of preoperative perforator mapping. Ann Plast Surg. 2007; 58(1):18–26

[35] Patel KM, Lin CY, Cheng MH. From theory to evidence: long-term evaluation of the mechanism of action and flap integration of distal vascularized lymph node transfers. J Reconstr Microsurg. 2015; 31 (1):26–30

[36] Vibhakar D, Reddy , Morgan-Hazelwood W, Chang E. Chimeric pedicled latissimus dorsi flap with lateral thoracic lymph nodes for breast reconstruction and lymphedema treatment in a hypercoagulable patient. J Plast Reconstr Surg. 2014; 134(3):494e–495e

[37] Inbal A, Teven CM, Chang DW. Latissimus dorsi flap with vascularized lymph node transfer for lymphedema treatment: technique, outcomes, indications, and review of literature. J Surg Oncol. 2017; 115(1):72–77

[38] Masia J, Pons G, Nardulli ML. Combined surgical treatment in breast cancer-related lymphedema. J Reconstr Microsurg. 2016; 32(1):16–27

[39] Nguyen AT, Suami H. Laparoscopic free omental lymphatic flap for the treatment of lymphedema. Plast Reconstr Surg. 2015; 136(1): 114–118

12 Nodo-Venal Shunt Microsurgery

Gurusamy Manokaran and Leela Praveen Kumar

Summary

This chapter describes the surgical technique of nodo-venal shunts as they are regularly performed by the first author. The surgery essentially consists of an anastomosis between the "low pressure" lymphatic vascular system and the "high pressure" vascular system of the superficial veins to conduct a physiological bypass. Accordingly, a connection is established surgically between a well-functioning and draining lymph node in the inguinal region and a patent superficial vein, usually in the draining area of the greater saphenous. Most of the cases that are treated using this technique suffer from chronic lymphedema resulting from filariasis affecting almost always the lower limb.

Keywords: conservative treatment, lymphatic filariasis, lymphovenous anastomosis, microvascular lymph node transfer, nodo-venal shunt, physiological bypass surgery

12.1 General Considerations

Lymphatic filariasis is a common problem in emerging and low-income countries such as India (see **Chapter 3**). Unfortunately, most of the patients present at a late stage of the disease, most often due to lack of education and knowledge, poverty, and unavailability of adequate medical treatment and personnel. More recently, people have started to understand the disease itself and the fact that there is potentially a definitive cure for any stage of filariasis-associated lymphedema.

The cases that present early can be managed conservatively[1] (see **Chapter 6**), but the ones which present a little late will need some kind of surgery to improve the quality of life of affected patients. According to the lymphedema stage, surgical procedures to be offered can be classified as reconstructive or physiological (see **Chapters 7–12**) and lymphoablative (see **Chapters 13** and **14**).

In vivo and experimental lymphovenous shunts have already been described in the early 1960s.[2] The first clinical cases have been performed only little later.[3,4] Since that time, various surgical modifications of lymphovenous shunts have been described, including nodo-venal (NV) shunts.[5,6,7,8,9,10]

Accordingly, this chapter will describe the surgical technique that concerns the NV shunt in the inguinal region.

12.2 Indications and Contraindications

- NV shunt is one reconstructive option of treatment to improve complete blockage or significant functional impairment of the afferent lymphatics.
- NV shunt is indicated in irreversible stages of lymphedema graded II (according to the Gerusa Dreyer classification[11]) or higher (see **Chapter 3**).
- In grade II lymphedema, NV shunt alone can be sufficient, whereas in higher grades, often additional surgical procedures using lymphoablative or excisional techniques are needed (see **Chapters 13** and **14**). Obviously, surgery is accompanied by conservative measures before and after the procedure of NV shunts, including periodic antibiotics, pressure garments, and meticulous hygiene of the feet.
- The NV shunt is contraindicated in primary lymphedema and in secondary lymphedema with progressive malignancies.
- For acute infections such cellulitis and/or lymphangitis, an infection-free interval of at least 6 weeks is recommended following successful treatment with antibiotics.
- Any infection at the surgical site such as the groin needs to be treated before surgery.
- It is contraindicated if there is no visible lymph node on lymphoscintigraphy or ultrasound.
- Incompetent drainage between superficial and deep venous system at sapheno-femoral junction (SFJ), diagnosed by Duplex ultrasound.
- No reduction of limb size or volume, even after 1 week of intensive manual lymph drainage (MLD).
- Patients with significant comorbidities with renal, cardiac, or pulmonary insufficiency, diabetes mellitus, as well as active smoking present with relative contraindications.

12.3 Preoperative Assessment

- Prior to NV shunt surgery, a competent SFJ junction has to be confirmed using ultrasound color Doppler.
- Lymphoscintigraphy should confirm the presence of a healthy and functional lymph node in the inguinal region.
- Preoperative ultrasound should identify and allow to mark a functional lymph node in case lymph nodes are not palpable.
- Finally, preoperative measurement of the limb's circumference is performed in a standardized manner,

using the Jobst measuring scale, taking measures every 4 cm from ankle to inguinal crease. This measurement serves as an objective baseline value to monitor the efficacy of the surgical treatment.

12.4 Preoperative Preparation

When surgery is indicated, the patient is informed in detail about the surgery and the potential benefits and drawbacks, including complications. After consenting to surgery, the patient is admitted a couple of days prior to surgery in order to guarantee best possible result. Therefore, conservative treatment including MLD, compressive bandaging, respiratory physiotherapy and physical exercises, and low-fat diet are initiated. This helps to drain the lymph proximally toward the groin, and eventually "bloats" the lymph nodes in the groin on the day of surgery. Accordingly, identification of the draining and hence functioning lymph node is much easier.

The inguinal region is depilated the evening prior to surgery, whereas antiseptic wash is recommended both on the day prior to and the morning of surgery. Antibiotic prophylaxis is administered briefly before initiating surgery.

12.5 Surgical Technique

Surgery is usually performed under general anesthesia but can also be executed under regional anesthesia in select cases.

The patient is positioned in supine, with the hip of the affected extremity slightly flexed and externally rotated and the knee in mild flexion.

After disinfection and draping, the markings are made, first identifying the inguinal crease and the femoral artery. If ultrasound marking of the lymph node has not been made preoperatively, the surgeon tries to identify a "bloated" lymph node by palpation, if possible, and marks it. Surgery is generally performed using loupe magnification (3.2 to 4 ×). In rare cases the microscope is indicated. Further, using microsurgical instruments is highly advised.

A vertical skin incision of 3 to 4 cm is made medial to the course of the femoral artery. Thereafter, gentle retraction of the skin allows progressive incision of the subcutaneous tissue up to the level of the superficial fascia of the fat, where the great saphenous vein (GSV) can be identified. Particular care is taken to cut the fat in order to least traumatize lymphatics adjacent to the incision. Thereafter, the small side branches of the GSV are ligated to obtain a segment of 4 to 5 cm proximally to the SFJ if a lymph node has been identified in the proximity. If needed, the skin incision can be extended distally for better identification and isolation of the GSV.

The identification of the lymph node is usually performed by gentle palpation within the surgical wound, whereas visual identification needs some experience. If the surgeon neither sees, nor palpates a lymph node, further dissection is performed medial to the GSV. Basically, an afunctional lymph node usually appears slightly pinkish, embedded in the surrounding yellow fat. Once a potential lymph node has been identified, a self-retaining retractor is placed into the surgical access. Thereafter, minimal dissection is performed around the lymph node to free it from its peri-nodal fat, as unnecessary dissection can damage the afferent and efferent lymphatics to the node. Then the capsule of the lymph node is exposed at its surface in order to excise a circular patch of capsule and underlying nodular tissue. The resected tissue of the lymph node is sent for histopathological examination. After truncating the lymph node, the surgeon should see adequate punctual bleeding from the lymph node that stops with gentle pressure with a gauze after 2 to 3 minutes. Once bleeding stops, oozing of milky fluid indicating lymph flow may be seen from the lymph node's truncated and exposed surface.

The GSV is then clamped distally and competence at the SFJ is checked, excluding the presence of backflow (anterograde and retrograde streaking of the vein). Thereafter, the vein is transected at an adequate distance from the SFJ, which allows to reach the selected lymph node to be shunted easily (▶ Fig. 12.1 and ▶ Fig. 12.2). The venous end is then prepared by trimming the adjacent adventitia and enlarged by a longitudinal incision creating a "fish mouth"-like vascular opening. The venous end is then placed over the lymph node and a microvascular anastomosis is performed using the "heal-to-toe" technique (also known as the "open-book" technique) with a continuous suture using 6–0 or 7–0 nonresorbable monofilament suture. Care is taken to precisely set the stich including the full thickness of the venous wall and the breached capsule of the lymph node in order to put over the transected vein over the truncated lymph node (▶ Fig. 12.3, ▶ Fig. 12.4, ▶ Fig. 12.5, ▶ Fig. 12.6, ▶ Fig. 12.7, ▶ Fig. 12.8, ▶ Fig. 12.9, ▶ Fig. 12.10). After completion of the anastomosis, the clamp is released to free lymph flow. Following adequate hemostasis, the wound is closed in a layered manner using usually resorbable monofilament suture. Most often, the surgical wound is left without drains, but in select cases, a drain is inserted and generally removed on postoperative day 2.

Previously, NV shunts were performed using an end-to-side technique in order to leave the veins in continuity. The author modified the technique describing an end-to-end method, "connecting and attaching" the vein to the

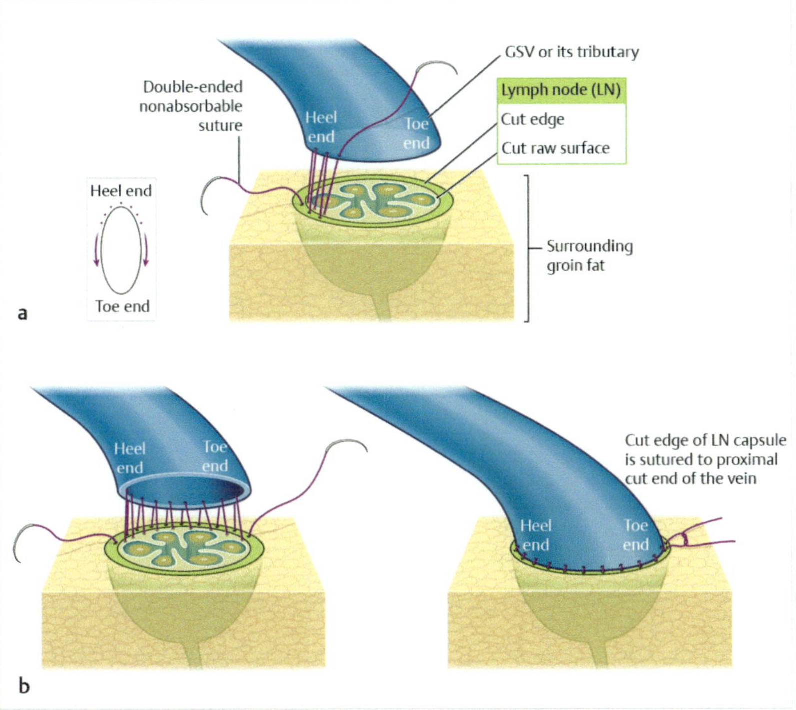

Fig. 12.1 (a, b) The author's (Dr. Manokaran) modified technique of nodo-venal shunt where it is done in an end-to-end style.

truncated lymph node. The end-to-end technique enables minimal dissection of the lymph node, and the freed venous "stump" reached the ideal node that is not always close to the GSV more easily. Accordingly, improved reduction of the limb volume could be achieved when compared to the end-to-side lymph node shunt technique.

12.6 Postoperative Care

Mild compression with a compressive and adhesive plaster such as dynaplast is applied to the wound. Compression bandage is put around the legs. The patient is maintained on strict bedrest for 24 hours after surgery. Thereafter, the patient starts mobilization with full weight-bearing. Further, the patient executes respiratory physiotherapy with breathing exercises using a spirometer.

The surgical wound is first inspected after 48 hours, while dressings are usually changed and drains removed, if in place, in order to discharge the patient. On day 2 or 3 after surgery, the compression bandage is replaced by a customized compression garment up to mid-thigh long.

The patient is maintained on periodic oral antibiotics and antiparasitic treatment including doxycycline 100 mg twice daily and Banocide Forte thrice daily for 5 days a month for at least 2 years, followed 5 days a year for another 5 years. The patient is seen in an outpatient clinic at 4 weeks and 6 months after surgery, during which circumferential measurements of the extremities are taken. Further clinical controls are scheduled every 6 months.

12.7 Patient Education

- All patients are put on low-fat diet to reduce the load on the lymphatics in the early stages.
- All patients are best educated on how to maintain general hygiene.
- Patients are advised to maintain good oral hygiene to ideally avoid recurrent lymphangitis.
- Fungal infections in between the toes and intertrigo in the skinfolds need to be prevented and treated if present to reduce the risk of recurrent lymphangitis.
- Patients are advised to wear compression stockings throughout the day and elevate the lower extremity at rest. No nocturnal bandage is indicated.
- In cases of skin changes like thickening and discoloration, unidirectional massage using a cream or ointment containing 1% salicylic acid should be used for external massage at bedtime to take away the hyperpigmentation and small nodules for at least 3 months. If necessary, it can be extended to 6 months. Prolonged usage can induce vitiligo-like depigmentation.

12.8 Complications

- Wound dehiscence
- Seroma
- Lymphocele
- Lymphorrhea

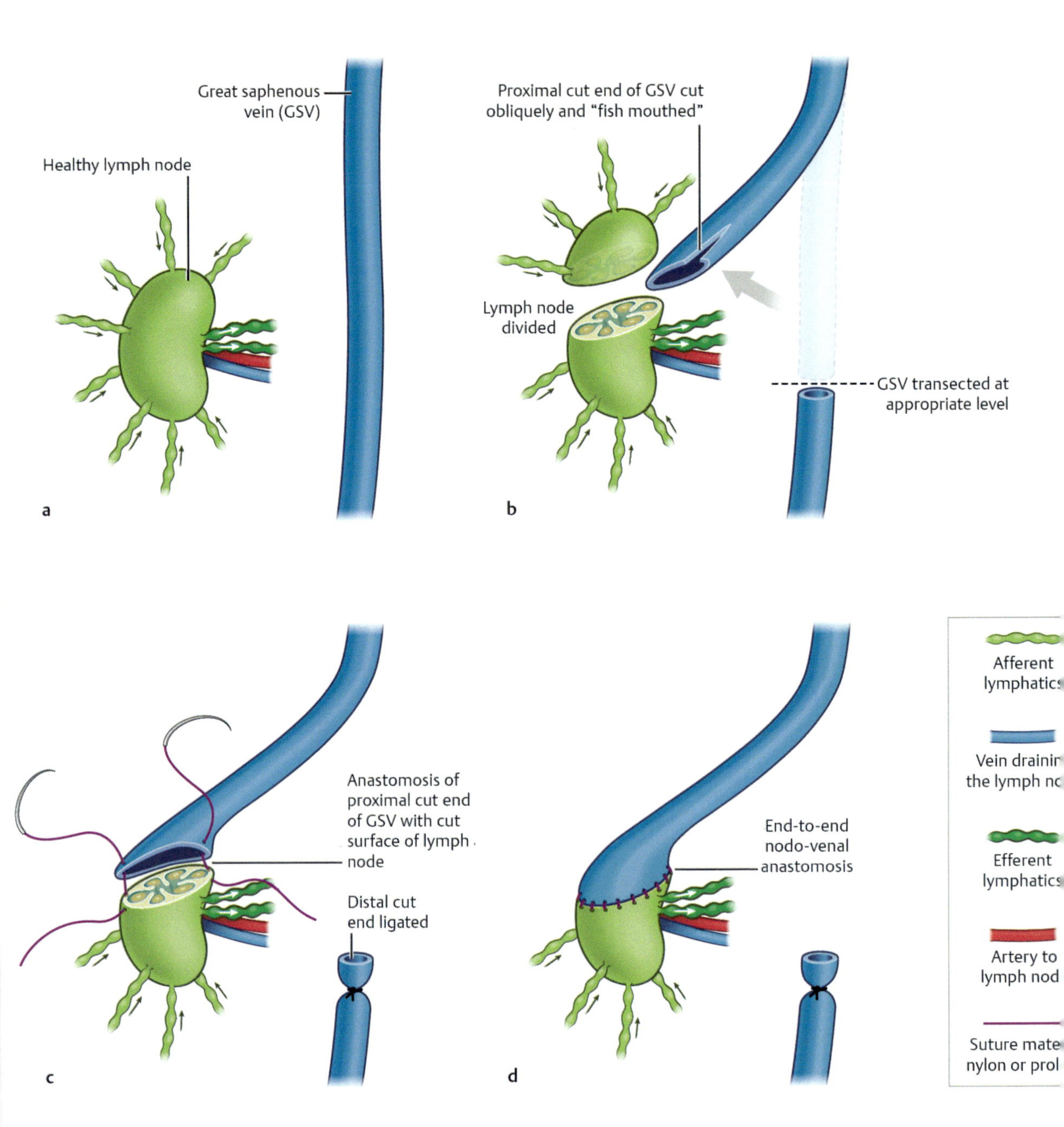

Fig. 12.2 Schematic diagram of an end-to-end nodo-venal shunt or anastomoses modified by Gurusamy Manokaran: **(a)** Healthy inguinal lymph node adjacent to great saphenous vein or its tributary. **(b)** Lymph node is minimally dissected to avoid destruction of afferent and efferent lymphatics. Truncation of the lymph node followed by ligation and transection of the vein distally. The proximal venous stump is transected obliquely and "fish-mouthed" to best match the size of the circumference of the lymph node at the truncation site. **(c)** Anastomosis between great saphenous vein and lymph node is performed with 6–0 or 7–0 nonresorbable, monofilament, continuous suture using the "heel-to-toe" technique. **(d)** Presentation of a lymph node shunt after completing the anastomoses.

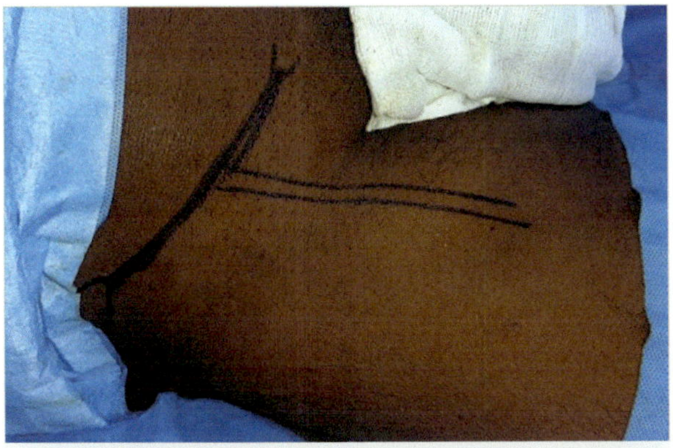

Fig. 12.3 Preoperative markings of the landmarks.

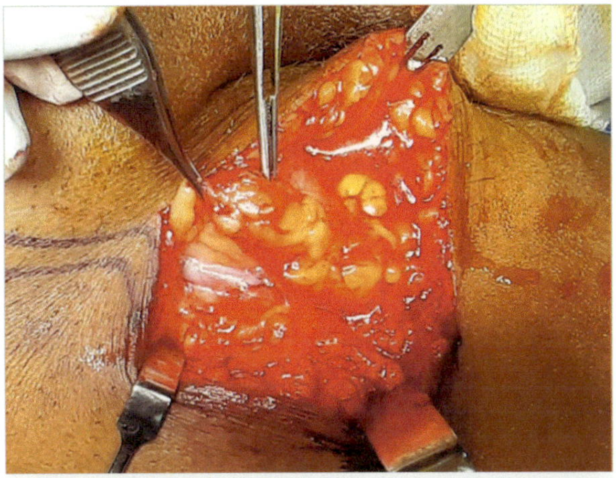

Fig. 12.4 Identification of great saphenous vein and a functioning lymph node (forceps).

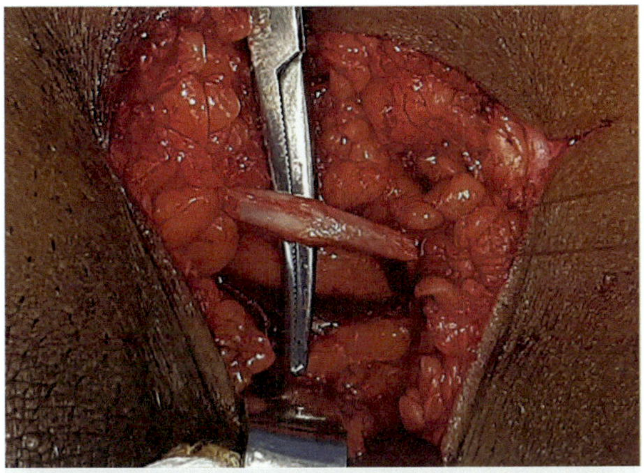

Fig. 12.5 Isolation and distal ligation of great saphenous vein.

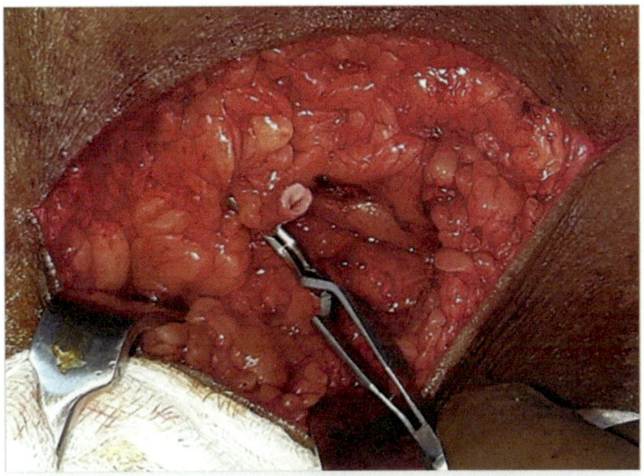

Fig. 12.6 Proximal transection of great saphenous vein.

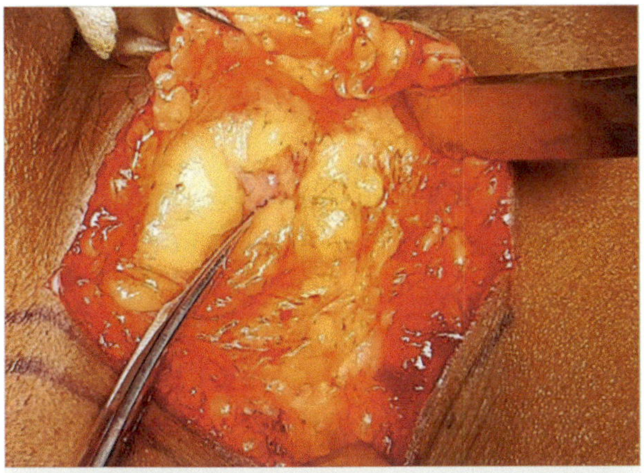

Fig. 12.7 Trimming of the fat to expose the lymph node (purple tissue adjacent to the tip of the scissor).

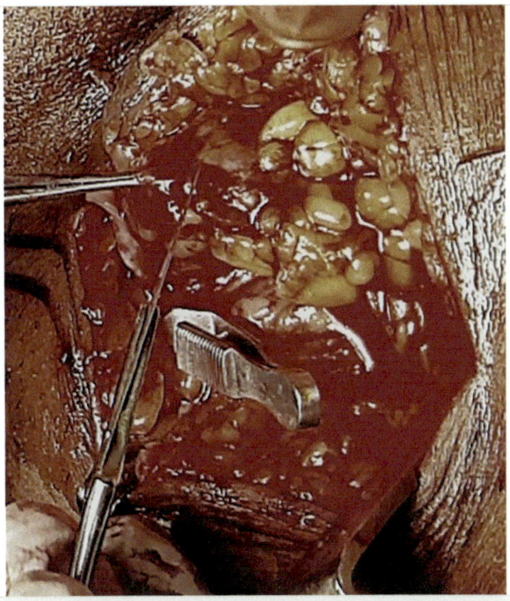

Fig. 12.8 The capsule of the lymph node is picked with the forceps and cut with an # 11 blade.

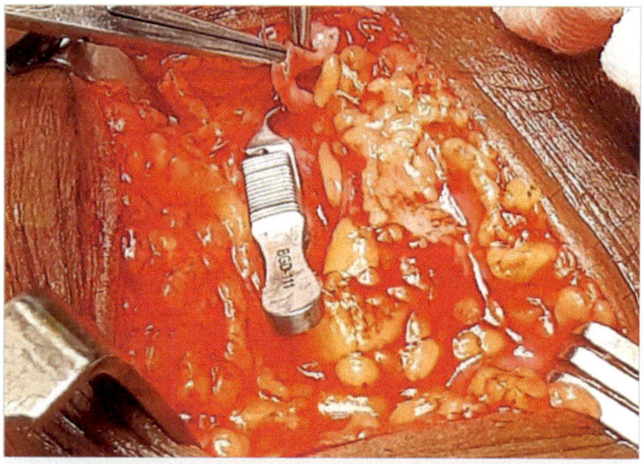

Fig. 12.9 The great saphenous vein has been fish-mouthed and the first suture of the anastomosis is being placed.

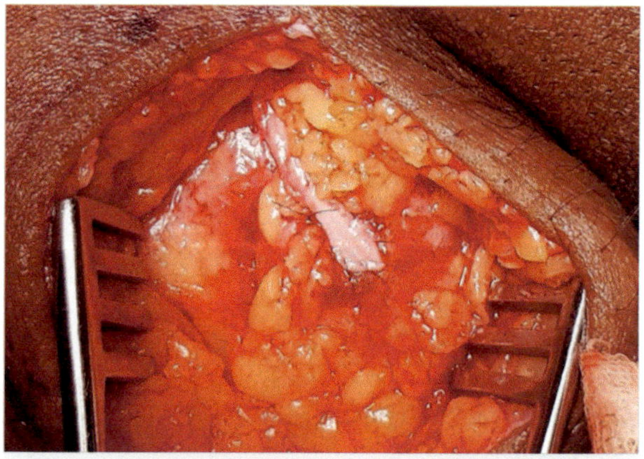

Fig. 12.10 After completion of nodo-venal shunt, "cobra-hood" appearance of the great saphenous vein is seen.

References

[1] Lee BB, Bergan J, Rockson SG, eds. Lymphedema: A Concise Compendium of Theory and Practice. USA: Springer; 2011:11–564

[2] Nielubowicz J, Olszewski W. Experimental lymphovenous anastomosis. Br J Surg. 1968; 55(6):449–451

[3] Nielubowicz J, Olszewski W. Surgical lymphaticovenous shunts in patients with secondary lymphoedema. Br J Surg. 1968; 55(6):440–442

[4] Sedlácek J. Lymphovenous shunt as supplementary treatment of elephantiasis of lower limbs. Acta Chir Plast. 1969; 11(2):157–162

[5] Gilbert A, O'Brien BM, Vorrath JW, Sykes PJ. Lymphaticovenous anastomosis by microvascular technique. Br J Plast Surg. 1976; 29(4): 355–360

[6] Bresadola F, Mannella P, Sortini A, et al. Peripheral lymphatico-venous anastomosis. New surgical technic. [in Italian]. Minerva Chir. 1978; 33(23–24):1711–1718

[7] Degni M. New microsurgical technique of lymphatico-venous anastomosis for the treatment of lymphedema. Lymphology. 1981; 14(2):61–63

[8] al Assal F, Cordeiro AK, De Souza e Castro I. A new technique of microlympho-venous anastomoses. Experimental study. J Cardiovasc Surg (Torino). 1988; 29(5):552–555

[9] Campisi C. Use of autologous interposition vein graft in management of lymphedema: preliminary experimental and clinical observations. Lymphology. 1991; 24(2):71–76

[10] Kinjo O, Kusaba A. Lymphatic vessel-to-isolated-vein anastomosis for secondary lymphedema in a canine model. Surg Today. 1995; 25(7): 633–639

[11] Dreyer G, Coutinho A, Albuquerque R. [Clinical manifestations of lymphatic bancroftian filariasis]. AMB Rev Assoc Med Bras. 1989; 35(5):189–196

Section VII

Lymphoreductive Procedures, Secondary Procedures, and Tips and Tricks

Edited by Christoph Hirche, Katrin Seidenstücker, and Moustapha Hamdi

VII

13 Suction-Assisted Lipectomy

Arin K. Greene, Jeremy A. Goss, and Håkan Brorson

Summary

Chronic lymphedema results from a protein-rich fluid accumulation in the interstitial tissues and presents as a soft tissue swelling of the extremities. The accumulation of protein-rich fluid causes an increasing fibrotic alteration and enlargement of the subcutaneous tissue compartment. Once these morphological tissue changes have occurred, the only way to reduce size and volume of the affected extremity is to resect the hypertrophic tissue. Preoperatively, all accumulation of free fluid must be eliminated by maximizing manual lymphatic drainage and compression. Patients that undergo suction-assisted lipectomy are educated that the procedure will not cure lymphedema. Therefore, a prerequisite to maintaining the effect of suction-assisted lipectomy is the lifelong continuous use of compression garments to reduce the risk of recurrence. Patients who are not compliant with compression therapy are not candidates for surgery. Suction-assisted lipectomy can be performed using a tourniquet or with tumescent solution. Custom made compression garments (class 3) need to be ordered in advance based on the measurements of the healthy leg/arm.

Keywords: adipose tissue, excision, extremity, fat, lipectomy, lymphedema

13.1 Indications and Contraindications

In primary and secondary lymphedemas, the high-protein fluid causes the production of subcutaneous adipose tissue and fibrosis and enlarges the subcutaneous compartment.[1,2,3] Once fibro-adipose deposition has occurred and chronic lymphedema in the end stage, the only way to reduce the size and volume of the arm or leg is to resect the overgrown tissue.

In addition to a standalone technique as it has been successfully applied, suction-assisted lipectomy nowadays is increasingly a surgical tool in conjunction with preceding lymphoreconstructive procedures to improve the reduction of volume (see **Chapters 8, 10** and **Subchapter 15.2**).

In the present chapter, the technique of suction-assisted lipectomy is illustrated as standalone technique.

The preferred lymphoablative technique to remove excess fibro-adipose tissue is lipectomy (suction-assisted lipectomy). This procedure is equally effective for both primary and secondary disease. It was popularized by Brorson who performed the first lipectomy in severe lymphedema in 1987.[1,4,5] The excess volume of the extremity can be reduced by 70% to 100% or more.[1,4,5,6,7,8,9,10] Compared to staged skin/subcutaneous excision, lipectomy can be often performed on an outpatient basis and in one stage and is associated with fewer surgery-induced complications (e.g., dehiscence of surgical wound, skin necrosis, iatrogenic injury to deeper structures, bleeding). The procedure has been shown to increase blood flow to the extremity,[11] does not injure the lymphatics,[13] and reduces the incidence of erysipelas by 87%.[12]

Liposuction can be used for mild to severe overgrowth of the subcutaneous tissue by fat accumulation and hypertrophy and fibrosis. Patients must be symptomatic (e.g., lowered self-esteem, infections, difficulty fitting clothing, limited activities of daily living, social stigmatization) despite being compliant with compression therapies. Liposuction is not used for patients with penile or scrotal lymphedema; these patients are treated with resection of the excess skin and subcutaneous tissue since excess volume consists of accumulated lymph and fibrosis only and not fat (see **Chapter 14**).

13.2 Preoperative Evaluation and Planning

Approximately 95% of patients with lymphedema are successfully managed using conservative treatments (e.g., compression garments, pneumatic pump, complete decongestive therapy).[16] When nonoperative therapies have failed and there is significant morbidity, then the patients are candidates for operative intervention. Potential surgical candidates undergo lymphoscintigraphy to definitively determine whether they have lymphedema (25% of referrals to a lymphedema program have another disease).[16,17] A color Doppler investigation is recommended to rule out any perforating veins or deep venous insufficiency. Patients undergo MRI to assess the amount of subcutaneous adipose tissue. If minimal fat is observed and the extremity is primarily enlarged because of free fluids, the patient is counseled to further maximize his/her compression regimen (see **Chapter 6**). It is relevant for the indication for suction-assisted lipectomy to clinically estimate the amount of fluid with the *pitting test*. "Pitting" refers to the depression formed after pressure is applied to the edematous tissue. A thumb is pressed as hard as possible on the affected extremity for at least 1 minute; sometimes 3 to 4 minutes are needed if the extremity is very congested. The amount of depression is estimated in millimeters (see **Chapter 4** and **Fig. 4.1**).

Edema that is mainly characterized by hypertrophied adipose tissue and/or fibrosis shows little or no pitting. In the authors' experience, it usually takes at least 5 years following the onset of edema for significant subcutaneous adipose to develop, but the deposition of fat starts within the first year after lymphedema begins.[2]

Prior to the surgery, patients are educated that:

- the procedure is not a cure for lymphedema;
- patients must continue compression postoperatively to reduce the risk of recurrence of adipose tissue; and
- patients who are not compliant with compression preoperatively are not candidates for surgery.

Even subjects with severe overgrowth will have adequate skin retraction postoperatively and usually do not require resection of excess skin. Patients with bilateral arm or lymphedema of the leg undergo treatment of one extremity followed by a procedure on the contralateral extremity 6 to 12 weeks later.

Note:

Performing surgery on both extremities simultaneously significantly affects the course of postoperative recovery. In the event of simultaneous surgery of the lower extremities, ambulation will be significantly hindered, increasing the risk of postoperative deep vein thrombosis.

13.3 Surgical Technique

Suction-assisted lipectomy can be performed using a tourniquet or with tumescent solution, or a combination of both. If tumescence is used, 35 mg/kg of lidocaine is not to be exceeded. If a tourniquet is applied, tumescent solution is injected only where the tourniquet has been applied, and this area is aspirated after completing the rest of the limb.[15] In the relaxed-skin tension lines of the extremity, 10 to 15 incisions measuring 4 to 7 mm are made. The direction of the lipectomy is strictly longitudinal due to the course of the lymphatics. For the upper extremity, 3- or 4-mm cannulas are used and 3- to 5-mm cannulas for the lower extremity. Power-assisted lipectomy can preferably be used for both the upper and lower extremity because it is faster than conventional suction-assisted lipectomy. As much subcutaneous adipose tissue as possible is removed, and the limb undergoes circumferential suctioning from the wrist/ankle to the shoulder/hip.

Note:

Neither hands nor feet need to be treated, because these anatomical areas do not develop significant deposition of adipose tissue.

If only tumescent solution is used, the procedure is stopped once the aspirate becomes significantly bloody and/or when the aspirate volume equals the amount that was infused ("superwet technique"). The incisions are either left open to drain or closed loosely with one suture each. A soft ace-wrap dressing is applied or a custom-made flat-knitted compression garment (compression class 3), which has been previously ordered based on the measurements of the healthy leg/arm. Patients undergoing leg lipectomy are admitted for at least 1 night to ensure they are ambulating and have adequate pain control before discharge. Patients having arm lipectomy can be discharged on the same day as the procedure. Alternatively, compression garments are ordered 2 weeks before surgery based on the measurements of the healthy extremity and put on at the time of surgery. When the arm distal to the tourniquet has been treated, a sterilized made-to-measure compression sleeve is applied (compression class 2) to the arm to stem bleeding and reduce postoperative edema. A sterilized, standard interim glove, in which the tips of the fingers have been cut to facilitate gripping, is put on the hand. The tourniquet is removed, and the most proximal part of the upper arm is treated using the tumescent technique. This involves infiltration of 1 liter of tumescence solution.

Finally, the proximal part of the compression sleeve is pulled up to compress the proximal part of the upper arm. The incisions are left open to drain through the sleeve. The arm is lightly wrapped with a large absorbent compress covering the whole arm (e.g., 60 × 60 cm). The arm is kept at the level of the heart on a large pillow. The compress is changed when needed. On the following day, a standard gauntlet (i.e., a glove without fingers, but with a thumb, compression class 2) is put over the interim glove after the thumb of the gauntlet has been cut off to ease the pressure on the thumb. If the gauntlet is put on straight after surgery, it can exert too much pressure on the hand when the patient is still not able to move the fingers after the anesthesia.

13.4 Intraoperative Position

Patients being treated for both upper and lower extremity lymphedema are placed in supine position. The entire extremity is prepped and draped. Antithrombotic prophylaxis is typically given to reduce the risk of deep venous thrombosis, especially in patients with obesity. Pneumatic compression can be used after surgery to facilitate removal of postoperative edema. Perioperative antibiotics are given. An assistant is needed to help position the limb intraoperatively to allow circumferential lipectomy.

13.5 Postoperative Management

Patients are mobilized immediately after the procedure to reduce the risk of thromboembolism. The operative dressing is removed in a few days postoperatively, and the patient may shower. The patient continues ace bandaging for 4 to 6 weeks postoperatively while the edema resolves and skin retraction occurs. Once the patients achieve their new steady-state volume, they are re-fitted for new, smaller compression garments. Full activity is encouraged as the patient's recovery allows. The patient undergoes repeated volume measurements and photography to assess the improvement 3 months postoperatively.[18]

Alternatively, garments are removed 2 days postoperatively so that the patient can take a shower. Then, the other set of garments is put on and the used set is washed and dried. The patient repeats this process after another 2 days before discharge. The standard glove and gauntlet are usually changed to the made-to-measure glove at the end of the hospital stay.

The patient alternates between the two sets of garments (one set = one sleeve and one glove) during the 2 weeks postoperatively, changing them daily or every other day so that a clean set is always put on after showering and lubricating the arm. After the 2-week control, the garments are changed every day after being washed. Washing "activates" the garment by increasing the compression due to shrinkage.

Rare major complications from suction-assisted lipectomy include deep venous thrombosis, pulmonary embolism, fat embolism, and lidocaine toxicity. Minor complications include infection, bleeding requiring transfusion, and localized area of skin loss. Patients are informed that there may be contour abnormalities and decreased sensation that improve in time.

Patients undergoing suction-assisted lipectomy for severe lower extremity lymphedema have a higher likelihood of skin loss or bleeding when only tumescent lipectomy is used. For these patients a tourniquet is recommended which minimizes blood loss.[15]

A prerequisite to maintaining the effect of suction-assisted lipectomy is the lifelong continuous use of compression garment.[1,4] Compression therapy is crucial, and its application is therefore thoroughly described and discussed with the patient at the first clinical evaluation.

> **Note:**
>
> If the patient expresses any doubt about continued compression therapy following surgery, they should not be considered a candidate for suction-assisted lipectomy.

During the visit in the third month, the arm is measured for new custom-made garments (two sets). This procedure is repeated at 6, 9, and 12 months. If complete reduction has been achieved at 6 months, the 9-month control may be omitted. When the excess volume has decreased as much as possible and a steady state is achieved, new garments can be prescribed using the latest measurements. In this way, the garments are renewed three or four times during the first year. Two sets of sleeve-and-glove garments are always at the patient's disposal, one being worn while the other is washed. Thus, a garment is worn permanently, and treatment is interrupted only briefly when showering and, possibly, for formal social occasions. The life span for two custom-made compression garments worn alternately is usually 4 to 6 months. Furthermore, the patient is informed about the importance of hygiene and skin care, as all patients with lymphedema are susceptible to infections, and keeping the skin clean and soft is a prophylactic measure.[1,4]

After the first year, the patient is seen again after 6 months (1.5 years after surgery) and then at 2 years after surgery. Then the patient is seen once a year only, when new garments are prescribed for the coming year, usually four garments and four gloves (or four gauntlets). For very active patients, six to eight garments and the same amount of gauntlets/gloves a year are needed. Patients without preoperative swelling of the hand can usually stop using the glove/gauntlet after 6 to 12 months postoperatively.

For legs, up to two, sometimes three, compression garments, on top of each other, are used depending on what is needed to prevent pitting. A typical example is a panty with a leg-long garment of compression class 2. After complete reduction has been achieved, usually by around 12 months, the patient is seen once a year when all new garments are prescribed for the coming year. After complete reduction, the panty with a leg-long garment can be changed to one without a panty. During night, only one leg-long garment is used.

13.6 Patient Education

Patients are advised that suction-assisted lipectomy does not cure their lymphedema and that they must continue their preoperative compression regimen postoperatively. Patients do not exhibit significant recurrence of subcutaneous adipose tissue after the procedure, which might be explained by improved lymphatic function because of the operation.[14] We also advise patients that although the hand and foot are not operated on, they may experience reduced swelling in these after the procedure.[14] Patients are advised to exercise the extremity and maintain a normal body mass index (BMI) to prevent worsening of their disease. Patients with a lymphedema of the leg who have a high BMI, when the excess volume in kilogram has been deducted from the weight, are encouraged to lose weight before the operation since it is difficult to get optimal compression when the diameter of the leg is large according to Laplace's law.

13.7 Clinical Cases

13.7.1 Lymphedema of the Lower Extremity

An adult female with adolescent-onset primary lymphedema was unhappy with the appearance of her extremity and was having difficulty in fitting clothing despite being compliant with her compression regimen (▶ Fig. 13.1). Prior to her procedure, she underwent lymphoscintigraphy to confirm her disease and MRI to ensure she had enough subcutaneous adipose tissue to benefit from suction-assisted lipectomy. Intraoperatively, 15 to 20 incisions measuring 1 cm were made along the limb in relaxed skin-tension lines and joint creases. Tumescent solution (1-liter saline + 50-cc 1% lidocaine + 1-cc epinephrine [1:000]) was infused circumferentially throughout the extremity not exceeding 35 mg/kg of lidocaine. Standard lipectomy was used for the upper extremity (3- to 4-mm cannulas) while power-assisted lipectomy was employed for the lower limb (4- to 5-mm cannulas). The aspirate typically equals the volume of the tumescent solution that is infused. The incisions were closed loosely with one suture to allow drainage, and the limb was dressed with gauze and an ace wrap. Large lower extremity operations often require a short inpatient hospital stay; patients ambulate immediately following the procedure. The saturated operative dressings were changed in the office 2 to 3 days postoperatively. The patient then showered each day and wrapped the extremity with ace wraps. Pneumatic compression was resumed approximately 2 weeks following the procedure. In 6 to 12 weeks postoperatively, when the limb had obtained a new steady-state volume and the skin had contracted, the patient was measured for smaller custom-fitted garments and discontinued the ace wraps.

13.7.2 Lymphedema of the Lower Extremity Preceded by Conservative Treatment

The patient is a 27-year-old man who underwent surgery as a newborn because of congenital left-sided chylothorax (▶ Fig. 13.2). At the age of 12, he had an incipient swelling in the left leg and 2 years later, in the right leg. He received conservative treatment with elastic bandages that had some effect. When he was 22 years old, he had surgery because of seminoma of the left testicle followed by radiation therapy. Then there was a rapid progression of the edema in the left leg. At the age of 26, he was referred to the plastic surgery clinic. He showed pronounced edema, elephantiasis, with severe pitting edema of several centimeters. The excess volume measured by plethysmography was 14,310 ml. Since the edema was dominated by lymph, conservative treatment was started using compression garments that were decreased in size regularly by taking in the garments using a sewing machine as well as ordering of new compression garments. The edema decreased from 10,120 to 4,190 ml (71% reduction) after a year. Persistent swelling consisted of clinical adipose tissue and fibrosis. For the first time in many years the patient could buy a pair of normal pants. After 2 years of conservative treatment, suction-assisted lipectomy was performed to decrease adipose tissue and complete reduction was achieved. He now works full time as a fitter.

13.7.3 Lymphedema of the Upper Extremity

Typical outcome after lipectomy of lymphedema of the arm is shown in ▶ Fig. 13.3. The patient is a 74-year-old

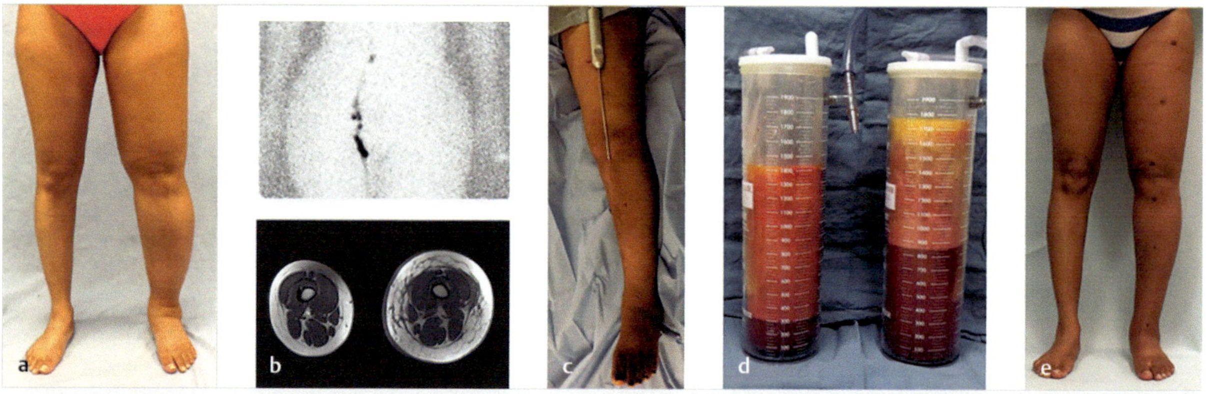

Fig. 13.1 Operative treatment of lymphedema of the leg using lipectomy. **(a)** Preoperative appearance. **(b)** Lymphoscintigram shows absence of radiolabeled tracer in the left inguinal lymph nodes confirming the diagnosis of lymphedema. Magnetic resonance imaging demonstrates an increase in subcutaneous adipose tissue. **(c)** Intraoperative view. **(d)** Lipoaspirate. **(e)** Appearance at 6 weeks postoperatively. (Reproduced with permission from Greene AK. Operative Management of Vascular Anomalies. Thieme; 2017.)

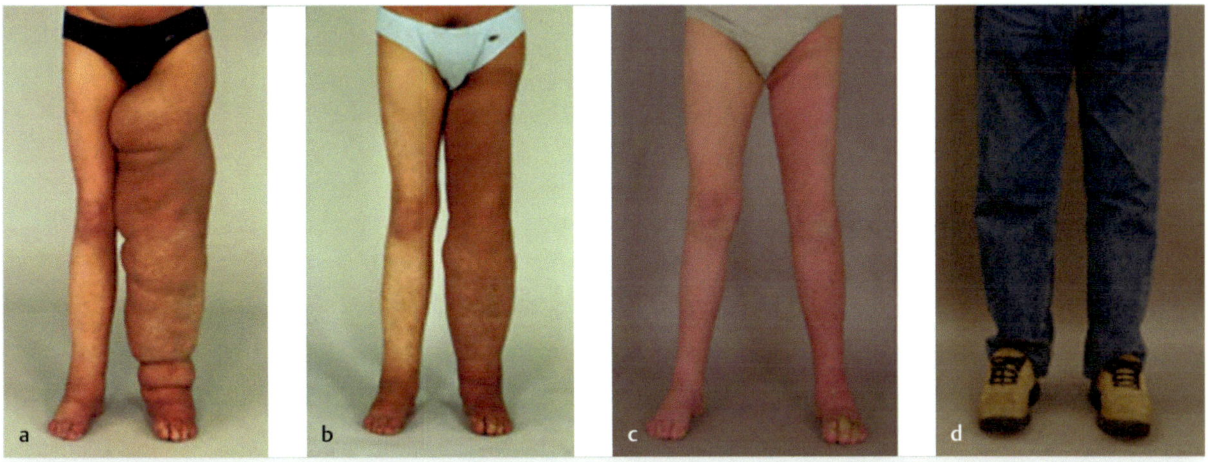

Fig. 13.2 **(a)** Before treatment with controlled compression therapy, significant excess volume of approx. 14,000 ml. **(b)** After 2 years of complete decongestive therapy and before lipectomy, a 75% reduction of the excess volume was achieved. **(c)** Complete reduction was achieved 4 years after surgery: Excess volume was -865 ml, i.e., the treated leg was somewhat smaller than the contralateral (106%). **(d)** He can now wear jeans, which was impossible before treatment. (Reproduced with permission from Brorson, H. et al., Controlled Compression and Liposuction Treatment for Lower Extremity Lymphedema. Lymphology 41(2); 2008, pp. 52–63.)

woman with a nonpitting lymphedema of the arm for 15 years following breast cancer treatment including radiotherapy. The edema started 5 years after surgery. She received conservative treatment for 15 years, including combined decongestive treatment and pneumatic compression, without any effect due to adipose tissue deposition. Measurements were taken 2 weeks before surgery for compression garments based on the healthy arm. Preoperative excess volume was 3,090 ml. After 1 year of suction-assisted lipectomy complete reduction was achieved with a remaining excess volume of –110 ml, that is, the treated arm became somewhat smaller than that of the nonaffected arm.

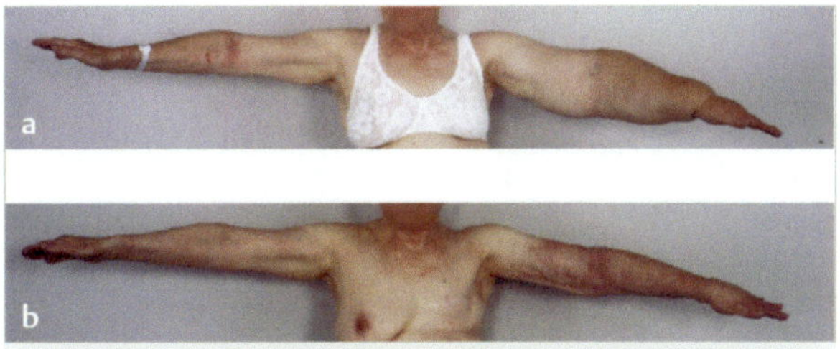

Fig. 13.3 **(a)** A 74-year-old woman with a nonpitting lymphedema of the arm for 15 years. Preoperative excess volume was 3,090 ml. **(b)** Postoperative result after 1 year. The treated arm is smaller than the healthy one: –110 ml.

13.8 Pearls and Pitfalls

Prior to performing suction-assisted lipectomy, it is critical to ensure the patient will benefit from the procedure by documenting increased subcutaneous adipose tissue with the clinically negative pitting test and proven by MRI. As much fat as possible is removed during the operation because repeat resection is more difficult after additional interstitial scar tissue has been developed. Patients with long-standing, severe disease remain candidates for suction-assisted lipectomy, although more effort may be required to remove the tissue because of increased fibrosis in the lower extremity. Patients must be educated that lipectomy does not cure their disease, and that they must remain compliant with postoperative compression to limit recurrent adipose deposition.

References

[1] Brorson H, Svensson H. Liposuction combined with controlled compression therapy reduces arm lymphedema more effectively than controlled compression therapy alone. Plast Reconstr Surg. 1998; 102(4):1058–1067, discussion 1068

[2] Brorson H, Ohlin K, Olsson G, Nilsson M. Adipose tissue dominates chronic arm lymphedema following breast cancer: an analysis using volume rendered CT images. Lymphat Res Biol. 2006; 4(4):199–210

[3] Brorson H, Ohlin K, Olsson G, Karlsson MK. Breast cancer-related chronic arm lymphedema is associated with excess adipose and muscle tissue. Lymphat Res Biol. 2009; 7(1):3–10

[4] Brorson H, Svensson H. Complete reduction of lymphoedema of the arm by liposuction after breast cancer. Scand J Plast Reconstr Surg Hand Surg. 1997; 31(2):137–143

[5] Brorson H. Liposuction in lymphedema treatment. J Reconstr Microsurg. 2016; 32(1):56–65

[6] Greene AK, Slavin SA, Borud L. Treatment of lower extremity lymphedema with suction-assisted lipectomy. Plast Reconstr Surg. 2006; 118(5):118e–121e

[7] Brorson H, Ohlin K, Olsson G, Svensson B, Svensson H. Controlled compression and liposuction treatment for lower extremity lymphedema. Lymphology. 2008; 41(2):52–63

[8] Greene AK, Maclellan RA. Operative treatment of lymphedema using suction-assisted lipectomy. Ann Plast Surg. 2016; 77(3):337–340

[9] Lamprou DA, Voesten HG, Damstra RJ, Wikkeling OR. Circumferential suction-assisted lipectomy in the treatment of primary and secondary end-stage lymphoedema of the leg. Br J Surg. 2017; 104(1):84–89

[10] Stewart CJ, Munnoch DA. Liposuction as an effective treatment for lower extremity lymphoedema: a single surgeon's experience over nine years. J Plast Reconstr Aesthet Surg. 2018; 71(2):239–245

[11] Brorson H, Svensson H. Skin blood flow of the lymphedematous arm before and after liposuction. Lymphology. 1997; 30(4):165–172

[12] Lee D, Piller N, Hoffner M, Manjer J, Brorson H. Liposuction of postmastectomy arm lymphedema decreases the incidence of erysipelas. Lymphology. 2016; 49(2):85–92

[13] Brorson H, Svensson H, Norrgren K, Thorsson O. Liposuction reduces arm lymphedema without significantly altering the already impaired lymph transport. Lymphology. 1998; 31(4):156–172

[14] Greene AK, Voss SD, Maclellan RA. Liposuction for swelling in patients with lymphedema. N Engl J Med. 2017; 377(18):1788–1789

[15] Wojnikow S, Malm J, Brorson H. Use of a tourniquet with and without adrenaline reduces blood loss during liposuction for lymphoedema of the arm. Scand J Plast Reconstr Surg Hand Surg. 2007; 41(5):243–249

[16] Maclellan RA, Couto RA, Sullivan JE, Grant FD, Slavin SA, Greene AK. Management of primary and Secondary lymphedema: analysis of 225 referrals to a center. Ann Plast Surg. 2015; 75(2):197–200

[17] Schook CC, Mulliken JB, Fishman SJ, Alomari AI, Grant FD, Greene AK. Differential diagnosis of lower extremity enlargement in pediatric patients referred with a diagnosis of lymphedema. Plast Reconstr Surg. 2011; 127(4):1571–1581

[18] Brorson H, Höijer P. Standardised measurements used to order compression garments can also be used to calculate the arm volume in order to evaluate lymphoedema treatment. J Plast Surg Hand Surg. 2012; 46(6):410–415

14 Excisional Procedures

Vincenzo Penna and Nestor Torio

Summary

Modern surgical management of chronic lymphedema requires local excisional and lymphoablative surgery in selected cases of mid to end stage lymphedema (stages II–III). While highly invasive and often mutilating surgery, such as Charles' or Homans' procedures, is rarely indicated today, especially for genital lymphedema (stage II) or local fibrotic, dermal bulging can be functionally and effectively treated with local dermolipectomies followed by lifelong conservative therapy and compression. While lymphedema with a high degree of adipogenesis can be approached by suction-assisted lipectomy alone, lipectomy can be used in conjunction with local dermolipectomies for lymphoablative surgery to improve weight loss and wound healing. Experience is required for preoperative planning and marking with repetitive pinch tests. Patient education must include the noncausal character of the procedure, successfully addressing form, function, weight, quality of life, local infection control, and aesthetics.

Keywords: Charles' procedure, debulking, dermolipectomy, genital lymphedema, Homans procedure, lymphoablative surgery, lymphedema-related papilloma, scrotal lymphedema, suction-assisted lipectomy, Thompson procedure

14.1 Lymphoreductive Surgery

Light and moderate stages (stages I and II) of lymphedema can be successfully treated conservatively by complete decongestive physical therapy (CDT) (see **Chapter 6**) and/or lymphovenous anastomosis (LVA) (see **Chapter 8**) or vascularized lymph node transfer (VLNT) (see **Chapter 10**) in the event of refractory to conservative therapy. In severe cases (stage III) the conservative treatment is limited with regard to its efficacy, and often reconstructive or diverging procedures such as LVA and VLNT may not be indicated, so these patients require more invasive treatment options. These excisional procedures that have been described in the early 20th century aim at reducing excess skin and subcutaneous tissues that often present with morphological changes such a fibrosis and scaring.

Charles described excision of the affected tissue (skin, subcutaneous tissue) with consecutive split-thickness skin grafting[1] (▸ Fig. 14.1). Homans described a modification of the Charles' procedure that preserved the overlying skin[2] (▸ Fig. 14.2). Skin flaps were elevated, followed by excision of the subcutaneous tissue, followed by closure of the wound with trimming of the skin flap surplus. If needed, this procedure can be staged to avoid skin necrosis. The Homans' procedure is mainly used for the calf. Thompson modified these techniques for the upper extremity by using de-epithelialized dermal flaps as dermal bridges for lymphatic fluid transport enhancement[3] (▸ Fig. 14.3). To establish a connection between the superficial and deep lymphatic systems the de-epithelialized dermal flaps were fixed to the deep fascia around the muscle or even buried into the muscle after fascial incisions prior to wound closure.

The above-described lymphoablative techniques are associated with a high rate of complications, such as wound dehiscence, skin necrosis, nonhealing and chronic wounds, infection, lymphorrhea, worsening of lymphedema distal to the excision, etc.[4] Thus, these originally published techniques and there modifications should be considered historic and outdated and indicated only in very specific cases that present a very advanced stage of the disease and/or where "sophisticated" surgery such as LVA or VLNT is not available.

Modern approaches to lymphoablative surgery include *local dermolipectomies* and lipectomy instead of the above-mentioned techniques. It is paramount for these techniques to work that patients are adequately treated for their lymphedema. CDT is a crucial step for tissue preparation prior to surgery, as edematous tissue lacks a respectable surplus and due to high tissue tension, it is prone to postoperative wound healing problems. In addition, chronic edema causes fibrotic tissue reactions, which makes lipectomy hard, if not impossible.

Local dermolipectomies are indicated based on functional limitations and prognosis, and mostly performed at the upper arm, thigh region, genital region, and abdomen, while lipectomy are reserved for the upper and lower extremities.[5,6,7]

Patients with stage III lymphedema always present with enlargement of the affected area—sometimes even with elephantiasic changes such as Papillomatosis Cutis Lymphostatica (see ▸ Fig. 14.8 and ▸ Fig. 14.9). Presentation of stage III patients is not uniform but can involve fatty degeneration (treatable with lipectomy on) or massive edema (adequate CDT results in skin surplus that can then be approached by an lymphoablative procedure).

14.2 Indications and Contraindications

Dermolipectomies is mainly reserved for stage III lymphedema patients presenting with tissue surplus resulting after adequate decongestion of the tissue through CDT. Often the skin surplus leads to hygienic problems and reduced mobility. Dermolipectomies should not be performed in patients

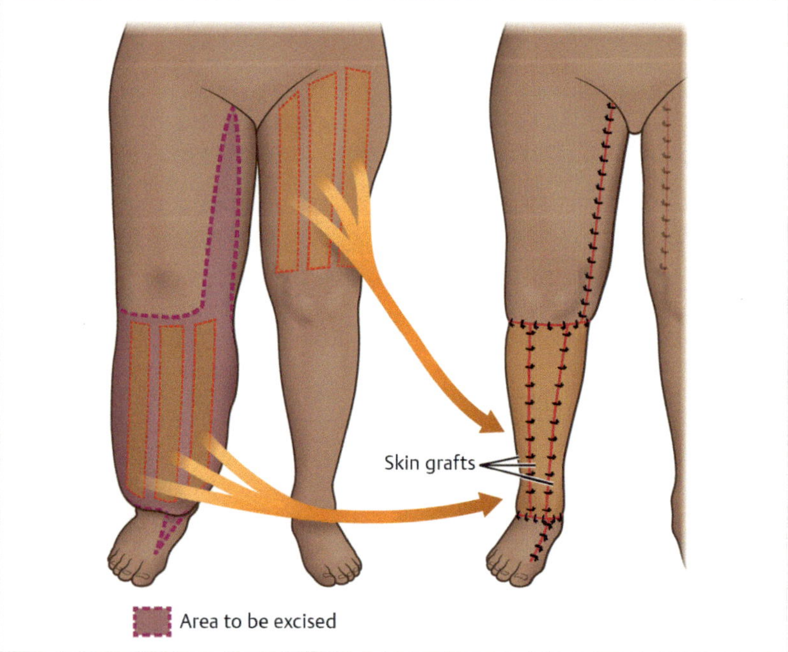

Fig. 14.1 Charles' procedure: Skin, subcutaneous tissue, and deep fascia are excised circumferentially in the affected area and then covered with skin graft.

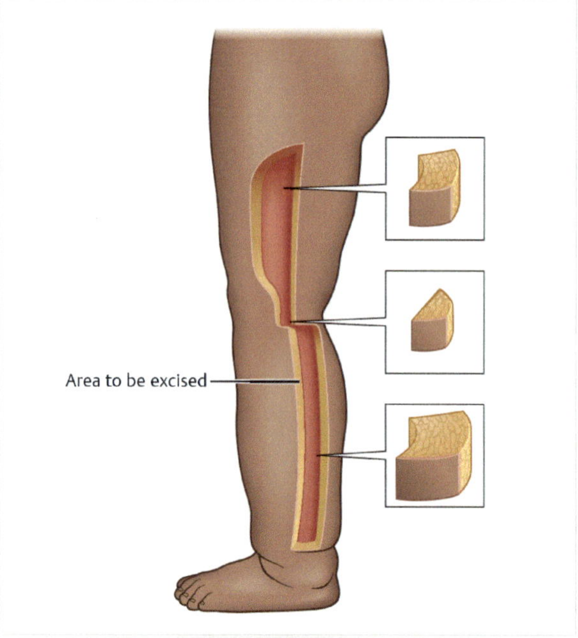

Fig. 14.2 Homans' procedure: Skin flaps in the affected area are elevated; subsequently, the subcutaneous tissue in the same region is excised, and the skin flap trimmed and closed.

with pitting edema and without sufficient skin surplus following intensive CDT. If a postoperative CDT treatment cannot be guaranteed, the decision for dermolipectomy procedures should be thoroughly reconsidered. In patient with genital lymphedema, lymphoablative operations can be recommendable even in early stages (e.g., stage II), as these patients often present with recurrent erysipelas, lymphatic cysts, and chronic lymphorrhea.

Indications and Contraindications

Indications:

- Mainly stage III lymphedema (stage II in genital lymphedema)
- Tissue surplus after adequate decongestion of the tissue through CDT
- Hygienic and mobility impairment due to tissue surplus
- Recurrent erysipelas, lymphatic cysts, and chronic lymphorrhea with genital lymphedema

Contraindications:

- Pitting edema patient
- Absence of skin surplus
- Impossibility to perform conservative treatment postoperatively (lifelong need of CDT)

14.3 Preoperative Evaluation and Planning

Patient management is always an integrated surgical and conservative lymphological strategy. Prior to surgery—which is a general recommendation in all patients undergoing surgery for lymphedema—patients undergo intensive CDT at a specialized lymphological clinic for 3 weeks. This therapy involves manual lymph drainage

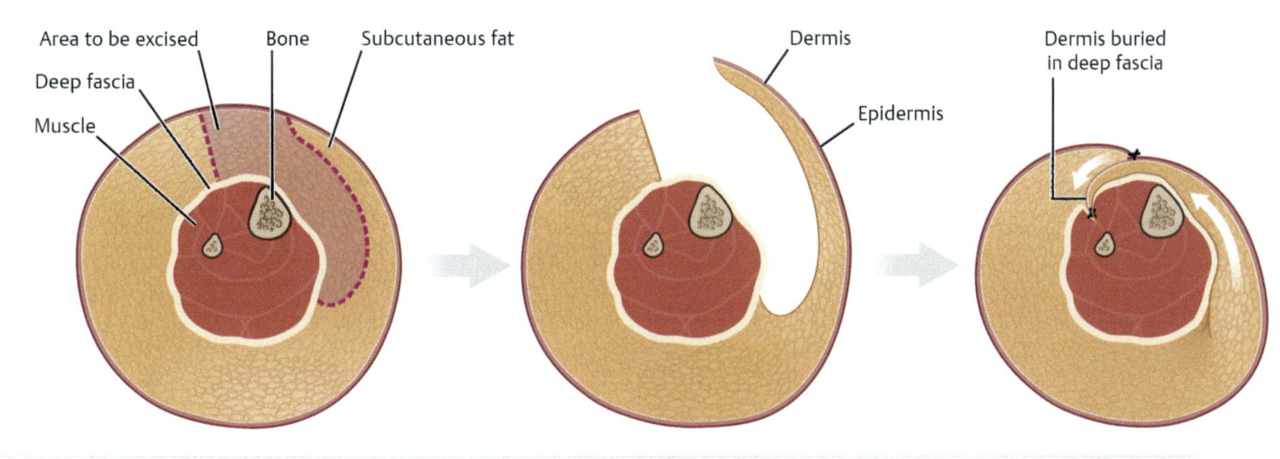

Fig. 14.3 Thompson procedure: After excision of the affected subcutaneous tissue, a de-epithelialized skin flap is formed, buried, and sutured to the deep fascia in order to establish a connection between the superficial and deep lymphatic system.

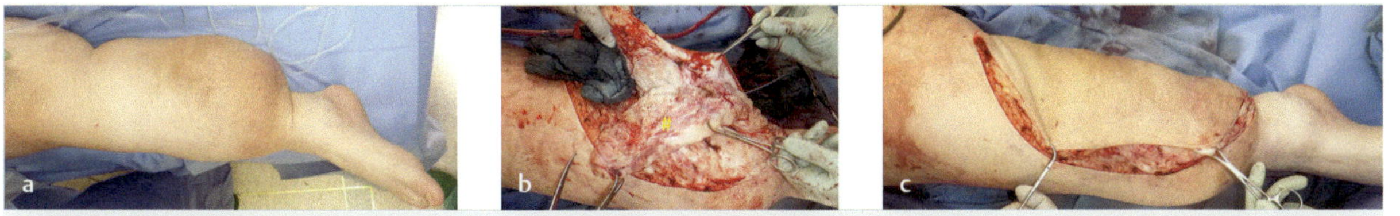

Fig. 14.4 57-year-old male patient with stage III lymphedema to the right distal lower extremity (calf) secondary to a bilateral lipedema associated with hypotesteronemia. Initial suction-assisted lipectomy yielded moderate success. Due to anticipated high degree of fibrosis and functional impairment, the patient was scheduled for a local debulking procedure by excision with dermolipectomy and deep tissue thinning. The excision to the calf **(a)** was performed with multiple pinch tests and incision with repetitive adjustments with resection of the fibrotic tissue **(b)** and final excision **(c)**. (Courtesy of Christoph Hirche.)

twice daily, compression bandaging, physical exercises, and skin care. This results in reduction of tissue volume, softening of the skin, and partial recovery of skin elasticity, thus facilitating and improving surgery (▶ Fig. 14.5). Patients who suffer from concomitant conditions (diabetes mellitus, hypoproteinemia, cardiac and respiratory diseases, etc.) are treated by the medical team and are prepared for anesthesia and surgery.

14.4 Surgical Technique

14.4.1 General Remarks

There is no standard planning of skin resection and markings in lymphedema patients. Thus, a good preoperative evaluation of the skin surplus by pinch test is paramount and intraoperatively the amount of resection must be carefully performed in order to avoid the risk of wound complications. Patients who undergo dermolipectomies without pre- and postoperative CDT have a higher risk for complications.[6] Pre- and postoperative CDT in a specialized lymphedema rehabilitation center is recommended for a period of around 3 weeks in cases of lymphoablative lymphedema surgery.

Following disinfection and sterile covering, a third-generation cephalosporin is administered intravenously. Then, the tissue is infiltrated with a diluted solution containing a local anesthetic (e.g., prilocaine) and epinephrine, for example, 50 ml of prilocaine with 1,200,000 epinephrine in 1,000 ml of saline. Skin incision is done with scalpel; further preparation is undertaken with electrocautery. It is often required to ligate dilated vessels; meticulous coagulation is mandatory.

14.4.2 Dermolipectomies in Extremities

In extremities, excision is performed starting ventrally, and then preparing the dorsal aspect of the tissue surplus. The dissection plane is down to the deep fascia. The amount of skin resection is determined by pulling the tissue surplus ventrally and pushing towel clamps, which are fixed at the dermis of the anterior wound site, dorsally and transcutaneously. This step prevents over- and under-excision (▶ Fig. 14.4a–c and 14.6 a–c).

Multiple Charrière (Ch) 18 drains are inserted, and the wound is closed with Donati single stitches (2–0 nylon). An elastic compression is applied.

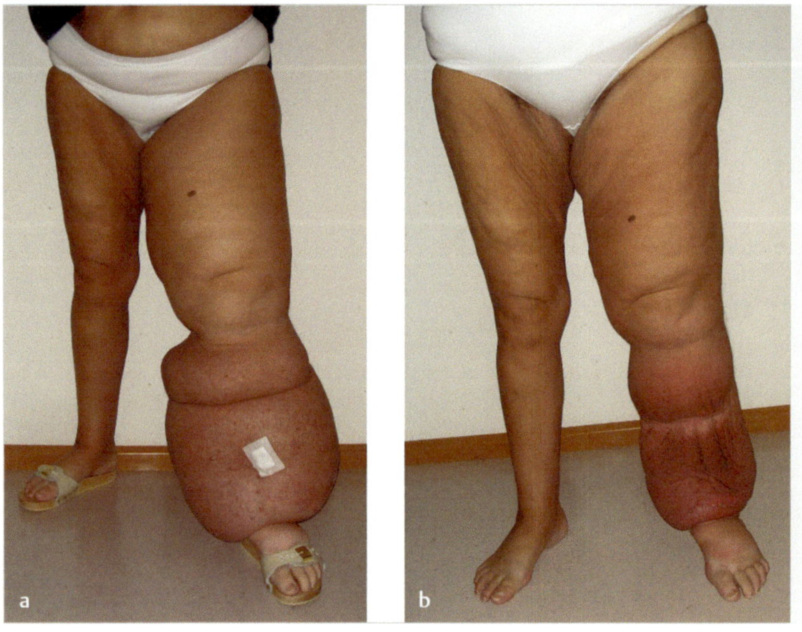

Fig. 14.5 Patient with a severe stage III primary lymphedema on the left lower extremity. **(a)** Result after 4 weeks of intensive complete decompression therapy. **(b)** Tissue surplus on the lower leg, which must be surgically resected in order to avoid further accumulation of lymphatic fluid. (Courtesy of the Földi Klinik.)

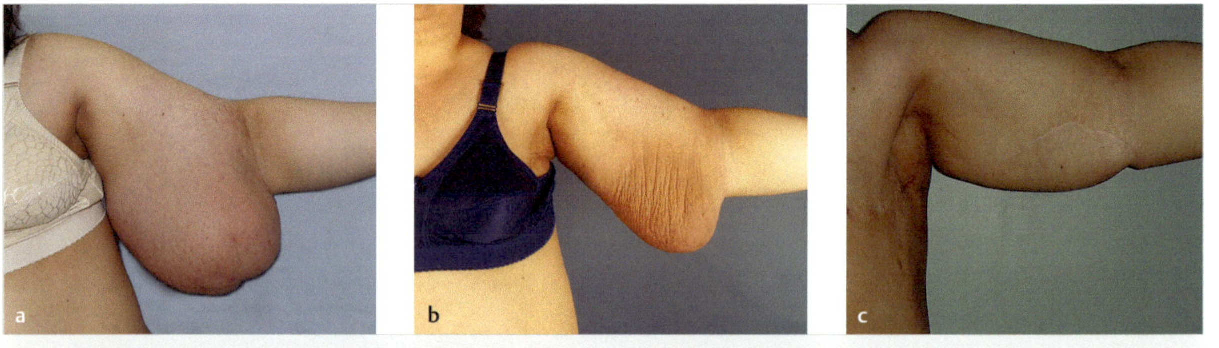

Fig. 14.6 36-year-old patient with stage III secondary lymphedema after mastectomy and lymphadenectomy to the upper extremity. Volume before complete decompression therapy was 7,100 ml **(a)**, after complete decompression therapy **(b)**, and extremity 1 year postoperatively **(c)** after dermolipectomy on the upper arm. Weight of excised tissue: 1.5 kg. (Courtesy of Christoph Hirche.)

14.4.3 Scrotal Dermolipectomies

In cases of less pronounced scrotal lymphedema, a median incision of the scrotum and, if necessary, the penis, is performed, allowing sufficient exposure of the scrotal contents during debulking. The incision lines are marked laterally at the border of elephantiastic and normal skin, taking care to preserve enough skin for closure. The lateral incision lines meet dorsally at the perineum. If excess skin is present at the mons pubis, a fishtail-shaped excision is planned to include a transversal dermolipectomy of this region (▸ Fig. 14.7). The dissection plane is directly underneath the dartos fascia, and lymphedema-related papilloma are included in the excision pattern. It is important to quickly identify spermatic cords and the testes. These structures are dissected bluntly and preserved (▸ Fig. 14.8). If encountered, a hydrocele is released and resected. Following meticulous hemostasis, easy flow drains are inserted, and lateral flaps are joined in the midline. The wound closure is achieved using 3–0 and 4–0 nylon interrupted sutures.

In patients with the penis skin affected by multiple lymphatic cysts, this tissue cannot be preserved. A reconstruction of the skin can be performed using the preserved and unaffected foreskin as a foreskin flap (▸ Fig. 14.8).

14.4.4 Vulvar Dermolipectomies

The affected areas of the labia are marked—excision patterns and drawings are similar to reduction plasty of labia majora—and excision is performed just at the border between the affected and healthy skin. Care must be taken not to over-resect and thus risk distortion of the vulva. After thorough coagulation, drains are normally not

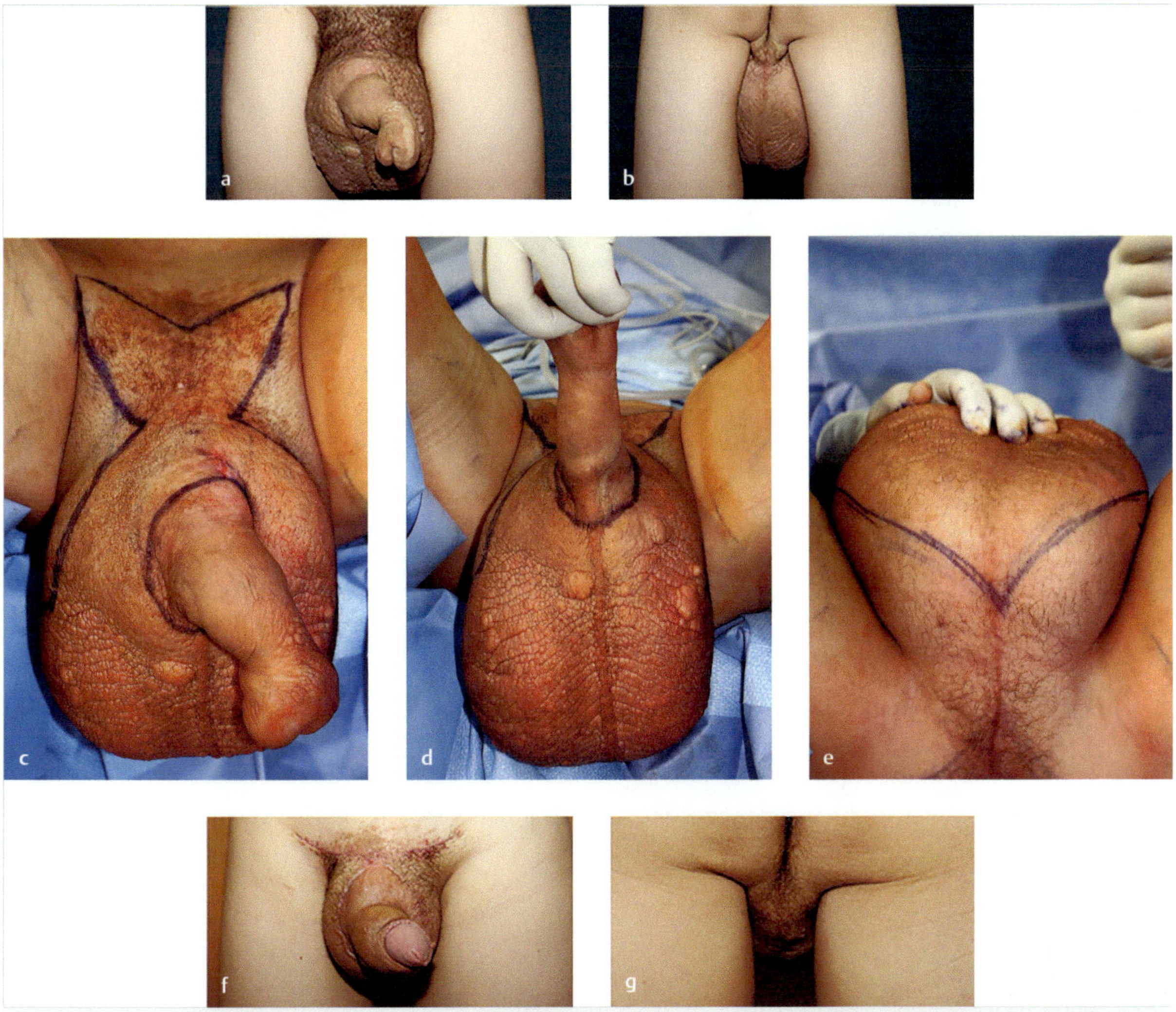

Fig. 14.7 Preoperative view of patient with stage III scrotal primary lymphedema prior to scrotal dermolipectomy **(a, b)**, intraoperative markings for reduction dermolipectomy **(c–e)**, and 5 weeks after scrotal dermolipectomy, circumcision, and resection of hydrocele testis **(f, g)**.

needed. The wound is closed with 4–0 nylon running suture (▶ Fig. 14.9).

14.5 Intraoperative Position

Upper extremities:

- Supine position with affected upper extremity on arm table

Lower extremities:

- Liposuction: Supine position
- Dermolipectomies: Supine position or lithotomy position (if possible)

Genital:

- Lithotomy position

14.6 Additional Intraoperative Tools

- Power-assisted lipectomy device
- Electrocautery
- Tourniquet

14.7 Surgical Equipment

Standard surgical instruments:

- Metzenbaum dissecting scissors
- Adson tissue forceps
- Needle holder
- Towel clamps
- Electrocautery

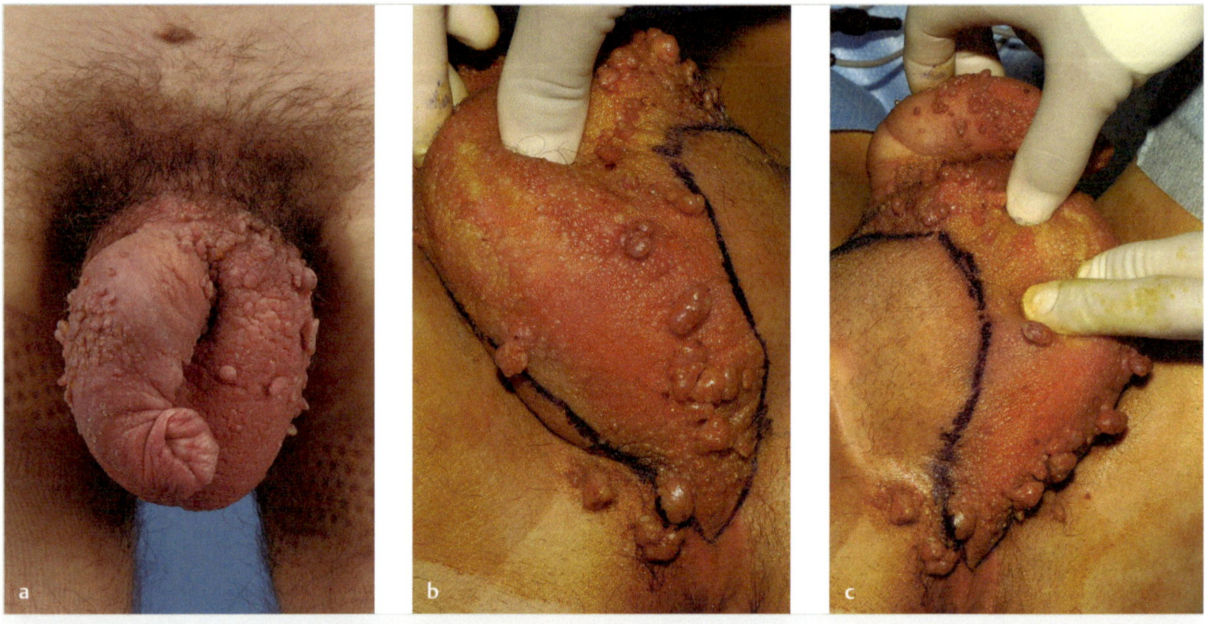

Fig. 14.8 (a) 15-year-old patient suffering from stage III primary lymphedema with multiple lymphatic cysts and recurrent erysipelas. **(b, c)** Intraoperative markings.

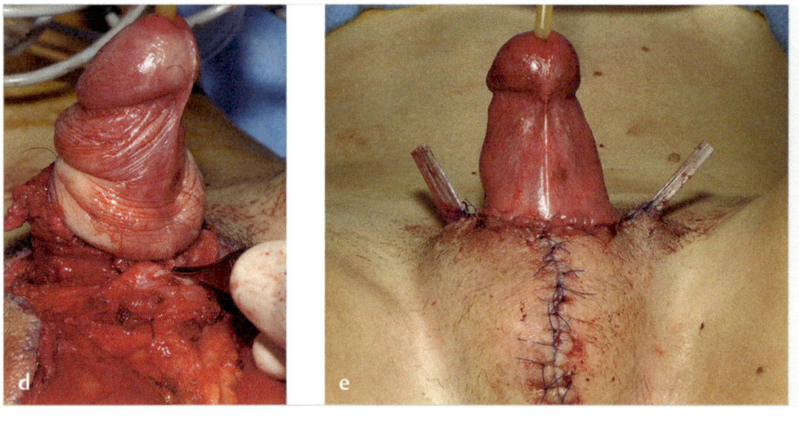

Fig. 14.8 *(Continued)* **(d, e)** After reduction dermolipectomy of the scrotum and resection of the affected skin on the penis with the lymphatic cysts; a foreskin flap was performed in order to reconstruct the penis skin.

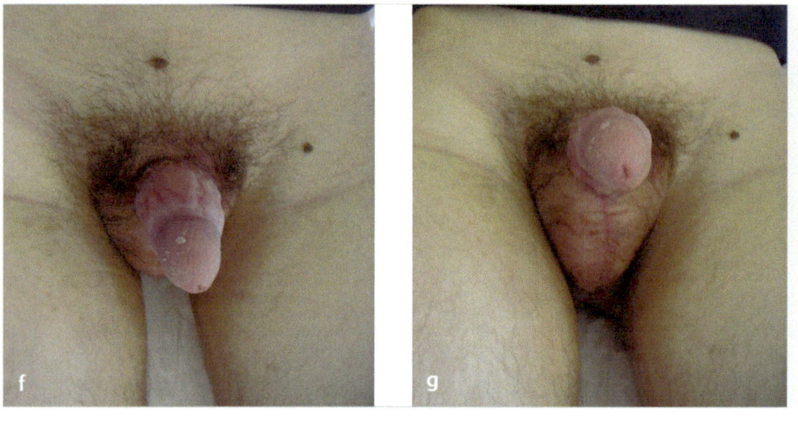

Fig. 14.8 *(Continued)* **(f, g)** Result 5 weeks after scrotal dermolipectomy and circumcision.

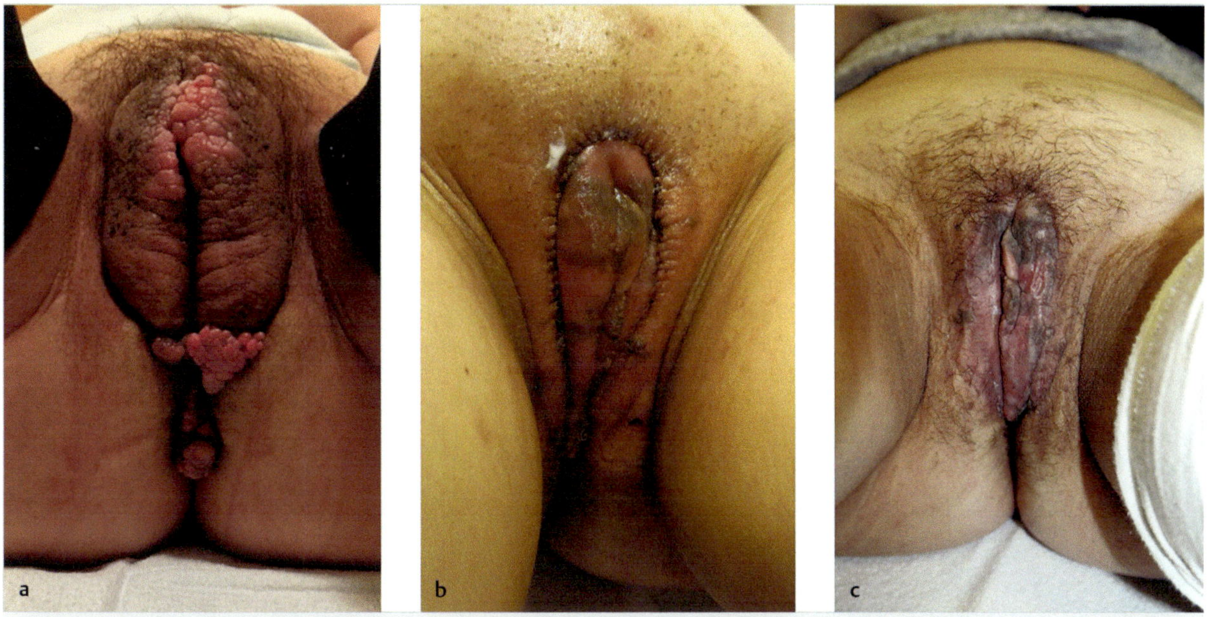

Fig. 14.9 **(a)** 29-year-old patient with a stage III vulvar primary lymphedema preoperatively. The affected tissue of the labia majora was excised bilaterally and the wounds were closed using the healthy surrounding tissue areas. A total of 1.1 kg of tissue was excised. **(b)** Result 2 weeks **(c)** and 5 weeks after surgery.

14.8 Postoperative Management

Postoperatively the patients are mobilized as soon as possible. Extremities remain bandaged and antithrombotic prophylaxis is given. The patients are hospitalized for 2 to 3 days postoperatively due to high bleeding risk and the necessity of adequate intravenous (i.v.) analgesia. Then they are ideally transferred back to the lymphological clinic, where intensive CDT is continued until the wounds are healed. Sutures are removed at 2 to 3 weeks postoperatively. Patients are discharged from the lymphological clinic after 3 weeks with made-to-measure compression garments and are followed up by the lymphologist on an outpatient basis. The compression garments must be adapted to the continuous volume loss over the following months.

14.9 Patient Education

Patients undergoing dermolipectomies due to lymphedema require regular CDT to prevent recurrence.

In general, lifelong use of compression garments is necessary in these patients.

After liposuctions, the continuous use of compression garments is mandatory. In case edema progresses, manual lymphatic decongestion can also become necessary.

In instances of recurrence, the plastic surgeon is involved again.

14.10 Pearls and Pitfalls

Thorough patient selection is a key element for successful surgery. This is even more appropriate in lymphoablative lymphological surgery. Surgical strategy in lymphoablative lymphological surgery can be broken down to the following statements:

- Patients with nonpitting edema and fatty hypertrophy qualify more for primary lipectomy, whereas patients presenting with skin surplus after adequate CDT need dermolipectomies.
- Patients with pitting edema need preoperative CDT to reduce complication rate and improve outcome for lymphoablative surgery.
- Complications after operations can be avoided by postoperatively allocating the patients to a facility providing high-quality CDT and by ensuring long-term lymphological monitoring.

References

[1] Charles RH. Elephantiasis Scroti. London: Churchill; 1912

[2] Homans J. The treatment of elephantiasis of the legs. A preliminary report. N Engl J Med. 1936; 215:1099–1104

[3] Thompson N. Buried dermal flap operation for chronic lymphedema of the extremities. Ten-year survey of results in 79 cases. Plast Reconstr Surg. 1970; 45(6):541–548

[4] Doscher ME, Herman S, Garfein ES. Surgical management of inoperable lymphedema: the re-emergence of abandoned techniques. J Am Coll Surg. 2012; 215(2):278–283

[5] Torio-Padron N, Stark GB, Földi E, Simunovic F. Treatment of male genital lymphedema: an integrated concept. J Plast Reconstr Aesthet Surg. 2015; 68(2):262–268

[6] Kiefer J, Koulaxouzidis G, Stark GB, Foeldi E, Torio-Padron N, Penna V. An integrative therapeutic concept for surgical treatment of severe cases of lymphedema of the lower extremity. Obes Surg. 2016; 26(7): 1436–1442

[7] Brorson H. Liposuction in lymphedema treatment. J Reconstr Microsurg. 2016; 32(1):56–65

15 Secondary Procedures after Reconstructive Microsurgery

Summary

In late-stage lymphedema or in nonevolutive lymphedema after reconstructive microsurgical treatment, various procedures could still be done in order to improve the quality of life of patients. Suction-assisted lipectomy is an efficient surgical method to reduce excess subcutaneous tissue in patients with chronic lymphedema of the extremities following microsurgical reconstruction of the lymphatic outflow, including vascularized lymph node transfer and lymphovenous anastomoses. It is important to respect the longitudinal arrangement of the lymphatic vessels. In the event of any limb lymphedema with ICG-positive lymphangiography, lymphovenous anastomosis is still considered as the first-line therapy. However, vascularized lymph node transfer as a second procedure could follow the lymphovenous anastomosis surgery and could follow excisional suction-assisted lipectomy to improve lymphatic drainage. In the event of chronic lymphocele formation with compromised wound healing and development of a cutaneous lymphatic fistula, revisional surgery including ICG lymphangiography and lymphovenous anastomosis, if possible, and/or microscopic lymphatic ligation will be necessary. Combined surgical procedures encompass one-stage and sequential utilization of lymphovenous anastomosis, vascularized lymph node transfer, suction-assisted lipectomy, and excisional debulking surgery in various combinations and sequences. Evidence-based assessment and treatment algorithms should be established to individualize treatment for each patient. This chapter will discuss using different options of surgical treatment of reluctant chronic lymphedema or chronic lymphocele.

Keywords: debridement, debulking, excisional surgery, indocyanine green (ICG) lymphangiography, lipolymphoaspiration, suction-assisted lipectomy (SAL) lymphosuction, lymphocele, lymphorrhea, lymphovenous anastomosis (LVA), vascularized lymph node transfer (VLNT)

15.1 Suction-Assisted Lipectomy

Amir K. Bigdeli, Andreas Frick, and Christiane G. Stäuble

Suction-assisted lipectomy is a minimally invasive surgical method to reduce excess subcutaneous tissue in patients with chronic lymphedema of the extremities (see **Chapter 13**). It can also been used following microsurgical reconstruction of the lymphatic outflow, including LVA, autologous lymph vessel transfer (ALVT), and vascularized lymph node transfer (VLNT).

In order to avoid suction-associated damage to the lymphatic vessels, it is important to respect the longitudinal arrangement of the lymphatic vessels. Frick et al. demonstrated in cadaver studies that lymphatic vessel features a certain tensile strength if the mechanical stress of negative pressure is applied parallel to the axis of the vessels when compared to suction-assisted lipectomy perpendicularly to the lymphatic vessel that resist only little forces.[1]

Additionally, dry suction has shown to result in more severe lesions when compared to suction using tumescent solution, which is currently performed. Interestingly, the addition of tumescent solution to reduce excess of fat tissue also reduce suction-associated damage to the lymphatic vessels when performed perpendicularly to the vessels rather than longitudinally nowadays.[2]

Lymphatic anatomy is important, especially the course of the collectors and possible ways, to protect them. Different interactions between lipectomy and lymphatics were evaluated in various studies. Lymphatics of lower limbs transport Patent Blue V, a lympho-trope dye of 583 Da, even post-mortally. Thereafter, lipectomy using dry technique without preceding fluid instillation was performed using a blunt 4-mm cannula. In 10 lower extremities, sequential regions were defined in which either longitudinal or transverse suction was performed.[2] Lymphatics have an axial tensile strength of up to a certain limit in contrast to low transverse tension. If suction is performed in the axes (0–10 degrees) of the extremities and the lymphatics, there was no or only a small damage to the lymphatics in the cadaver study. In addition, only moderate extravasation of Patent Blue V into the surrounding tissues was observed. In regions where suction-assisted lipectomy was performed vertical (80–90 degrees) to the direction of the lymphatics, lesions were significantly increased.[2]

In an experimental study using the dry technique, we could demonstrate that the risk of lymphatic lesions is decreased by longitudinal handling of the cannula and increased by transverse lipectomy. In a second anatomical study using the tumescent technique, the lymphatic lesions were significantly reduced, even with transverse handling of the cannula when compared to the dry technique.

For the therapeutic strategy, possibilities of microsurgical reconstructive procedures should be clarified first. In these patients an autogenous lymphatic transplantation can be performed if required. Derived procedures including autogenous lymph node transplantations or LVAs are possible microsurgical alternatives. A resting surplus of tissue in arms and especially in legs may be treated by suction-assisted lipectomy later on.

Conventional, blunt, straight cannulas and water-jet-associated vacuum pumps (body-jet, Human Med AG, Schwerin, Germany) are used, which produce a negative atmospheric pressure of 750 mmHg (1 bar). The direction of the suction cannula is mainly longitudinal to the axes of the extremities and lymphatics or at an angle of 10 degrees. Currently, transverse lipectomy is avoided as far as possible.

Brorson and coworkers performed only a resection procedure in lymphedemas by lipo-lymphoaspiration resulting in lower circumferences than the healthy contralateral extremity.[3] Long-term follow-up (7–15 years) did not show any recurrence of the edema.

Other surgical colleagues performed suction-assisted lipectomy as a staged procedure after VLNT or LVA. In the literature so far, only one series of short-term results of up to 12 months after simultaneous lipectomy and LVAs has been published by Chang et al.[4]

In a clinical series[4] involving autologous lymph vessel interposition and transposition in patients suffering from arm lymphedema, a significant volume reduction of the treated extremities was observed which could be further reduced significantly by performing secondary suction-assisted lipectomy (▸ Fig. 15.1 and ▸ Fig. 15.2).

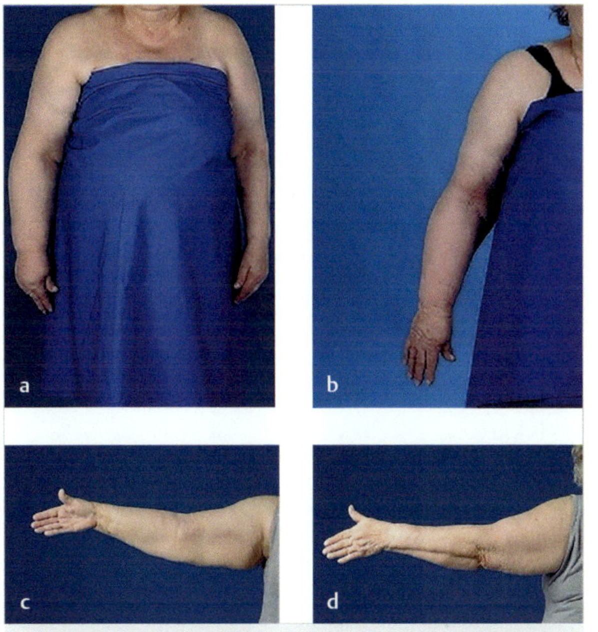

Fig. 15.1 Autologous lymph vessel transfer to treat breast cancer-related chronic lymphedema after mastectomy, axillary dissection, and adjuvant radiotherapy: **(a)** Preoperative view: Patient 12 years after treatment showing chronic lymphedema of the upper extremity. **(b)** Postoperative view 1 year after autologous lymph vessel transfer, with persistent lipedema; therefore, the patient was candidate for upper extremity lipectomy. **(c, d)** The result after lipectomy.

15.2 Secondary Lymph Node Transfer

Katrin Seidenstücker

If we apply the principle of the reconstructive ladder utilized in reconstructive surgery to lymphatic surgery, VLNT would come after LVA due to its surgical invasiveness and the potential for donor site morbidity. Accordingly, it would represent the first-line therapy if due to an advanced stage of lymphedema and secondary fibrotic alteration of the subcutaneous tissues, LVA is no longer possible (see **Chapter 8**).

VLNT as a second procedure could follow LVA surgery and suction-assisted lipectomy to further improve lymphatic drainage. In secondary lymphedema following lymph node resection of the axilla (level I and II) or superficial groin, despite the presence of intra-abdominal iliac or pelvic nodes, a surgical scar release and obliteration of the defect with a well-perfused flap may also improve the lymphatic flow due to spontaneous development and rearrangement of lympholymphatic and lymphovenous anastomoses. Scar release after lymph node resection and/or radiotherapy of the lymph node basin is an important component of VLNT in view of an anatomical reconstruction of the recipient site and can provide patients with a rather rapid improvement both of the severity of the lymphedema, and the patient's range of motion of the affected extremity.

Studies have shown that over time previously performed LVAs might spontaneously obstruct or impair lymphedema after primary improvement. Patency rates between 66% and 72% are described at least 12-month postoperatively for the upper extremity by Wolfs et al.[7] and Winters et al.[8] For the lower extremity, the patency rates after 6 to 12 months range from 44% to 75%.[9]

Lymphedema, as a chronic disease, can often be improved using surgical methods. Unfortunately, in many cases, the lymphatic function cannot be restored completely, except when the disease is in its very early stages.[10]

Fortunately, lymphedema surgery and its understanding has developed considerably in the last two decades, and suction-assisted lipectomy, LVA or lymph vessel transfer is not considered a contraindication for subsequent or secondary VLNT. Though, after harvesting of a lymphatic collector from the thigh or arm for autologous lymph-vessel transfer or interposition, the donor site for the lymph node flap should be considered carefully and VLNT performed as a second procedure should not further impair lymphatic flow of the donor site extremity.[14] Nevertheless, in any instance of harvesting subcutaneous lymph nodes in the area of the groin or lateral thoracic wall for VLNT, reverse mapping is mandatory (see **Sub Chapter 4.7**). Particularly in cases of secondary surgery, intra-abdominal nodes should be considered for donor site.

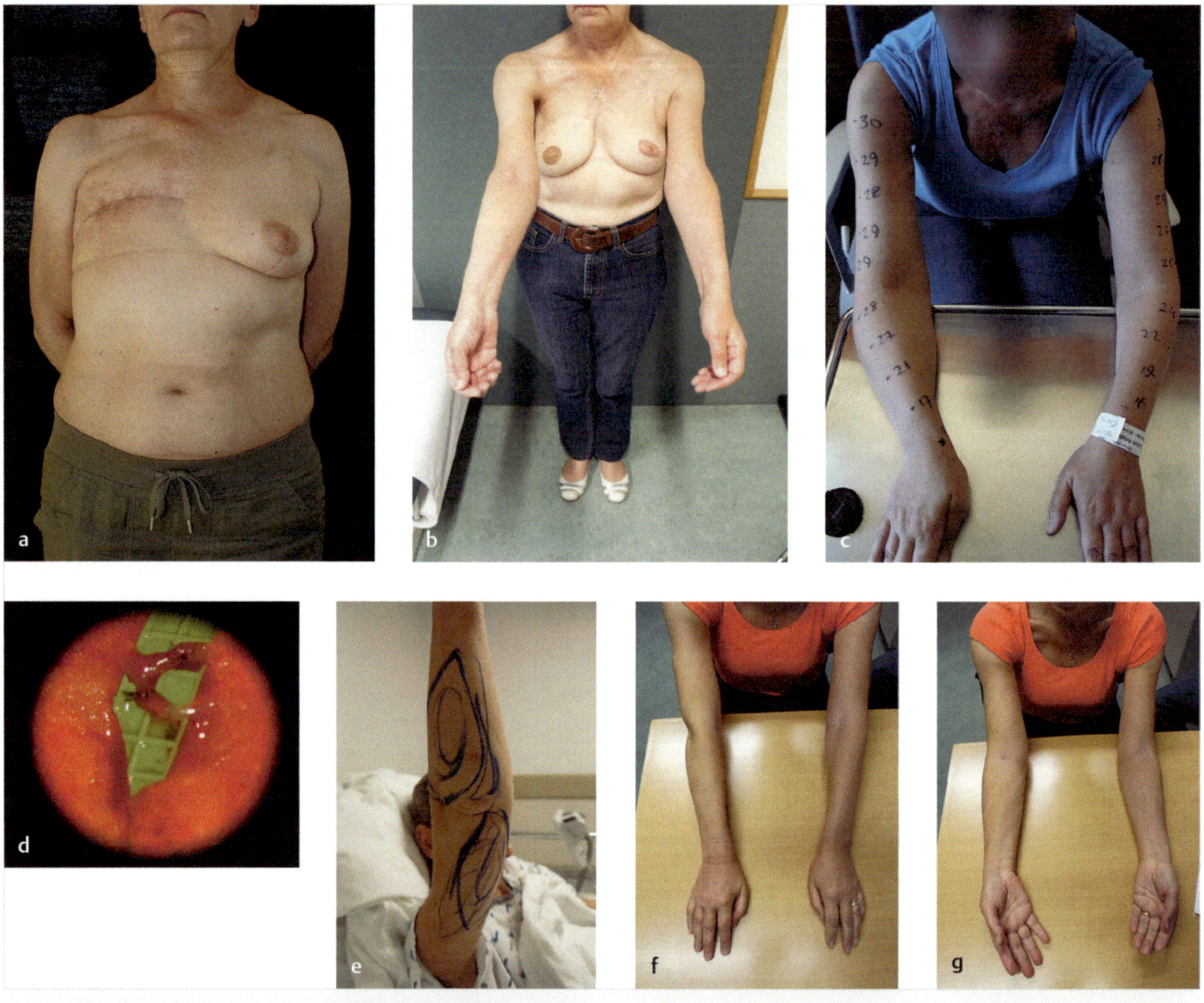

Fig. 15.2 55-year-old patient who underwent right breast reconstruction with a deep inferior epigastric artery perforator flap combined with vascularized lymph node transfer from the groin for stage 2 lymphedema. Residual lymphedema of the forearm was treated secondarily with two lymphovenous anastomoses. However, lipedema was still present at the latero-posterior aspect of the arm and forearm; therefore, selected suction-assisted lipectomy was performed 1 year later. **(a)** Preoperative view. **(b)** Postoperative view after DIEP flap and inguinal vascularized lymph node transfer. **(c)** Residual forearm lymphedema. **(d)** Two lymphovenous anastomoses were performed 6 months later. **(e)** Localized suction-assisted lipectomy 6 months later. **(f, g)** Outcome at 1 year follow-up after suction-assisted lipectomy. (Courtesy of Moustapha Hamdi.)

In case of lower limb lymphedema with ICG-positive lymphatics, LVA is the first-line therapy (see **Chapter 18**). If you merely achieve a partial improvement, secondary VLNT to the groin combined with scar release, in the event of previous inguinal surgery, could bring about further improvements. Distal placement of the lymph node flap in the event of primary lymphedema or previous pelvic or iliac node surgery could improve the results, too. To monitor the postoperative improvement of the treated region, a follow-up examination should be carried out after one year, before additional procedure.

Granzow et al. offered VLNT after suction-assisted lipectomy after volume reduction had stabilized to reduce the amount of postoperative compression required.[5] Two of the patients in this series went on to have VLNT after so-called suction-assisted lipectomy. The patients were able to maintain their improved volumes with compression only in the evening and at night, instead of continuous compression as advised by Brorson. After suction-assisted lipectomy and ICG-negative lymphangiography, detection of the recipient vessel with color flow duplex or MRL should be considered.

15.3 Lymphovenous Anastomosis for Chronic Lymphocele After Lymph Node Excision and/or Vascularized Lymph Node Transfer

Nicole Lindenblatt and Semra Uyulmaz

Chronic postsurgical lymphocele increases morbidity and health care costs. Based on the anatomy of the lymphatic system and distribution of lymphatic vessels throughout the human body, many surgical procedures may cause lymphatic vessel injury. In general, if dead space occurs as a result of surgery, drainage systems should be placed before wound closure to allow for sufficient wound healing. In order to close dead space, flaps can be used primarily or secondarily. If primary wound healing is uneventful, percutaneous puncturing should be performed no more than three times. If lymphocele persists, sclerotherapy should be performed. Reconstructive methods should be integrated into the overall treatment plan whenever possible. ICG lymphangiography navigated LVAs are preferable to lymphatic vessel ligation alone because these will reduce the pressure within the lymphatic system and lead to a physiological drainage of the lymphatic fluid into the venous system. If only microscopic lymphatic vessel ligation is performed, rising pressure in the lymphatics may cause a relapse due to rupture or renewed opening of the ligated lymphatic vessel. However, the extent of the resulting lymphocele is usually much smaller than the initial one and can be handled better by, for example, another course of sclerotherapy. Revisional surgery including reconstructive microsurgery should be performed early in immunocompromised patients, after radiotherapy, and for percutaneous lymphatic fistula.

While the formation of symptomatic lymphocele after sentinel lymph node biopsy (SLNB) is less than 7%, the incidence following lymph node dissection of the axilla or the groin is significantly higher and is repeatedly reported to be between 40% and 50%.[13] The incidence of chronic fluid accumulation following surgery for excision of a soft tissue tumor varies between 10% and 36%.[12] The incidence of lymphocele at the donor site area after lymph node harvest for transfer varies between 11% and 30%. However, as lymphocele formation itself is associated with a higher predilection for developing lymphedema, which requires additional therapies and further increases the health and financial burden, reconstructive options should be preferred whenever possible.

It has been hypothesized that bypassing lymphatic vessels to veins prophylactically could minimize lymphatic dysfunction, such as lymphedema, seen following lymphadenectomy. A systematic search by Jørgensen et al. yielded 12 articles, 4 of which were eligible to be included in the quantitative analysis.[15] Patients treated with prophylactic LVA had a significant reduction in lymphedema incidence when compared to patients receiving no prophylactic treatment. Low-quality studies and a high risk of bias halt the formulating of strong recommendations in favor of prophylactic lymphovenous anastomosis, despite preliminary reports theoretically indicating that they may significantly decrease the incidence of cancer-related surgery lymphedema.[16]

Prophylactic LVA might also prevent chronic lymphocele. Prophylactic LVAs in patients with soft tissue sarcoma of the proximal medial thigh necessitating neoadjuvant radiation therapy and tumor excision with transection of the lymphatic vessels of the medial thigh can be applied to prevent chronic lymphocele and lymphedema.

LVAs have been described as useful in lymphocele treatment and seem to be a potent reconstructive option. The technique was used successfully by Todokoro et al. for pelvic lymphocele after gynecologic cancer treatment combined with lymphocele capsule resection.[17] The lymphocele was completely resolved in six patients and partially resolved in the remaining five patients. In localized subcutaneous groin lymphoceles after sentinel node biopsy for skin melanoma and vulvar cancer, this technique was successfully used in 16 patients by Boccardo et al.[18] Subcutaneous LVA to a collateral branch of the great saphenous vein after lymphocele capsule excision was effective in one patient for treating postoperative groin lymphocele as reported by Gentileschi et al.[19] One patient with chronic lymphocele after inguinal hernia repair was treated successfully by Ayestaray et al. using a surrounding LVA.[20] In this case, lymphocele capsule excision was not required, and MRI revealed a gradient lymphocele volume reduction 5 days after surgery. The advantage of surrounding LVA based on small incisions was to minimize the length of surgical scars.

In conclusion, LVA should be considered as a potent therapy for the treatment of lymphocele because of its low invasiveness and its effectiveness in reestablishing circulation of lymphatic flow. Further prospective and large-scale studies are mandatory to confirm and compare results with other minimally invasive techniques, such as percutaneous catheter and sclerotherapy.

Chronic lymphocele in our patients most frequently occurs after lymph node dissections of axilla and groin due to cancer and after vascular access to the femoral vessels in the groin (e.g., cannulation for cardiopulmonary bypass pumps). Immunosuppression after cardiac or lung transplantation often represents an aggravating factor in these patients. In addition, severe lymphocele occurs in patients after soft tissue sarcoma resection of the leg, especially the medial thigh.

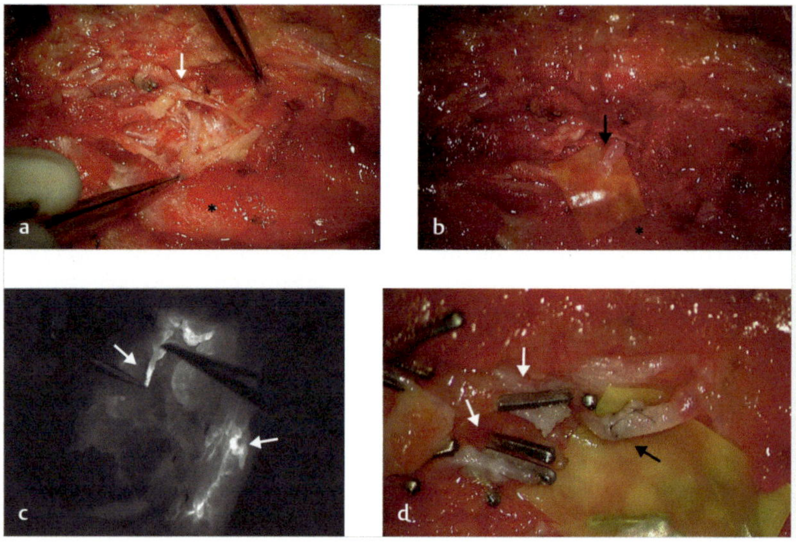

Fig. 15.3 **(a)** Intraoperative microscopic images of a chronic lymphocele 5 weeks after vascular access to the femoral artery (asterisk). Multiple severed lymphatic vessels are detected within the wound (white arrow). **(b)** Transected high-flow lymphatic collector (approximately 0.8 mm) with visible lymphatic flow (black arrow). Magnification × 12.5. **(c)** ICG lymphangiography of a chronic lymphocele showing visible lymphatic flow from two transected lymphatic vessels (white arrows). Magnification × 12.5. **(d)** Multiple microscopic micro-clip ligations of severed lymphatic vessels (white arrows) and lymphovenous anastomosis of a high-flow lymphatic collector (black arrow). Magnification × 30.

The following recommendations were established based on the authors' experience:

- Investigate the wound bed after initial tissue resection or LND and before primary wound closure with ICG lymphangiography in order to detect severed high-flow lymphatics and implement preferably LVA if a suitable vein is present or microscopic lymphatic vessel ligature as an alternative. Presently, we perform this approach in patients with a high risk for severe lymphocele, which will be difficult to treat by sclerotherapy alone. This applies to patients under immunosuppression and with soft tissue sarcoma of the medial thigh, with our without radiotherapy (▶ Fig. 15.3a,b).
- If dead space occurs as a result of surgery, place drains before wound closure and leave them 10 to 12 days *in situ* to allow for sufficient wound healing. Pedicled muscle flaps have been described as a primary or secondary strategy to close dead space successfully in some cases.
- If primary wound healing is uneventful and the wound is closed, the drain can be removed after 10 to 12 days and a developing lymphocele can be punctured percutaneously. This should be performed no more than three times.
- If lymphocele persists, sclerotherapy by interventional radiologists with potent agents such as OK-453 should be planned. It induces a localized inflammatory[21] reaction, as seen in bacterial infection, and causes apoptosis of lymphatic endothelium with promising results. In the authors' experience, sclerotherapy (one to three sessions) alone will be successful in 92% of the outpatient collective if there is no additional complicating factor. OK-453 should not be used in immunocompromised patients because tissue reaction and adhesion are reduced and therefore the effect is limited.
- In the event of chronic lymphocele formation with compromised wound healing and development of a cutaneous lymphatic fistula, revisional surgery including ICG lymphangiography and LVA, if possible, and/or microscopic lymphatic ligation will be necessary (▶ Fig. 15.3c,d).

15.4 One Stage versus Staged-Combined Surgical Procedures to Treat Lymphedema

Holger Engel

At the beginning of lymphatic surgery, most of the surgical procedures focused on a single treatment modality per patient, e.g., solely LVA, VLNT, suction-assisted lipectomy or further excisional debulking procedures (see **Chapters 8, 10, 13** and **14**). It is not always the case that one single operation using only one treatment modality would achieve top clinical results, especially in progressed stages with existing fat deposition and fibrosis. Currently, it is clear that all available treatment options (surgical and nonsurgical) have to be utilized to achieve the best possible outcome for the patient, taking into account, their clinical staging.

Combined surgical procedures encompass one stage and sequential utilization of LVA, VLNT, suction-assisted lipectomy, and excisional debulking surgery in various combinations and sequences (▶ Fig. 15.2). The goal of combined surgical procedures is to achieve a maximum outcome for each patient by perfectly adapting to the specific lymphedema stage and condition. There is heterogeneity regarding the sequences of treatment modalities even within a one-stage approach (e.g., suction-assisted lipectomy before or after VLNT and/or LVA). Additionally, within one single treatment modality, there are many differences regarding the type and technique of LVA (location, number or type of LVA, e.g., end-to-end, side-to-end, end-to-side: see **Chapter 8**),[11] of VLNT (donor site, recipient site, number: see **Chapter 10**), of suction-assisted lipectomy: see **Chapter 13**) and of excisional or debulking surgery (see **Chapter 14**).

Publications regarding combined surgical procedures are still limited but have rapidly increased in number over the last 5 years.

The authors also published a retrospective study on the usage of LVAs in conjunction with ultrasound suction-assisted lipectomy in 24 patients. Preoperative ICG lymphangiography was performed to detect the LVA location. The procedure began with Vaser based, suction-assisted lipectomy, followed by one to two LVAs per extremity. The mean CRR was 90%. The postoperative infection rate decreased to zero in all patients.

Chang et al. performed simultaneous suction-assisted lipectomy with LVA on 49 patients with secondary lymphedema, which was published in 2017.[4] Lower limb circumference was monitored at 7 days, 6 months, and 12 months postoperatively, and showed significant decrease. Campisi et al. also described this approach in 2017.[26]

Leppäpuska et al. compared[31] a group of 21 patients treated with combined VLNT and suction-assisted lipectomy with 27 patients who were treated with VLNT only. The average arm volume excess decreased postoperatively to 87.7% (27.5% with VLNT only). The number of cellulitis episodes was reduced in 7 out of 10 patients and was better than in the VLNT only group. They concluded that suction-assisted lipectomy could safely be performed with lymph node transfer in a one-stage approach. Ciudad et al.[25] described their own technique (CHAHOVA) combining excisional surgeries such as Charles and Homans procedures with reconstructive surgery using the VLNT.

Engel et al.[22] discussed the outcomes of lymphedema microsurgery for breast cancer-related lymphedema with or without microvascular breast reconstruction. The authors could show that there was no further improvement regarding recurrent infection and decrease of arm circumference in the cases that benefit from a combined reconstruction of the axillary lymph node basin (LVA or VLNT) and the breast after mastectomy when compared to lymphedema surgery alone. Though, they could show an increased improvement of the lymphedema after VLNT when compared to LVA. In 2016, Masia et al. described their standardized assessment and treatment algorithm based on a combined surgical approach, using both LVA and VLNT in selected patients with breast cancer-related lymphedema.[27] Out of 106 patients, 40 were treated with one-stage lymph node transplants from the groin area and, on average, 3.4 LVAs per patient. Circumference as an outcome parameter decreased by 39.7% on average. The number of cellulitis episodes decreased from 1.8 to 0.2 per year. No further clinical improvement was noted after 18 months. The decision for a one-stage combined surgical treatment was mainly based upon residual lymphatic functionality, which was assessed by ICG and MRL. Patients with no functional lymphatic system underwent an excisional procedure or vibroliposuction/power-assisted liposuction (PAL), so-called suction-assisted lipectomy.

Sequential combined surgical procedures were published by Agko et al. in 2018.[28] In a prospective study with 12 patients, a dual gastroepiploic VLNT was performed, followed 6 to 8 months later by suction-assisted lipectomy (▶ Fig. 15.1). The overall CRR was, on average, 37.8%. After suction-assisted lipectomy, the overall CRR increased to 97.8%. No infection was registered after suction-assisted lipectomy. All patients continued with daytime compression garments.

Ito et al. described[32] their case report results of bilateral submental VLNT after excisional Charles procedure of the lower extremity, which was done 2 years before. The female patient had CRR of 23%, 50%, and 22% above the knee, below the knee, and above the ankle, respectively. The patient discontinued the use of compression garment. At 5-month follow-up, no relapsing cellulitis was detected.

In 2015, Nicoli et al. described the results of 10 patients with either supraclavicular or groin VLNT followed 1 to 3 months later by laser-based suction-assisted lipectomy.[29] At the 6-month follow-up, the reduction in arm circumference was 90% compared to preoperative measurements. Skin tonicity was also significantly improved. No reason was mentioned why suction-assisted lipectomy was performed after VLNT.

Both one-stage and sequential combined procedures demonstrate significant improvements in treating lymphedema patients. To date, it has not been possible to state whether one approach is superior to the other due to the limited literature and wide variability in study designs with different outcome parameters, methods in patient selection, and techniques.

Knowledge and evolution in lymphatic surgery has been rapidly increasing, but there are still ongoing debate and open questions regarding the significance of each single treatment modality and pathophysiology. Basta et al. published a meta-analysis of 27 studies, which

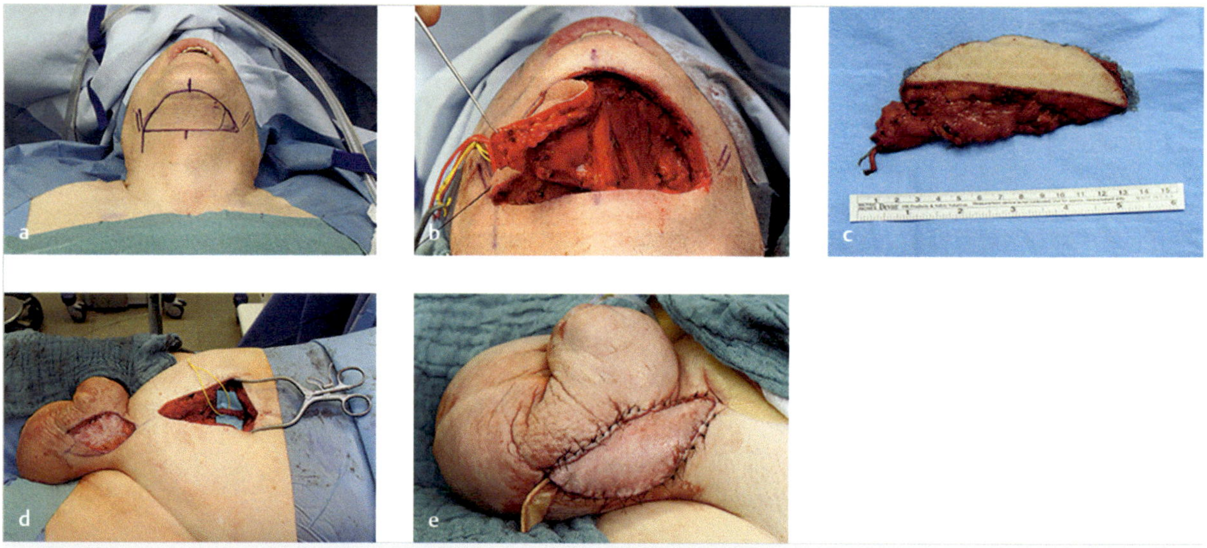

Fig. 15.4 66-year-old patient with scrotal lymphedema stage III. Before lympho-reconstructive surgery with lymph node flap from the submental region: **(a)** Planning of submental lymph node flap harvesting. **(b)** Flap dissection. **(c)** Submental flap ex vivo after surgical harvesting. **(d)** Preparation of recipient vessels (deep inferior epigastric vessels). **(e)** The flap sit-up.

included 1,610 patients, to quantify the efficacy and safety of microsurgery for lymphedema.[30] They concluded that operative interventions provided quantitative improvements but lacked high evidence levels (24 studies out of 27 offering only level IV evidence).

In 2018, a consensus paper of the German-speaking Society for Microsurgery of Peripheral Nerves and Vessels concluded that one-stage combined surgical procedures were promising but not the gold standard.[23] The consensus was that an approach with the "core" treatment modalities such as LVA, VLNT, etc., should first gather sufficient data to improve the overall level of evidence. Sequential surgical procedures were excluded from the discussion. With more evidence-based data in the upcoming future, combined surgical procedures will be established as the new gold standard.

15.5 Pearls and Pitfalls

Holger Engel

In general, it is advisable to establish a setting where the patients are referred to the lymphedema center as early as possible. Professional networking with other faculties and health care providers, such as departments of gynecology and surgery, breast centers, medical supply stores, self-support groups, etc., is critical.

Evidence-based assessment and treatment algorithms should be established to individualize treatment for each patient. To assess patients with lymphedema, thorough clinical examination, history, and imaging examinations are obligatory as diagnostic and staging tools, including ICG lymphangiography, dynamic ultrasound, and MRI. Facultative examinations are MRL or lymphoscintigraphy. Local fat depositions detected with MRI could be treated with lipectomy, e.g., using the Brorson technique. ICG lymphangiography and ultrasonography (US) investigation of lymphatic vessel will conclude if LVAs are feasible. Each procedural step should have defined outcome parameters to enhance the data and evidence levels further.

LVA is a less invasive procedure than VLNT or suction-assisted lipectomy and should be the first step in a sequential surgical plan. Suction-assisted lipectomy theoretically has the potential to violate LVAs or VLNT that were previously transplanted. Therefore, for safety reasons suction-assisted lipectomy should be considered before that.

In failed cases, excisional debulking surgery or even amputation is the final option which can be adequate (▶ Fig. 15.4 and ▶ Fig. 15.5).

For sequential and secondary procedures, the following sequence of treatment modality selection offers a risk-adjusted method with predictable outcomes:

- MRI and ICG/US-positive patients would be treated with suction-assisted lipectomy first, followed by LVA and VLNT.
- MRI-positive and ICG/US-negative patients would undergo suction-assisted lipectomy followed by VLNT only.

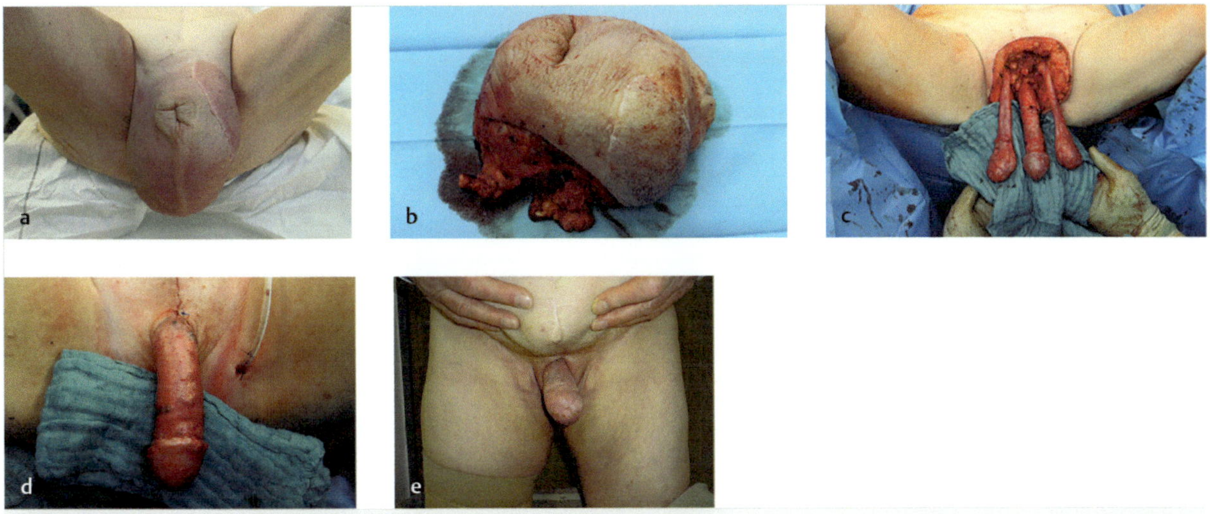

Fig. 15.5 Persisting lymphedema after vascularized lymph node transfer from the submental region. Indication for excisional surgery: **(a)** Preoperative situation with stage 3 lymphedema after submental vascularized lymph node transfer. **(b, c)** After scrotal debulking. **(d)** Skin grafts were used to resurface the penile shaft. **(e)** Long-term result.

References

[1] Frick A, Hoffmann JN, Baumeister RGH, Putz R. Liposuction technique and lymphatic lesions in lower legs: anatomic study to reduce risks. Plast Reconstr Surg. 1999; 103(7):1868–1873, discussion 1874–1875

[2] Hoffmann JN, Fertmann JP, Baumeister RG, Putz R, Frick A. Tumescent and dry liposuction of lower extremities: differences in lymph vessel injury. Plast Reconstr Surg. 2004; 113(2):718–724, discussion 725–726

[3] Brorson H, Ohlin K, Olsson G, Svensson B. Long term cosmetic and functional results following liposuction for arm lymphedema: and eleven year study. Lymphology. 2007; 40:253–255

[4] Chang K, Xia S, Sun YG, Xin JF, Shen WB. [Liposuction combined with lymphatico-venous anastomosis for treatment of secondary lymphedema of the lower limbs: a report of 49 cases] (in Chinese). Zhonghua Wai Ke Za Zhi. 2017; 55(4):274–278

[5] Granzow JW, Soderberg JM, Dauphine C. A novel two-stage surgical approach to treat chronic lymphedema. Breast J. 2014; 20 (4):420–422

[6] Chang EI, Masià J, Smith ML. Combining autologous breast reconstruction and vascularized lymph node transfer. Semin Plast Surg. 2018; 32(1):36–41

[7] Wolfs JAGN, de Joode LGEH, van der Hulst RRWJ, Qiu SS. Correlation between patency and clinical improvement after lymphaticovenous anastomosis (LVA) in breast cancer-related lymphedema: 12-month follow-up. Breast Cancer Res Treat. 2020; 179(1):131–138

[8] Winters H, Tielemans HJP, Verhulst AC, Paulus VAA, Slater NJ, Ulrich DJO. The long-term patency of lymphaticovenular anastomosis in breast cancer-related lymphedema. Ann Plast Surg. 2019; 82(2): 196–200

[9] Suzuki Y, Sakuma H, Yamazaki S. Comparison of patency rates of lymphaticovenous anastomoses at different sites for lower extremity lymphedema. J Vasc Surg Venous Lymphat Disord. 2019; 7(2):222–227

[10] Boccardo F, De Cian F, Campisi CC, et al. Surgical prevention and treatment of lymphedema after lymph node dissection in patients with cutaneous melanoma. Lymphology. 2013; 46(1):20–26

[11] Maegawa J, Yabuki Y, Tomoeda H, Hosono M, Yasumura K. Outcomes of lymphaticovenous side-to-end anastomosis in peripheral lymphedema. J Vasc Surg. 2012; 55(3):753–760

[12] McCaul JA, Aslaam A, Spooner RJ, Louden I, Cavanagh T, Purushotham AD. Aetiology of seroma formation in patients undergoing surgery for breast cancer. Breast. 2000; 9(3):144–148

[13] Greuter L, Klein J, Rezaeian F, Giovanoli P, Lindenblatt N. Evaluation of factors in seroma formation and complications in sentinel and radical lymph node dissections in skin cancer patients. Eur J Plast Surg. 2017; 40(1):39–46

[14] Viitanen TP, Mäki MT, Seppänen MP, Suominen EA, Saaristo AM. Donor-site lymphatic function after microvascular lymph node transfer. Plast Reconstr Surg. 2012; 130(6):1246–1253

[15] Jørgensen MG, Toyserkani NM, Sørensen JA. The effect of prophylactic lymphovenous anastomosis and shunts for preventing cancer-related lymphedema: a systematic review and meta-analysis. Microsurgery. 2018; 38(5):576–585

[16] Ciudad P, Escandón JM, Bustos VP, Manrique OJ, Kaciulyte J. Primary Prevention of Cancer-Related Lymphedema Using Preventive Lymphatic Surgery: Systematic Review and Meta-analysis. Indian J Plast Surg. 2022 Feb 25;55(1):18–25.

[17] Todokoro T, Furniss D, Oda K, et al. Effective treatment of pelvic lymphocele by lymphaticovenular anastomosis. Gynecol Oncol. 2013; 128(2):209–214

[18] Boccardo F, Dessalvi S, Campisi C, et al. Microsurgery for groin lymphocele and lymphedema after oncologic surgery. Microsurgery. 2014; 34(1):10–13

[19] Gentileschi S, Servillo M, Salgarello M. Supramicrosurgical lymphatic-venous anastomosis for postsurgical subcutaneous lymphocele treatment. Microsurgery. 2015; 35(7):565–568

[20] Ayestaray B, Esnault M, Godard M, Picquot S. Treatment of refractory groin lymphocele by surrounding supermicrosurgical lymphaticovenous anastomosis. Arch Plast Surg. 2018; 45(3):290–291

[21] Uyulmaz, Semra; Puippe, Gilbert; Büyükakyüz, Nilgün; Giovanoli, Pietro; Pfammatter, Thomas; Lindenblatt, Nicole (2020). *Sclerotherapy with OK-432 for the treatment of symptomatic lymphocele after lymph node dissection.* Annals of Plastic Surgery, 85(4):407–412.

[22] Engel H, Lin CY, Huang JJ, Cheng MH. Outcomes of lymphedema microsurgery for breast cancer-related lymphedema with or without microvascular breast reconstruction. Ann Surg. 2018; 268 (6):1076–1083

[23] Hirche C, Engel H, Seidenstuecker K, et al. [Lympho-reconstructive microsurgery for secondary lymphedema: consensus of the

German-Speaking Society for Microsurgery of Peripheral Nerves and Vessels (DAM) on indication, diagnostic and therapy by lymphovenous anastomosis (LVA) and vascularized lymph node transfer (VLNT)]. Handchir Mikrochir Plast Chir. 2019; 51(6):424–433

[24] Ciudad P, Manrique OJ, Adabi K, et al. Combined double vascularized lymph node transfers and modified radical reduction with preservation of perforators for advanced stages of lymphedema. J Surg Oncol. 2019; 119(4):439–448

[25] Ciudad P, Agko M, Huang TCT, et al. Comprehensive multimodal surgical treatment of end-stage lower extremity lymphedema with toe management: the combined Charles', Homan's, and vascularized lymph node transfer (CHAHOVA) procedures. J Surg Oncol. 2019; 119 (4):430–438

[26] Campisi CC, Ryan M, Boccardo F, Campisi C. Fibro-lipo-lymph-aspiration with a lymph vessel sparing procedure to treat advanced lymphedema after multiple lymphatic-venous anastomoses: the complete treatment protocol. Ann Plast Surg. 2017; 78(2):184–190

[27] Masia J, Pons G, Nardulli ML. Combined surgical treatment in breast cancer-related lymphedema. J Reconstr Microsurg. 2016; 32 (1):16–27

[28] Agko M, Ciudad P, Chen HC. Staged surgical treatment of extremity lymphedema with dual gastroepiploic vascularized lymph node transfers followed by suction-assisted lipectomy—a prospective study. J Surg Oncol. 2018; 117(6):1148–1156

[29] Nicoli F, Constantinides J, Ciudad P, et al. Free lymph node flap transfer and laser-assisted liposuction: a combined technique for the treatment of moderate upper limb lymphedema. Lasers Med Sci. 2015; 30(4):1377–1385

[30] Basta MN, Gao LL, Wu LC. Operative treatment of peripheral lymphedema: a systematic meta-analysis of the efficacy and safety of lymphovenous microsurgery and tissue transplantation. Plast Reconstr Surg. 2014; 133(4):905–913

[31] Leppäpuska I-M, Suominen E, Viitanen T, et al. Combined Surgical Treatment for Chronic Upper Extremity Lymphedema Patients: Simultaneous Lymph Node Transfer and Liposuction. Ann Plast Surg. 2019; 83(3):308–317

[32] Ito R, Lin MC, Cheng MH. Simultaneous Bilateral Submental Lymph Node Flaps for Lower Limb Lymphedema Post Leg Charles Procedure. Plast Reconstr Surg Glob Open. 2015; 3(9):e513

16 Tips and Tricks for Modern Surgical Management of Chronic Lymphedema

Summary

In surgery, indications can only be determined with certainty through extensive experience and evidence, and one of the avoidable missteps is to choose the wrong technique for the wrong patient and the wrong stage. It is of foremost interest for us to prevent the future generation of lymphedema surgeons from falling foul to the same oversights that might have occurred in treating patients in the last decades. Therefore, an open-minded summary of the most relevant tips and tricks of modern surgical management of lymphedema for reconstructive surgery with lymphovenous anastomosis or vascularized lymph node transfer, in conjunction with breast reconstruction or lymphoablative surgery with suction-assisted lipectomy, reflects the value of this chapter. Recognizing and dealing with therapeutic failure and decision-making for secondary procedures is a necessary part of a surgeon's portfolio.

Keywords: adipose tissue, excision, extremity, fat, lymphoablative surgery, lymphoreconstructive surgery and breast reconstruction, lymphovenous anastomosis (LVA), lymphedema, secondary procedures, suction-assisted lipectomy, therapeutic failure, tips and tricks, vascularized lymph node transfer (VLNT), wrong technique for wrong stage

16.1 How to Avoid the Wrong Surgical Technique in the Wrong Patient for the Wrong Lymphedema Stage

Christoph Hirche and Yves Harder

The most important advice for modern surgical management of lymphedema and pitfalls at the same time, is to avoid the wrong surgical technique for the wrong patient for the wrong stage of lymphedema. What may sound obvious, but nonetheless fundamental, in medical treatment in general has unfortunately not been applied for several decades in lymphedema surgery. In particular, surgical treatment of lymphedema has been performed based on individual experience of experts in the field, rather than scientific evidence.

In other words, very often, one particular surgical technique was offered for all stages of lymphedema by one surgeon capable of technically executing this technique very well, regardless of the etiology and the stage of lymphedema, as well as the damage to the lymphatic structures. Furthermore, preoperative diagnostics were limited for a long time or even misinterpreted.

It is quite significant that nowadays modern surgical management of lymphedema implies an individual and targeted, stage-dependent decision-making process to choose the right surgical technique for the right stage and patient in the correct anatomical region that is based on an interprofessional and multidisciplinary decision-making (see **Chapter 5**). This means that a surgeon who consults patients for surgical management of lymphedema—when indicated—should either offer all relevant reconstructive and lymphoablative surgeries with his or her team or consult patients clearly that they are only offering surgery for a particular stage and that treatment success will depend on multiple factors, including patient compliance.

Therefore, thorough diagnostic evaluation of the affected region—always in comparison with the healthy side, if possible—has to define the location and extent of damage of lymphatic vessels and nodes, which results in correct grading of lymphedema stage. This will without any doubt facilitate a decision on the right surgical technique to be offered to the patient.

Interprofessional evaluation helps to further decide on the ideal preoperative patient preparation, including complete decongestive therapy (CDT) (see **Chapter 6** and **Subchapter 7.3**) to get "the best out" of the affected extremity or region for the surgery itself and thereafter.

Modern surgical treatment of lymphedema can only be as good as the therapeutic concept. Fortunately, even in countries where CDT with continuous conservative treatment is not achievable, correct surgical technique applied to the affected region, taking into account the correct lymphedema stage, can successfully and long-lastingly reduce the burden of lymphedema and stage progression.

A standardized and thorough evaluation of the lymphedema patient with re-evaluation after 6 months of intense conservative treatment is the key to choose the right surgical technique for the right stage and patient.

Finally, only correct assessment of one's own ability, skills, and competences does justice to the patient who deserves an individualized and stage-dependent multidisciplinary treatment, which is often long-lasting. Therefore, we encourage the readers of this book to proceed with the reading of any special tips and tricks. They include lymphoablative surgery such as suction-assisted lipectomy and excisional procedures, as well as reconstructive surgery, such LVA and VLNT with and without synchronous breast reconstruction, secondary procedures, and management of therapeutic failure.

A network of surgeons, lymphologist, and specialized therapists working hand-in-hand in a multidisciplinary and interprofessional way is the key to success for both lymphedema patients and doctors that can popularize sustainable and recognized modern surgical lymphedema treatment.

16.2 Local Dermolipectomy and Lymphoreductive Surgery

Vincenzo Penna and Nestor Torio

Prior to performing dermolipectomies (see **Chapter 14**), thorough patient selection is mandatory. Patients with reduced or questionable compliance should not be operated as the success of the operation is partly dependent on good patient–surgeon partnership. If the patient's general condition is impaired due to multiple diseases, indications for dermolipectomies should be considered with caution. The necessity of postoperative therapeutic anticoagulation is a contraindication, as the bleeding risk is extremely high and coagulation in fibrotic tissue is impaired.

If the CDT is inadequate or has been performed only for a short period, the tissue is not well prepared for surgery resulting in poor results and/or wound healing problems. If you have any doubts about the decongestion, postpone the surgery and try to improve or prolong the CDT. A good interaction between the surgeon and CDT facility is very helpful and important in lymphedema surgery. After surgery a fast return to CDT is crucial as the underlying pathology causing the lymphedema has not been cured by surgery. After complete wound healing, customized compression garments must be prescribed so that the new reduced tissue shape can be maintained.

Impaired lymphedema tissue is more vulnerable to infections. Perioperative intravenous antibiotics (broad spectrum such as Cephalexin) and postoperative oral antibiotics (e.g., Clindamycin) should be administered in the first 2 weeks.

Use nonresorbable sutures and perform single stitches. In the event of local infection limited removal of the stitches prevents large wound dehiscence.

When performing tissue resection, it is paramount to be cautious not to under- or over-resect. Under-resection leads to insufficient reduction of the affected tissue which may lead to additional surgical procedures after a short time. Over-resection causes immediate and severe complications necessitating further plastic surgical techniques, resulting in longer hospital stays.

Lymphoablative surgery still has its role in select patients with extended fibrotic lymphedema disease (stage III) to improve the quality of life by weight reduction and debulking. The procedure is invasive and requires several preoperative, perioperative, and postoperative considerations:

- Evaluate the stage of CDT regarding tissue decongestion around 1 week prior to planned surgery. Postpone surgery if unsatisfied with the edema status and pitting edema is still predominant.
- Start CDT within the first 2 to 3 days after the operation.
- Keep the patients on intravenous or oral antibiotics for the first 2 weeks postoperatively (or till sutures are removed).
- In dermolipectomies be cautious with the amount of tissue resected; do not over- or under-resect and frequently reevaluate the resection margins with pinch testing.
- Synchronous suction-assisted dermolipectomy may improve the total amount of tissue to be debulked.
- Use a tourniquet to reduce blood loss.
- Compression therapy is essential after lymphoablative surgery as a life-long modality to maintain the surgical outcome.

16.3 Suction-Assisted Lipectomy

Håkan Brorson, Arin Greene, and Jeremy Goss

16.3.1 Preoperative

The surgeon should *not* agree to perform suction-assisted lipectomy on a patient unless the surgeon has confirmed that the individual has lymphedema with a considerable degree of adipose hypertrophy.[1] Subjects with an equivocal diagnosis should undergo lymphoscintigraphy to document they have lymphedema.[2] In addition, the patient must exhibit excess subcutaneous adipose tissue by pitting test and/or MRI.[2,3,4] Most patients with lymphedema are successfully managed without any type of surgical intervention. To be a candidate for the procedure, individuals must be symptomatic with a considerable level of suffering, e.g., recurrent infections, psychosocial morbidity, difficulty using the extremity, and/or inability to fit clothing despite maximal conservative therapy.[6] Suction-assisted lipectomy is not effective for penile/scrotal lymphedema which is managed better open surgical skin/ subcutaneous resection. Suction-assisted lipectomy should also not be performed on subjects with obesity-induced lymphedema unless they have lost weight and reduced degree of adipositas and achieved the lowest body mass index (BMI) possible. Patients must be compliant with their preoperative compression regimen to be a potential candidate for the procedure. Patients should have reasonable expectations and understand that the procedure does not cure the disease and that lifelong compression following the operation is needed. If patients have bilateral extremity disease, operating on the limbs should be staged at least 3 months apart. Performing lipectomy on both arms or legs at the same time would significantly limit postoperative function and recovery, as well as increase the risk for complications. Suction-assisted lipectomy is effective for both primary and secondary lymphedemas and is independent of the etiology of the disease (e.g., familial, nonfamilial, lymphadenectomy, trauma, infection, etc.).[5,6]

Obesity aggravates lymphedema. Especially for suction-assisted lipectomy in legs, a maximum of BMI 30 is recommended. If the excess volume is 4 liters, 4 kg is deducted from the patient's weight before BMI is calculated. The reason for a maximum BMI of 30 is that with increasing BMI, the diameter or radius of the extremity increases, and thus the circumference of the extremity, eventually significantly decreasing the efficacy of the compression garments according to Laplace's law. Compression class (CCL) 3 is used for legs 24/7 and an additional CCL 2 during daytime (see **Chapter 6**).

16.3.2 Intraoperative

We avoid operating on the hand or foot because these areas have no or minimal adipose tissue. Thus, patients with swelling of the dorsum of the hand should be told that this will probably not change after lipectomy since it is caused by accumulated lymph. Since the hand is oval in shape, most of the compression exerted by the garment is exerted on the sides of the hand, and not where you want it, that is, on the dorsum. Even if foam rubber is put between the glove and skin to improve compression, when it is removed the swelling will recur quickly. The same goes for the foot, ankles, and area around the patella. After complete reduction when patients point out that they want a nice dorsum of the foot, ankles, and patella, they are told that it is not possible since the compression garment cannot exert compression in the groove that is normally seen in the front and behind the ankles and around the patella. These matters are pointed out before the surgery. If it gets better, it will be a bonus for the patient, and this often happens. Since double garments are used on legs, loose measurements are taken around the ankle by putting two fingers beneath the tape measure at this level since compression will be too high here due to the small radius. Also, while measuring the foot we put one finger between tape measure and skin. The compression will be enough anyhow since the radius of these areas is small.

It is important to place the incisions in relaxed-skin tension lines to make them as inconspicuous as possible. Many incisions are placed so that suction-assisted lipectomy can be performed at different angles to help prevent contour abnormalities. We use regular or power-assisted lipectomy, which is adequate to remove the adipose tissue especially in more fibrotic areas in the distal part of the lower leg. We have not found other types of liposuctions (e.g., power-, water-, laser-, ultrasound-assisted) necessary or helpful to remove the adipose tissue. Also, techniques that generate heat at the tip of the cannula are a possible risk for skin necrosis. A cannula, where the holes in a line point in the same direction, is preferred so that suction can be controlled and not exerted toward the skin. In power-assisted cannulas, the use of two machines at the same time can facilitate the operation particularly for large lower extremity cases. As much fat as possible is removed during the operation because repeating resections are more difficult after additional scar tissue has been produced. The incisions are either left open or closed loosely with one to two simple interrupted dissolvable sutures to allow drainage. Facilitating drainage reduces ecchymosis and swelling, which expedites recovery.

16.3.3 Postoperative

Individuals are encouraged to use the extremity as tolerated and elevate the limb as much as possible. It takes several weeks for swelling to resolve and for the skin to contract to achieve the new volume. Pneumatic compression can be initiated, if needed, as soon as tolerated (usually after 1 week). Patients can wrap the extremity with elastic bandage wraps for 2 to 4 weeks postoperatively before being fitted for a new garment. Alternatively, the contralateral, nonaffected limb may be used to produce a garment preoperatively that can then be applied postoperatively.[3] Patients are advised that although their lymphatic function and risk of infection may be improved following lipectomy, their disease is not cured and they must continue their conservative treatments.

16.4 Lymphovenous Anastomosis

Johnson Chia-Shen Yang and Christoph Hirche

Lymphovenous anastomosis (LVA) using supermicrosurgical instruments, equipment, and techniques can be optimized by tips and tricks for the surgeon, during surgery, and with regard to the patient.

16.4.1 For the Surgeon

- For the supermicrosurgeon, finding a comfortable posture is essential. It helps the surgeon to endure a long operation with less tremor and better instrument control.
- During supermicrosurgery, having well-cushioned hands on rolled-up drapes is critical to minimize tremor.

- Personally, I use waist compression to maintain my upright posture during supermicrosurgery. It also helps to reduce fatigue.
- Whether to have coffee or not before supermicrosurgery is surgeon dependent.

16.4.2 During Surgery

- Protect the soft tissue. The operative field can dry up quickly especially under high magnification.
- Small disposable hooks with elastic fixation are the best at keeping the operative field open instead of having assistant retract the wound by hand. No tremor can come from the hooks (▶ Fig. 16.1).
- Use foot paddle for controlling microscope is highly recommended. The paddle is very useful at fine tuning the zoom and adjusting the focus, especially at very high magnification.
- For LVA, use temporary intraluminal stenting[7] of the lymphatic vessel and recipient vein. It is very helpful to visualize the lumen during the anastomoses.

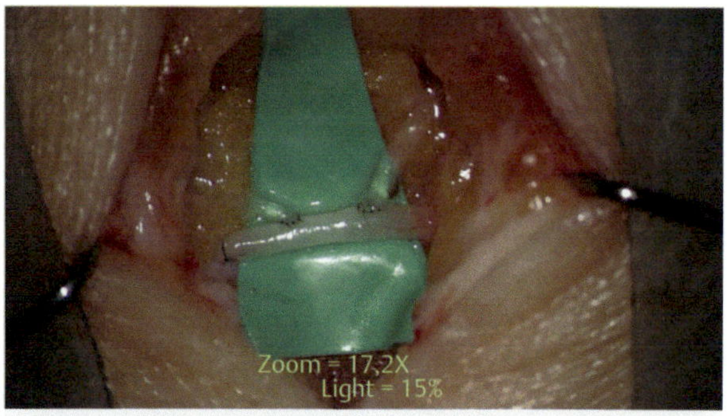

Fig. 16.1 Intraoperative use of hook for LVA.

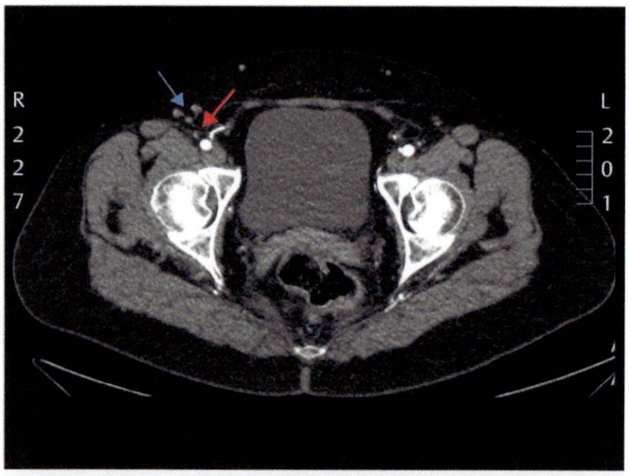

Fig. 16.2 Axial view of CT angiography showing the right superficial inguinal lymph nodes (blue arrow) and the nourishing superficial circumflex iliac vessels (red arrow). It permits to locate the lymph nodes to be harvested and their nourishing vessels using a combination of coordinates in a system of cartesian axis.

- If no supermicrosurgical instrument is available, a wide tip micro-forceps can replace microsurgical needle holder.
- Open and close the wound with microscope to avoid injuring the LVA.
- Use of a blunt microsurgery dissector is helpful during dissection.

16.4.3 Regarding the Patient

- Thorough explanation before the operation is essential. Occasionally, the unrealistic expectations of the patients need to be identified.

16.5 Vascularized Lymph Node Transfer

Holger Engel

- The donor area that we use most often is the groin region with a VLN flap from the superficial inferior epigastric area pedicled to the superficial circumflex iliac vessels. We prefer to use this site because it has low morbidity, and the final cosmetic result is satisfactory.
- Before surgery, we study these areas using CT-based angiography to assess the location of the superficial nodes and their vascular pedicle. We also check the number and distribution of the deep lymph nodes, trying to make sure that the nodes we are removing are not disturbing normal lymphatic drainage of the lower limb (▶ Fig. 16.2).
- The use of reverse lymphatic mapping techniques with an additional dye/tracer is recommended to avoid harvesting essential (sentinel) nodes to prevent secondary lymphedema of the donor site. Reverse mapping helps in identifying nodes that are draining the ipsilateral limb downstream from the lymph node donor site. Subsequently, these nodes are avoided in the harvest, decreasing the chances of donor site lymphedema.[9,10]
- A skin island of approximately 8 × 4 cm is included in the flap design and the compound flap is harvested above the inguinal region and its vascular pedicle is dissected gently up to the femoral vessels. The skin island makes postoperative monitoring easier and increases the contact surface for lymphangiogenesis, especially with partial de-epithelialization, as even the de-epithelialized skin is a lymphatic organ. In addition, it reduces dermal tension in extra-anatomical positioning when lymphedema is present at the recipient site.
- The donor site is closed primarily with a continuous spiral suture, avoiding dead spaces and after spraying a tissue sealant, to reduce the risk of seroma. A suction drain is left in the donor area until the drainage is less

than 15 ml/day and external compression is applied for 2 to 3 weeks.

- Anastomosis of the VLN flap in the axilla is usually performed to a branch of the circumflex scapular system after debridement of fibrotic tissue and scar release.
- It is critical to position the lymph node flap on the apex of the axilla and in contact with the axillary tissue where the afferent dominant lymphatic channels arrive from the arm—respecting the dermal insertion of the skin island without intraflap traction. The adipose tissue surrounding the lymph nodes and the skin island included in the flap is useful to replace the fibrotic tissue in the axillary region and facilitate lymph absorption through the physiologic lymphovenous shunts.[11]

16.6 Autologous Breast Reconstruction in Conjunction with Vascularized Lymph Node Transfer

Moustapha Hamdi, Elena Rodríguez-Bauza, and Jaume Masia

- The principle refers to the combination of autologous reconstruction of the breast in conjunction with scar release of the axilla, VLNT with or without lympho-lymphatic anastomosis (LLA), and/or LVA. This procedure is most frequently done with adipocutaneous flaps derived from lower abdomen and VLN transplants from the groin, but several alternative donor sites of adipocutaneous tissue for breast reconstruction and VLN flap are possible.[8] Technically, two separate flaps (for breast and lymphatic reconstruction) can be harvested with separate anastomosis, or a compound abdominal flap containing the VLNT with double vascularization (conjoined flap) can be harvested.
- The nodes are inserted into the previous adenectomy site, which has received considerable scar release for recipient bed preparation. Next, the abdominal skin is folded to rebuild the breast. The anastomosis of the vessels of the abdominal flap (normally deep inferior epigastric vessels) to the internal mammary vessels is performed.
- Anastomosis of the vessels of the lymph node flap (superficial inferior epigastric or superficial circumflex iliac vessels) is performed additionally to the vessels of the circumflex scapular system.

An additional anastomosis for the lymph nodes is recommended to ensure that the nodes are well perfused, as a conjoined compound flap of the lower abdomen and VLN flap of the groin clinically shows reduced perfusion at the VLN part of the flap.

  - If good lymphatic channels from the arm are found during the dissection of the fibrotic tissue on axilla, one could add an LLA to the afferent lymphatic channels from the transplanted skin–adipose–VLN transplant.
  - Placement of the VLN transplant on the real, deep apex of the axilla in contact with the axillary tissue, where the afferent dominant lymphatic channels are arriving from the arm, is as important as for isolated VLNT (see **Chapter 10**), and more convenient and safer with separated flaps and anastomosis.
  - The selection of recipient vessels especially for the second VLNT may also remain a challenge to the surgeon following an axillary dissection in which often the lateral thoracic vessels have been ligated and are not available to serve as recipient vessels. The thoracodorsal vessels may even have been divided during the node dissection, but if they have been preserved, they are reliable vessels that can be used to perfuse the lymph nodes. An end-to-side anastomosis to the main pedicle of the thoracodorsal vessels or end to end to a branch of the thoracodorsal vessels is recommended preferably as the latissimus dorsi flap remains a versatile fallback option in the event of free flap failure in breast reconstruction. As an alternative, the circumflex scapular system can be used, with an improvement in the clinical course.[13,14]

16.7 Dealing with Therapeutic Failure

Holger Engel

The types of therapeutic failure in lymphatic surgery can be manifold and should always be taken into consideration to provide the best, individualized, stage-dependent patient care and strategy.

To measure therapeutic failure or a lack of response, the patient's feedback has to be highlighted less the surgeon's objective criteria.[15]

What is a therapeutic failure in lymphatic surgery, and how is it related to an absent or low therapeutic response rate?

As a general definition, therapeutic failure can be defined as a failure to accomplish the goals of treatment resulting from inadequate or inappropriate therapy or technical failure and is not related to the natural progression of the disease. That said, a discussion of therapeutic failure is dependent on the goals of treatment, which were predetermined. There is a fluid transition from a lack of response to therapeutic failure. If one expects a complete reversion of pitting edema as a goal of LVA, a "therapeutic failure" would occur if pitting edema was only 50% resolved. However, the procedure would still have a clinical impact, despite being considered a lack of response.

The ultimate goal in lymphatic surgery is a stable cure through the restoration of transport capacity and/or rerouting of the lymphatic load. At least, LVA procedures should lead to a long-lasting significant drop in lymphatic load, resulting in a measurable decrease in indocyanine green (ICG) dermal backflow, volume, weight, and circumference, episodes of cellulitis, and tissue tension. The same conditions apply to VLNT with partial restoration of the lymphatic network. Reductive surgery, including suction-assisted lipectomy, should decrease a high percentage of volume, weight, and circumference through excision and removal of fibrotic tissue or deposited fat.

Therefore, all available modalities of lymphatic surgery fail if whether objective nor subjective outcome parameters are improved. Additionally, worsening of the lymphedema condition is a therapeutic failure, e.g., producing lymphedema at the donor site.

All modalities should lead to discontinued use or reduced frequency or compression level of compression garments and, importantly, to a noticeable improvement in life of quality for the patient. Either subjective and/or objective outcome parameters should lead to improved quality of life for the patient.

16.7.1 Analysis of Causes

A lack of therapeutic effects should always lead to a critical review of the performed procedure and the setting.

Procedural failures in LVA could have their origin in an improper selection of location, an afunctional lymph collector, choice of an inadequate venule or mistaken arterial perforator, incorrect execution of supermicrosurgical anastomosis with lack of patency, backflow of blood into the lymph collector due to untreated/uncovered vein insufficiency, or tension on wound closure. A large number of LVAs should be closely examined due to a high occlusion rate of approximately 50% after 2 years.[16,17]

Faulty execution VLNT could be due to a free tissue transplant without the inclusion of lymph nodes (e.g., possible with gastroepiploic transplants) or too few lymph nodes (< 3), insufficient preparation of the recipient site without scar removal or enough space, inadequate preparation of the recipient's vein, incorrect anastomosis leading to a nonperfused transplant, or wound closure with tension compromising venous outflow. Under all circumstances, donor site lymphedema should be avoided, which is also a therapeutic failure.

Incorrect handling and technique of suction-assisted lipectomy or noncompliance in adhering to compression garments can additionally harm the last functioning lymph collectors, worsening the lymphedema. Precise anatomic knowledge and intraoperative lymphatic mapping decrease the risk of damage.

Another reason for therapeutic failure could be an inadequate patient assessment algorithm, choosing the wrong patients with the wrong stage for the selected treatment. Additionally, the postoperative treatment protocol could be a source of error regarding wound care, timing, and strength of reapplication of compression garments, mobilization, and start of lymphatic drainage, e.g., the patient could be a source of failure: noncompliant patients incapable of following adequate postoperative protocols or conservative treatment modalities do not recommend themselves for further treatment.[18]

In the event of obvious failure, a case discussion with other experts or referral to gain a second opinion for both the patient and the surgeon including evaluation by a lymphatic therapist is highly recommended, as the field requires ongoing experience and evidence to provide the best patient care.

16.7.2 Secondary Procedures

After the identification of possible reasons for therapeutic failure or a lack of response, available secondary options should be considered to improve the outcome.

In **Chapter 18** an algorithmic approach with the sequential use of surgical procedures is proposed. Further, based on **Subchapter 16.4** secondary options depend on a thorough re-evaluation of the patient's needs with all available modalities for diagnostic workup (see **Chapter 4**).

In select cases with decreased dermal backflow due to previous lymphatic surgery as a partial therapeutic response, it is possible to detect additional lymph collectors available for LVA, which were not found in the initial assessment but can be proven by a modality for deep collectors such as MRI or lymphoscintigraphy. It is also possible to perform a "blind" LVA guided by anatomical landmarks.[19,20] After skin incision, fluorescent imaging, e.g., with a microscope, could also reveal additional lymph collectors. The more the number of LVAs performed, the better the outcome should be, as the occlusion rate of 50% should be taken into consideration.[16,17]

Additional second or third lymph node transplants can be performed distal or proximal to the primary location after VLNT or as a primary VLNT transfer after initial LVA without a significant or expected response.[21,22,23,24] Choosing a transplant with a large number of lymph nodes, scar removal at the recipient site, vein preparation, and tensionless wound closure is crucial. Gustafsson et al. demonstrated that transplants with more than three lymph nodes have a significant better effect on the clinical outcome.[25]

In some stages of progression, with or without significant adipose cell hypertrophy, reductive or lymphoablative surgery is inevitable. Although suction-assisted lipectomy is increasingly added as an effective tool after partial response or therapeutic failure to reduce volume, lymphoablative procedures such as the Charles or Homans procedure are still rarely indicated and should be considered very carefully due to its associated high surgery-induced morbidity (see **Chapters 13** and **14** and **Subchapter 15.2**).[26] In rare cases with acute life-threatening conditions, such as uncontrolled or repetitive infections of the extremity or possible erosion of vessels, amputation is inescapable.

References

[1] Schook CC, Mulliken JB, Fishman SJ, Alomari AI, Grant FD, Greene AK. Differential diagnosis of lower extremity enlargement in pediatric patients referred with a diagnosis of lymphedema. Plast Reconstr Surg. 2011; 127(4):1571–1581

[2] Maclellan RA, Couto RA, Sullivan JE, Grant FD, Slavin SA, Greene AK. Management of primary and secondary lymphedema: analysis of 225 referrals to a center. Ann Plast Surg. 2015; 75(2):197–200

[3] Brorson H, Svensson H. Liposuction combined with controlled compression therapy reduces arm lymphedema more effectively than controlled compression therapy alone. Plast Reconstr Surg. 1998; 102(4):1058–1067, discussion 1068

[4] Brorson H, Ohlin K, Olsson G, Nilsson M. Adipose tissue dominates chronic arm lymphedema following breast cancer: an analysis using volume rendered CT images. Lymphat Res Biol. 2006; 4(4):199–210

[5] Brorson H, Ohlin K, Olsson G, Karlsson MK. Breast cancer-related chronic arm lymphedema is associated with excess adipose and muscle tissue. Lymphat Res Biol. 2009; 7(1):3–10

[6] Greene AK, Maclellan RA. Operative treatment of lymphedema using suction-assisted lipectomy. Ann Plast Surg. 2016; 77(3):337–340

[7] Narushima M, Mihara M, Yamamoto Y, Iida T, Koshima I, Mundinger GS. The intravascular stenting method for treatment of extremity lymphedema with multiconfiguration lymphaticovenous anastomoses. Plast Reconstr Surg. 2010; 125(3):935–943

[8] Nguyen AT, Suami H. Laparoscopic free omental lymphatic flap for the treatment of lymphedema. Plast Reconstr Surg. 2015; 136(1): 114–118

[9] Pons G, Masia J, Loschi P, Nardulli ML, Duch J. A case of donor-site lymphoedema after lymph node-superficial circumflex iliac artery perforator flap transfer. J Plast Reconstr Aesthet Surg. 2014; 67(1): 119–123

[10] Viitanen TP, Mäki MT, Seppänen MP, Suominen EA, Saaristo AM. Donor-site lymphatic function after microvascular lymph node transfer. Plast Reconstr Surg. 2012; 130(6):1246–1253

[11] Miranda Garcés M, Mirapeix R, Pons G, Sadri A, Masià J. A comprehensive review of the natural lymphaticovenous communications and their role in lymphedema surgery. J Surg Oncol. 2016; 113(4):374–380

[12] Hadamitzky C, Pabst R, Gordon K, Vogt PM. Surgical procedures in lymphedema management. J Vasc Surg Venous Lymphat Disord. 2014; 2(4):461–468

[13] Masià J, Pons G, Rodríguez-Bauzà E. Barcelona lymphedema algorithm for surgical treatment in breast cancer-related lymphedema. J Reconstr Microsurg. 2016; 32(5):329–335

[14] Chang EI, Masià J, Smith ML. Combining autologous breast reconstruction and vascularized lymph node transfer. Semin Plast Surg. 2018; 32(1):36–41

[15] Fish ML, Grover R, Schwarz GS. Quality-of-life outcomes in surgical vs nonsurgical treatment of breast cancer-related lymphedema: a systematic review. JAMA Surg. 2020; 155(6):513–519

[16] Maegawa J, Yabuki Y, Tomoeda H, Hosono M, Yasumura K. Outcomes of lymphaticovenous side-to-end anastomosis in peripheral lymphedema. J Vasc Surg. 2012; 55(3):753–760

[17] Tourani SS, Taylor GI, Ashton MW. Long-term patency of lymphovenous anastomoses: a systematic review. Plast Reconstr Surg. 2016; 138(2):492–498

[18] Ha Dinh TT, Bonner A, Clark R, Ramsbotham J, Hines S. The effectiveness of the teach-back method on adherence and self-management in health education for people with chronic disease: a systematic review. JBI Database Syst Rev Implement Reports. 2016; 14(1):210–247

[19] Seki Y, Kajikawa A, Yamamoto T, Takeuchi T, Terashima T, Kurogi N. Single lymphaticovenular anastomosis for early-stage lower extremity lymphedema treated by the superior-edge-of-the-knee incision method. Plast Reconstr Surg Glob Open. 2018; 6(2):e1679

[20] Seki Y, Kajikawa A, Yamamoto T, Takeuchi T, Terashima T, Kurogi N. Real-time indocyanine green videolymphography navigation for lymphaticovenular anastomosis. Plast Reconstr Surg Glob Open. 2019; 7(5):e2253

[21] Ciudad P, Manrique OJ, Adabi K, et al. Combined double vascularized lymph node transfers and modified radical reduction with preservation of perforators for advanced stages of lymphedema. J Surg Oncol. 2019; 119(4):439–448

[22] Ciudad P, Manrique OJ, Date S, et al. Double gastroepiploic vascularized lymph node tranfers to middle and distal limb for the treatment of lymphedema. Microsurgery. 2017; 37(7):771–779

[23] Ito R, Lin MC, Cheng MH. Simultaneous bilateral submental lymph node flaps for lower limb lymphedema post leg Charles procedure. Plast Reconstr Surg Glob Open. 2015; 3(9):e513

[24] Kenworthy EO, Nelson JA, Verma R, Mbabuike J, Mehrara BJ, Dayan JH. Double vascularized omentum lymphatic transplant (VOLT) for the treatment of lymphedema. J Surg Oncol. 2018; 117 (7):1413–1419

[25] Gustafsson J, Chu SY, Chan WH, Cheng MH. Correlation between quantity of transferred lymph nodes and outcome in vascularized submental lymph node flap transfer for lower limb lymphedema. Plast Reconstr Surg. 2018; 142(4):1056–1063

[26] Park KE, Allam O, Chandler L, et al. Surgical management of lymphedema: a review of current literature. Gland Surg. 2020; 9(2): 503–511

Section VIII

Training, Treatment Algorithm, Outcomes, and Further Developments

Edited by Christoph Hirche, Yves Harder, and Moustapha Hamdi

VIII

17 Teaching and Training in Lymphoreconstructive Surgery

Amir Bigdeli and Christoph Hirche

Summary

Lymphovenous anastomosis and vascularized lymph node transfer have been demonstrated to be efficient and inevitable for the treatment of lymphedema. However, the management of lymphatic vessels based on supermicrosurgical techniques is even more difficult as they are smaller, thinner, less visible, and more fragile than blood vessels. Although microsurgical techniques are routinely taught to plastic surgeons, supermicrosurgery, which is regularly not part of this training, demands an even higher skill set. In addition, magnification extenders and special instruments and sutures are necessary. Thus, several training models have been developed for training supermicrosurgical techniques. They can be divided into nonbiological or biological in vivo and ex vivo training models as well as simulators using virtual reality or augmented virtual reality. The demand of an even higher level of dexterity and surgical precision for successful handling of lymphatic vessels has opened the way for robotic-assisted surgery. The ultraprecision of robotic-assisted surgery by minimizing the surgeon's tremor as well as its superior imaging system can be of great benefit and thus improve supermicrosurgery.

Keywords: competences, lymphedema, lymphedema surgery, microsurgery, next generation, robotics, robotic-assisted surgery (RAS), robotic supermicrosurgery, skills, surgeon's tremor, teaching, training, training models

17.1 Introduction

Advances in microsurgery have paved the way for new surgical options for the treatment of lymphedema. Classified as physiologic methods, lymphovenous anastomosis (LVA) and vascularized lymph node transfer (VLNT) have revolutionized the causative treatment of lymphedema.[1,2,3] Especially, supermicrosurgical LVA and multiple LVA (see **Chapter 8**) have been demonstrated to be efficient for the treatment of lymphedema.[4] However, the management of lymphatic vessels is even more difficult because they are thinner, smaller, less visible, and more fragile than blood vessels. The necessary skills differ from that required for conventional microsurgery.[5] In particular, an even higher level of dexterity and surgical precision with reduced tremor for successful supermicrosurgical dissection and anastomosis of lymphatic vessels, which normally range from 0.3 to 0.8 mm in diameter, is needed.[6]

Microsurgical techniques are routinely taught to plastic surgeons. However, supermicrosurgery demands meticulous eye–microscope–hand coordination, more dexterous tissues handling, and even more refined motor skills and control, which are not part of this basic training.[7] It is obvious that these technical skills can only be acquired through extensive training and practice before they can be appropriately applied on humans.[3] Consequently, there is an increased need for supermicrosurgical training to enable microsurgeons to rapidly acquire the needed skill set to overcome the demand for lymphatic surgery.

Until now, there are several training models available for supermicrosurgical techniques. They can be divided into *nonbiological* or *biological, in vivo* and *ex vivo* training models.[3]

17.2 Supermicrosurgical Training Models without the Use of Lymphatic Vessels

Matsumura et al. developed a practice card model for gaining basic supermicrosurgical skills.[8] Small-caliber silicone tubes with an external diameter of 0.3, 0.5, or 0.7 mm and a tube wall thickness of 0.05 mm are fixed to the pocketbook-size practice card (14 cm × 7.5 cm). It is ideally suited for repeatedly practicing basic supermicrosurgical techniques and for warming up before surgery. This nonbiological, ex vivo training model can be used either outside of the operating room (OR) or with the operating microscope in the OR in order to practice or warm up supermicrosurgical techniques.[8] Consequently, nonbiological, ex vivo synthetic models are suited for acquiring fundamental supermicrosurgical skills, for example, handling of supermicrosurgical tools and learning of microscopic adjustments, but do not leave room to train supermicrosurgical dissection.[3] When the microsurgeons have achieved basic skills and have become comfortable with the microscope and supermicrosurgical instruments, they can proceed to biological, ex vivo training models for advanced skill acquisition.[3] The chicken thigh model has been introduced by Chen et al. for this purpose.[7] It was developed to terminate the use of the established live rat models with ongoing ethical discussion as the biological, ex vivo model is more accessible and less expensive for training. Using overall available chicken thighs, the ischiatic neurovascular bundle is identified where the branching pattern of the ischiatic artery and vein shows vessel diameters in the range of 0.3 to 0.8 mm. Using these branches, supermicrosurgical anastomoses can be successfully performed. Thus, the chicken thigh is a convenient and economical model for supermicrosurgical training with appropriate vessel diameters. This nonliving biologic model is suitable for developing or refining supermicrosurgical skills. Its major advantage over nonbiological, ex vivo models is that the surgeon receives tactile feedback similar to human tissue and allows dissection training.[7] Recently, Cifuentes and colleagues presented a new biological, ex vivo training model using a chicken leg.[9] A musculocutaneous perforator vessel whose source vessel is the medial tibial artery, a branch of the popliteal artery, is identified and dissected until arterial diameters reach 0.7, 0.5, and 0.3 mm. Under 22.5 times microscope magnification, arterial anastomoses are performed on 0.3- and 0.5-mm diameter arteries using nylon 11–0 and 12–0 sutures. The investigators pronounced the chicken leg model as a simple alternative training model for acquisition and training of supermicrosurgical skills, which is reproducible and easily accessible.[9]

After sufficient development of supermicrosurgical skills using ex vivo training models, practicing on in vivo models is the next step. To date, several in vivo animal training models have been introduced for training handling of submillimeter vessels. In 2008, Yamashita and colleagues introduced the superficial inferior epigastric artery (SIEA) flap in the rat for supermicrosurgical training and concluded that the SIEA flap was an ideal model for developing supermicrosurgical skills including dissection.[10] In 2011, Sakrak et al. described the rat tail revascularization model as a time-saving microsurgical exercise for advanced microsurgical training and research.[11] They stated that the rat tail revascularization model provided practical training for advanced microsurgical training.[11] Liu published another in vivo rat model for the training of anastomosis of submillimeter vessels using the segment of the femoral vessels which was lying on the ventral muscle group of the hind limb.[5] The mean diameters of the femoral artery and vein were 0.54 and 0.56 mm, respectively. The author reports that the consistent anatomy and size of the femoral vessels makes the model suitable for training supermicrosurgical anastomosis of submillimeter vessels.[5]

17.3 Supermicrosurgical Training Models with the Use of Lymphatic Vessels

In 2016, Onoda and colleagues introduced a novel in vivo training model for LVA, as only a few models that used lymphatics for direct handling for supermicrosurgical training were available.[12] Their relatively simple LVA model using the lumbar lymphatic duct (mean diameter of 0.61 mm) and iliolumbar veins (mean diameter of 0.81 mm) of rats showed that the diameter, nature, and placement of the end-to-end anastomosis were very similar to surgery in human.[12] Another supermicrosurgical lymphaticovenular anastomosis in vivo model was introduced by Yamamoto and colleagues.[13] Using ICG lymphangiography, lymphatic vessels in the posteromedial aspect of the rat high are identified and dissected. The largest lymphatic vessel is then anastomosed to the short saphenous vein or its branch in an end-to-end manner. Patency of the anastomosis is evaluated intraoperatively and, on the 7th, postoperative day. The investigators found that the course of lymphatic vessels in the rat thigh was constant, running along the short saphenous vein. The mean diameter of lymphatic vessels and the short saphenous vein were 0.240 ± 0.057 mm and 0.370 ± 0.146 mm, respectively, and thus ideally suitable for a supermicrosurgical LVA training model. They concluded that rat lymphatic vessels were thin, translucent, and fragile similar to human lymphatic vessels and thus stated that the presented in vivo LVA model is useful for the training of supermicrosurgical LVA.[13]

17.4 Supermicrosurgical Training Models with the Use of Lymphatic Vessels for Different Types of Lymphovenous Anastomosis and for Vascularized Lymph Node Transfer

Recently, Campisi et al. presented an adaptable living porcine model, which is suitable for training to practice several advanced lymphatic microsurgical techniques, including LVA and VLNT, in the same animal.[14] Due to the limited number of models for lymphatic microsurgical training, Leuzzi and colleagues developed a training model for MLVAs in rats.[15] Using Patent Blue V injection in lumbar lymph nodes, two to four lymphatic vessels were identified in the region. MLVAs were then established through anastomosing end-to-end to the right lumbar vein. They concluded that their simple and reliable MLVA in vivo model could be very useful for supermicrosurgical training.[15] However, as the limited number of LVA training models implemented only end-to-end LVA, Malagón-López and colleagues recently presented a new in vivo training model in rats to practice both end-to-end and end-to-side lymphovenous anastomoses using the iliolumbar vein and ureter.[16] They promoted their model for LVA training because of the similarity in the color, fragility, and diameter of the vessels (rat ureter: 0.3–0.5 mm, human lymphatic vessel: 0.2–0.8 mm).[16]

Lastly, several models have been developed to acquire supermicrosurgical skills, but there is a relative lack of validation and standardization in education and training.[17]

As the clinical relevance, purpose, and validation of these training models have not been addressed yet, Pafitanis and colleagues recently reviewed the available literature in order to summarize the existing supermicrosurgical training models and their impact on training for supermicrosurgical anastomosis of submillimeter vessels.[17] A total of 36 out of 390 identified articles were included in the reviewing process, wherein 15 supermicrosurgery training models could be identified. The simulation models were classified as nonbiological or biological and as ex vivo or in vivo.[17] Being the first review to highlight the clinical relevance of supermicrosurgery training models and the need for validation, a variety of training models were identified to enable the acquisition of the specific skills.[17] Furthermore, a ladder-based curriculum for supermicrosurgical training was established.

17.5 Robotic-Assisted Lymphedema Surgery

Robotic-assisted surgery (RAS) is defined as a surgery which is performed by a human surgeon through the use of a robotic instrument.[18] RAS has already revolutionized the field of minimally invasive surgery. It has further made its way into various surgical specialties, including plastic and reconstructive surgery. It is obvious that the unique features of RAS predestine the technique for microsurgery as no other surgical field requires that level of precision.[18] Consequently, this microsurgical specialty is extremely technically demanding and challenging and may exceed the limits of human precision.

RAS has been validated to improve the radius of movements for the surgical hand, providing access to deep, difficult to approach regions and significantly reducing the surgeon's tremor, thus addressing reliability and reproducibility in microsurgery.

Note:

For lymphatic surgery, RAS can be applied both to assist harvest of intraabdominal VLNT as a minimally invasive procedure or to improve ergonomy and handling by reducing the surgeon's tremor in modern lymphatic (super-)microsurgery.

Accordingly, the ultraprecision of RAS as well as its superior imaging system can be of great benefit and thus facilitate a more reliable use of supermicrosurgery.[18]

Recently, Ibrahim and colleagues presented an overview of clinical applications of RAS.[18] They evaluated the Da Vinci robot for LVA surgery and found it promising for this application.[18] Not only did they recommend the robotic system because of its tremor elimination, but also found that it allowed fast transitioning between normal bright field and near-infrared laser vision, which provided a dynamic method for mapping the lymphatic vascular network and the visualization of ICG diffusion patterns.[18] Furthermore, they reported that the setup for robotic lymphatic microsurgery was relatively straightforward.[18] Nevertheless, the Da Vinci platform has not been primarily designed for microsurgery or supermicrosurgery, when using the moveable instruments. Size and relation do not perfectly match demands of needles and instruments for vessels of 0.3 mm and sutures of 12–0 size. That is why the search for additional platforms exclusively designed for microsurgery has continued and revealed two remarkable platforms:

- The MUSA robotic system (MicroSure, Eindhoven, The Netherlands) has been exclusively designed for reconstructive microsurgery and has been validated in a first human randomized pilot trial in breast cancer-related lymphedema for LVA. The MUSA is designed to aid in stabilizing movements of the microsurgeon by filtering tremors and scaling down motions. The platform is added to the classical OR microscope and uses classical microinstruments connected to the robotic arms.
- The Symani microsurgical robotic platform with specific, paired, disposable, sterile microinstruments (MMI S.p.A., Calci-Pisa, Italy) has been exclusively developed for microsurgery and supermicrosurgery. The robotic platform includes an ergonomic OR chair with input devices for the control of the paired instruments; the suspension arms with adapters for the paired instruments are placed around the classical OR microscope in this platform (▶ Fig. 17.1). The robotic platform has already been validated for LVA surgery (see **Chapter 8** and **Fig. 8.3**).[19]

Both the platforms have different technical features and concepts for the surgeon (e.g., input devices, instruments), but share the common feature of using the preexisting OR microscope, improving the radius of movements for the surgical hand and reducing the surgeon's tremor, thus addressing reliability and reproducibility in microsurgery.

Training for robotic platforms and supermicrosurgery in general can be successfully addressed with VR simulation, which has the strength to provide training without the use of specific physical models, and allows trainer supervision, video recall of training, and 24-hour access (▶ Fig. 17.2).

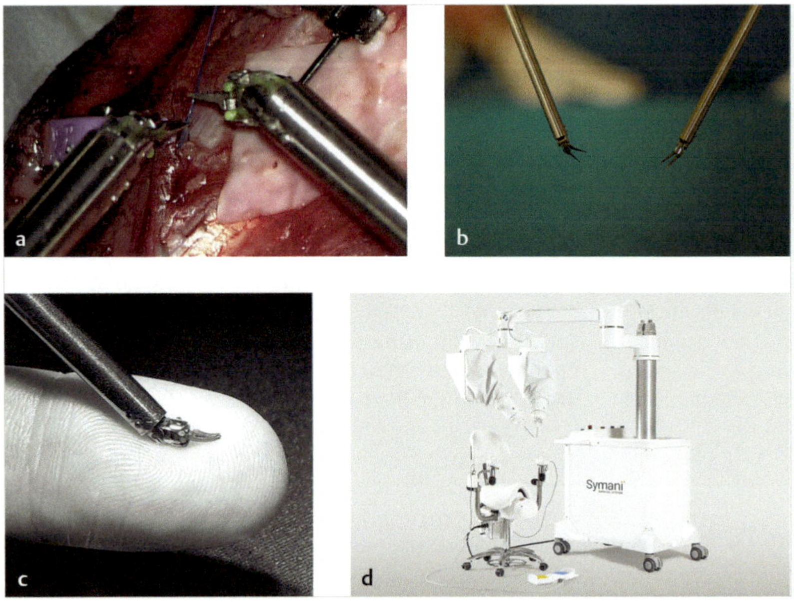

Fig. 17.1 **(a)** Cannulation of lymphatic vessel with a segment of 6/0 nylon suture using the robotic platform. (Courtesy of Marco Innocenti and Gerardo Malzone.) **(b, c)** Frontal view of the paired disposable, sterile microinstruments, which have a great range of motion, and in relation to a fingertip. **(d)** The complete robotic platform includes an ergonomic chair for the operating room with input devices for the remote control of the paired instruments; the suspension arms include adapters to fix the paired instruments around the classical microscope included in this platform. (Microsurgical robotic platform and microinstruments by Medical Microinstruments, S.p.A., Calci-Pisa, Italy).

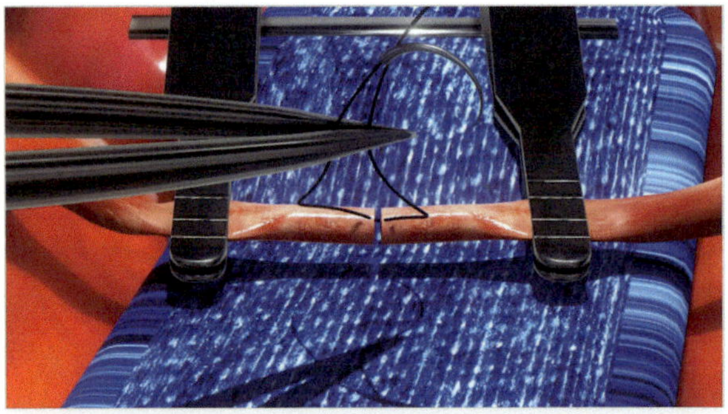

Fig. 17.2 Screen of a virtual reality microsurgical training full simulator (VR Magic, Mannheim, Germany), addressing training of residents without animal models using an electromagnetically tracked input device. The full simulator facilitates curriculum training, trainer supervision, as well as the video recall of the sessions.

References

[1] Scaglioni MF, Fontein DBY, Arvanitakis M, Giovanoli P. Systematic review of lymphovenous anastomosis (LVA) for the treatment of lymphedema. Microsurgery. 2017; 37(8):947–953

[2] Lee BB, Andrade M, Antignani PL, et al. International Union of Phlebology. Diagnosis and treatment of primary lymphedema. Consensus document of the International Union of Phlebology (IUP)-2013. Int Angiol. 2013; 32(6):541–574

[3] Badash I, Gould DJ, Patel KM. Supermicrosurgery: history, applications, training and the future. Front Surg. 2018; 5:23

[4] Boccardo F, Valenzano M, Costantini S, et al. LYMPHA technique to prevent secondary lower limb lymphedema. Ann Surg Oncol. 2016; 23(11):3558–3563

[5] Liu H-L. Microvascular anastomosis of submillimeter vessels—a training model in rats. J Hand Microsurg. 2013; 5(1):14–17

[6] Koshima I, Yamamoto T, Narushima M, Mihara M, Iida T. Perforator flaps and supermicrosurgery. Clin Plast Surg. 2010; 37(4):683–689, vii–iii

[7] Chen WF, Eid A, Yamamoto T, Keith J, Nimmons GL, Lawrence WT. A novel supermicrosurgery training model: the chicken thigh. J Plast Reconstr Aesthet Surg. 2014; 67(7):973–978

[8] Matsumura N, Horie Y, Shibata T, Kubo M, Hayashi N, Endo S. Basic training model for supermicrosurgery: a novel practice card model. J Reconstr Microsurg. 2011; 27(6):377–382

[9] Cifuentes IJ, Rodriguez JR, Yañez RA, et al. A novel ex vivo training model for acquiring supermicrosurgical skills using a chicken leg. J Reconstr Microsurg. 2016; 32(9):699–705

[10] Yamashita S, Sugiyama N, Hasegawa K, Namba Y, Kimata Y. A novel model for supermicrosurgery training: the superficial inferior epigastric artery flap in rats. J Reconstr Microsurg. 2008; 24(8): 537–543

[11] Şakrak T, Köse AA, Karabağli Y, Koçman AE, Ozbayoğlu AC, Cetin C. Rat tail revascularization model for advanced microsurgery training and research. J Reconstr Microsurg. 2011; 27(7):391–396

[12] Onoda S, Kimata Y, Matsumoto K. A novel lymphaticovenular anastomosis rat model. Ann Plast Surg. 2016; 76(3):332–335

[13] Yamamoto T, Yamamoto N, Yamashita M, Furuya M, Hayashi A, Koshima I. Establishment of supermicrosurgical lymphaticovenular anastomosis model in rat. Microsurgery. 2017; 37(1):57–60

[14] Campisi CC, Jiga LP, Ryan M, di Summa PG, Campisi C, Ionac M. Mastering lymphatic microsurgery: a new training model in living tissue. Ann Plast Surg. 2017; 79(3):298–303

[15] Leuzzi S, Maruccia M, Elia R, et al. Lymphatic-venous anastomosis in a rat model: a novel exercise for microsurgical training. J Surg Oncol. 2018; 118(6):936–940

[16] Malagón-López P, Carrasco-López C, Vilà J, Pi-Folguera J, Higueras-Suñe C. Supermicrosurgery training model for lymphaticovenous anastomosis in advanced lymphedema by iliolumbar vein and ureter anastomosis in the rat. Microsurgery. 2019; 39(5):480–481

[17] Pafitanis G, Narushima M, Yamamoto T, et al. Evolution of an evidence-based supermicrosurgery simulation training curriculum: a systematic review. J Plast Reconstr Aesthet Surg. 2018; 71(7): 976–988

[18] Ibrahim AE, Sarhane KA, Selber JC. New frontiers in robotic-assisted microsurgical reconstruction. Clin Plast Surg. 2017; 44(2): 415–423

[19] Innocenti M. Robotics in super-microsurgery: making a more reliable and reproducible surgery. Oral presentation, World Society of Lymphatic Surgery, Barcelona, Spain, October 2020

18 Treatment Algorithm for the Surgical Management of Lymphedema

Christoph Hirche, Moustapha Hamdi, Katrin Seidenstücker, and Yves Harder

Summary

Individualized, stage-dependent treatment of lymphedema requires both decisive diagnostic workup of the affected tissue and the remaining function of the lymphatic system as well as provision of various surgical techniques. Reconstructive procedures are promising and improve the outcome if functional lymphatic collectors are visible and approachable (lymphovenous anastomosis) or at least the tissue of the affected extremity has a chance to partly recover and promote rearrangement of the lymphatic flow by vascularized lymph node transfer. If not indicated, suction-assisted lipectomy in patients with predominant adipogenesis during stage progression without major fibrosis can help to permanently resolve the weight and circumference, and improve quality of life in conjunction with lifelong complete decongestive therapy and compression therapy. Lymphoreductive or local excisional surgery is indicated when fibrotic tissue changes are predominant to reduce the burden of weight and functional limitation. A treatment algorithm enabling the reader to provide the patients a decisive diagnostic workup followed by individual, stage-dependent surgical decisions is provided, addressing lower and upper extremity lymphedema, breast cancer-related lymphedema and lymphedema characterized by fibrosis of fat hypertrophy.

Keywords: algorithm, autologous lymph vessel transfer (ALVT), breast cancer-related lymphedema, functional collectors, lymphedema, lymphoablative, lymphovenous anastomosis (LVA), lymph node to vein anastomosis (LNVA), lymphangiography, lower extremity, reconstructive, treatment, vascularized lymph node transfer (VLNT)

18.1 Introduction

A patient who undergoes surgery for chronic lymphedema deserves individual, stage-dependent treatment, including specific pre- and postsurgical measures, both related to diagnostic (see **Chapter 4**) and therapeutic procedures (see **Chapters 8–14**).

Essentially, primary and secondary lymphedemas should be approached in the same way regarding diagnostic measures, although treatment options may vary depending on lymphedema stage and presence or absence of a functional lymphatic system, i.e., lymphatic collectors and lymph nodes.

As a matter of course, the cornerstone of surgical lymphedema treatment is conservative treatment defined as complete decongestive therapy (CDT). Surgery that is offered to treat chronic lymphedema consists of a wide range of different procedures that are classified into reconstructive or derivative and reductive or lymphoablative techniques. The latter includes suction-assisted lipectomy (see **Chapter 13**) and reductive or ecsisional surgeries of different kinds (see **Chapter 14**). Reconstructive or derivative procedures comprise lymphovenous anastomosis (see **Chapter 8**), autologous lymph vessel transfer (see **Chapter 9**), vascularized lymph node transfer (see **Chapters 10** and **11**), and in rare cases lymph node venous anastomosis, usually performed in emerging countries for postinfectious lymphedema (see **Chapter 12**).

Worldwide, all these techniques are offered and performed according to personal habits and experience and local conditions and requirements, most often as a consequence of existing and available competence and infrastructure. The following chapter presents the current use of surgical techniques that have gained most popularity worldwide based on the number of treated cases and underlying evidence.

Currently, reconstructive surgery to address chronic lymphedema has become quite popular. Accordingly, an increasing number of surgeons are starting to treat cases without always having neither the multiprofessional setting nor the surgical skills to correctly perform this type of surgery on these patients. It is therefore of particular importance that surgical standards should be defined based upon registries to be created, and outcome-related quality should be evaluated in order to progressively create scientific evidence.

Every patient with chronic lymphedema requires CDT, which is effective in reducing the burden of lymphedema and hence improving the functional outcome and eventually quality of life in up to 90% of all patients. Prior to reconstructive surgery, it is advisable to undergo CDT for a period of at least 6 months in order to "get the best out" of the affected extremity and to significantly reduce the pitting component of the edema, i.e., to improve lymphatic decongestion and reduce filtration by lymphatic drainage, respectively, through compression.

For patients who do not respond well to CDT despite continuous application, including stagnation of decongestion or even increase of edema, persistent functional impairment, and reduced quality of life or simply desire for improvement, the lymphatic therapist and lymphologist should direct the patient to plastic surgeons and microsurgeons specialized in reductive and/or reconstructive lymphedema surgery and collaborate within their network (see **Chapters 5, 8, 9, 10** and **11**).

18.2 Diagnostics

Besides thorough patient history and clinical examination, imaging plays a crucial role, which nowadays consists mainly of MRI and ICG lymphangiography (see **Chapter 4**).

ICG lymphangiography is regarded as the workhorse and "screening tool" to visualize the condition of the superficial lymphatic system, since it may demonstrate both the existence of functional lymphatic collectors as well as define areas of damaged and nonfunctional lymphatic network.[1,2] Due to its limitation to visualize lymphatic vessels in the depth of the subcutaneous tissues, especially in areas of pronounced dermal backflow, lymphoscintigraphy may still play a role as the standard diagnostic tool because it can visualize lymph collecting structures in the depth of the subcutaneous tissues. However, lymphoscintigraphy has limitations when it comes to defining functionality and/or localizing lymphatic vessels. Accordingly, there is an increasing request for MRI with MIP, which is indicated when examining an affected extremity or region of the body in an integral way. MRI with or without contrast agent has the advantage of not only assessing lymph collecting vessels, but also venules in their vicinity, free fluid within the soft tissues, and fat hypertrophy, and finally quantifying volume of the affected extremity, always in comparison to the contralateral side that in many cases is nonaffected. Of interest, MRI with a contrast agent allows for a three-dimensional visualization of a potential postsurgical lymphovascular remodelling.[3] High-frequency ultrasound can be additionally used as an investigator-dependent modality to both localize and evaluate lymph collectors and veins, and their flow characteristics using color-coded duplex.[4,5]

The minimal diagnostic assessment should therefore include standardized circumferential measurements, ideally every 4 cm of the extremity, always in comparison to the contralateral side, using tables to calculate volume as a valuable alternative to water displacement or MRI volumetry. Lymphedema-related quality of life questionnaires with defined scores that are presented to the patients in their native language should complete diagnostical workup.

This diagnostic approach should be applied before surgical treatment to define a sort of baseline for the long-term follow-up in order to objectify surgery-related outcome.

Thereby, it is crucial to always take into consideration not only the regional swelling that is resistant to conservative treatment, but also the existence or nonexistence of functional lymphatic collectors in order to indicate the most appropriate treatment to every single patient that should be personalized to every individual case. This can be objectified by ICG lymphangiography or MRL and helps to understand the individual disease state and its underlying morphological changes (▶ Fig. 18.1).

According to personal experience of the editors and based on currently available scientific evidence mostly described in this textbook, surgical treatment of lymphedema should be offered as follows in the text and with reference to ▶ Fig. 18.2.

18.3 Modern Surgical Management of Chronic Lymphedema

18.3.1 Surgery for Lymphedema Presenting with Functional Lymphatic Collectors

Lymphedema stage I and II according to ISL with the presence of functional lymph collectors detected following preoperative imaging or surgical exploration and after exclusion of chronic venous insufficiency that may aggravate lymphedema due to compromised venous drainage should be treated with LVA (see **Chapter 8**). LVA is regarded a less invasive surgery when compared with (see **Chapter 10**). Technically, LVA can be performed with local anesthesia, and is associated with a comparable outcome when compared to VLNT, assuming that surgery has been indicated correctly.[6,7]

If functionality of lymphatic collectors is unclear after preoperative imaging, surgical exploration for LVA can be indicated in select cases, clearly informing the patient that the procedure has a certain risk to end up in the impossibility of performing LVA due to absent or nonfunctional lymphatic collectors and/or adjacent draining veins.[8] Accordingly, surgery can be terminated without performing LVA or continued by converting to VLNT, depending upon how the patient has decided and consented to undergo surgery (▶ Fig. 18.2).

18.3.2 Surgery for Lymphedema Lacking Functional Lymphatic Collectors

For patients who present with a nonreversible and even progressive stage II or higher lymphedema, which is determined by an absence of functional lymphatic collectors according to preoperative imaging, as well as for patients who do not consent to surgical exploration for LVA with increased risk for unsuitable collectors,[8] VLNT is recommended straight away.

VLNT has demonstrated to have a slightly superior outcome when compared to all other reconstructive procedures in advanced stages of lymphedema; nevertheless, it bears the risk of a collateral damage at the donor site, including impaired lymphatic function without visible

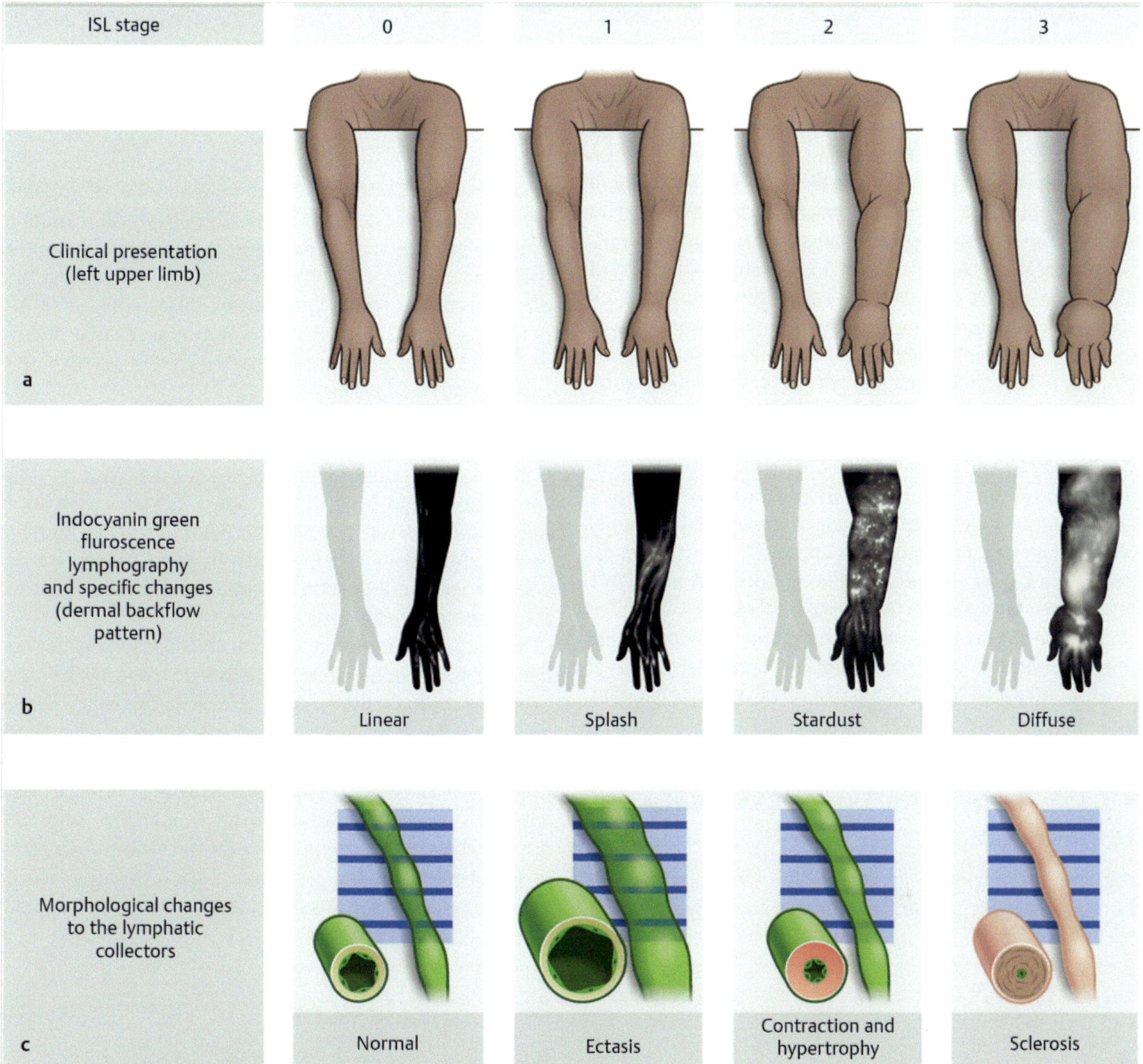

Fig. 18.1 The International Society of Lymphology stages 1–3 of lymphedema are in direct correlation with the stage-dependent alterations seen in ICG green lymphangiography and the underlying morphological changes of the lymphatic collecting vessels. The correlation between clinical stage, functional alteration, and morphological changes helps to understand the necessity of an algorithmic approach to diagnose and eventually treat each individual lymphedema stage.

swelling and with visible swelling in 10% and 2%, respectively (see **Chapter 10**).[9,10,11]

This is one of the reasons to continuously search for the ideal donor site, the optimal surgical technique to prepare the lymph node flap, and future approaches that are based upon tissue engineering (▶ Fig. 18.2).

18.3.3 Surgery for Breast Cancer-Related Lymphedema

Patients who have undergone breast cancer-associated tumorectomy or mastectomy and/or axillary surgery (sentinel lymph node biopsy, axillary sampling, lymph node clearance) and/or adjuvant radiotherapy of the chest wall and/or adjacent lymph node basins and eventually develop secondary lymphedema of the upper extremity should be offered the following therapeutic treatment.

Usually, *de novo* breast reconstruction ideally using autologous tissue as well as axillary scar release and VLNT is recommended (see **Chapter 11**).[12,13] In these cases, the groin is an attractive donor site for VLNT (see **Chapter 10**) due to its vicinity to the abdominal adipocutaneous tissue that is the most common donor site for autologous breast reconstruction (deep inferior epigastric perforator [DIEP] flap). This approach allows anatomical reconstruction of the breast and partial restoration of lymphatics to the axilla. In these cases, it is advisable to completely separate the abdominal flap from the lymph node flap to best place the flap for breast reconstruction and hence shape the new breast and best place the lymph node flap to the axilla, eventually requiring two sets of arteriovenous microsurgical anastomoses. Whether a one-step or a two-step procedure using one or two individual flaps has to be offered is currently a matter of discussion within the scientific community. However, an orthotopic reconstruction should be offered in all cases that undergo synchronous scar release in the axillary region, i.e., the axilla being the recipient site, followed by heterotopic or combined ortho- and heterotopic reconstruction (see **Chapter 11**).

In select cases, some patients who undergo mastectomy and sentinel lymph node biopsy and axillary lymph node clearance with or without adjuvant radiotherapy with a high risk for secondary lymphedema can benefit from prophylactic surgery, including both LVA and VLNT during primary oncological surgery. Patients who have undergone mastectomy and suffer from subclinical lymphedema of the upper extremity despite conservative treatment can benefit from early reconstructive surgery including LVA or VLNT with scar release.

18.3.4 Surgery for Upper Extremity Lymphedema

For lymphedema in the upper extremity without any past history of surgery and/or radiotherapy to the lymph node basins adjacent to the axilla, one can indicate LVA in the presence of functional lymphatic vessels (stages I and II) and/or VLNT with heterotopic positioning of the flap usually at the wrist (for stages II and III) (▸ Fig. 18.2).

18.3.5 Surgery for Lower Extremity Lymphedema

If lymphedema results from inguinal lymph node dissection and/or radiotherapy, scar release surgery in combination with LVA in instances of functional lymphatic vessels and/or VLNT with orthotopic placement is recommended analogous to lymphatic reconstruction for breast cancer-related lymphedema. If proximal lymphatic damage is extensive, such as after iliacal and/or para-aortic lymphadenectomy, LVA is indicated in the event of functional lymphatic vessels and/or VLNT with heterotopic placement of the lymph node flap is recommended (▸ Fig. 18.2).

18.3.6 Surgery for Lymphedema with Fat Hypertrophy and/or Tissue Fibrosis

Some patients who have been successfully evaluated and would qualify for some kind of lymphoreconstructive procedure such as LVA or VLNT may refuse reconstructive surgery in favor of a debulking procedure that will guarantee a much quicker and more effective volume reduction of the affected arm or leg. These patients can be successfully offered *suction-assisted lipectomy* in the presence of fat hypertrophy (see **Chapter 13**). This technique can be offered as a stand-alone procedure requiring lifelong compression using customized garments.

Suction-assisted lipectomy further plays a major role in areas of the extremity refractory to LVA or VLNT, especially in cases after recurrent erysipelas (cellulitis). Accordingly, suction-assisted lipectomy can also accompany a microsurgical reconstructive procedure in a synchronous way or after about 3 to 6 months in order to increase the effect of volume reduction and eventually further improve the outcome of reconstructive surgery.

Reductive surgery using surgical ablation, such as dermolipectomy, should be limited to selected cases only, i.e., very advanced cases (stage IV and more or cases clearly refractory to reconstructive measures) (see **Chapter 14**). These cases are usually affected by a high amount of tissue fibrosis rather than fat hypertrophy, confirming the chronicity and advanced stage of the disease. These lymphoablative procedures still have a high significance for the surgical treatment of lymphedema of the genital area, the extremity, and in emerging countries that cannot always offer highly sophisticated surgeries (▸ Fig. 18.2).

18.4 Conclusions

We believe that it is of outmost importance to offer staged surgery, if the therapeutical approach consists of multiple procedures, in order to gain experience and hence foster scientific evidence that will allow to better define an adequate stage-dependent surgical treatment of chronic lymphedema. This is not possible if different surgical treatments are offered simultaneously. Furthermore, it is of outmost importance to evaluate preoperative imaging in great detail and address the whole extremity with the therapeutic plan.

One technique only fits to one stage, region, or extremity, not all. Accordingly, in selected cases, it may be useful to approach the distal part of the extremity with LVAs and the proximal part with VLNT, including scar release.

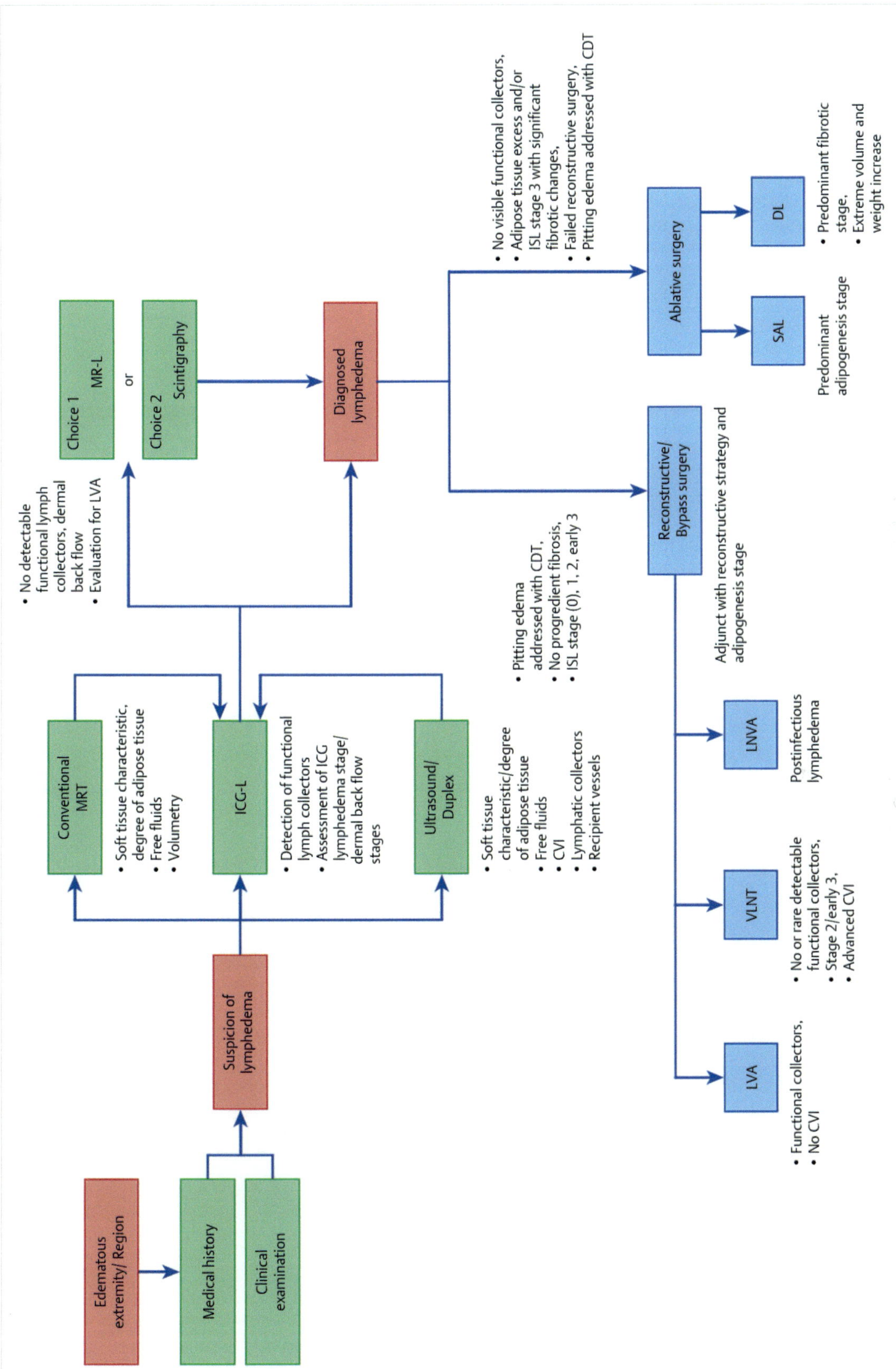

Fig. 18.2 Treatment algorithm for diagnostic workup and modern surgical management of lymphedema for lower and upper extremity lymphedema, breast cancer-related lymphedema, and lymphedema characterized by fibrosis of fat hypertrophy.

References

[1] Mihara M, Hara H, Araki J, et al. Indocyanine green (ICG) lymphography is superior to lymphoscintigraphy for diagnostic imaging of early lymphedema of the upper limbs. PLoS One. 2012; 7(6):e38182

[2] Yamamoto T, Yamamoto N, Doi K, et al. Indocyanine green-enhanced lymphography for upper extremity lymphedema: a novel severity staging system using dermal backflow patterns. Plast Reconstr Surg. 2011; 128(4):941-947

[3] Bae JS, Yoo RE, Choi SH, et al. Evaluation of lymphedema in upper extremities by MR lymphangiography: comparison with lymphoscintigraphy. Magn Reson Imaging. 2018; 49:63–70

[4] Hayashi A, Visconti G, Yamamoto T, et al. Intraoperative imaging of lymphatic vessel using ultra high-frequency ultrasound. J Plast Reconstr Aesthet Surg. 2018; 71(5):778–780

[5] Hayashi A, Yamamoto T, Yoshimatsu H, et al. Ultrasound visualization of the lymphatic vessels in the lower leg. Microsurgery. 2016; 36(5): 397–401

[6] Bianchi A, Salgarello M, Hayashi A, Yang JC, Visconti G. Recipient venule selection and anastomosis configuration for lymphaticovenular anastomosis in extremity lymphedema: algorithm based on 1,000 lymphaticovenular anastomosis. J Reconstr Microsurg. 2021

[7] Yang JC, Wu SC, Chiang MH, Lin WC, Hsieh CH. Intraoperative identification and definition of "functional" lymphatic collecting vessels for supermicrosurgical lymphatico-venous anastomosis in treating lymphedema patients. J Surg Oncol. 2018; 117(5):994–1000

[8] Yang JC, Wu SC, Lin WC, Chiang MH, Chiang PL, Hsieh CH. Supermicrosurgical lymphaticovenous anastomosis as alternative treatment option for moderate-to-severe lower limb lymphedema. J Am Coll Surg. 2020; 230(2):216–227

[9] Basta MN, Gao LL, Wu LC. Operative treatment of peripheral lymphedema: a systematic meta-analysis of the efficacy and safety of lymphovenous microsurgery and tissue transplantation. Plast Reconstr Surg. 2014; 133(4):905–913

[10] Hirche C, Engel H, Seidenstuecker K, et al. [Lympho-reconstructive microsurgery for secondary lymphedema: consensus of the German-Speaking Society for Microsurgery of Peripheral Nerves and Vessels (DAM) on indication, diagnostic and therapy by lymphovenous anastomosis (LVA) and vascularized lymph node transfer (VLNT)]. Handchir Mikrochir Plast Chir. 2019; 51(6):424–433

[11] Viitanen TP, Mäki MT, Seppänen MP, Suominen EA, Saaristo AM. Donor-site lymphatic function after microvascular lymph node transfer. Plast Reconstr Surg. 2012; 130(6):1246–1253

[12] Saaristo AM, Niemi TS, Viitanen TP, Tervala TV, Hartiala P, Suominen EA. Microvascular breast reconstruction and lymph node transfer for postmastectomy lymphedema patients. Ann Surg. 2012; 255(3):468–473

[13] Becker C, Assouad J, Riquet M, Hidden G. Postmastectomy lymphedema: long-term results following microsurgical lymph node transplantation. Ann Surg. 2006; 243(3):313–315

19 Review of the Current Literature

Mario F. Scaglioni and Matteo Meroni

Summary

This chapter will highlight the current scientific evidence available that describes the different surgical procedures to be used to treat lymphedema. Since comparative studies are still infrequent, most studies available nowadays are more or less big case series and expert opinion based on personal experience and, therefore, the level of evidence is rather low. Yet, over the last years, the surgical management of lymphedema has undergone a true revival, particularly with regard to reconstructive microsurgery and therefore resulted in a continuous increase in scientific evidence. This chapter summarizes the current state of pre-, intra-, and postoperative visualization and monitoring of the lymphatic vascular system. Further, it highlights the currently used surgical procedures, both when offering lymphoablative surgery and reconstructive surgery, as a standalone procedure or in combination. It also highlights reconstructive surgery in a prophylactic setting, i.e., while performing lymph node dissection during oncological surgery, and finally describes potential therapeutical approaches based on scientific consensus.

Keywords: diagnostics in lymphedema, lymphoablative surgery, lymphovenous anastomosis (LVA), lymph node vein anastomosis (LNVA), nonvascularized lymph vessel transfer, reconstructive surgery, suction-assisted lipectomy, vascularized lymph node transfer (VLNT)

19.1 Introduction

Lymphedema is characterized by an accumulation of fluid and protein in the interstitial space of subcutaneous tissues caused by obstruction or impairment of lymphatic fluid transport. This may result in swelling of the affected limb with discomfort, sometimes pain, impaired range of motion, and recurrent infections. If this potentially progressive and debilitating condition becomes chronic, irreversible changes, such as tissue fibrosis and excess of adipose tissue, will inevitably occur[1,2] (see **Chapters 1** and **2**). Its first-line treatment is dictated by conservative measure of complete decongestive therapy (CDT) that is crucial as a stand-alone treatment as well as before and after a surgical procedure (see **Chapter 6** and **Subchapter 7.3**. Unfortunately, many cases are resistant to conservative measures, i.e., CDT maintains the stage of lymphedema rather than truly improving it.

Accordingly, a variety of surgical measures have been described that aim at reducing, almost always, the excess subcutaneous tissue and sometimes skin or at least somehow restoring the circulation of lymphatic fluid. They include suction-assisted lipectomy (see **Chapter 13**) and surgical techniques aiming at excising excess of skin and/or subcutaneous fat (see **Chapter 14**). Yet, both approaches treat the symptoms rather than really the cause. This is why lately more sophisticated microsurgical and potentially causal approaches have become more and more popular. These so-called physiological procedures aim at reducing the lymphatic fluid burden by improving lymphatic circulation by diverting (see **Chapter 8**) and bypassing (see **Chapter 9**) lymphatic blockage and/or creating alternate outflow pathways by developing new lymphatic drainage pathways (see **Chapter 10**).

The increasing popularity of this surgery is not only reflected in a continuous increase of colleagues who perform congresses and courses that promulgate this type of surgery, but also the increase in number and level of evidence (LoE) in the literature.

This chapter shall highlight the current status of the literature with regard to new diagnostic tools that have been implemented in microsurgical reconstructive procedures to treat lymphedema. Further, it will highlight the actual status of the two most popular surgical procedures used to treat lymphedema, i.e., lymphvenous anastomosis (LVA) and vascularized lymph node transfer (VLNT).

19.2 Lymphoreductive Surgery

Surgical procedures that aim at reducing the tissue excess were mainly used historically. However, they may be used in advanced stages of lymphedema or in remote areas of the world where they lack microsurgical equipment or as a concomitant or staged adjunct to reconstructive microsurgery of the lymphatic system (see **Chapters 8–12**).

The forerunner of this type of surgery was the Charles' procedure first described in 1912. The procedure involved circumferential excision of skin, subcutaneous tissue, muscle fascia, followed by grafting of the excised skin to finally cover the iatrogenic defect resulting from the excision. Later on, modifications have been described by Sistrunk in 1927 and Homan-Miller in 1936 to decrease the invasiveness of the method. Approximately 30 years later, Thompson further modified the technique in order to induce spontaneous lympho-lymphatic and lymphovenular connections by transposing thin and deepithelialized superficial flaps of the surrounding skin excess into the deeper muscular tissue eventually linking superficial adipo-dermal lymphatic drainage system to the deep muscular system.

Unfortunately, all these procedures are associated with a rather high rate of complications, including pain, wound healing complication, infections, hypertrophic and retractile scars, and lymphatic fistulas.[2] Therefore, this type of surgery is used only occasionally in developed countries in cases of severely voluminous extremities, whereas it might be used on regular basis in filariasis-associated severe forms of lymphedema (see **Chapters 3** and **12**).

Another far less invasive surgical approach that reduces the volume of tissue excess is lipectomy. The feasibility is based on the fact that subcutaneous tissues exposed to chronic lymphedema progressively converts first into excessive fatty tissue and eventually fibrotic tissue. Accordingly, Brorson took advantage of that pathophysiological change of tissues in order to remove subcutaneous tissue excess and reduce the volume of the affected extremity, propagating suction-assisted lipectomy (see **Chapter 13**). In recent years many promising results have been published. Brorson reported in a prospective study with 56 patients diagnosed with lymphedema (29 primary and 27 secondary lymphedemas) that the volume of the lower extremity treated by suction-assisted lipectomy had significantly been reduced after 10 years, but the wearing of compression garments had to be continued. The same author confirmed his findings in another prospective study, including 146 breast cancer patients with upper limb lymphedema. Importantly, risk of suction-associated damage to the lymphatic vessels has not yet been observed, either experimentally or clinically. In order to avoid cardiovascular impairment, the author, however, insists on the shift of electrolytes, and therefore recommends a maximum extraction of 4 liters that should not be exceeded.[3,4]

19.3 New Tools to be Used for Pre-, Intra-, and Postoperative Visualization of Lymphatic Structures

Today, lymphoscintigraphy is still most commonly used to assess the lymphatic system and therefore considered as the standard procedure. Further technical progresses have allowed to develop various methods, including three-dimensional imaging techniques and video-based tools that seem to be superior when compared to lymphoscintigraphy.[5] ICG lymphangiography is currently used to objectively display in real-time a precise map of the lymphatics in the layers of dermal and superficial subcutaneous tissue indicating the stage of lymphedema.

Furthermore, ICG lymphangiography is able to assess the function of the lymphatic vessels, both qualitatively and quantitatively, enabling new avenues for diagnosis and classification. Currently, it delivers accurate data for preoperative planning, intraoperative assessment of functionality and vascular patency, and postoperative follow-up.[6,7] It also allows for intraoperative reversed lymphatic mapping in order to clearly define which lymphatic structures need to be saved to best avoid surgery-induced donor-site lymphedema as well as display lymphatic collectors and/or lymph nodes to be used as donor tissue[8] (see **Chapter 4**).

Bioimpedance spectroscopy (BIS) is another rather new diagnostic tool that that is based on altered electrical conductance of extracellular fluid. BIS is able to accurately assess the extracellular fluid compartment, particularly in cases of early-stage lymphedema where structural changes are not yet present. Unfortunately, accuracy of BIS decreases with progression of lymphedema.

MRL is currently used to demonstrate the water content within the subcutaneous tissues and under certain circumstances lymphatic vascularization to map the course of lymphatics. It is used with or without contrast media. Moreover, another advantage specific to MRL is the possibility to create three-dimensional images.

19.4 Lymphoreconstructive Surgery

Improved understanding of the pathophysiological processes of lymphedema and the continuous amendment of micro- and even supermicrosurgery have allowed to further develop specific surgical techniques with a potentially curative approach. They include predominantly LVAs (see **Chapter 8**), less frequently autologous lymph vessel transfer (ALVT) (see **Chapter 9**), and in particular vascularized lymph node transfer (VLNT) (see **Chapter 10**). They all have in common the potential to restore physiological lymphatic flow, aiming at alleviating functional complaints preventing recurrent infection and eventually reducing lymphedema stage. If the outcome is modest, the aim should at least be to stop the progression of the disease. Ideally, patients undergoing this type of surgery should be able to live without being dependent on CDT, compression garment included.[9,10]

The concept of LVAs was first introduced in the 1960s.[5,11] Since then, a variety of studies have described the mechanism of function of these physiological bypasses, that is, the outflow of a low-pressure vascular network of lymphatic vessels into a high-pressure vascular network of venous vessels following microsurgical anastomosis distal to the actual lymphatic blockage.[12] Usually, LVAs are performed under general anesthesia for better patient comfort, but its execution is also possible under local anesthesia. Current literature displays a large variety of surgical techniques, number of anastomoses to be performed, and additional procedures that can be offered, including debulking procedures. The efficacy of LVAs seems to present if a minimum of three anastomoses are performed per affected extremity per patient.[13] Although many authors claim that the number of anastomoses is of paramount importance in lymphedema treatment, no current consensus is currently available that may predict edema reduction and eventually decrease of tissue excess. Despite the description of many techniques of vascular anastomosis (end-to-end, end-to-side, side-to-end, "octopus," parachute, and so on), no clear benefit of one technique over the other is currently known.[13]

This technique is effective with reports of high patient satisfaction when it comes to edema-associated relief of symptom and a 35% to 60% reduction in circumference. About 83% of patients who were assessed using some sort of extremity index consisting of multiple circumference measurements at defined anatomical points of reference on the upper and/or lower extremity showed significant improvements after LVA surgery. Patient-reported subjective symptom relief, including reduced occurrence of cellulitis (erysipelas) following LVA, ranges from 50% to 100%. Additional surgical debulking have shown to further improve the rate of soft tissue infection and symptom relief reported by the patients. However, all in all the level of evidence is still rather weak due to small sample size, heterogeneity, and retrospective character of the data[13,14]. The currently relevant data are summarized in ▶ Table 19.1 and refer exclusively to the treatment of secondary lymphedema.

LVA surgery is also a potent tool to reduce episodes of cellulitis. The relationship between lymphedema and cellulitis episodes is well established. Frequently, cellulitis-induced lymphedema results from the obstruction of superficial lymphatic vessels caused by tissue inflammation. Tissue inflammation results in fibrotic changes in the lymphatic vessels and subcutaneous tissue, with subsequent worsening of lymphedema, resulting in a vicious cycle of lymphatic vessel destruction, lymphedema, and recurring cellulitis episodes. The restoration of lymphatic flow back into the circulation and subsequent reduction in pressure on the lymphatic channels as well as less stasis are plausible explanations for the reduction of cellulitis episode frequency.

Hara and colleagues were the only to focus on patients with primary lymphedema undergoing LVA surgery. Interestingly, they demonstrated efficacy of technique to improve postoperative extremity circumference only in patients over 11 years of age. If operated before that age, lymphedema symptoms clearly worsened.[15]

Another promising microsurgical technique to treat lymphedema is the transfer of vascularized lymph nodes (VLNT). In recent years an increase in literature addressing the developing field of VLNT for lymphedema treatment has been noticed. Since the first descriptions aiming at popularizing the concept of VLNT in lymphedema treatment, lately a number of studies have demonstrated promising results, most often popularizing the transfer of inguinal lymph nodes to treat secondary lymphedema of the upper extremity following breast cancer treatment.

The concept of VLNT consists of transferring vascularized lymph nodes, usually included into an adipo-fascial, adipo-dermal, or adipo-cutaneous flap, to the recipient site of the affected extremity in order to restore lymphatic drainage function. The detailed physiologic mechanisms are still speculative. One explanation is that the transferred lymph nodes act as a sponge to absorb lymphatic fluid, while another theory suggests that the transferred lymph nodes induce lymphangiogenesis in order to newly create lympho-lymphatic and lymphovenous channels and eventually improve drainage.[16] A recent review of the literature evaluated more than 270 VLNTs, mostly performed using microsurgical techniques. Of interest, follow-up time range from 1 to 96 months and therefore renders comparability difficult.

Assessment of postoperative subjective and objective improvement is usually based on the measurement of circumference and volumetry, the assessment of functionality and patency of the lymphatics, and quality of life. A prospective study with a follow-up of more than 3 years revealed significantly greater edema reduction in patients following VLNT when compared to CDT only. Another study demonstrated a 24% and 35% reduction in arm lymphedema and leg lymphedema, respectively, 1 year after VLNT. It is of interest that patients undergoing VLNT for upper extremity lymphedema report superior outcomes when compared to those undergoing lymph node transfer for lower extremity lymphedema[1,17,18] ▶ Table 19.2 provides overview of the currently available relevant data in the field of VLNT.

Iatrogenic lymphedema due to lymph node harvesting at the donor extremity is a devastating complication. Careful preoperative assessment of potential donor sites for lymph node transfer is therefore crucial. A number of potential donor sites for VLNT have been described, including the inguinal, the submental, the supraclavicular, the lateral thoracic areas, and the gastroepiploic lymph nodes (see **Chapter 10**). Although the inguinal lymph nodes are most commonly used as a donor site, they are associated with the highest risk for surgery-induced lymphedema, especially when inguinal nodes are harvested in the deep tissue layers and medial to the femoral vessels. Furthermore, it is critical to spare the sentinel lymph node in the groin and axilla for potential oncological reasons. The use of donor sites for VLNT were as follows: groin (72%; also in combination with microvascular abdominal flap for breast reconstruction), lateral thoracic area (15%), supraclavicular region (7%), omentum (4%), and submental region (3%). The supraclavicular and the submental flaps are not yet well supported by literature, but their donor sites are associated with a minimal risk of iatrogenic lymphedema. However, they may have more obvious scars and potential risks for other important structures, such as the marginal mandibular nerve during the harvesting of submental nodes, in addition to variable anatomy of the pedicle vessels, particularly as concerns supraclavicular lymph nodes.

Additionally, there is some risk of harming the marginal mandibular branch of the of the facial nerve (submental flap) and the thoracic duct (right supraclavicular flap).

Table 19.1 Overview of the literature on lymphovenous anastomosis in lymphedema surgery

Authors	Year of publication	Number of included patients	Number of included extremities (n)	Affected extremities	Lymphedema type	Mean duration of lymphedema before surgery (months)	Type of surgery	Number of anastomoses/ patient (mean)	Measurement method	Mean postoperative follow-up time (months)	Objective outcomes in % of patients	P-values of objective outcomes	Subjective symptoms in % of patients
Akita et al.	2014	96	192	LE	SL	12	LVA + compressive treatment	4.4	LEL index and ICG	20.9	100	$p < 0.001$	44.8 (elimination of compressive therapy)
Auba et al.	2012	10	13	UE and LE	PL and SL	110	LVA + compressive treatment	3.2	Circumference measurement	18	80	$p = 0.04$	100
Chang	2010	20	20	UE and LE	SL	57.6	LVA + compression treatment	3.5	Volumetry (optoelectronic limb volumeter)	18	65	n/a	95
Chang et al.	2013	100	100 UE: 89 LE: 11	UE and LE	SL	UE: 42 LE: 79.2	LVA (n = 35 without ICG, n = 65 with ICG)	n/a	Volumetry (optoelectronic limb volumeter)	UE: 30 LE: 18.2	74	$p = 0.032$	UE: 96 LE: 57
Chen et al.	2016	18	18	UE and LE	PL and SL	≥6	LVA + compressive treatment (ICG or along anatomic courses of cephalic vein/ great saphenous vein)	10	LEL and UEL index and ICG	12	83	$p < 0.01$	n/a
Chen et al.	2015	9	9	UE and LE	PL and SL	81.6	LVA + compressive treatment ("octopus" method)	39 ("octopus" method)	LEL and UEL index and ICG	7.6	100	$p = 0.0003$	100

(Continued)

Table 19.1 (*Continued*) Overview of the literature on lymphovenous anastomosis in lymphedema surgery

Authors	Year of publication	Number of included patients	Number of included extremities (n)	Affected extremities	Lymphedema type	Mean duration of lymphedema before surgery (months)	Type of surgery	Number of anastomoses/ patient (mean)	Measurement method	Mean postoperative follow-up time (months)	Objective outcomes in % of patients	P-values of objective outcomes	Subjective symptoms in % of patients
Damstra et al.	2009	10	11	UE	SL	63.6	LVA + compression treatment (7–10 cm above elbow)	3.5	Volumetry (inverse water volumetry)	12	2	n/a	n/a
Hara et al.	2015	62	79	LE	PL	127.2	LVA (with ICG)	4.5	Circumference measurement	20	76 (only in subgroup C, n = 22)	p = 0.001	n/a
Ito et al.	2016	5	n/a	LE	PL and SL	≥6	LVA (with ICG) with or without compressive treatment	2	Circumference measurement and ICG	10	63.8	p < 0.05	100
Koshima et al.	2000	27	12	UE	SL	98.4	LVA (with or without indigo carmine)	4.1	Circumference measurement	26.4	47.3	n/a	n/a
Koshima et al.	2003	25	n/a	LE	PL and SL	80.4	LVA (with or without indigo carmine)	n/a	Circumference measurement	55.2	55.6	n/a	n/a
Mihara et al.	2014	95	n/a	UE and LE	PL and SL	n/a	LVA + compression treatment (n = 92), LVA with excessive tissue resection + compression treatment (n = 3)	≥3	Cellulitis episodes (1 year before and 1 year after surgery)	27.3	100 Mean pre-op vs. post-op: 1.46 vs. 0.18	p < 0.001	n/a

(Continued)

Table 19.1 (*Continued*) Overview of the literature on lymphovenous anastomosis in lymphedema surgery

Authors	Year of publication	Number of included patients	Number of included extremities (n)	Affected extremities	Lymphedema type	Mean duration of lymphedema before surgery (months)	Type of surgery	Number of anastomoses/ patient (mean)	Measurement method	Mean postoperative follow-up time (months)	Objective outcomes in % of patients	P-values of objective outcomes	Subjective symptoms in % of patients
Mihara et al.	2016	84	162	LE	PL and SL	n/a	LVA + compression treatment	n/a	ICG and limb lymphoscintigraphy	18.3	47.7	n/s	61.5
O'Brien et al.	1977	62	n/a	UE and LE	SL	n/a	LVA + conservative treatment	4	Volumetry (water displacement)	5	19	n/a	66
O'Brien et al.	1990	90	n/a	UE and LE	SL	96	LVA only (n = 52), LVA plus segmental or radical reduction (n = 38)	n/a	Volumetry (water displacement)	50.4	44 vs. 60 (LVA only vs. LVA plus debulking)	n/a	75
Seki et al.	2015	30	30	LE	SL	LVA-SEKI: 41.4 LVA: 63.5	LVA + conservative treatment	LVA: 2.1 LVA (SEKI): 2	LEL index, ICG and lymphoscintigraphy	12	53	p = 0.006	n/a
Yamamoto et al.	2013	48	n/a	LE	PL and SL	66	LVA (with ICG non-SEATTLE, n = 23), LVA (with ICG SEATTLE, n = 25)	Non-SEATTLE-LVA: 1.6 SEATTLE-LVA: 1.8	LEL index	6	100	p < 0.001	n/a
Yamamoto et al.	2013	14	14	LE	SL	n/a	LVA (modified)	1.7	LEL index	6	100	p < 0.001	n/a

Abbreviations: ICG, indocyanine green; LE, lower extremity; LEL, lower extremity lymphedema index; LVA, lymphovenous anastomosis; PL, primary lymphedema; SL, secondary lymphedema; UE, upper extremity; UEL, upper extremity lymphedema index.

Table 19.2 Overview of the literature on vascularized lymph node transfer (VLNT) in lymphedema surgery

Authors	Year of publication	Number of included patients (n) Number of VLNT flaps	Flap type (n)	Recipient site	Mean follow-up time (months)	Measurement method	Concomitant nonreconstructive surgery (n)	Reduction of lymphedema or improvement (%)
Attash et al.	2013	4	Pedicle omental flap	Groin, lower leg	12	Circumference, volumetry	None	50%–75%
Barreiro et al.	2014	7	Lateral thoracic lymph node flap (1 free and 6 pedicle)	Axilla and shoulder (6), dorsum foot (1)	6, 8	Lymphoscintigraphy	None	n/a
Becker et al.	2006	24	Inguinal flap	Axilla	60	Circumference, lymphoscintigraphy	Second VLNT inguinal to elbow (7)	Return to normal (10), unchanged (2), > 50% decrease (6), < 50% decrease (6)
Chen et al.	2014	10	DIEP with inguinal lymph nodes based on SCIV	Axilla	12	Circumference, lymphoscintigraphy	None	88.9% improvement
Cheng et al.	2012	6 (7)	Submental flap	Ankle	2–22	Circumference, lymphoscintigraphy	None	64.9%
Cheng et al.	2013	10	Inguinal flap based on SCIV	Wrist (8), elbow (2)	12–54	Circumference	Cosmetic deepithelialization flap (4)	40.4%
Ciudad et al.	2016	6	Free omental flap	Ankle (4), wrist (2)	12	Circumference, lymphoscintigraphy	None	All improved
Dancey et al.	2013	18	DIEP with inguinal lymph nodes flap based on SIEA	Axilla	4–22	LYMQOL score	None	100% improvement
Dayan et al.	2014	35	Inguinal flap (19) and lateral thoracic lymph node flap (16)	n/a	1–30	n/a	None	n/a
Fanzio et al.	2011	1	Lateral thoracic lymph node flap	Thigh: 6 cm above patella	8	n/a	Excision	n/a
Gharb et al.	2011	21	Inguinal flap based on SCIV standard (11) and hilar perforators (10)	Wrist, forearm	23–50	Circumference	Debulking surgery (1), lipectomy (2)	Hilar perforators (10) significant difference
Gómez Martin et al.	2013	1 (2)	Inguinal flap and lateral thoracic lymph node flap	Knee and groin	5	Circumference	None	Foot = 86% Ankle = 57% Leg = 40% Knee = 14% Thigh = 100%

Table 19.2 (*Continued*) Overview of the literature on vascularized lymph node transfer (VLNT) in lymphedema surgery

Authors	Year of publication	Number of included patients (n) Number of VLNT flaps	Flap type (n)	Recipient site	Mean follow-up time (months)	Measurement method	Concomitant nonreconstructive surgery (n)	Reduction of lymphedema or improvement (%)
Granzow et al.	2014	2	Inguinal flap	Axilla	n/a	Volumetry	Liposuction	75%–90% (1), 108–113% (1)
Granzow et al.	2014	8	Inguinal flap	Axilla	18–50	n/a	None	n/a
Lin et al.	2009	13	Groin flap based on SCIV	Wrist	6–96	Circumference, Lymphoscintigraphy	Wedge excision or suction-assisted lipectomy (2)	50.5% reduction
Nguyen et al.	2015	29	Inguinal nodes with abdominal free flap	Axilla	3–33	Volumetry, perometer	None	52.4% improvement
Pons et al.	2013	1	Inguinal flap	Axilla	24	Circumference, volumetry, lymphoscintigraphy	None	9.8% reduction
Qiu et al.	2014	1	Submental flap	Ankle	3	Circumference, lymphoscintigraphy	None	61%–67%
Sapountzis et al.	2014	2	Supraclavicular flap (2)	Foot dorsum	6–7	Circumference, lymphoscintigraphy	None	100% improvement
Saaristo et al.	2012	9	DIEP with inguinal lymph nodes based on SIEA/SCIV	Axilla	6	Circumference, lymphoscintigraphy	None	32.2%
Sapountzis et al.	2014	24	Supraclavicular flap (13) and groin flap (11)	Dorsum foot	3–26	n/a	Charles procedure	100%
Vignes et al.	2013	26 (34)	Inguinal flap (20) and lateral thoracic lymph node flap (14)	Inguinal, axilla	14–72	Circumference, volumetry	Liposuction (4)	n/a
Vibhakar et al.	2014	1	LD with lateral thoracic lymph nodes	Axilla	n/a	Volumetry	None	44%
Yeo et al.	2014	1 (2)	Supraclavicular flap	Ankle bilaterally	1–2	Circumference	Charles procedure one side	n/a

Abbreviations: VLNT, autologous lymph node transfer; DIEP, deep inferior epigastric perforator; LD; LYMQOL; SCIV, superficial circumflex iliac vein; SIEA, superficial inferior epigastric artery.

Furthermore, scarring—at least in the face—is more obvious and prone to pathological scarring when compared to the inguinal or axillary region. The gastroepiploic or omental flap in contrast has a very specific risk of complication that is due to the intra-abdominal approach and may result in intestinal adhesions and subsequent bowel obstruction as well as incisional hernias.

Of interest, the lateral thoracic lymph nodes seem to be the least effective ones and have the highest complication rates when compared to the other donor sites.

▶ Table 19.3 and ▶ Table 19.4 show reported complications, both of the donor and the recipient sites after VLNT harvesting.[9]

Similar to the ideal donor site in VLNT surgery, currently there is no clear consensus about the best recipient site for VLNT. Many studies describe that recipient site does not appear to have a significant impact on overall outcome; nevertheless, it is important to consider the specific anatomy of the affected extremity. For upper extremity lymphedema, VLNT can be transferred to the axilla, the elbow, or the wrist. Extensive scar release is necessary in secondary lymphedema to create an adequate space to correctly place and insert the vascularized lymph nodes. Bear in mind that identification of patent recipient vessels may be challenging in a scarred area resulting from infection, previous surgery, and/or radiotherapy to the axilla. Many vessels may serve as potential recipient vessels, including the lateral thoracic, the thoracodorsal, or the serratus vessels or side branches.

Some microsurgeons recommend performing VLNT more distally at the level of the elbow or even at the wrist, in areas that have not been affected by prior surgery or radiation. For lymphedema treatment of the upper extremity, currently the most frequent treatment procedure is the transfer of inguinal lymph nodes to the axilla. In more than one-third of these cases, inguinal VLNT has been associated with an abdominal free flap for simultaneous breast reconstruction.

For lower extremity lymphedema, there is a similar debate regarding whether the lymph nodes should be transferred proximally or distally. The groin, the popliteal fossa, and the ankle have been described as potential recipient sites. Analogous to the axillary region, dissection of the inguinal region can be difficult following a previous surgery such as inguinal lymph node clearance and/or radiotherapy. More distally, the branches of the medial genicular artery or saphenous vein can be used as recipient vessels around the knee, whereas VLNT to ankle region will most likely depend on branches of the anterior tibial or dorsalis pedis artery and concomitant veins.[19]

The majority of VLNT from the lateral thoracic area have been predominantly used for lower extremity lymphedema, including the supraclavicular and submental lymph node flap. Interestingly, all these vascularized lymph nodes were transferred distally to the ankle or the dorsum of the foot. Submental VLNT was most effective with 100% of patients (n = 58) reporting improvement of symptoms followed by the supraclavicular VLNT reporting 88% improvement in 515 patients. Inguinal VLNT did not improve the symptomatology (0.4%; 5,138 patients).[20]

Although VLNT has been recommended for early-stage lymphedema, this technique can also be effectively applied in more advanced stages of lymphedema and may be combined with debulking procedures, nowadays usually suction-assisted lipectomy. In cases with diffusely swollen and fibrotic extremities, VLNT and subsequent lipectomy may need to be performed in a staged manner. This approach is advisable since the assessment of the true utility and efficacy of one or the other technique is confounding when combining VLNT with suction-associated lipectomy, hence potentially overestimating the efficacy of VLNT in reducing volume.

Recently there have been studies describing simultaneous VLNT and abdominal-based microvascular flap (deep inferior epigastric perforator [DIEP] flap) for concomitant treatment of arm lymphedema and breast reconstruction. The simultaneous restoration of lymphatic flow in the upper extremity and reconstruction of the breast seems appealing since 79% of the patients reported improvement of lymphedema-associated symptoms. Currently literature is not clear on whether to perform a single pedicle composite flap or two separated flaps with two independent pedicles. The latter is more time consuming, yet placement of the groin flap to the axilla is easier and shaping of the breast more predictable.[8,21]

Complications at the recipient site include wound infection and wound dehiscence, delayed wound healing, prolonged flap edema, and partial or total flap loss. The latter is more common when VLNT is associated with an oncoplastic procedure of the breast (▶ Table 19.3). Total complication rate at the donor site of inguinal lymph nodes is approximately 10% as demonstrated in a series of 5,195 flaps (▶ Table 19.4). In detail, following complications were observed: seroma formation or lymphocele (approximately 8%), pain at the donor site (approximately 2%), hydrocele of the testes and delayed wound healing (approximately 1%).

When harvesting the lateral thoracic flap, total complication rate of approximately 28% has been described in a series of 540 flaps, whereas harvesting of 518 supraclavicular flaps revealed one case of lymphorrhea. No complications were reported in patients undergoing submental or omental flap harvesting.[1,21]

19.5 Combined Surgical Approaches

All the previously described procedures present their own advantages and disadvantages. For this reason, in some cases it has been proposed to use more than one surgical technique at the same time in order to increase the surgery-associated drainage potential and effect of

Table 19.3 Recipient and donor site complications following vascularized lymph node transfer (VLNT)

Authors	Year of publication	Numbers of lymph node flaps	Type of lymph node flap (n)	Complications at recipient site (n)	Complications at donor site (n)
Barreiro et al.	2014	7	Lateral thoracic lymph node flap (1 free and 6 pedicle)	Prolonged flap edema (1)	Prolonged donor site edema (1), minor donor area dehiscence (1)
Becker et al.	2006	24	Inguinal flap	None	Lymphorrhea (8)
Cheng et al.	2012	7	Submental flap	None	None
Chen et al.	2014	10	DIEP with inguinal lymph nodes based on SCIV	None	None
Cheng et al.	2013	10	Inguinal flap based on SCIV	None	None
Ciudad et al.	2016	6	Free omental flap	None	None
Dancey et al.	2013	18	DIEP with inguinal lymph nodes flap based on SIEA	Flap necrosis (1)	Donor seroma (2)
Dayan et al.	2014	35	Inguinal flap (19) and lateral thoracic lymph node flap (16)	None	None
Gharb et al.	2011	21	Inguinal flap based on SCIV standard (11) and hilar perforators (10)	Forearm cellulitis (1)	None
Lin et al.	2009	13	Inguinal flap based on SCIV	Wound infection (1), venous congestion (1)	None
Nguyen et al.	2015	29	Inguinal node with abdominal free flap	Delayed wound healing (3), mastectomy skin flap necrosis (1), venous thrombosis (1)	Delayed wound healing (1), abdominal hernia (1)
Pons et al.	2013	1	Inguinal flap	None	Lymphedema (1)
Saaristo et al.	2012	9	DIEP with inguinal lymph nodes based on SIEA/SCIV	Delayed wound healing (2)	Seroma drainage (1)
Sapountzis et al.	2014	11 but 2 fully described	Supraclavicular flap (1)	None	Lymphorrhea (1)
Sapountzis et al.	2014	24	Supraclavicular flap (13) and inguinal flap (11)	Partial loss of skin paddle in 1 flap, partial loss of STSG on flap (6)	None
Vignes et al.	2013	34	Inguinal flap (20) and lateral thoracic lymph node flap (14)	None	Inguinal: Lymphedema (2) Lymphocele (3) Donor site pain (3) Hydrocele (1) Axilla: Lymphedema (4) Lymphocele (1) Donor site pain (1)
Vibhakar et al.	2014	1	LD with lateral thoracic lymph nodes	None	None

Abbreviations: DIEP, deep inferior epigastric perforator; SCIV, superficial circumflex iliac vein; SIEA, superficial inferior epigastric artery; STSG, split-thickness skin graft; VLNT, autologous lymph node transfer.

Table 19.4 Overall complication rates based on the flap's donor site

Type of flap and donor region	Total number of flap n (%)	Total complication rate n (%)	Complication rate at donor site (in general: n (%))	Lymphedema rate at donor site n (%)	Lymphocele or seroma n (%)	Hydrocele n (%)	Pain at donor site n (%)
Inguinal region	195 (71.9)	20 (10.3)	17 (8.7)	3 (1.5)	15 (7.7)	1 (0.5)	3 (1.5)
Lateral thoracic region	40 (14.8)	11 (27.5)	6 (15)	5 (12.5)	1 (2.5)	0	1 (2.5)
Supraclavicular region	18 (6.5)	1 (5.6)	1 (5.6)	0	1 (5.6)	0	0
Omentum	10 (3.8)	0	0	0	0	0	0
Submental region	8 (3)	0	0	0	0	0	0

decongestion. Different combinations are possible including, most of the times, physiological and lymphoablative procedures (LVA and SAL or a VLNT and SAL). The combination of LVA with VLNT is poorly described. These solutions are particularly indicated in difficult cases, where a massive refractory lymphedema is present and the result reachable with one technique alone is considered not sufficient to obtain an adequate amount of fluid drainage. While physiological procedures are mostly effective in early stages, the addition of lymphoablative therapy can make them effective therapeutic options for late stages as well.

A retrospective study by Granzow et al., published in 2014,[22] demonstrated significant improvements for early and chronic lymphedema by means of either VLNT or suction-assisted lipectomy and LVA. Besides the usual parameters such as volume reduction and compressive therapy discontinuation, they highlighted a dramatic reduction of cellulitis episodes after surgery. This is an interesting result in terms of patient morbidity and health costs, since many lymphedema patients are often hospitalized for intravenous antibiotic therapies. This work showed better results with VLNT than with LVA; however, this should be balanced with the higher donor site risks related to the lymph nodes harvest. In 2020, a study by Di Taranto et al.[23] compared the results obtained by gastroepiploic VLNT alone and combined VLNT and LVA. Also in this case, in both groups additional suction lipectomy was performed. The patients were then prospectively evaluated through clinical examination, circumference measurement, and skin tonicity. The results showed that the improvements obtained in patients who received the combined approach were significantly superior to those who received only VLNT. Even if it is not clear which procedure is more responsible for the result, this work adds further evidence about the enhanced outcome of the synergistic approach. An additional procedure worth mentioning is the simultaneous microsurgical breast reconstruction with VLNT. This consists in the harvest of some lymph nodes close to the superficial inferior epigastric vein (SIEVs) on the contralateral side of the deep inferior epigastric vessels used for the flap. The SIEV can be then anastomosed to vessels in the axilla, thus improving the blood supply and, more importantly, mimicking the physiologic drainage of the axillary lymph nodes. Results from this approach are limited due to the lack of data currently available, but some improvement has been noted. Nguyen et al.[21] proposed a geometric arrangement for various scenarios; however, the right positioning of the lymph nodes in the axilla remains a challenging aspect of this procedure.

A systematic review of contemporary peer-reviewed literature by Carl et al.[24] included the most relevant works in lymphatic surgery setting. It also evaluated the combined procedures according to the methodological index for randomized studies (MINORS) scoring system[25] and it proved that the effectiveness of lymphedema surgery is consistently enhanced in combined approaches for the treatment of either upper or lower extremities lymphedema.

19.6 Prophylactic Surgery

A protocol to be followed for lymphedema prevention when an increased risk of developing lymphatic complications is recognized has been established. This procedure, described first in 2009 by Boccardo et al.[26] with the acronym LYMPHA (lymphatic microsurgical preventive healing approach), consists in performing multiple LVAs at time of lymph node dissection. It was originally intended for primary prevention of arm lymphedema following breast cancer, but then it showed encouraging results also in patients presenting with trunk melanoma or other tumor/lymphatic dissections throughout the body.[27] The risk evaluation must be done preoperatively and relies on different clinical and lymphoscintigraphic parameters (age, body mass index [BMI], number of lymph nodes retrieved, number of metastatic lymph nodes, types of surgery, radiotherapy, cellulitis). Obesity is a strong risk factor; therefore, patients with BMI of over 30 were all considered eligible, while the others were evaluated with lymphoscintigraphy. In this case LYMPHA was performed in patients with transport index of > 10. The learning curve is estimated at about 30 operations. Another study from different authors[28] added further evidence for the efficacy of this approach analyzing the postoperative course of 37 women over a period of 26 months. The evaluation in this case were made by means of pre- and postoperative lymphoscintigraphy, arm measurements, and BIS.

Even if the original authors stated that this procedure can be performed during axillary lymph node dissection in only 15 to 20 minutes, it remains technically demanding for less experienced surgeons. For this reason, a simplified approach named S-LYMPHA has been proposed in 2019.[29] It consists in identifying the leaking transected lymphatic vessels at the end of the dissection which are then invaginated using sleeve technique into the cut end of a neighboring vein with two 7–0 nonabsorbable stitches. In this case no microscope is required. This procedure showed interesting results over a median follow-up time of 15 months; however, some criticisms were raised over the surgical technique because the invaginating sutures left in place may essentially occlude the lymphatic channels.

19.7 Consensus for Treatment Indication

Lymphatic sequelae are complex conditions whose management remains delicate. In particular, secondary lymphedema might be a devastating problem that can deeply affect the quality of life of patients who have often already faced serious diseases such as tumors. As previously described, many different lymphatic presentations are possible; thus, a clear and uniform classification is essential in order to guarantee the best therapy. The varying degrees of clinical features can be characterized according to the lymphedema staging system from the International Society of Lymphology (ISL) and the Campisi scale,[30,31] or according to lymphoscintigraphy transport index (TI). The management must be tailored, conforming to the specific conditions and the needs of the patient. In this respect, many studies have been done but there is still a lack of consensus over a common algorithm for total patient care. Physical therapy and compression such as CDT are overall accepted as initial treatment; however, when no improvement is reported, the choice between LVA, VLNT, or a combined procedure is more difficult. A recent article by Hirche et al.[32] summarized the indications for LVA and VLNT, pointing out the advantages of each of these procedures. LVA is normally considered the ideal treatment for initial stages (I and II), while the VLNT demonstrated a slight superiority for stages II and III. However, when treating moderate forms of lymphedema, other features should also be taken into account. First of all, the morbidity of the procedure, which is different (4% for LVA and 10% for VLNT) in terms of infection, lymphorrhea, and re-exploration requirement. The circumference reduction is almost identical, while discontinuation of compressive therapy is better for VLNT (78% versus 56.3%). For excessive volumes, the suction is still very relevant since it is the only procedure that guarantees a large volume reduction. Nevertheless, it is almost always recommended to combine it with a physiologic procedure that allows an improvement of the tissue quality and a better patient feeling. Further evidence of physiological lymphatic reconstructions efficacy, and specifically of LVA and VLNT, was provided by a couple of recent studies. From an objective point of view, Beederman et al.[33] showed that a detectable volume reduction is retained over a period of more than 4 years, with an improvement of the Lymphedema Life Impact Scale (LLIS) scores in 86% of cases involving the upper limbs and 75% in the lower limbs. Then, another work from Grünherz et al.[34] made an interesting large systematic review of literature, which reported a significant improvement in the quality of life in patients with lower limb lymphedema after reconstructive lymphatic surgery. In the last few years, the number of studies reporting the long-terms effects of these procedures is continuously growing and they are almost evenly giving solid result to support their reliability and remarkable benefits for the patients.

19.8 Conclusions

Current tools used to diagnose and quantify lymphedema and evaluate functionality of the lymphatic system, before, during, and after surgery, are powerful and efficient. ICG lymphangiography seems to have become the standard to be used before, during, and after surgery. Water displacement is still probably the most accurate, yet cumbersome and complicated, tool to measure volume. MR lymphangiography may reproduce the affected anatomical region in three dimensions and often compare it with normal anatomy in instances of unilateral affliction of an extremity.

LVA may provide both subjective and objective improvement of lymphedema-associated symptoms, including decrease of tissue excess, in particular in early-stage lymphedema.

VLNT offers promising results in early and intermediate stage lymphedemas. It seems to be more efficient when addressing lymphatic edema of the upper extremity when compared to the one of the lower extremities. Although the groin seems to be the preferred donor site, it has the highest risk of surgery-associated lymphedema. Therefore, the ideal donor site for VLNT continues to remain an area of considerable debate. Otherwise, complication rate of lymph node flap harvesting is acceptable, particularly if the surgery respects the anatomical landmarks. Further, standardization of quantification parameters for lymphedema is necessary as some studies relied on circumferential measurements while others used volumetric measurements or perometric measurements. However, high level of evidence data is still limited and requires further prospective and comparative studies, ideally based on national and international registries. A prerequisite must be to best standardize parameters to be collected when it comes to diagnosis and quantification of lymphedema.

References

[1] Scaglioni MF, Arvanitakis M, Chen YC, Giovanoli P, Chia-Shen Yang J, Chang EI. Comprehensive review of vascularized lymph node transfers for lymphedema: outcomes and complications. Microsurgery. 2018; 38(2):222–229

[2] Charles H. Elephantiasis of the leg. In: Latham A, English TC, eds. A System of Treatment. Vol. 3. London: Churchill; 1912

[3] Brorson H. Liposuction normalizes lymphedema induced adipose tissue hypertrophy in elephantiasis of the leg—a prospective study with a ten-year follow-up. Plast Reconstr Surg. 2015; 136(4) Suppl: 133–134

[4] Brorson H. Complete reduction of arm lymphedema following breast cancer—a prospective twenty-one years' study. Plast Reconstr Surg. 2015; 136(4) Suppl:134–135

[5] Danese C, Bower R, Howard J. Experimental anastomoses of lymphatics. Arch Surg. 1962; 84:6–9. Discussion following

[6] Yamamoto T, Yoshimatsu H, Koshima I. Navigation lymphatic supermicrosurgery for iatrogenic lymphorrhea: supermicrosurgical lymphaticolymphatic anastomosis and lymphaticovenular anastomosis under indocyanine green lymphography navigation. J Plast Reconstr Aesthet Surg. 2014; 67(11):1573–1579

[7] Li K, Zhang Z, Nicoli F, et al. Application of indocyanine green in flap surgery: a systematic review. J Reconstr Microsurg. 2018; 34 (2):77–86

[8] Saaristo AM, Niemi TS, Viitanen TP, Tervala TV, Hartiala P, Suominen EA. Microvascular breast reconstruction and lymph node transfer for postmastectomy lymphedema patients. Ann Surg. 2012; 255(3): 468–473

[9] Scaglioni MF, Suami H. Lymphatic anatomy of the inguinal region in aid of vascularized lymph node flap harvesting. J Plast Reconstr Aesthet Surg. 2015; 68(3):419–427

[10] Agko M, Ciudad P, Chen HC. Staged surgical treatment of extremity lymphedema with dual gastroepiploic vascularized lymph node transfers followed by suction-assisted lipectomy—a prospective study. J Surg Oncol. 2018; 117(6):1148–1156

[11] Sedlácek J. Lymphovenous shunt as supplementary treatment of elephantiasis of lower limbs. Acta Chir Plast. 1969; 11(2):157–162

[12] Chang EI, Skoracki RJ, Chang DW. Lymphovenous anastomosis bypass surgery. Semin Plast Surg. 2018; 32(1):22–27

[13] Scaglioni MF, Fontein DBY, Arvanitakis M, Giovanoli P. Systematic review of lymphovenous anastomosis (LVA) for the treatment of lymphedema. Microsurgery. 2017; 37(8):947–953

[14] Chang DW, Suami H, Skoracki R. A prospective analysis of 100 consecutive lymphovenous bypass cases for treatment of extremity lymphedema. Plast Reconstr Surg. 2013; 132(5):1305–1314

[15] Hara H, Mihara M, Ohtsu H, Narushima M, Iida T, Koshima I. Indication of lymphaticovenous anastomosis for lower limb primary lymphedema. Plast Reconstr Surg. 2015; 136(4):883–893

[16] Suami H, Scaglioni MF, Dixon KA, Tailor RC. Interaction between vascularized lymph node transfer and recipient lymphatics after lymph node dissection—a pilot study in a canine model. J Surg Res. 2016; 204(2):418–427

[17] Cheng MH, Chen SC, Henry SL, Tan BK, Chia-Yu Lin M, Huang JJ. Vascularized groin lymph node flap transfer for postmastectomy upper limb lymphedema: flap anatomy, recipient sites, and outcomes. Plast Reconstr Surg. 2013; 131(6):1286–1298

[18] Ciudad P, Manrique OJ, Bustos SS, et al. Comparisons in long-term clinical outcomes among patients with upper or lower extremity lymphedema treated with diverse vascularized lymph node transfer. Microsurgery. 2020; 40(2):130–136

[19] Chen WF, McNurlen M, Ding J, Bowen M. Vascularized lymph vessel transfer for extremity lymphedema—is transfer of lymph node still necessary? Int Microsurg J. 2019; 3(3):1

[20] Raju A, Chang DW. Vascularized lymph node transfer for treatment of lymphedema: a comprehensive literature review. Ann Surg. 2015; 261(5):1013–1023

[21] Nguyen AT, Chang EI, Suami H, Chang DW. An algorithmic approach to simultaneous vascularized lymph node transfer with microvascular breast reconstruction. Ann Surg Oncol. 2015; 22(9):2919–2924

[22] Granzow JW, Soderberg JM, Kaji AH, Dauphine C. An effective system of surgical treatment of lymphedema. Ann Surg Oncol. 2014; 21(4): 1189–1194

[23] Di Taranto G, Bolletta A, Chen SH, et al. A prospective study on combined lymphedema surgery: gastroepiploic vascularized lymph nodes transfer and lymphaticovenous anastomosis followed by suction lipectomy. Microsurgery. 2021; 41(1):34–43

[24] Carl HM, Walia G, Bello R, et al. Systematic review of the surgical treatment of extremity lymphedema. J Reconstr Microsurg. 2017; 33 (6):412–425

[25] Slim K, Nini E, Forestier D, Kwiatkowski F, Panis Y, Chipponi J. Methodological index for non-randomized studies (minors): development and validation of a new instrument. ANZ J Surg. 2003; 73(9):712–716

[26] Boccardo F, Casabona F, De Cian F, et al. Lymphedema microsurgical preventive healing approach: a new technique for primary prevention of arm lymphedema after mastectomy. Ann Surg Oncol. 2009; 16(3):703–708

[27] Boccardo F, De Cian F, Campisi CC, et al. Surgical prevention and treatment of lymphedema after lymph node dissection in patients with cutaneous melanoma. Lymphology. 2013; 46(1):20–26

[28] Feldman S, Bansil H, Ascherman J, et al. Single institution experience with lymphatic microsurgical preventive healing approach (LYMPHA) for the primary prevention of lymphedema. Ann Surg Oncol. 2015; 22(10):3296–3301

[29] Ozmen T, Lazaro M, Zhou Y, Vinyard A, Avisar E. Evaluation of simplified lymphatic microsurgical preventing healing approach (S-LYMPHA) for the prevention of breast cancer-related clinical lymphedema after axillary lymph node dissection. Ann Surg. 2019; 270(6):1156–1160

[30] International Society of Lymphology. The diagnosis and treatment of peripheral lymphedema: 2013 Consensus Document of the International Society of Lymphology. Lymphology. 2013; 46(1):1–11

[31] Campisi C, Boccardo F, Zilli A, Macciò A, Napoli F. Long-term results after lymphatic-venous anastomoses for the treatment of obstructive lymphedema. Microsurgery. 2001; 21(4):135–139

[32] Hirche C, Engel H, Seidenstuecker K, et al. Rekonstruktive Mikrochirurgie des sekundären Lymphödems: Konsensus der Deutschsprachigen Arbeitsgemeinschaft für Mikrochirurgie der peripheren Nerven und Gefäße (DAM) zur Indikation, Diagnostik und Therapie mittels Lymphovenöser Anastomosen (LVA) und vaskularisierter Lymphknotentransplantation (VLKT). [Lympho-reconstructive microsurgery for secondary lymphedema: Consensus of the German-Speaking Society for Microsurgery of Peripheral Nerves and Vessels (DAM) on indication, diagnostic and therapy by lymphovenous anastomosis (LVA) and vascularized lymph node transfer (VLNT)]. Handchir Mikrochir Plast Chir. 2019; 51(6):424–433

[33] Beederman M, Garza RM, Agarwal S, Chang DW. Outcomes for physiologic microsurgical treatment of secondary lymphedema involving the extremity. Ann Surg. 2020.. DOI: 10.1097/SLA.0000000000004457

[34] Grünherz L, Hulla H, Uyulmaz S, Giovanoli P, Lindenblatt N. Patient-reported outcomes following lymph reconstructive surgery in lower limb lymphedema: a systematic review of literature. J Vasc. 2021; 9 (3):811–819.e2

20 Experimental Research and Future Directions

Summary
Secondary lymphedema, caused by oncologic surgery, radiation, and chemotherapy, is one of the most relevant, non-oncological complications affecting cancer survivors. In the last decades, lymphatic surgery has been revolutionized by significant technical concepts and advances, especially procedures such as lymphovenous anastomosis and vascularized lymph node transfer. However, some patients have unsuitable or nonfunctional lymphatic vessels, lymph node harvesting is associated with risks, and some patients are non-responders to the microsurgical techniques. Experimental research to define future directions with a focus on lymphatic tissue engineering has included animal models mimicking the human lymphedema pathophysiology, cell harvesting, nutrient supply of engineered tissue, biocompatibility, and hydrostatic properties of the future transplants. Clinical translation is a relevant issue and is in focus for lymph nodes and complex microarchitecture of the lymphatic network. Lymphatic tissue engineering has the potential to be the next step for microsurgical treatment of secondary lymphedema.

Keywords: animal model, artificial organs, biocompatibility, biomaterials, clinical application, growth factors, lymphatic system, lymph nodes, lymphatic network, lymphedema, non-responder, research, scaffolds, tissue engineering, translation

20.1 Animal Models

Florian Früh

20.1.1 Introduction

In industrialized countries, the surgical treatment of cancer is the most common etiology of secondary lymphedema.[1] In particular, the combined damage and ablation of the lymphatic system using radiation and surgery is associated with high rates of lymphatic complications. Up to 55% of women treated for breast cancer and patients undergoing treatment of melanoma develop lymphedema of the extremities depending on the oncological treatment.[2,3,4,5] Because secondary lymphedema is a complex disease involving several tissue components, its exploration by means of *in vitro* models is not feasible.[6] Consequently, reliable animal models are of paramount importance to dissect the pathophysiology of the disease and to develop novel treatment strategies. Although primary lymphedema and secondary postinfectious lymphedema also contribute to the burden of lymphedema, the latter especially in the third world, most models focus on the pathophysiology of secondary, postoncologic lymphedema.

The demand for solid preclinical models is currently increasing due to the emerging clinical application of reconstructive microsurgical techniques, such as lymphovenous anastomoses (LVA[7]) and vascularized lymph node transfer (VLNT[8,9]). Even though the clinical results of these reconstructive approaches are promising, the majority of lymphedema patients still depend on lifelong supportive decongestion therapy to control the disease. Animal models are not only crucial to understand the underlying biological mechanisms of lymphatic dysfunction and stage progression, but also to explore technical refinements of reconstructive lymphatic microsurgery. Moreover, animal models provide a unique opportunity for microsurgical training before performing these procedures on patients. In recent years, several innovative approaches in large as well as small animal models have been introduced.

This chapter will provide a summary of selected large and small animal models with a focus on novel and useful developments. For detailed historical and technical information on preclinical lymphedema models, the interested reader is referred to a previously published systematic review.[6] Finally, specific challenges of the popular rodent lymphedema models, such as induction modality and technique, limb versus tail model, limb volumetry, lymphatic imaging, and role of immunohistochemical analyses and translational approaches will be discussed.

20.1.2 Lymphedema Models in Large Animal

The initial phase of lymphatic research in the early 20th century was characterized by experiments on dogs. Hindlimb lymphedema was induced with combined ablation of the lymphatic system by means of ligation and intralymphatic injection of a sclerosing solution.[10] Later, this approach was replaced by lymphatic resection and pre- or postoperative radiation, resulting in chronic hindlimb swelling.[11,12] The dog hindlimb model has been discontinued due to ethical concerns and a long latency until lymphedema develops.[13] However, recent experiments by Suami et al. comparing the canine and human lymphatic territories ("lymphosomes") revealed that the canine model may still be suitable for the evaluation of lymphatic regeneration in translational means.[14] Their canine lymphosome map has been used for the observation of lymphatic collateral formation after lymph node dissection[15] (▶ Fig. 20.1).

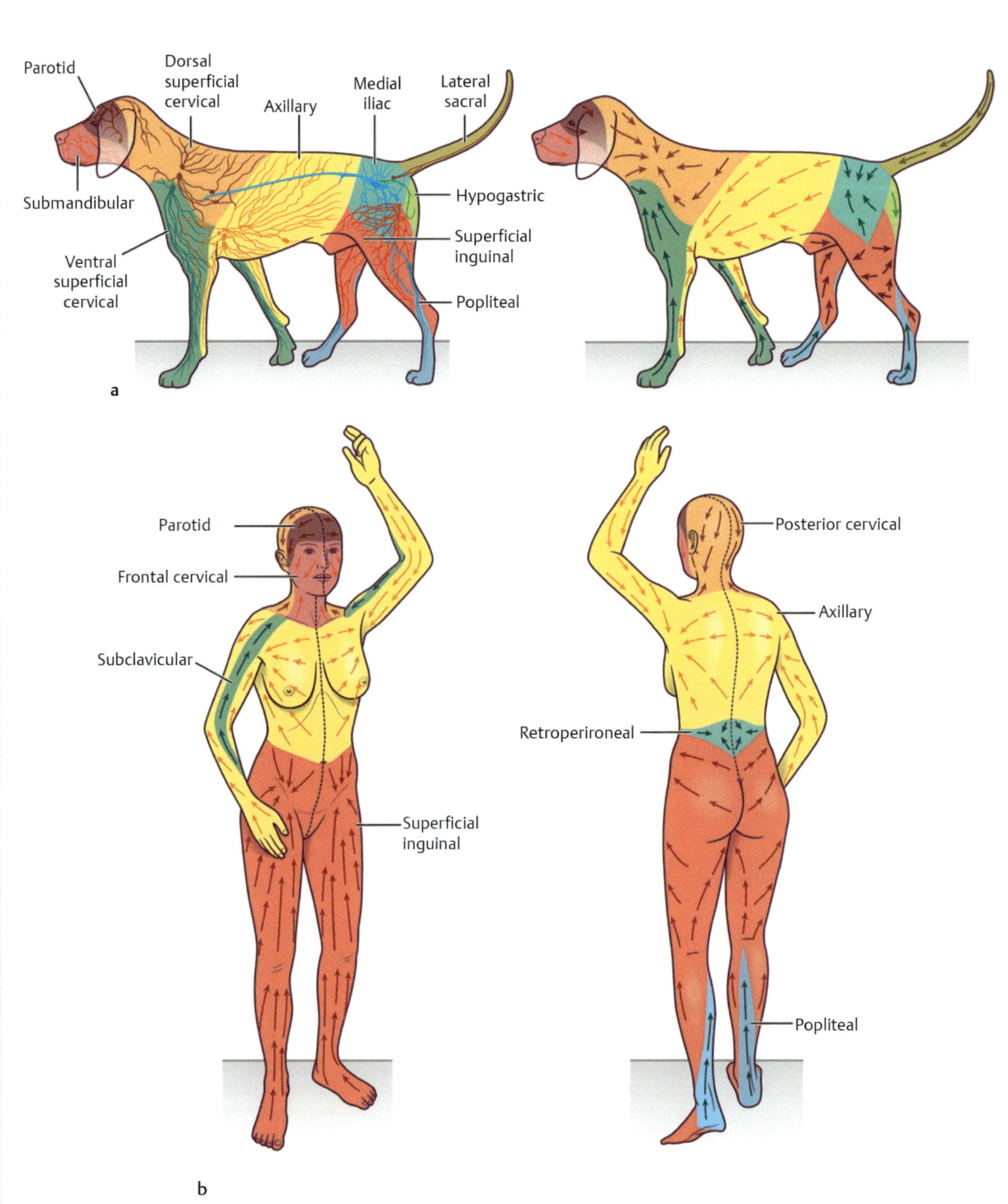

Fig. 20.1 Canine **(a)** versus human **(b)** lymphatic lymphosomes. (Redrawn with permission from Suami et al.[15])

Lymphedema has also been induced in sheep, pigs, and monkeys.[16,17,18] The lymphatic anatomy of the sheep is thought to be particularly suitable for the surgical induction of lymphedema.[16] Besides a "human-sized," translational perspective, this species offers the possibility of disrupting the lymphatic drainage of the whole limb by a single lymph node excision. Due to their anatomical features, sheep and pigs are interesting models for the experimental evaluation of VLNT and other reconstructive lymphatic surgeries. Accordingly, they have been used to study the effect of VLNT.[16,17] Of special interest, the porcine model revealed the efficacy of additional pro-lymphangiogenic growth factor treatment to enhance the functional integration of transplanted lymph nodes.[19] Based on these experimental findings, perinodal growth factor delivery was suggested for future clinical trials in lymphedema patients. Despite these promising investigations, it has to be noted that the findings on VLNT in the current large animal models suffer from important limitations: (i) The experimental data are based on short- or mid-term (< 6 months) follow-up, not giving consideration to the lifelong course of human lymphedema and (ii) the evaluation of the therapeutic approach is not consistent, including frequent absence of histologic or immunohistochemical analyses of the specimens.[6] In addition, the use of large animal models requires resources and is costly. Interestingly, recent experiments in the porcine model have revealed that a relatively long timeframe is necessary for the establishment of chronic lymphedema features in the tissues.[20] Even though lymphedema research has markedly advanced based on large animal model investigations, they have been mostly abandoned in the last decade in favor of small animal models (i.e., rodents), which are easier to breed and less expensive to handle.

20.1.3 Lymphedema Models in Rodents

After their introduction in the 1980s, rodent lymphedema models have gained increasing popularity for several reasons. The small animals are uncomplicated to handle and allow a broadly available, cost-effective, and reliable investigation of different pathologies of the lymphatic system. From the reconstructive surgeon's perspective, rodent models are particularly appealing because they also offer a unique opportunity for microsurgical training and teaching. In the following, characteristics of selected rodent lymphedema models are introduced (▶ Fig. 20.2).

Despite limited knowledge on the anatomy of the rodent lymphatic system, the hindlimb lymphedema model in rats was introduced back in 1985.[21] Originally, the induction of secondary lymphedema was achieved by resection of the main lymphatic trunk as well as the popliteal lymph node and the edges of the circumferential skin incision were sutured to the muscle to reduce the neoformation of lymphatic collaterals. However, most techniques based on surgery alone resulted in a spontaneous decrease of hindlimb swelling. Thereafter, a multitude of technical modifications was suggested to achieve a more durable hindlimb lymphedema, mimicking the chronic disease of human patients. Altogether, the combined ablation of the lymphatic system with surgery and radiation resulted in a reliable and sustained induction of hindlimb swelling in rats.[22] More recent investigations of the rat hindlimb model with dedicated lymphatic imaging and immunohistochemical assessment revealed that the combination of surgery and radiation is also associated with typical histopathological hallmarks of chronic lymphedema.[23] From a physiological point of view, the ideal hindlimb rat model would be based on isolated surgical ablation of the lymphatic system because high radiation doses might interfere with the natural development of secondary lymphedema due to unspecific, further inflammatory triggers and actinic fibrosis despite the original pathophysiology of lymphedema. In line with this, Will et al. recently suggested a promising modification of the hindlimb model.[24] Using ICG pre- and intraoperative mapping and resection of the popliteal and inguinal lymphatic vasculature and lymph nodes, they achieved a stable and immunohistochemically proven secondary lymphedema throughout the course of a 45-day experiment. Based on these findings, the surgical rat hindlimb model appears more suitable for the investigations of chronic lymphedema as previously thought.

To unravel the pathophysiology of secondary lymphedema and to enhance the understanding of therapeutic

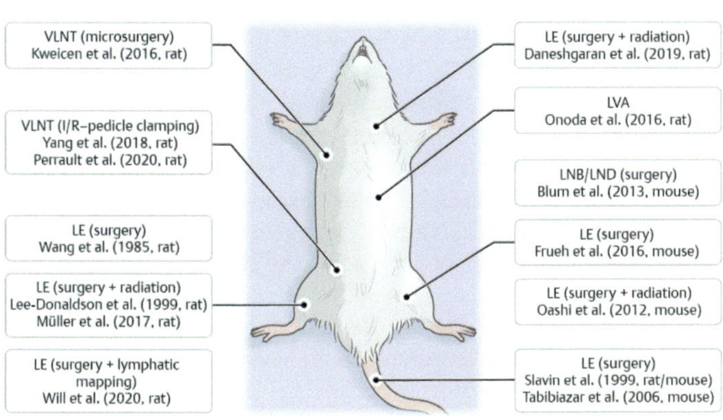

Fig. 20.2 Selection of rodent models for the study of lymphatic dysfunction. LE, lymphedema; LNB, lymph node biopsy; LND, lymph node dissection; LVA, lymphovenous anastomosis; VLNT, vascularized lymph node transfer. (Original drawing by Isabel Zucal)

strategies, different mouse models of lymphedema have been introduced. Experiments using mice have opened the field to a wide range of molecular biology tools, including specific antibodies and transgenic, knock-out animals, allowing a more sophisticated approach to understand lymphatic dysfunction and to mimic primary lymphedema. A powerful model is the mouse tail model, which is technically easy and robust.[25] Briefly, the lymphatic vasculature of the mouse tail is ligated, cauterized, or excised over a circular skin incision with resection of 3- to 5-mm skin. This results in tail swelling, impairment of lymphatic function, and histopathological findings consistent with clinical lymphedema for as long as 10 weeks postoperatively.[26,27] Recently, investigations based on the mouse tail model markedly contributed to our understanding of secondary lymphedema.[27,28] Furthermore, promising preclinical therapeutic strategies with the potential for clinical translation were introduced.[29,30,31] Potential drawbacks of the tail model are the intra-individual lack of comparison to an unaffected “extremity” by volumetry and translational research.

Besides the mouse tail, also its hindlimb has been used for the investigation of secondary lymphedema. Oashi et al. reported hindlimb lymphedema after irradiation of the groin with 30 Gy and resection of the deep lymphatics and subiliacal as well as popliteal lymph nodes.[32] To induce sustained swelling of the hindlimb with the development of chronic lymphedema, it is commonly accepted to resect a small portion of the circular skin incision and suture the wound edges down to the muscle. Without irradiation and skin resection, the lymphatic ablation is not radical enough, only resulting in “acute” lymphedema with spontaneous regression of the swelling.[33] However, the hindlimb model with isolated popliteal lymph node removal contributed to our understanding of lymphatic damage and regeneration after diagnostic procedures such as sentinel lymph node biopsies.[34]

Surgical lymphedema models traditionally tackle lymphatic dysfunction of the extremities while there is a lack of research identifying preventative or curative agents for the progression of head and neck lymphedema. Daneshgaran et al. recently introduced a rat model for secondary head and neck lymphedema.[35] They were able to induce sustained lymphedema by a cervical lymphadenectomy followed by adjuvant radiation therapy. This model may pave the way to study head and neck lymphedema in greater depth and could serve as a platform to evaluate future therapeutic approaches specific to this debilitating disease. Besides lymphedema research, rodent models are valuable tools for the investigation of reconstructive microsurgical techniques, such as LVA or VLNT. For instance, recent ischemia-reperfusion studies using lymph node flaps in the rat groin contributed to our understanding of VLNT.[36,37] Remarkably, this model relies on *in situ* clamping of the flap pedicle, eliminating a potential bias of microvascular complications, which is a matter of concern when evaluating VLNT in small animal models. Finally, from an educational point of view, the axillary VLNT model[38] and the abdominal LVA model[39] are useful microsurgical training opportunities before performing reconstructive lymphatic surgery in the clinical setting.

20.1.4 Challenges of Small Animal Models

During the last decades, mice and rats have gained great popularity for experimental lymphedema studies. Breeding and animal handling is easy and affordable and rodent tissue can be analyzed with a multitude of molecular biology tools, allowing deep insights into the pathophysiology of lymphedema. However, rodent lymphedema models exhibit important technical hurdles that should be mastered for flawless experiments, particularly when the hindlimb model is used.

Hindlimb Volumetry

A reproducible and reliable assessment of hindlimb volumes in rats and mice is challenging. In the beginning of rodent lymphedema research, volumetry was commonly performed using simple techniques, such as water displacement or the assessment of limb circumference. However, these methods are unprecise and prone to measuring errors due to small animal size and lack of standardization.[33] To enhance precision, hindlimb volumetry based on three-dimensional imaging was proposed.[33,40,41] Volumetry based on three-dimensional imaging (i.e., CT or MRI) allows for the determination of hindlimb volumes by means of (i) manual outlining of parallel axial slices with volume calculation by integrating the outlined areas[33] or (ii) software-based volume calculation in a manually selected area.[41] Both techniques are characterized by high precision and low inter- as well as intra-rater variability. The key to reliable volumetry based on three-dimensional imaging is the limitation of volume calculation to a clearly defined area of the limb. The distal tibio-fibular joint is a reliable landmark to determine the proximal border of hindlimb volumetry in mice.[33] Using this easily reproducible anatomical landmark, volumetry can be limited to the distal limb, resulting in comparable volumes with neglectable measuring errors (▶ Fig. 20.3a–e). Another technically feasible and cost-effective tool for the assessment of hindlimb volumes is the measurement of paw thickness with an electronic caliper (▶ Fig. 20.3f). This technique evaluates the swelling of the paw as a surrogate parameter for the limb volume. Remarkably, caliper-measured paw thickness correlated well with CT ($r = 0.861$) and MRI ($r = 0.821$).[33] Therefore, it may be ideally suited for the quantification of rodent hindlimb lymphedema.

An important advantage of the rodent hindlimb compared to the rodent tail is the availability of a contralateral, non-operated limb which serves as an intraindividual

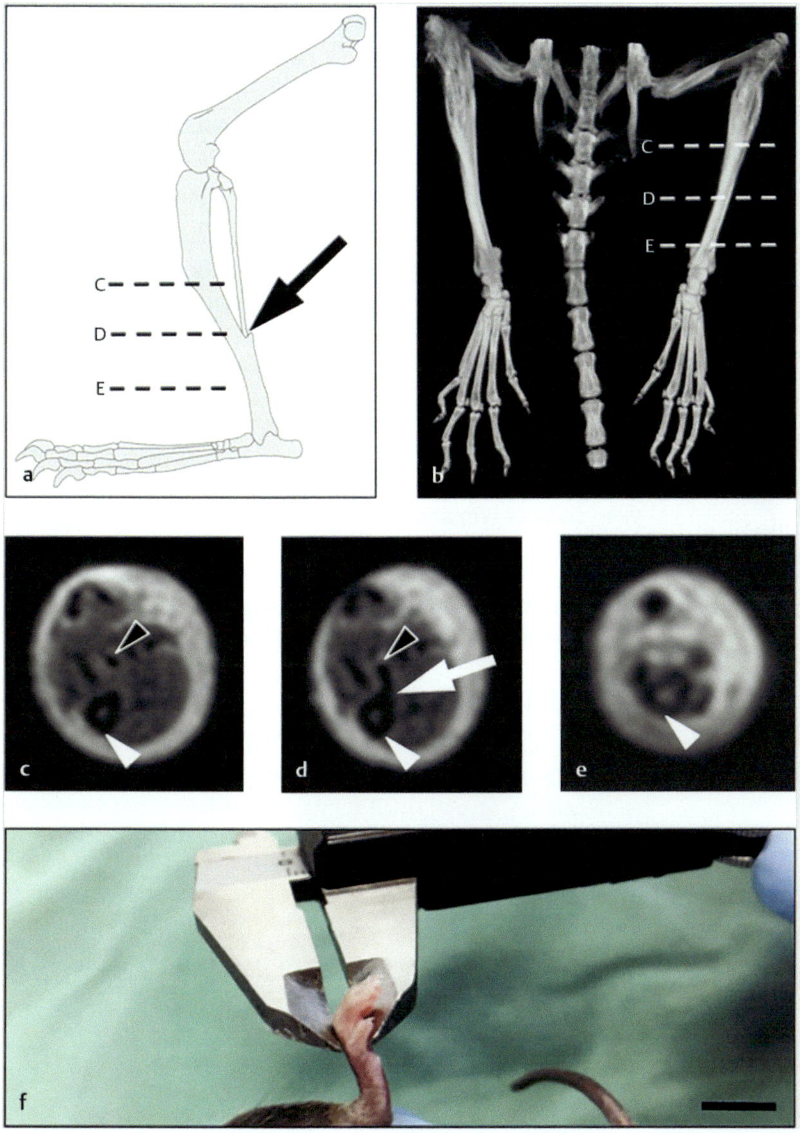

Fig. 20.3a–e Volumetry of the mouse hind limb. **(a,b)** Standardization of three-dimensional, imaging-based volumetry using the distal tibio-fibular joint (arrow). **(c–e)** Localization of the tibio-fibular joint in axial magnetic resonance images. **(c)** Proximal to the joint, both tibia (white arrowhead) and fibula (black arrowhead) are detectable. **(d)** At the joint level, one recognizes a fusion between tibia and fibula (arrow). **(e)** More distally, only the tibia is identifiable (white arrowhead). **(f)** Caliper-based measurement of murine paw thickness as surrogate parameter for hind limb volume; scale = 7 mm. (f reproduced with permission from Früh et al.[33])

control for experimental lymphedema research. Even though no generally accepted definition of experimental lymphedema exists, it may be reasonable to use clinically established human diagnostic criteria, such as the increase of > 10 % volume of an extremity compared with the contralateral one. The use of clinical diagnostic lymphedema criteria enhances the comparability and clarity of experimental lymphedema research and has recently been applied on the rat hindlimb model.[24]

Lymphatic Imaging

The visualization of the lymphatic system is crucial when performing rodent lymphedema experiments. Due to the small size of the animals and the absence of specific contrast agents for the lymphatic vasculature, imaging of the lymphatic system was considered difficult in the beginning of surgical lymphedema research. Importantly, direct lymphangiography in small animals is challenging and intralymphatic cannulation ("direct lymphangiography") is not feasible for repetitive *in vivo* analyses.[42] Therefore, the logical solution consists of contrast deposition in the interstitial space with subsequent transport through lymphatic capillaries ("indirect lymphangiography").[23] For this purpose, several techniques have been introduced, but ICG lymphangiography[41,43] and MRL[23,44] may be most suitable for preclinical lymphatic imaging. However, Food and Drug Administration (FDA)-approved and clinically established contrast agents, such as ICG or Gd-DOTA, are limited by nonspecific uptake from the interstitium through venous capillaries, resulting in suboptimal lymphatic imaging. Cutting-edge experimental ICG lymphangiography can be performed using an optimized liposomal formulation of ICG.[43] This contrast agent is specifically taken up by lymphatic vessels due to its modified molecular structure and weight and is also suitable for improved visualization of deep lymph nodes. Moreover, ICG lymphangiography allows for dynamic and objective, real-time analyses, such as the evaluation of lymphatic vessel contractility and lymphatic transport capacity.[28]

Similarly, interstitial MRI using Gd-DOTA is limited by possible venous contamination. A novel and promising contrast agent is the nanoparticle AGuIX, which consists of 10 Gd-DOTA species binding to a polysiloxane core, yielding a higher molecule size with a rigid structure.[45] AGuIX was recently introduced for interstitial MRL at 9.4 T in a secondary hindlimb lymphedema model in rats.[23] Remarkably, AGuIX injection allowed high-resolution depiction of the lymphatic vessel anatomy *in vivo* with good correlation to *ex vivo* dissection after methylene blue injection (▶ Fig. 20.4). Moreover, it yielded a clear depiction of the collecting lymphatic vessels on the dorsum of the paw and a precise three-dimensional reconstruction of the lymphatic vessel configuration around the popliteal lymph node, indicating the high potential of AGuIX for the assessment of the rodent lymphatic system.

Histology and Immunohistochemistry

Along with volumetry and lymphatic imaging, histological and immunohistochemical analyses play an integral role when working with experimental lymphedema models. Conventional hematoxylin-eosin staining can be used for the quantification of epidermal thickness. Moreover, chronic lymphedema is characterized by histopathological hallmarks, such as fibro-adipose tissue accumulation and dermal inflammatory cell infiltration.[46] A thorough quantification of these tissue alterations is crucial to verify the efficacy of an animal model and of therapeutic approaches. It can be achieved by means of Sirius red (collagen), BODIPY (lipid droplets) as well as different immunohistochemical staining targeting infiltrating inflammatory cells. Finally, lymphatic vessels are stained using antibodies against lymphatic endothelial cells, such as lymphatic vessel endothelial hyaluronan receptor 1 (LYVE-1). The quantification of lymphatic vessel density or lymphatic vessel area/total tissue area completes the immunohistochemical workup and increases the scientific value of preclinical lymphedema investigations.

20.1.5 Conclusions

Secondary lymphedema is a quickly evolving field of experimental research, and since the first experiments in canines, several small animal models have been developed.

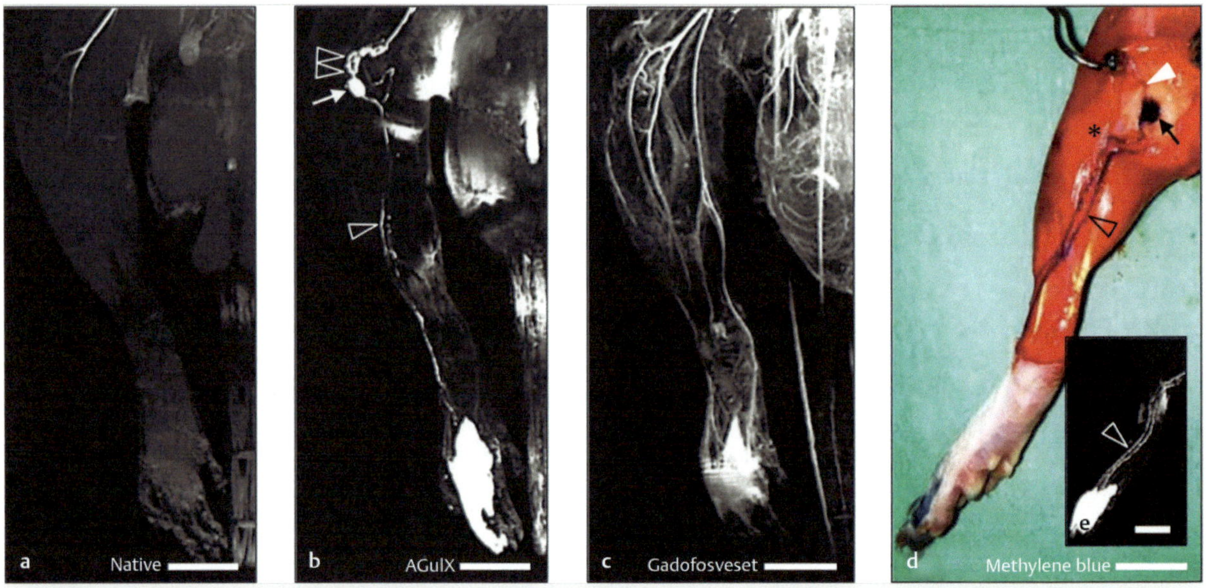

Fig. 20.4 Nanoparticle-based interstitial magnetic resonance lymphangiography of rat hindlimb. **(a, b)** Magnetic resonance lymphangiography before **(a)** and after **(b)** intradermal AGuIX injection in the paw (arrowhead = afferent lymphatic vessels, arrow = popliteal lymph node, double arrowhead = efferent lymphatic vessel). **(c)** Magnetic resonance angiography with intravenous Gadofosveset injection. **(d)** Corresponding dissection of the hindlimb lymphatic system after methylene blue injection. The afferent lymphatic vessels (arrowhead) pierce the fascia of the biceps femoris muscle (asterisk). Arrow = popliteal lymph node. White arrowhead = vascular lymph node pedicle. **(e)** Dorsolateral view of the paw after AGuIX injection highlighting the paired collecting lymphatic vessels (arrowhead). Scales: **a–d** = 8 mm, **e** = 6.5 mm. (Reproduced with permission from Müller et al.[23])

Taken together, animal models are continuously expanding our understanding of how secondary lymphedema develops and how we might be able to tackle this debilitating disease. Even though the translational value of experimental lymphedema investigations remains somewhat unclear, they may pave the way to take future therapeutic strategies from bench to bedside.

20.2 Tissue Engineering and Replacement of Lymphatic Vascular Network

Anja M. Boos, Andreas Spörlein, and Patrick A. Will

20.2.1 Introduction

Tissue engineering describes the bioengineered construction of tissues and organs, either in vitro or in vivo, in order to enhance or replace the body's own tissues. Cells as well as scaffolds or matrices are necessary, thus combining techniques of the fields of biology and engineering. The difficulty lies in developing a graft with ideal biomechanical properties, while at the same time having good biocompatibility, i.e., causing no adverse reactions such as inflammation and local cell degeneration after insertion.

Successful clinical applications have in the past been approved for replacement or regeneration of skin, bone, cartilage, as well as the improvement of wound healing and nerve repair.[47] There have also been substantial advances in establishing a tissue-engineered blood vessel. However, equivalent research on lymphatic vessels is scarcer.

With such a tissue-engineered lymphatic vessel graft for the development of a lymphatic vascular network, surgical therapy for lymphedema and other diseases would no longer be dependent on the patient's own vessels, which are often of poor quality due to oncologic therapy including radiation, chemotherapy, and surgery. In the following sections of this chapter, current approaches, limitations, and possible applications will be discussed.

20.2.2 Cells and Growth Factors for Lymphatic Tissue Engineering

Cell Source

The first key milestone for tissue engineering a certain organ is establishing a suitable cell source, with lymphatic endothelial cells (LECs), endothelial progenitor cells, and/or stem cells. They are mostly of venous origin and physiologically, they align in a single layer of overlapping cells connected by button-like junctions to form lymphatic capillaries, which lack pericytes and do not have a basement membrane.[48] Multiple tissue types—dermal, vascular, and adipose—have been used as a source material for the direct acquisition of LECs or for harvesting pluripotent cells for differentiation into LECs (▸ Table 20.1).

Dermal tissue can easily be acquired during routine circumcisions and is a suitable source for direct acquisition of LECs. The cells can be isolated with magnetic activated cell sorting (MACS) or fluorescence activated cell sorting (FACS), both of which require the utilization of antibodies against LEC markers like vascular endothelial growth factor receptor 3 (VEGFR-3), Podoplanin, Prox-1, and LYVE-1.[53]

Dermal tissue can also be used in order to isolate human dermal microvascular endothelial cells (HDMECs). Because isolates of HDMEC contain both blood and lymphatic endothelial cells, they are particularly useful for experimental settings in which both cell types are required. It allows for the growth of separate blood and lymphatic vascular networks under in vitro conditions, which is particularly relevant for the prevascularization of grafts.

Alternative methods do not rely on primary isolation but on the differentiation of stem cells. Human blood

Table 20.1 Source of endothelial cells and methods of isolation and cultivation

Cell source	Obtained cell type	Isolation method	Cultivation	Reference
Blood	hMSCs	Density gradient centrifugation and selective growth	Supernatant from isolated LECs	Conrad[51]
Dermis	LECs	Magnetic beads (anti-LYVE-1)	EC basal medium in collagen-coated flask	Podgrabinska[49]
Dermis	HDMECs	Magnetic beads (anti-podoplanin)	VEGF-C and ASC coculture	Knezevic[50]
Adipose tissue	ASCs	Density gradient centrifugation after collagenase treatment	VEGF-C and bFGF	Yang[52]

Abbreviations: ASC, adipose-derived stem cell; bFGF, basic fibroblast growth factor; EC, endothelial cell; hMSC, multipotent mesenchymal stem cells; HDMEC, human dermal microvascular endothelial cell; LEC, lymphatic endothelial cell; LYVE-1, lymphatic vessel endothelial hyaluronan receptor 1; VEGF-C, vascular endothelial growth factor C.

contains multipotent mesenchymal stem cells (hMSC), which can be differentiated into LECs by treatment with supernatant from previously isolated LECs, as shown by an endothelial-like morphology and the expression of common lymphatic markers.[51] The phenotype could not be achieved by treatment with vascular endothelial growth factor (VEGF)-C only, which suggests that other paracrine factors secreted by LECs as well as the exposure to VEGFR-2 and -3 might play a role in this differentiation. The exact cues that are necessary remain to be determined, however. Contemplating a future clinical application, it is always preferable to use specific growth factors instead of supernatant because the risk of adverse immunologic reactions is smaller.

Adipose-derived stem cells (ASCs), which are easily obtainable during lipectomy, can be differentiated into LECs as well. The differentiation was successful after incubation with VEGF-C156S and basic fibroblast growth factor (bFGF), as confirmed by immunofluorescent staining against the lymphatic markers LYVE-1 and VEGFR-3.[52]

In conclusion, the ideal cell source for clinical application of a tissue-engineered lymphatic vessel remains to be established. Good availability, a cost-efficient standardized isolation, and patient safety need to be considered. The procedures vary in invasiveness between the different sources—while blood is routinely drawn in a clinical setting, the isolation from dermal or adipose sources require additional procedures.

Once LECs are primarily isolated or differentiated from precursor cell, their growth needs to be sustained, either by external addition of growth factors or by coculturing them with different cell types that provide an adequate environment.

External Growth Factors

The central mediator of lymphatic vessel growth is VEGF-C, which is a part of the larger group of VEGFs. VEGF-C sustains the growth of LEC and is particularly significant for LEC migration and would healing.[54] It is essential for growing LEC in vitro despite the use of serum. There are multiple VEGF-C isoforms with varying affinity to VEGFR-3 (almost exclusively on LEC) and VEGFR-2 (also present on blood endothelium), including VEGF-C156S which was developed to activate VEGFR-3 only, thus being more specific to LEC.[55]

VEGF-D is a paralog to VEGF-C and has similar features. The lymphangiogenic potential is even higher, but it is less suitable than VEGF-C for LEC cultures because of difficulties in controlling the proteolytic environment.[55] In contrast to VEGF-C, knock-out mice lacking VEGF-D can survive, indicating a less critical role in lymphatic development.[55]

As shown by Gibot et al.,[54] hepatocyte growth factor (HGF) is important for LEC tubulogenesis and proliferation and shows synergistic effects with VEGF-C by activation of extracellular signal-regulated kinase 1/2 (ERK1/2) signaling.[54]

Avraham et al. found that by blockage of transforming growth factor β1 (TGF-β1) with a monoclonal antibody in a mouse model of lymphedema, lymphatic growth and regeneration could significantly be increased. The effects were independent of VEGF-A, VEGF-C, and HGF, thus identifying TGF-β1 as a potent anti-lymphangiogenic cue (► Table 20.2).[56]

There are further external growth factors which play a role in the regulation, which are not discussed in detail in this chapter but listed in terms of completeness of content: basic fibroblast growth factor (bFGF), angiopoietin-1 and its receptor Tie-2, ephrin-B2 and its tyrosine kinase receptor EphB4, endothelial hyaluron receptor Lyve 1, fibronectin, and C-chemokine ligand 21 (CCL21).

Cocultures: Fibroblasts and Adipose-Derived Stem Cells

A tissue environment that is favorable for LEC growth can be provided by different cell types in a coculture. Of all

Table 20.2 Lymphangiogenic Growth Factors: Corresponding receptors and effects

Growth factor	Pathway/Receptor	Effect	Reference
VEGF-C	VEGFR-2 and -3	Key regulator of lymphangiogenesis and important component of LEC cultures	Knezevic[50]
VEGF-D*	VEGFR-2 and -3	Strongly induces lymphangiogenesis, but handling of cultures difficult due to proteolysis	Rauniyar[55]
HGF	c-Met	Fibroblast-derived HGF induces lymphatic network formation in together with VEGF-C	Gibot[54]
TGF-β1*	TGF-βR	Blockage leads to increased lymphatic growth and regeneration	Avraham[56]
IFN-γ*	IFN-γR	Inhibits proliferation and migration of LEC in vitro, most likely due to induced apoptosis	Shao[57]

Abbreviations: HGF, hepatocyte growth factor; IFN, interferon; LEC, lymphatic endothelial cell; TGF, transforming growth factor; VEGF, vascular endothelial growth factor; VEGFR, vascular endothelial growth factor receptor.
*Note: Not yet specifically used for lymphatic tissue engineering.

the options, two are of note and have been used to sustain lymphatic growth in vitro: fibroblasts and ASCs and bone marrow-derived stem cells (MSCs).[58]

Fibroblasts can be found in connective tissue and are capable of synthesizing extracellular matrix and growth factors; they play a central role in wound healing and regulate inflammation and differentiation of epithelial cells.[59] In vitro co-cultivation of fibroblasts with LECs allows for the spontaneous organization of a three-dimensional capillary network without externally added growth factors.[54,60] This is most likely due to the fibroblasts' endogenous production of VEGF-C and HGF.[54,61]

ASCs are a useful tool for culturing LECs, as their proliferation and migration are enhanced in a coculture.[62] The effect is dependent on direct cell–cell interaction and cannot be traced back to the production of certain growth factors.[50] However, ASCs may produce enough VEGF-C to sustain LEC growth independently and the addition of the growth factor significantly augments lymphatic growth, but in some settings require external VEGF-C stimulation.[63,64]

20.2.3 Scaffolds for Lymphatic Tissue Engineering—Translational Concepts

De- and Recellularized Scaffolds

Decellularizing existing tissue is a common approach in tissue engineering. Cells and genetic material are removed from the donor tissue by treating with a detergent or by physical means. This reduces the immunogenicity of the tissue, but the residue of the detergents often makes subsequent recellularization challenging. The specialized tissue structure, i.e., extracellular matrix, remains largely unmodified, thus providing stability and a suitable scaffold.

Yang et al.[65] have used arteries decellularized with Triton X in order to engineer a large lymphatic vessel. The collagen and elastic fiber structure remained intact during decellularization and LECs could successfully be attached afterwards. In the future, venous scaffolds could be used, as they resemble the biomechanical properties of lymphatic vessels more closely and the existing valves would likely prevent lymphatic backflow, as parts of the valve structure remain and in addition provide cell growth during recellularization.

Hydrogels: the Use of Fibrin and Collagen

Hydrogels, which consist of water and a polymer, can be used as a matrix that provides a suitable environment for network formation of LECs. They can be easily modified, for example, by integrating growth factors. Helm et al., in search of the ideal hydrogel for lymphatic tissue engineering, used matrices with covalently bound VEGF-A and varying amounts of fibrin and collagen.[66] The most extensive network of lymphatic capillaries was formed in a fibrin-only matrix. In contrast, blood capillaries could be best grown in matrices with a higher collagen content. This shows that not all proceedings applied in the field of blood vessel engineering can be transferred to lymphatic vessel engineering. In a different study in which LECs were cocultured with fibroblasts, the formation of lymphatic capillaries was better in collagen matrices than in those that only contained fibrin.[60]

Matrigel, a hydrogel that consists of proteins secreted by murine Engelbreth-Holm-Swarm sarcoma cells, is a basement membrane substitute frequently used for in vitro cell cultivation. However, its suitability for lymphatic tissue engineering proved controversial as no tube formation was found when LECs were cultured in Matrigel with VEGF-C, even in combination with ASCs.[62] This might be due to the fact that lymphatic vessels physiologically do not rely on a basement membrane.[67]

20.2.4 Current Achievements and Limitations

Multiple preliminary studies have succeeded in tissue engineering lymphatic vessels or capillaries. Marino et al.[60] engineered a prevascularized full-thickness skin graft based on a coculture of fibroblasts and HDMECs in a fibrin hydrogel. Since HDMECs contain both blood vascular endothelial cells (BECs) and LECs, this resulted in the formation of two separate vascular networks. With the addition of keratinocytes, a substitute for full-thickness skin was created ready for transplantation on immunodeficient rats. The graft did not contain nerves or dermal appendages. However, for the first time, there was a functioning lymphatic capillary network that connected to the animal's proper lymphatic system (observable in confocal microscopy after immunofluorescent staining) and had an intact clearance capability as determined after Evans blue injection.

Dai et al.[68] used multiple sheets of polyglycolic acid (PGA) that were seeded with human dermal LECs and were wrapped around a silicone canal that measured 3 mm in diameter in order to create a lymphatic vessel. The LECs attached successfully and 6 weeks after transplantation on nude mice, the PGA scaffold was resorbed. Although there were no valves, and no layers of media or adventitia, the group proved that it was feasible to engineer a large lymphatic vessel in the laboratory with three layers mimicking intima for cell growth, media, and adventitia, and to transplant it on an animal model.

Will et al. used dandelion (*Taraxacum officinale*) haulms as a scaffold and successfully decellularized the haulms, which showed long-term storage characteristics prior to rehydration. The dandelion scaffold was evaluated on relevant physical attributes for further use as a lymphatic vessel scaffold, including tensile strength, patency, and kinking, with excellent results. Diameters ranged from 1 to 9 mm. Recellularization with LECs was

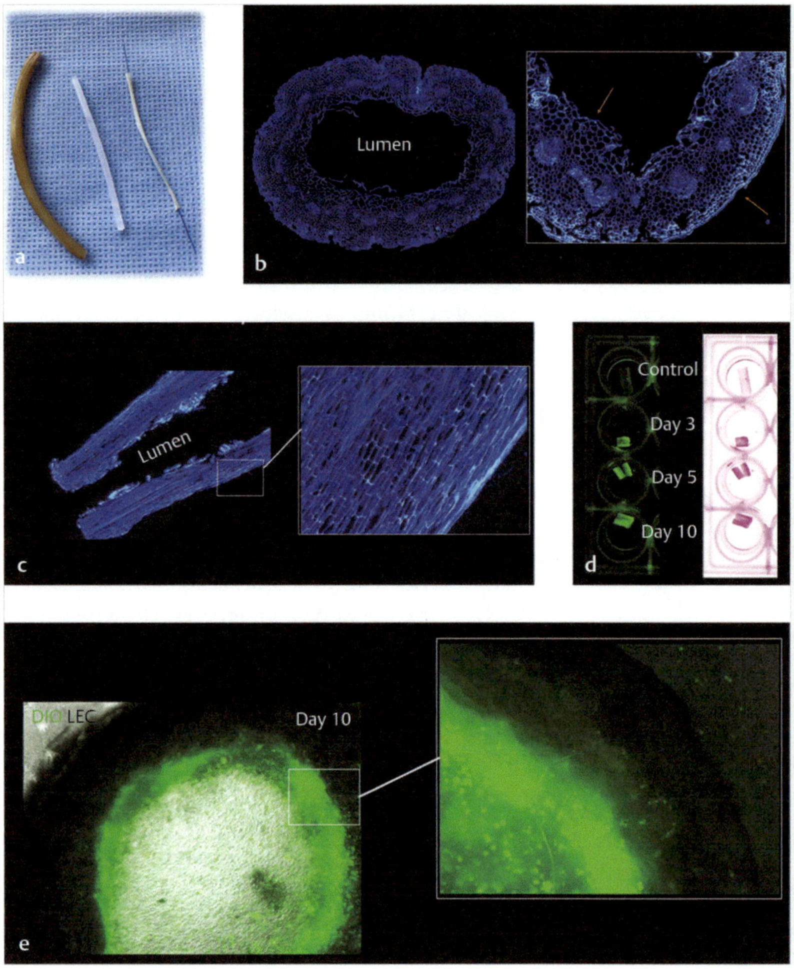

Fig. 20.5 Decellularization of dandelion (*Taraxacum officinale*) haulms with a standardized protocol. **(a)** The native haulm is seen on the left site, the decellularized haulm with remaining innate three-dimensional structure in the middle, the dehydrolyzed and splinted haulm (polyfil surgical suture) prior to rehydration on the right site. The scaffolds are shown to have a structural polarization with space for recellularization and growth in cross sections **(b)** and longitudinal sections **(c)**. During recellularization with DiO-labeled lymphatic endothelial cells, the tubes demonstrated *in vitro* proliferation and organization of the cells continuously until day 10 (longitudinal section; **d**). Here LECs were shown to endothelialize into a multilayer within the tube **(e)**.

successful, and further tests including the value without the valves are necessary (▶ Fig. 20.5).[69]

Kanapathy et al.[70] used polyhedral oligomeric silsesquioxane poly(carbonate-urea) urethane (POSS-PCU) as a scaffold in a similar approach. It showed good physical attributes in terms of kinking, suture retention, and tensile strength. Human dermal LECs adhered well; however, a complete endothelial lining could not be achieved. Like the vessel engineered by Dai et al.,[68] the one from Kanapathy et al. had a relatively large diameter of 2 mm, which results in low capillarity. In combination with the lack of valves, it is therefore questionable whether such a graft would prevent backflow of lymphatic fluid in clinical applications.[51,71,72]

20.2.5 Conclusions

No replacement graft for lymphatic vessels is available for clinical use yet. Although there are multiple good sources for LECs, endothelial progenitor cell (EPC), or stem cells, further work is required to establish a procedure that allows for high-quality, reproducible, and safe harvesting with minimal invasiveness and low cost. Concerning scaffolds, there are promising candidates that are highly biocompatible, allow attachment and growth of cells, and can be easily implanted. Further challenges are providing an ongoing and effective growth environment, initial and long-term functionalization of the grafts, and control of growth, proliferation, and lymphangiogenesis beyond the experimental in vitro and in vivo concepts.

A design challenge lies in ensuring anterograde flow by capillary forces and local tissue gradients, and the possible integration of valves in collectors and distinction of smaller lymphatic vessels such as capillaries. Results and insights on biomaterial technologies from tissue engineering of blood vessels can often be transferred to lymphatic vessels, because the requirements are similar, albeit not identical. Three-dimensional printing of the scaffold prior to recellularization may also be another experimental track in this ongoing and promising field.

After successful engineering in the laboratory and in vivo testing on rodents, the next step toward clinical translation for promising approaches will be large animal models like pigs and sheep. In comparison to rodent lymphedema models, they provide physiological lymphatic structures in human-equivalent dimensions. Additionally, the induced secondary lymphedema of large animal models is more stable over long periods, while lymphedema in rodents often shows spontaneous remission.[73]

20.3 Tissue Engineering for the Replacement of Lymph Nodes

Min-Seok Kwak and Hans-Günther Machens

20.3.1 Introduction

In recent years scientists and clinicians focus more and more on the lymphatic system and its disorder in clinical settings, which has been neglected besides the vascular network for some decades. The lymphatic system is complex in structure and its function, but the potential of regeneration was discovered early on by different authors. Lymphedema is still difficult to cure, but several surgical approaches were described in the past. Tissue engineering aims at replacing damaged or diseased tissues and organs using different kinds of modern biomaterials and scaffolds in combination with cells and tissue types. Biomaterials should provide suitable mechanical properties and high biocompatibility to ensure effective tissue engineering. The micro-architecture of a healthy lymph node is very sophisticated due to the different functions, cell types, and lymph node sections. Therefore, bioengineering functional lymph nodes is still challenging and some obstacles have to be overcome. Several groups presented artificial lymphoid organs in vitro and in vivo to mimic lymph node function. The aim is either to generate adequate immune response or to restore the lymphatic network for effective lymph drainage.

20.3.2 The Lymphatic System

In 2017, Suami presented the lymphosome concept in humans after several studies in animals to better understand the lymphatic pathways with regard to the lymph nodes.[74] It is estimated that human beings have roughly 600 to 700 lymph nodes in their body.[75] Every day, 2 to 4 liters of interstitial fluid is drained by the lymphatic vessels containing 20 to 30 g protein per liter of lymph.[76] The velocity of lymphatic fluid drainage is not well known, but Fischer et al.[77] published a study with 15 healthy individuals to determine the flow velocity in lymphatic capillaries using fluorescein isothiocyanate-dextran, which was injected intradermally (subepidermal) in the foot dorsum. They initially measured a median velocity of 0.51 mm/s (initial network filling) and afterwards a resting velocity of 9.7 µm/s—in which all the lymph node has its essential role. The lymph node itself has a quite complex architecture and is divided into cortex, paracortex, and medulla with different clusters of B and T lymphocytes.[78] Afferent lymphatic vessels enter the lymph node, and the lymph passes a complex labyrinth before leaving it via efferent lymphatic vessels in the hilum where blood vessels also enter to nourish the lymph node.[79] B cells form follicles in the cortex region (B-zone) whereas T cells mainly reside in the paracortex (T-zone). Specialized endothelial cells, called high endothelial venules (HEVs), are also located in the paracortex which are important for lymphocyte homing and recirculation (▶ Table 20.3).[78]

20.3.3 Regeneration of Lymphatic Tissue

The potential of lymphatic and lymph node–like tissue regeneration was already described by Gottesman and Jaffe in 1926. They used small fragments (3 mm) of thymus to implant them into the abdominal muscle of 53 rats. After several time points the transplants were examined histologically for regeneration (212 transplants). Initially, they observed tissue necrosis, but on day 10 the transplants showed complete regeneration with thymic lobules and Hassall's corpuscles.[82] Later Jaffe found similar results using thymus lobules for avascular transplantation in guinea pigs. Complete regeneration was observed on day 21.[83] After 2 years, Jaffe and Richter reported the regeneration of autologous lymph node transplants. In that study they used 31 albino rats and transplanted two nodes in each rat. After initial partial necrosis on day 6, the nodes showed complete regeneration.[84] In

Table 20.3 Allocation of lymphocytes and other cell types in a lymph node (from Nosenko et al.[80] and Lippert[81])

Lymph node sections	Lymphocytes	Stromal and dendritic cells	Cell–cell interactions
Cortex (B-zone)	B-lymphocytes	MRCs, FDC	Maturation of B-lymphocytes
Paracortex (T-zone)	T-lymphocytes	FRCs, DCs	Antigen presentation to T-lymphocytes
Medulla (B-zone)	B-lymphocytes		

Abbreviations: DC, dendritic cells; FDC, follicular dendritic cells; FRC, fibroblast reticular cells; MRC, marginal zone reticular cells.

1965, Tilak and Howard used popliteal lymph nodes for autologous re-transplantation by processing whole lymph node fragments, medulla fragments, and lymph node capsules alone. Their study revealed no regeneration of entire lymph node slices and medulla fragments, whereas an intact capsule without medulla seemed to regenerate.[85]

In the 1980s, Pabst et al. performed several animal studies using lymph node fragments and splenic tissue to prove the regeneration potential of lymphatic tissue. In 1988, they presented a minipig study using superficial inguinal and mesenteric lymph nodes which were cut into small pieces (2 mm) and transplanted into different anatomic regions (greater omentum, groin region, and mesentery of the terminal ileum). All animals received antigen stimulation 1 month before explanation by injection of dead bacteria (*Pasteurella multocida*, *Bordetella bronchiseptica*) into the hindlimb to induce germinal center formation. After 6 months no regeneration was found in the greater omentum, but interestingly lymph node fragments in the groin region showed good regeneration. Antigen stimulation improved regeneration of lymph node fragments in the groin region.[86] In 1990, they conducted a second pig study to investigate more locations of transplantation. Among other things they found improved regeneration of fragments after subcutaneous than subfacial transplantation and inguinal lymph nodes seemed to better regenerate than mesenteric lymph nodes.[87] Shih et al.[88] could show survival and regeneration of human fetal lymph nodes in etoposide-treated severe combined immunodeficiency (SCID) mice. Human fetal lymph nodes were transplanted into three different regions: mammary fat pad (MFP), ear pouch, and kidney capsule. The subcutaneous ear pouch was found to be a region of significant engraftment rate (> 80%) and extensive growth in size (> 200-fold). This SCID-hu mouse model provides the possibility to study extrathymic T-cell development, lymphocyte proliferation and differentiation, and even HIV-1-mediated immunosuppression. The positive effect of platelet-rich plasma (PRP) in autotransplanted avascular lymph node fragments (Lewis rats) was also examined in 2009 by Hadamitzky et al.[89] They also observed B-cell proliferation in lymph nodes of the control group after PRP injection. The authors stated the accelerated potential of lymphangiogenesis and angiogenesis through growth factors contained in platelets. After 1 year, a minipig study was conducted by Blum et al.[90] A total of 26 minipigs underwent lymphadenectomy of both groin regions. The lymph nodes were sliced differently and were retransplanted into the groin region. The authors compared small versus large fragments and fragments with or without a capsule. Five months after transplantation most of the lymph node fragments could be localized with SPECT-CT. Isolated VEGF-C treatment seems to also improve regeneration of autotransplanted lymph node fragments and lymphatic reconnection in rats.[91,92]

20.3.4 Biomaterials

Tissue engineering and regenerative medicine encompasses a multidisciplinary field of cell biology, material science, and biomedical engineering which aims to restore damaged human tissue.[93] Three-dimensional scaffolds are necessary for tissue formation in vivo and in vitro. An ideal scaffold should have following characteristics:

- Porous structure
- Biocompatibility
- Suitable surface chemistry
- Mechanical properties
- Reproducibility

Several biomaterials are available for scaffold fabrication. They are mainly divided into synthetic (poly-glycolic/-lactic acid, polycaprolactone, polydioxane) and natural (collagen, alginate, agarose, polysaccharides, hyaluronan) polymers. Collagen, for example, which is generally derived from bovine origin, is used as suture material, wound dressings, hemostatic sponges, and cardiovascular implants. Hyaluronan is a polysaccharide of the extracellular matrix (ECM) with good biocompatibility and controlled biodegradability. Nevertheless, its fast resorption makes it unfavorable in hard tissue applications. In contrast, synthetic polymers like polycaprolactone offer different degradation parameters. Polycaprolactone is one of the earliest synthesized polymers in the 1930s. Its degradation and resorption are slow, which makes it suitable for hard and soft tissue applications as well. It is regarded as a nontoxic biocompatible material with a long track record. Polydioxanone is a homopolymer of p-dioxanone and is used as suture material. It was also applied in cartilage tissue engineering.[94] The advantage of natural polymers is biologic acceptance, whereas synthetic polymers can be reproduced on a large scale with controlled parameters. Several tissue sources for specific tissue engineering were introduced like urethra, bladder, genital tissues, blood vessels, and kidney. A third class of biomaterials are acellular tissue matrices like bladder submucosa and small intestinal submucosa. Consequently, biomaterials offer the possibility to replace damaged or diseased organs in patients in the future. Ideal biomaterials serve as an artificial ECM, and the three-dimensional structure of scaffolds enables cells to grow and to form new tissue.[93] Several techniques of scaffold fabrication were described in the past like gas foaming, solvent casting, and solution electrospinning. The main drawbacks of conventional scaffold fabrication techniques are the lack of control over pore size, pore geometry, and pore distribution. Moreover, some methods use organic solvents with the risk of toxic and carcinogenic residuals.[95] A possibility to engineer precise scaffold structures can

Table 20.4 Published tissue engineering approaches of lymph nodes or lymphoid organs by different groups

Authors	Year	Scaffold/Biomaterial	Cell/Tissue types	Model
Giese et al.	2006	Agarose, polyamide	Lymphocytes, DCs	In vitro, bioreactor
Hadamitzky et al.	2016	Collagen	Lymph node fragments	Pigs
Kwak et al.	2017	Polycaprolactone	Lymph node fragments	Immunodeficient nude mice
Okamoto et al.	2007	Collagen	TEL-2-LTα, DCs	BALB/c and SCID mice
Purwada et al.	2015	Gelatin, SiNP	Murine B cells, 40LB stromal cells	In vitro
Purwada et al.	2017	Gelatin, SiNP	Murine B cells, 40LB stromal cells	In vitro
Suematsu et al.	2004	Collagen	TEL-2-LTα, DCs	BALB/c* and SCID mice
Tomei et al.	2009	Polyurethane	Murine TRCs	In vitro

Abbreviations: DCs, dendritic cells; SCID, severe combined immunodeficiency; TRCs, T-zone fibroblastic reticular cells.
Note: * BALB/c is an albino, immunodeficient laboratory-bred strain of the common house mouse.

be achieved using the melt electrospinning technology. This method allows for the fabrication and design three-dimensional scaffolds with controllable parameters (fiber diameter, porosity etc.).[96,97] In addition, compared to solution electrospinning there is no risk of solvent residuals or release (biomedical safety).[98]

The cells or tissues are the second important component for successful tissue engineering. The use of native cells has the advantage of an autologous application after regeneration and expanding of the cell line. But not all human cell types can be cultivated and grown in vitro successfully. Conversely, stem cells have the ability to differentiate into many specialized cell types. They can be derived from human embryos, amniotic fluid, and placenta, or using stem cell technologies like cloning and reprogramming.[93]

Lastly, vascularization of the constructs is an important precondition for successful tissue engineering and cell survival. In 2012, Wiggenhauser et al.[99] demonstrated successful vascularization of adipose constructs using seeded and unseeded polyurethane and polycaprolactone scaffolds with human adipose tissue–derived precursor cells (hAPCs).

The requirements of lymphatic vessel and collector tissue engineering and the experimental results and further requirements are given in **Subchapter 20.3.**

20.3.5 Lymph Node Tissue Engineering

The architecture of healthy lymph nodes is complex, so engineering functional artificial lymph nodes is still challenging due to their vast number and density of different cell types, organized microstructure (B and T cell zones), and rapid cell motility. The extremely organized cell mass with different stromal cells, lymphocytes, and vascular network and its complex microenvironment makes it more difficult to engineer than other organs like the kidney or heart.[100] Until now several approaches were introduced combining different scaffolds/biomaterials and cell/tissue types in vivo and in vitro to generate functional lymph nodes (► Table 20.4).

Suematsu and Watanabe[101] developed a tissue-engineered secondary lymphoid tissue–like organoids using thymus-derived stromal cells (TEL-2-LTα) and sponge-like collagenous scaffolds to implant them into the renal subcapsular space of BALB/cAnNcrj and SCID mice. The regenerated organized tissue structure was similar to secondary lymphoid organs showing B-cell and T-cell clusters, HEV-like vessels, and follicular dendritic cell networks.[101] In 2006 Giese et al.[102] reported a very sophisticated approach to mimic lymph nodes using a bioreactor in vitro. Agarose and polyamide matrices were seeded with dendritic cells and cultivated in a bioreactor. Lymphocytes were inoculated subsequently. They observed lymphocyte cluster formation. T-cell activation and long-term reactivity of lymphatic tissue were proven by interleukin (IL)-2 and tumor necrosis factor (TNF)-α response.[102] After 1 year Okamoto et al.[103] could show an immune response using artificial lymphoid organs both in BALB/c and SCID mice after several immunizations with NP-OVA. There was also no difference in the ratio of $CD4^+$ to $CD8^+$ T cells between artificial lymph nodes and recipient lymph nodes in BALB/c mice. The cells migrated to the SCID mice spleen and bone marrow and generated a large number of antibody-forming cells.[103] Tomei et al.[104] regenerated a three-dimensional lymph node T-zone stromal network using murine T-zone fibroblastic reticular cells (TRCs) within polyurethane scaffolds. They could show a correlation between interstitial fluid flow, TRC organization, and secretion of the chemokine CCL21. When the flow through was blocked, the gene expression of CCL21 was downregulated. The chemokines CCL21 and

CCL19 play an important role in APC migration and T-cell extravasation.[104] Another interesting approach was introduced by Purwada et al.[105,106] using murine B cells and stromal 40LB cells cocultured in three-dimensional gelatin-based hydrogel matrices. They could show a phenotypical and functional germinal center reaction similar to other secondary lymphoid tissues. Compared to a two-dimensional coculture, they found a rapid differentiation of naive primary B cells with robust antibody class switching.[106] A combination of scaffolds and lymph node fragments was first presented by Hadamitzky et al.[107] in 2016. They used aligned nanofibrillar collagen scaffolds with or without lymph node fragments in a pig study after lymphedema development. A second group received VEGF-C-conjugated collagen scaffolds and a third group was untreated. The improvement of lymphedema was documented using bioimpedance measurements, a CT scan, and immunohistochemistry. The first group showed the best results in lymphedema improvement, which was confirmed by imaging and histological examination. Strictly speaking, the nanofibrillar scaffolds served rather as a splint for lymphangiogenesis than to engineer a lymphoid organ.

Based on the concept of vascularized lymph node transfer (VLNT), a similar approach, combining a scaffold and lymph node fragments, was presented by Kwak et al. in 2017.[108,109] The group used cylindrical, medical-grade polycaprolactone (mPCL) scaffolds, which were seeded with lymph node fragments to engineer artificial lymph nodes. These constructs can be cultivated in vitro or used as immediate implants for in vivo studies by placing them nearby a main vessel for angiogenesis and tissue regeneration. A first human study has already been performed and revealed an uptake of the radiotracer in the region of implantation after 1 year (not published). The PCL scaffolds, which use melt electrospinning technology and based on additive manufacturing (AM) principles, support cell migration, proliferation, and differentiation. Additive manufacturing allows to produce scaffolds following a computer programmed design with improved control over pore size, distribution, and precise three-dimensional micro-architectures using micro-to-nano scale polymer fibers. Over time the scaffold degrades, and the newly formed tissue takes its place. These scaffolds offer a very high surface to volume ratio which makes them favorable for tissue engineering and regenerative medicine.[95,110,111] Further research on this promising concept needs to be done in view of improved angiogenesis and revascularization of these bioartificially generated, avascular lymph nodes (▶ Fig. 20.6, ▶ Fig. 20.7, ▶ Fig. 20.8).

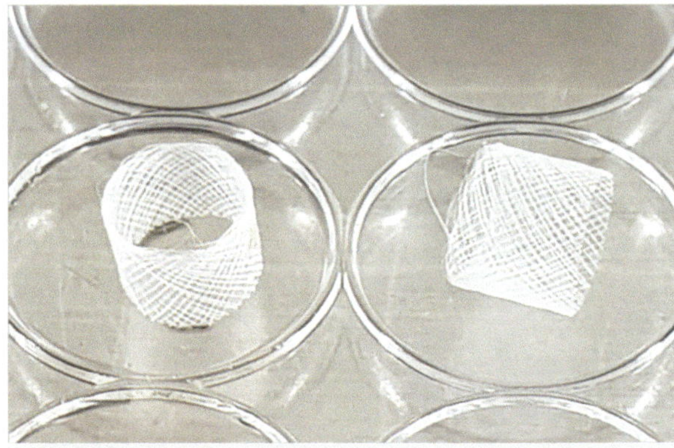

Fig. 20.6 Tubular scaffolds made from medical-grade polycaprolactone using the melt electrospinning technology to incorporate lymph node fragments. Computer-based precise manufacturing offers predetermined pore size, fiber diameter, and three-dimensional architecture.

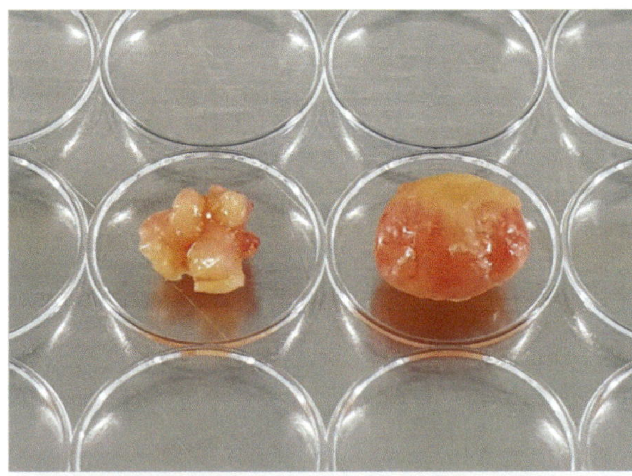

Fig. 20.7 Isolated lymph nodes prior to processing and incorporation into a scaffold: Intact (right) and after fragmentation (left).

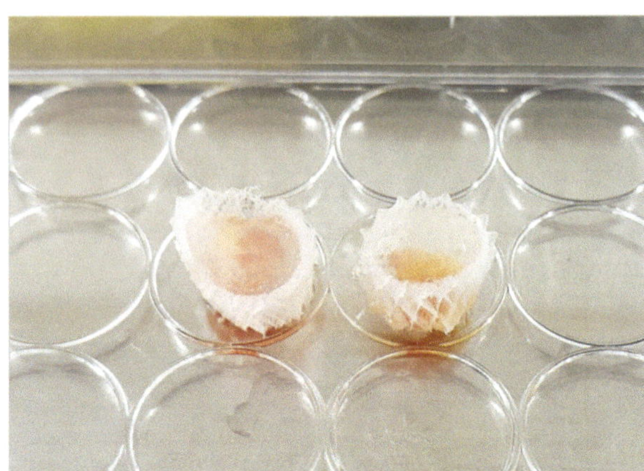

Fig. 20.8 Tissue-engineered lymph nodes integrated in the scaffold ready for in vitro cultivation or in vivo implantation for lymph node regeneration.

20.3.6 Conclusions

Compared to other organs like skin or bone, there are still some challenges to overcome for generating biologically adequate tissue-engineered lymphoid organs. Especially, lymph nodes with their sophisticated micro-architecture, diverse phenotype, and functional type, as well as different cell types are more difficult to be bioengineered.[112] Since 2004 several approaches were introduced using different scaffolds/biomaterials and cell types, but there is still no well-established method for translational medicine application to recreate effective immune response or a large-scale functional lymphatic network for lymph drainage.[101,102,103,104,105,106,107,109] Further work in cell biology and material science will be necessary to overcome these obstacles in future. Both the concepts of autologous ex vivo lymph node processing and scaffold implantation (organoid based) and the concept of recellularization (cell based) of scaffold, each with consecutive in vivo replantation, are promising and require further attention. In addition, both the concepts of vascularized and avascular tissue-engineered transplants should be addressed in future.

Conflict of interest

Submitted patent (PCT/EP 2015/080516) for an "Implant for Lymph Node Formation/Regeneration."

20.4 Vascularized Lymph Node Transfer and Growth Factors

Mikko Visuri, Pauliina Hartiala, and Anne Saaristo

20.4.1 Introduction

During the past few years, VLNT has gained widespread popularity as a surgical treatment for lymphedema, aiming to provide a physiological result and relieve the symptoms, e.g., decrease in swelling and incidence of infections.[113,114,115,116] This is in contrast to other surgical interventions (i.e., suction-assisted lipectomy), which focus on alleviating the symptoms instead of intervening with the underlying pathology.[116] In VLNT, healthy lymph nodes and surrounding lymphatic and adipose tissue are harvested from a remote area and transferred either into areas of lymph node dissection or, alternatively, extra-anatomically into distal lymphadematous tissue areas such as limbs, in order to restore lymphatic drainage function.[115,116]

Despite controversies, promising results, and need for further research, it is rather recommended to use microsurgical techniques for revascularization of the transplanted lymph node instead of implanting a nonvascularized lymph node transplant, as this increases the lymph node survival.[117] Although some mouse models have showed the transferred nonvascularized lymph nodes to retain their histology, in canine and pig models degeneration of even the vascularized lymph node has been observed in histological analyses, despite of integration to the recipient lymphatic vasculature.[115,116,118,119] According to current knowledge, this degeneration is less notable when the lymph node transfer is performed alongside with growth factor therapy.[117,118,119] The lymphatic vessels connecting the transplanted lymph node into the surrounding lymphatic network are thought to regenerate spontaneously via lymphangiogenesis, induced by the (re-)vascularized lymph node transfer, as such.[113,114,116] However, this process can be enhanced with growth factor therapy.[114,115,118,119,120,121,122,123] As survival of the VLNT is dependent on the lymph flow through them, increased lymphangiogenesis via growth factor therapy might contribute to their survival via this indirect route.[117]

In terms of lymphatic network regeneration, lymphangiogenesis-inducing growth factors have been utilized with promising results in various animal models.[114,124] VEGFs are considered as important regulators of both angiogenesis and lymphangiogenesis, stimulating cellular responses by signaling via receptor tyrosine kinases (RTKs) VEGFR-1, VEGFR-2, and VEGFR-3 (VEGFRs), expressed in the luminal surface of blood and lymphatic endothelial cells. The expression pattern of VEGFRs is not uniform across endothelial cells. VEGFR-1 and VEGFR-2 are expressed on BECs, while VEGFR-2 and VEGFR-3 are expressed on LECs.[121] Of all the prolymphangiogenic growth factors stimulating lymphangiogenesis through VEGFRs, VEGF-C holds an established position in the lymphedema research. It has been demonstrated to be an essential factor in adult lymphatic vessel network (re-)generation and is widely considered as the primary growth factor of choice for therapeutic applications involving LECs and lymphangiogenesis.[113,121] The affinity of VEGF-C is increased by proteolytic cleavage and only the fully processed form can bind to VEGFR-2, the main mediator of angiogenesis.[113,119] However, the affinity of processed mature VEGF-C for VEGFR-3 is four times higher than that for VEGFR-2.[122] VEGF-C therapy has been demonstrated to induce the growth of capillary lymph vessels, which are thought to stabilize into true collecting lymph vessels via an intrinsic differentiation and maturation program.[113,120]

VEGF-C has been shown to be beneficial in ameliorating lymphedema, inducing lymphangiogenesis and enhancing the survival, function, and lymphatic network integration of the transplanted lymph nodes. These studies have utilized mouse, rat, pig, and sheep models of lymphedema.[124] The use of VEGF-C therapy aims at restoring the normal anatomy and function of both collecting and capillary lymphatics. As a result, lymph fluid drainage increases, edema is alleviated, mechanical tension decreases, and inflammation is mitigated. The density of lymphatic capillaries is increased locally, accelerating immune cell trafficking to the draining lymph nodes. This enhances the immune protection around the surgical wound and availability of cytokines and growth factors.[122]

20.4.2 Application and Delivery of Growth Factors

VEGF-C can be delivered, for example, as a recombinant protein, viral vector, or naked plasmid. It can be administered directly or released on demand from bioengineered matrices or biodegradable microparticles.[124] Therapy with recombinant VEGF-C-expressing adeno-associated virus is considered as the most efficient method of delivering genes *in vivo* and it has been tested using various experimental animal models of lymphedema.[114,115,117,118,120,121,122,123] Although adenoviral VEGF-C therapy has been established to be safe in various animal models, VEGF-C-based lymphedema therapy can potentially also result in tumor growth or metastasis in cancer patients, as VEGF-C expression is known to contribute to these processes.[118,124] Therefore, patient safety is crucial. High VEGF-C levels are known to induce adverse side effects, such as blood vessel angiogenesis, enlargement, tortuosity, and leakage. Likewise, VEGF-C156S, a mutagenic modification of VEGF-C with lower VEGFR-2 specificity, has been demonstrated to accelerate the healing of diabetic wounds via nonspecific blood vessel angiogenesis stimulation. However, these undesirable vascular side effects have been attributed to a significantly and persistent increase in VEGF-C concentration and, in terms of adenoviral gene therapy, they can be minimized with transient expression, exerting only minimal effect on blood vessels.[122]

Nevertheless, reproducible and quantitative growth factor delivery might in some situations require administration of proteins as an alternative to gene therapy. Instead of direct injection of growth factors, generally resulting in protein clearance within hours, controlled release from bioengineered matrices or biodegradable microparticles, for example, could provide a long-lasting and local induction of lymphangiogenesis. In addition, several still rather unclear factors can influence the result of VEGF-C treatment. These include, for example, the subject's age and the presence of inflammatory stimuli, the level of VERGFr-3 expression, and endogenous proteolysis which might degrade growth factors in a certain milieu. Furthermore, as expression of even VEGFR-3, the main target receptor of lymphangiogenic therapy, is not exclusively confined to lymphatic endothelium, therapies via signaling it might influence vessels and structures beyond the lymphatic system. In addition, excessive stimulation can potentially also induce hyperplastic proliferation in collecting lymphatic vessel valve and lumen endothelium, resulting in lumen occlusion, valve hypertrophy, or otherwise abnormal valve development in collecting lymphatic vessels, responsible for blocking the drainage or inducing lymph backflow.[122]

In addition to VEGF-C, a number of other interesting and potentially usable growth factors and cytokines also exist, such as epidermal growth factor (EGF), fibroblast growth factor 2 (FGF2), HGF, insulin-like growth factor (IGF)-1/2, and platelet-derived growth factors (PDGFs).[121,123,124] EGF has been demonstrated to induce enhanced migration and tube formation of human lymphatic endothelial cells (HLECs) *in vitro* and result in increased lymphatic vessel area and size *in vivo*. In addition, tumor-produced EGF leads to lymphangiogenesis. The mechanism behind epidermal growth factor receptor (EGFR) signaling and lymphangiogenesis is currently not understood in full detail. FGF2, also known as basic fibroblast growth factor, increases the expression of VEGF-A, -C, and -D, inducing angiogenesis via VEGFR-2 signaling and lymphangiogenesis via VEGFR-3 signaling.[123] HGF has a potent synergistic effect with VEGF-C and has been utilized in gene therapy and demonstrated to stimulate the growth of lymphatic vascular system in a mouse model.[121] IGF-1 and IGF-2 have been shown to induce lymphangiogenesis, possibly as direct lymphangiogenic factors, regardless of VEGFR-3. PDGFs are also capable of stimulating lymphangiogenesis directly.[124]

20.4.3 Experimental Background

Despite the increasing popularity and some exciting clinical results, the relationship between VLNT and the resolution of lymphedema and other associated pathologies is yet unknown, as the pathophysiology of secondary lymphedema as such is still a subject for intensive research.[115,116] Studies conducted on animal models have suggested that the appearance of swelling, fibroadipose deposition, hyperkeratosis and fibrosis, the pathological skin changes following lymphedema, and, in addition, local immunosuppression can be reversed (and not merely prevented) with VLNT.[116]

It also remains unknown whether lymph node transfer has a direct effect on the impaired immune response associated with lymphedema. However, in a mouse model, lymph node transfer has been demonstrated to increase dendritic cell (DC) trafficking to regional lymph nodes and enhance T cell-mediated responses, suggesting an improvement in the adaptive immunity, which was impaired by an injury to the lymphatic system.[116] Furthermore, the clinical studies so far have not indicated whether the regenerated lymph vessels are capillaries or collecting vessels. The formation of collateral lymphatic vessels reconnecting the transplanted lymph nodes and decrease in the pathological changes in the collecting vessels due to lymphedema have, however, been demonstrated in animal model research.[116,118,119] It is also unclear if the collecting lymphatic vessels connect to the transplanted lymph node or to the next one in the regional lymph node chain, although an animal model has suggested formation of a direct connection to the transferred lymph node.[115,116,118,119]

An interesting canine study utilizing a forelimb lymphedema model and VLNT proposed that the lymphatic system has a homing mechanism, allowing the damaged lymph vessels to detect nearby lymph nodes and form connections with them. In this exploratory study, at 6 months after a unilateral axillary and lower neck node dissection and postoperative irradiation, a collateral lymphatic pathway connecting into the contralateral cervical node was observed. Furthermore, after VLNT, an additional collateral pathway formed a connection to the internal mammary node via the transferred axillary node, suggesting that the transferred lymph node can induce formation of new connections instead of bridging the original pathways.[115]

Regarding the recovery of lymph flow, two theories exist to explain the mechanism: The first theory proposes that the transferred lymph node and surrounding adipose tissue acts as a source of lymphangiogenic cytokines, thus inducing the formation of a lymphatic vessel bridge connecting the distal and proximal vessel ends.[125] The second theory suggests that the lymph node functions as a suction pump, draining a portion of lymph to the systemic circulation via the vascular pedicle through the connections with the high endothelial venules as a lymphovenous shunt.[115]

Furthermore, additional research is still needed in terms of growth factor therapy, alternatives for it, and the relationship between lymphangiogenesis, inflammation, and the immune system. It is known that during its synthesis, VEGF-C undergoes through multiple steps, during which its properties and affinities for different receptors change. However, the roles of these different forms have not been yet clarified thoroughly. Furthermore, most—if not all—current applications do not discriminate between the different forms, which are results of alternative splicing. Consequently, research focused on the different forms of VEGF-C might provide new modalities of therapy, possibly avoiding the adverse effects potentially associated with unprocessed VEGF-C. Furthermore, despite its essential role, there has been uncertainty whether VEGF-C alone is always sufficient for the successful reconstruction of lymphatic networks in certain situations. This has been partly clarified by the discovery of collagen and calcium binding epidermal growth factor domains 1 (CCBE1) protein and ADAMTS3 protease, obligatory cofactors required for the proteolytic activation of VEGF-C.[121] Using a mouse model, it has been demonstrated that adenoviral therapy with CCBE1 enhances both lymphangiogenesis and angiogenesis induced by VEGF-C adenoviral treatment in mouse skeletal muscle by enhancing VEGF-C's proteolytic cleavage into its mature form, resulting in increased VEGF-C receptor signaling.[126] Consequently, the presence or absence of these factors might provide an explanation for the differences in the lymphatic response.[121]

Interestingly, in some situations blocking lymphangiogenesis-inhibiting signals might provide a worthy alternative for VEGF-C and other lymphangiogenesis-inducing growth factors, especially considering the potential contribution to tumor growth or metastasis.[121,127] Based on multiple studies, it has turned out that despite the normal or increased expression of VEGF-C or other lymphangiogenic cytokines in certain pathological circumstances, lymphatic function can be impaired. Therefore, it has been suggested that other physiological mechanisms could either directly or indirectly inhibit lymphangiogenesis.[124] Worth mentioning is TGF-β1, a potent anti-lymphangiogenic agent, inducing decrease in LEC proliferation and migration, impaired formation of lymphatic tubules, and downregulation of lymphatic-specific gene expression.[121] TGF-β1 inhibition has been demonstrated to lead in increased lymphatic repair during wound healing and, in addition, to synergistic increase of the lymphangiogenic effect of VEGF-C.[124,127] Therefore, inhibition of TGF-β1 could promote lymphangiogenesis and provide a usable alternative for VEGF-C and other lymphangiogenesis-promoting growth factors in clinical situations.[121,124]

Furthermore, TGF-β1 also functions as an anti-inflammatory cytokine, regulating tissue fibrosis and scarring in the later stages of wound healing, thus linking lymphangiogenesis with inflammatory pathways. IL-10, an anti-inflammatory cytokine, has been shown to protect from TGF-β1-induced fibrosis. Increased IL-10 levels have been discovered after VLNT in humans and this could be one of the factors that define the effects of VLNT.[127]

An interesting application could utilize both prolymphangiogenic and anti-lymphangiogenic factors to trim the balance between these two in those situations, where the use of prolymphangiogenic growth factors alone is contraindicated.[124]

A relatively new approach for indirect lymphatic regeneration is based on the use of multipotent progenitor cells. Studies have shown that when the conditions are favorable, embryonic stem cells can differentiate into LECs *in vitro*. Furthermore, MSCs or adipose-derived mesenchymal stem cells can be stimulated with VEGF-C in cultured media *in vitro* to increase their prolymphangiogenic capabilities *in vivo*. In mouse tail and rat hindlimb models of lymphedema, stem cells injected directly or delivered in hydrogel improved lymphangiogenesis, restored lymph flow, and decreased tissue edema.[124] Similarly, ASCs provide a promising candidate for new modalities of lymphedema treatment. Utilizing a mouse model, they have been showed to express multidifferential capacities and to both enhance the spontaneous lymphangiogenesis associated with VLNT and alleviate the lymphedema in a more efficient way when compared to the VLNT alone—in the absence of VEGF-C.[125]

Also worth mentioning, previous research has demonstrated that histopathology in experimental lymphedema can be reversed with ketoprofen, a nonsteroidal anti-inflammatory drug (NSAID). This effect has been indicated to be specifically due to inhibition of 5-lipoxygenase metabolite, leukotriene B_4 (LTB_4). Low LTB_4 concentrations have been shown to promote lymphangiogenesis in both *in vitro* and *in vivo* experimental animal models, whereas lymphatic growth and function are impeded at high concentrations. Interestingly, LTB_4 concentrations are known to increase in both experimental animal model and human clinical lymphedema. It is speculated that in the first few days after surgery, during the initial wound-healing period, LTB_4 produced at low concentrations has an important function in promoting angiogenesis/lymphangiogenesis. However, with progression in lymphedema and concurrent increase in LTB_4 concentration, a shift from initial lymphangiogenesis-stimulating into anti-lymphangiogenic effect is seen. These findings have made LTB_4 a promising drug target in the treatment of acquired lymphedema.[128]

20.4.4 Clinical Application

Compared to the development of novel therapies in other areas of modern medicine, the situation in terms of the experimental treatment of lymphedema lags somewhat behind, as the molecular basis of lymphangiogenesis became a focus of attention only roughly two decades ago. However, current research has demonstrated the presence of lymphatic vessels in nearly all organs, including the central nervous system, and they are known to be essential for the survival of several organisms.[129] Thus, it is needless to say that we should continue the pursuit for the profound understanding of the whole lymphatic system in order to find a cure for the chronic lymphedema.

Surprisingly, the exact etiology of lymphatic diseases is poorly understood. For example, following mastectomy, the precipitating factors for developing lymphedema are not completely known. In addition, lymphedema in the late stages of lymphatic filariasis (see Chapter 3) is usually not occlusion of collecting lymphatic vessels but more likely at least partly a result of lymphatic backflow due to endothelial proliferation and lymphangiectasia. Furthermore, although lymphedema and elephantiasis are thought to develop due to recurrent infections and associated dermatolymphangioadenitis, it is also observed in individuals without signs of active infection or lymphatic occlusion. In addition, as inflammation involved in lymphedema development is a multifactorial process, several factors may contribute to its development and sustenance. Consequently, as the etiology of secondary lymphedema is not fully understood, developing reliable animal models has turned out to be challenging, resulting in difficulties in producing therapies beyond the selection currently available.[122]

Despite the fact that preclinical experience with VEGF-C in regrowth of lymphatic networks extends 15 years to the past, currently only one phase I and II clinical trial is underway. It exploits the combination of VLNT and VEGF-C-expressing adenovirus therapy (Lymfactin; Herantis Pharma, Espoo, Finland) in order to treat secondary lymphedema following breast cancer surgery. The concept and the clinical protocol with the steps of the study are summarized in ▶ Fig. 20.9a–f.[121] In addition, a clinical trial for treating lower limb secondary lymphedema using a LTB_4 blocker, bestatin, with already proven safety and high tolerability as chemotherapy adjuvant utilized in leukemia, is also underway at the moment.[128]

20.4.5 Conclusions

Our understanding of the roles of lymphatic vessels in both healthy and diseased subjects is constantly increasing. The significance of lymphatic circulation in internal organs and the way its disorders result in or are associated with different diseases are the subjects of ongoing research. Consequently, our perception of lymphatics has evolved from the role as an auxiliary circulation into a significant part of the human body homeostasis in terms of lipid transport, immunity, and fluid transport.[122]

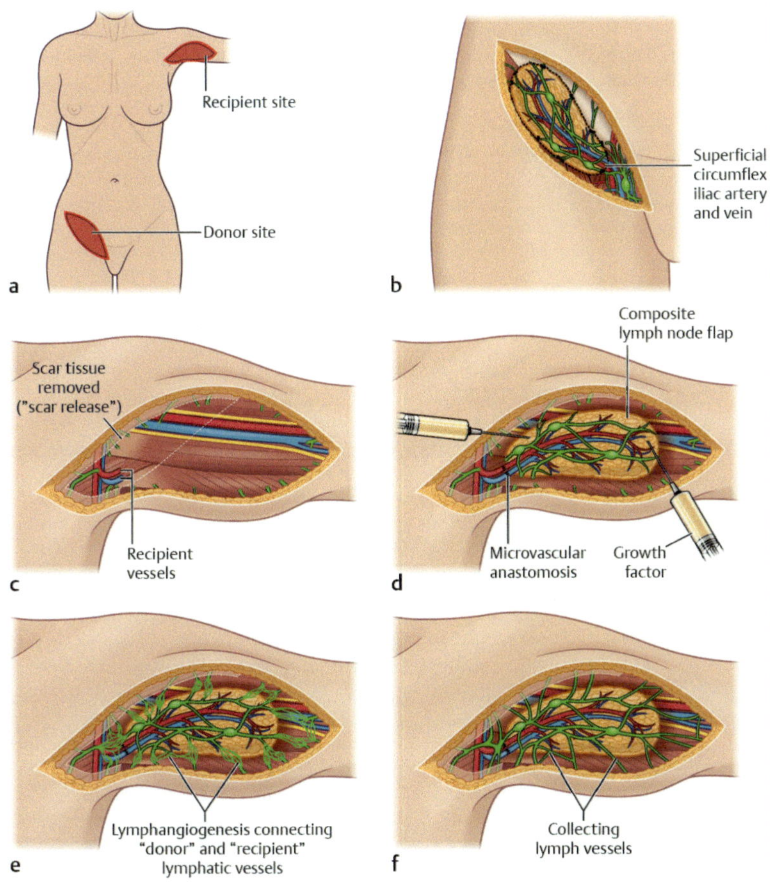

Fig. 20.9 In vascularized lymph node transfer, lymphatic tissue (lymph nodes and vessels) and surrounding fat are harvested as a vascularized free flap from a donor site and transferred to a recipient area, where microvascular blood vessel anastomosis is performed. The process is illustrated here as a transfer of a lymphatic flap from the right inguinal region into the left axilla **(a)**. An incision is made into the right groin area **(b)** and the flap is harvested using superficial circumflex artery and vein for the blood vessel supply. The recipient site, left axilla **(c)**, is prepared for the transfer. Old scar tissue is completely removed to enhance the therapeutic effect of the lymph node transfer. In addition, the recipient vessels, thoracodorsal artery, and vein or their branches are prepared. The vascularized lymphatic flap is then transferred into the left axilla **(d)**. The supplying artery and vein are anastomosed microsurgically (indicated by the black dashed line) with thoracodorsal vessels or their branches. Growth factor (e.g., adenoviral gene transfer vector encoding vascular endothelial growth factor C) is injected into the distal edges of the flap. Growth factor treatment induces a robust growth of new lymphatic vessels **(e)**, incorporating the transferred lymph nodes and vessels into the surrounding lymphatic network and enhancing lymphatic flow from the upper limb. After the initial lymphangiogenesis, the lymphatic vessel network regresses. However, the newly formed vessels with lymphatic flow will stabilize and mature into collecting lymphatic vessels **(f)**.

References

[1] Cormier JN, Askew RL, Mungovan KS, Xing Y, Ross MI, Armer JM. Lymphedema beyond breast cancer: a systematic review and meta-analysis of cancer-related secondary lymphedema. Cancer. 2010; 116 (22):5138–5149

[2] McLaughlin SA, Wright MJ, Morris KT, et al. Prevalence of lymphedema in women with breast cancer 5 years after sentinel lymph node biopsy or axillary dissection: objective measurements. J Clin Oncol. 2008; 26(32):5213–5219

[3] Williams AF, Franks PJ, Moffatt CJ. Lymphoedema: estimating the size of the problem. Palliat Med. 2005; 19(4):300–313

[4] DiSipio T, Rye S, Newman B, Hayes S. Incidence of unilateral arm lymphoedema after breast cancer: a systematic review and meta-analysis. Lancet Oncol. 2013; 14(6):500–515

[5] Bernas M, Thiadens SRJ, Smoot B, Armer JM, Stewart P, Granzow J. Lymphedema following cancer therapy: overview and options. Clin Exp Metastasis. 2018; 35(5–6):547–551

[6] Frueh FS, Gousopoulos E, Rezaeian F, Menger MD, Lindenblatt N, Giovanoli P. Animal models in surgical lymphedema research—a systematic review. J Surg Res. 2016; 200(1):208–220

[7] Khan AA, Hernan I, Adamthwaite JA, Ramsey KWD. Feasibility study of combined dynamic imaging and lymphaticovenous anastomosis surgery for breast cancer-related lymphoedema. Br J Surg. 2019; 106 (1):100–110

[8] Becker C, Assouad J, Riquet M, Hidden G. Postmastectomy lymphedema: long-term results following microsurgical lymph node transplantation. Ann Surg. 2006; 243(3):313–315

[9] Ito R, Suami H. Overview of lymph node transfer for lymphedema treatment. Plast Reconstr Surg. 2014; 134(3):548–556

[10] Homans J, Drinker CK, Field M. Elephantiasis and the clinical implications of its experimental reproduction in animals. Ann Surg. 1934; 100(4):812–832

[11] Clodius L, Wirth W. A new experimental model for chronic lymphoedema of the extremities (with clinical considerations). Chir Plastica. 1974; 2:115–132

[12] Das SK, Franklin JD, O'Brien BM, Morrison WA. A practical model of secondary lymphedema in dogs. Plast Reconstr Surg. 1981; 68(3): 422–428

[13] Hadamitzky C, Pabst R. Acquired lymphedema: an urgent need for adequate animal models. Cancer Res. 2008; 68(2):343–345

[14] Suami H, Shin D, Chang DW. Mapping of lymphosomes in the canine forelimb: comparative anatomy between canines and humans. Plast Reconstr Surg. 2012; 129(3):612–620

[15] Suami H, Yamashita S, Soto-Miranda MA, Chang DW. Lymphatic territories (lymphosomes) in a canine: an animal model for

investigation of postoperative lymphatic alterations. PLoS One. 2013; 8(7):e69222
[16] Tobbia D, Semple J, Baker A, Dumont D, Semple A, Johnston M. Lymphedema development and lymphatic function following lymph node excision in sheep. J Vasc Res. 2009; 46(5):426–434
[17] Lähteenvuo M, Honkonen K, Tervala T, et al. Growth factor therapy and autologous lymph node transfer in lymphedema. Circulation. 2011; 123(6):613–620
[18] Wu G, Xu H, Zhou W, et al. Rhesus monkey is a new model of secondary lymphedema in the upper limb. Int J Clin Exp Pathol. 2014; 7(9):5665–5673
[19] Honkonen KM, Visuri MT, Tervala TV, et al. Lymph node transfer and perinodal lymphatic growth factor treatment for lymphedema. Ann Surg. 2013; 257(5):961–967
[20] Hadamitzky C, Zaitseva TS, Bazalova-Carter M, et al. Aligned nanofibrillar collagen scaffolds—guiding lymphangiogenesis for treatment of acquired lymphedema. Biomaterials. 2016; 102: 259–267
[21] Wang GY, Zhong SZ. A model of experimental lymphedema in rats' limbs. Microsurgery. 1985; 6(4):204–210
[22] Lee-Donaldson L, Witte MH, Bernas M, Witte CL, Way D, Stea B. Refinement of a rodent model of peripheral lymphedema. Lymphology. 1999; 32(3):111–117
[23] Müller A, Fries P, Jelvani B, et al. Magnetic resonance lymphography at 9.4T using a gadolinium-based nanoparticle in rats: investigations in healthy animals and in a hindlimb lymphedema model. Invest Radiol. 2017; 52(12):725–733
[24] Will PA, Rafiei A, Pretze M, et al. Evidence of stage progression in a novel, validated fluorescence-navigated and microsurgical-assisted secondary lymphedema rodent model. PLoS One. 2020; 15(7): e0235965
[25] Slavin SA, Van den Abbeele AD, Losken A, Swartz MA, Jain RK. Return of lymphatic function after flap transfer for acute lymphedema. Ann Surg. 1999; 229(3):421–427
[26] Tabibiazar R, Cheung L, Han J, et al. Inflammatory manifestations of experimental lymphatic insufficiency. PLoS Med. 2006; 3(7):e254
[27] García Nores GD, Ly CL, Cuzzone DA, et al. $CD4^+$ T cells are activated in regional lymph nodes and migrate to skin to initiate lymphedema. Nat Commun. 2018; 9(1):1970
[28] Gousopoulos E, Proulx ST, Bachmann SB, et al. An important role of VEGF-C in promoting lymphedema development. J Invest Dermatol. 2017; 137(9):1995–2004
[29] Gardenier JC, Kataru RP, Hespe GE, et al. Topical tacrolimus for the treatment of secondary lymphedema. Nat Commun. 2017; 8:14345
[30] Tian W, Rockson SG, Jiang X, et al. Leukotriene B_4 antagonism ameliorates experimental lymphedema. Sci Transl Med. 2017; 9 (389):eaal3920
[31] Gousopoulos E, Proulx ST, Bachmann SB, et al. Regulatory T cell transfer ameliorates lymphedema and promotes lymphatic vessel function. JCI Insight. 2016; 1(16):e89081
[32] Oashi K, Furukawa H, Oyama A, et al. A new model of acquired lymphedema in the mouse hind limb: a preliminary report. Ann Plast Surg. 2012; 69(5):565–568
[33] Frueh FS, Körbel C, Gassert L, et al. High-resolution 3D volumetry versus conventional measuring techniques for the assessment of experimental lymphedema in the mouse hindlimb. Sci Rep. 2016; 6: 34673
[34] Blum KS, Proulx ST, Luciani P, Leroux JC, Detmar M. Dynamics of lymphatic regeneration and flow patterns after lymph node dissection. Breast Cancer Res Treat. 2013; 139(1):81–86
[35] Daneshgaran G, Lo AY, Paik CB, et al. A pre-clinical animal model of secondary head and neck lymphedema. Sci Rep. 2019; 9(1): 18264
[36] Yang CY, Ho OA, Cheng MH, Hsiao HY. Critical ischemia time, perfusion, and drainage function of vascularized lymph nodes. Plast Reconstr Surg. 2018; 142(3):688–697
[37] Perrault DP, Lee GK, Bouz A, et al. Ischemia and reperfusion injury in superficial inferior epigastric artery-based vascularized lymph node flaps. PLoS One. 2020; 15(1):e0227599
[38] Kwiecien GJ, Uygur S, Korn J, et al. Vascularized axillary lymph node transfer: a novel model in the rat. Microsurgery. 2015; 35(8): 662–667
[39] Onoda S, Kimata Y, Matsumoto K. A novel lymphaticovenular anastomosis rat model. Ann Plast Surg. 2016; 76(3):332–335
[40] Sommer T, Meier M, Bruns F, Pabst R, Breves G, Hadamitzky C. Quantification of lymphedema in a rat model by 3D-active contour segmentation by magnetic resonance imaging. Lymphat Res Biol. 2012; 10(1):25–29
[41] Wiinholt A, Gerke O, Dalaei F, Bučan A, Madsen CB, Sørensen JA. Quantification of tissue volume in the hindlimb of mice using microcomputed tomography images and analysing software. Sci Rep. 2020; 10(1):8297
[42] Sevick-Muraca EM, Kwon S, Rasmussen JC. Emerging lymphatic imaging technologies for mouse and man. J Clin Invest. 2014; 124(3): 905–914
[43] Proulx ST, Luciani P, Derzsi S, et al. Quantitative imaging of lymphatic function with liposomal indocyanine green. Cancer Res. 2010; 70 (18):7053–7062
[44] Kobayashi H, Kawamoto S, Star RA, Waldmann TA, Tagaya Y, Brechbiel MW. Micro-magnetic resonance lymphangiography in mice using a novel dendrimer-based magnetic resonance imaging contrast agent. Cancer Res. 2003; 63(2):271–276
[45] Lux F, Mignot A, Mowat P, et al. Ultrasmall rigid particles as multimodal probes for medical applications. Angew Chem Int Ed Engl. 2011; 50(51):12299–12303
[46] Dayan JH, Ly CL, Kataru RP, Mehrara BJ. Lymphedema: pathogenesis and novel therapies. Annu Rev Med. 2018; 69:263–276
[47] Hoffman T, Khademhosseini A, Langer R. Chasing the paradigm: clinical translation of 25 years of tissue engineering. Tissue Eng Part A. 2019; 25(9–10):679–687
[48] Betterman KL, Harvey NL. The lymphatic vasculature: development and role in shaping immunity. Immunol Rev. 2016; 271(1):276–292
[49] Podgrabinska S, Braun P, Velasco P, Kloos B, Pepper MS, Skobe M. Molecular characterization of lymphatic endothelial cells. Proc Natl Acad Sci U S A. 2002; 99(25):16069–16074
[50] Knezevic L, Schaupper M, Mühleder S, et al. Engineering blood and lymphatic microvascular networks in fibrin matrices. Front Bioeng Biotechnol. 2017; 5:25
[51] Conrad C, Niess H, Huss R, et al. Multipotent mesenchymal stem cells acquire a lymphendothelial phenotype and enhance lymphatic regeneration in vivo. Circulation. 2009; 119(2):281–289
[52] Yang Y, Chen XH, Li FG, et al. In vitro induction of human adipose-derived stem cells into lymphatic endothelial-like cells. Cell Reprogram. 2015; 17(1):69–76
[53] Kong L-L, Yang N-Z, Shi L-H, et al. The optimum marker for the detection of lymphatic vessels. Mol Clin Oncol. 2017; 7(4):515–520
[54] Gibot L, Galbraith T, Kloos B, et al. Cell-based approach for 3D reconstruction of lymphatic capillaries in vitro reveals distinct functions of HGF and VEGF-C in lymphangiogenesis. Biomaterials. 2016; 78:129–139
[55] Rauniyar K, Jha SK, Jeltsch M. Biology of vascular endothelial growth factor C in the morphogenesis of lymphatic vessels. Front Bioeng Biotechnol. 2018; 6:7
[56] Avraham T, Daluvoy S, Zampell J, et al. Blockade of transforming growth factor-β1 accelerates lymphatic regeneration during wound repair. Am J Pathol. 2010; 177(6):3202–3214
[57] Shao X, Liu C. Influence of IFN-α and IFN-γ on lymphangiogenesis. J Interferon Cytokine Res. 2006; 26(8):568–574
[58] Robering JW, Weigand A, Pfuhlmann R, Horch RE, Beier JP, Boos AM. Mesenchymal stem cells promote lymphangiogenic properties of lymphatic endothelial cells. J Cell Mol Med. 2018; 22(8):3740–3750
[59] Kalluri R, Zeisberg M. Fibroblasts in cancer. Nat Rev Cancer. 2006; 6 (5):392–401
[60] Marino D, Luginbühl J, Scola S, Meuli M, Reichmann E. Bioengineering dermo-epidermal skin grafts with blood and lymphatic capillaries. Sci Transl Med. 2014; 6(221):221ra14
[61] Alajati A, Laib AM, Weber H, et al. Spheroid-based engineering of a human vasculature in mice. Nat Methods. 2008; 5(5):439–445

[62] Strassburg S, Torio-Padron N, Finkenzeller G, Frankenschmidt A, Stark GB. Adipose-derived stem cells support lymphangiogenic parameters in vitro. J Cell Biochem. 2016; 117(11):2620–2629

[63] Rohringer S, Hofbauer P, Schneider KH, et al. Mechanisms of vasculogenesis in 3D fibrin matrices mediated by the interaction of adipose-derived stem cells and endothelial cells. Angiogenesis. 2014; 17(4):921–933

[64] Ahmadzadeh N, Robering JW, Kengelbach-Weigand A, Al-Abboodi M, Beier JP, Horch RE, Boos AM. Human adipose-derived stem cells support lymphangiogenesis in vitro by secretion of lymphangiogenic factors. Exp Cell Res. 2020; 388(2):111816:. Epub 2020 Jan 7

[65] Yang Y, Yang J-T, Chen X-H, et al. Construction of tissue-engineered lymphatic vessel using human adipose derived stem cells differentiated lymphatic endothelial like cells and decellularized arterial scaffold: a preliminary study. Biotechnol Appl Biochem. 2018; 65(3):428–434

[66] Helm C-LE, Zisch A, Swartz MA. Engineered blood and lymphatic capillaries in 3-D VEGF-fibrin-collagen matrices with interstitial flow. Biotechnol Bioeng. 2007; 96(1):167–176

[67] Pepper MS, Skobe M. Lymphatic endothelium: morphological, molecular and functional properties. J Cell Biol. 2003; 163(2):209–213

[68] Dai Tt, Jiang Zh, Li Sl, et al. Reconstruction of lymph vessel by lymphatic endothelial cells combined with polyglycolic acid scaffolds: a pilot study. J Biotechnol. 2010; 150(1):182–189

[69] Will et al. Decellularized dandelion [Taraxacum officinale] haulms as a scaffold for lymphatic tissue engineering. Submitted

[70] Kanapathy M, Patel NM, Kalaskar DM, Mosahebi A, Mehrara BJ, Seifalian AM. Tissue-engineered lymphatic graft for the treatment of lymphedema. J Surg Res. 2014; 192(2):544–554

[71] Shimizu Y, Shibata R, Shintani S, Ishii M, Murohara T. Therapeutic lymphangiogenesis with implantation of adipose-derived regenerative cells. J Am Heart Assoc. 2012; 1(4):e000877

[72] Maertens L, Erpicum C, Detry B, et al. Bone marrow-derived mesenchymal stem cells drive lymphangiogenesis. PLoS One. 2014; 9 (9):e106976

[73] Hadrian R, Palmes D. Animal models of secondary lymphedema: new approaches in the search for therapeutic options. Lymphat Res Biol. 2017; 15(1):2–16

[74] Suami H. Lymphosome concept: anatomical study of the lymphatic system. J Surg Oncol. 2017; 115(1):13–17

[75] Allen RJ, Jr, Cheng MH. Lymphedema surgery: patient selection and an overview of surgical techniques. J Surg Oncol. 2016; 113(8): 923–931

[76] Schaupper M, Jeltsch M, Rohringer S, Redl H, Holnthoner W. Lymphatic vessels in regenerative medicine and tissue engineering. Tissue Eng Part B Rev. 2016; 22(5):395–407

[77] Fischer M, Franzeck UK, Herrig I, et al. Flow velocity of single lymphatic capillaries in human skin. Am J Physiol. 1996; 270(1 Pt 2): H358–H363

[78] Katakai T, Hara T, Sugai M, Gonda H, Shimizu A. Lymph node fibroblastic reticular cells construct the stromal reticulum via contact with lymphocytes. J Exp Med. 2004; 200(6):783–795

[79] Ohtani O, Ohtani Y. Recent developments in morphology of lymphatic vessels and lymph nodes. Ann Vasc Dis. 2012; 5(2):145–150

[80] Nosenko MA, Drutskaya MS, Moisenovich MM, Nedospasov SA. Bioengineering of artificial lymphoid organs. Acta Naturae. 2016; 8 (2):10–23

[81] Lippert H, ed. Lehrbuch Anatomie. München, Jena: Urban & Fischer; 2000

[82] Gottesman JM, Jaffe HL. Studies on the histogenesis of autoplastic thymus transplantations. J Exp Med. 1926; 43(3):403–414

[83] Jaffe HL. Autoplastic thymus transplants: II. With particular reference to the regeneration of the reticulum cells and the formation of Hassall's corpuscles. J Exp Med. 1926; 44(4):523–532

[84] Jaffe HL, Richter MN. The regeneration of autoplastic lymph node transplants. J Exp Med. 1928; 47(6):977–980

[85] Tilak SP, Howard JM. Regeneration and autotransplantation of lymph nodes. Ann Surg. 1965; 161:441–446

[86] Pabst R, Rothkötter HJ. Regeneration of autotransplanted lymph node fragments. Cell Tissue Res. 1988; 251(3):597–601

[87] Rothkötter HJ, Pabst R. Autotransplantation of lymph node fragments. Structure and function of regenerated tissue. Scand J Plast Reconstr Surg Hand Surg. 1990; 24(2):101–105

[88] Shih C-C, Hu J, Arber D, LeBon T, Forman SJ. Transplantation and growth characteristics of human fetal lymph node in immunodeficient mice. Exp Hematol. 2000; 28(9):1046–1053

[89] Hadamitzky C, Blum KS, Pabst R. Regeneration of autotransplanted avascular lymph nodes in the rat is improved by platelet-rich plasma. J Vasc Res. 2009; 46(5):389–396

[90] Blum KS, Hadamitzky C, Gratz KF, Pabst R. Effects of autotransplanted lymph node fragments on the lymphatic system in the pig model. Breast Cancer Res Treat. 2010; 120(1):59–66

[91] Sommer T, Buettner M, Bruns F, Breves G, Hadamitzky C, Pabst R. Improved regeneration of autologous transplanted lymph node fragments by VEGF-C treatment. Anat Rec (Hoboken). 2012; 295(5): 786–791

[92] Schindewolffs L, Breves G, Buettner M, Hadamitzky C, Pabst R. VEGF-C improves regeneration and lymphatic reconnection of transplanted autologous lymph node fragments: an animal model for secondary lymphedema treatment. Immun Inflamm Dis. 2014; 2(3):152–161

[93] Atala A. Regenerative medicine strategies. J Pediatr Surg. 2012; 47(1): 17–28

[94] Hutmacher DW, Goh JCH, Teoh SH. An introduction to biodegradable materials for tissue engineering applications. Ann Acad Med Singap. 2001; 30(2):183–191

[95] Zaiss S, Brown TD, Reichert JC, Berner A. Poly(ε-caprolactone) scaffolds fabricated by melt electrospinning for bone tissue engineering. Materials (Basel). 2016; 9(4):1–15

[96] Brown TD, Dalton PD, Hutmacher DW. Direct writing by way of melt electrospinning. Adv Mater. 2011; 23(47):5651–5657

[97] Brown TD, Slotosch A, Thibaudeau L, et al. Design and fabrication of tubular scaffolds via direct writing in a melt electrospinning mode. Biointerphases. 2012; 7(1–4):13

[98] Lian H, Meng Z. Melt electrospinning vs. solution electrospinning: a comparative study of drug-loaded poly (ε-caprolactone) fibres. Mater Sci Eng C. 2017; 74:117–123

[99] Wiggenhauser PS, Müller DF, Melchels FPW, et al. Engineering of vascularized adipose constructs. Cell Tissue Res. 2012; 347(3): 747–757

[100] Cupedo T, Stroock A, Coles M. Application of tissue engineering to the immune system: development of artificial lymph nodes. Front Immunol. 2012; 3:343

[101] Suematsu S, Watanabe T. Generation of a synthetic lymphoid tissue-like organoid in mice. Nat Biotechnol. 2004; 22(12):1539–1545

[102] Giese C, Demmler CD, Ammer R, et al. A human lymph node in vitro —challenges and progress. Artif Organs. 2006; 30(10):803–808

[103] Okamoto N, Chihara R, Shimizu C, Nishimoto S, Watanabe T. Artificial lymph nodes induce potent secondary immune responses in naive and immunodeficient mice. J Clin Invest. 2007; 117(4):997–1007

[104] Tomei AA, Siegert S, Britschgi MR, Luther SA, Swartz MA. Fluid flow regulates stromal cell organization and CCL21 expression in a tissue-engineered lymph node microenvironment. J Immunol. 2009; 183 (7):4273–4283

[105] Purwada A, Singh A. Immuno-engineered organoids for regulating the kinetics of B-cell development and antibody production. Nat Protoc. 2017; 12(1):168–182

[106] Purwada A, Jaiswal MK, Ahn H, et al. Ex vivo engineered immune organoids for controlled germinal center reactions. Biomaterials. 2015; 63:24–34

[107] Hadamitzky C, Zaitseva TS, Bazalova-Carter M, et al. Aligned nanofibrillar collagen scaffolds—guiding lymphangiogenesis for treatment of acquired lymphedema. Biomaterials. 2016; 102:259–267

[108] Kwak MD, Machens HG. The lateral intercostal artery perforator as an alternative donor vessel for free vascularized lymph node transplantation. Arch Plast Surg. 2018; 45(3):275–279

[109] Kwak MSD, Balmayor ER, Schantz JT, Chhaya M. Implantation of tissue-engineered lymph nodes using polycaprolactone scaffolds in immunodeficient nude mice. Lymph Forsch. 2017; 21(2):68–73

[110] Wunner FM, Wille ML, Noonan TG, et al. Melt electrospinning writing of highly ordered large volume scaffold architectures. Adv Mater. 2018; 30(20):e1706570

[111] Muerza-Cascante ML, Haylock D, Hutmacher DW, Dalton PD. Melt electrospinning and its technologization in tissue engineering. Tissue Eng Part B Rev. 2015; 21(2):187–202

[112] Weitman E, Cuzzone D, Mehrara BJ. Tissue engineering and regeneration of lymphatic structures. Future Oncol. 2013; 9(9):1365–1374

[113] Hartiala P, Saaristo AM. Growth factor therapy and autologous lymph node transfer in lymphedema. Trends Cardiovasc Med. 2010; 20(8): 249–253

[114] Frueh FS, Gousopoulos E, Rezaeian F, Menger MD, Lindenblatt N, Giovanoli P. Animal models in surgical lymphedema research—a systematic review. J Surg Res. 2016; 200(1):208–220

[115] Suami H, Scaglioni MF, Dixon KA, Tailor RC. Interaction between vascularized lymph node transfer and recipient lymphatics after lymph node dissection—a pilot study in a canine model. J Surg Res. 2016; 204(2):418–427

[116] Huang JJ, Gardenier JC, Hespe GE, et al. Lymph node transplantation decreases swelling and restores immune responses in a transgenic model of lymphedema. PLoS One. 2016; 11(12):e0168259–e0168259

[117] Cornelissen AJ, Qiu SS, Lopez Penha T, et al. Outcomes of vascularized versus non-vascularized lymph node transplant in animal models for lymphedema. Review of the literature. J Surg Oncol. 2017; 115(1): 32–36

[118] Honkonen KM, Visuri MT, Tervala TV, et al. Lymph node transfer and perinodal lymphatic growth factor treatment for lymphedema. Ann Surg. 2013; 257(5):961–967

[119] Visuri MT, Honkonen KM, Hartiala P, et al. VEGF-C and VEGF-C156S in the pro-lymphangiogenic growth factor therapy of lymphedema: a large animal study. Angiogenesis. 2015; 18(3):313–326

[120] Tammela T, Saaristo A, Holopainen T, et al. Therapeutic differentiation and maturation of lymphatic vessels after lymph node dissection and transplantation. Nat Med. 2007; 13(12):1458–1466

[121] Rauniyar K, Jha SK, Jeltsch M. Biology of vascular endothelial growth factor C in the morphogenesis of lymphatic vessels. Front Bioeng Biotechnol. 2018; 6:7

[122] Kilarski WW. Physiological perspective on therapies of lymphatic vessels. Adv Wound Care (New Rochelle). 2018; 7(7):189–208

[123] Yamakawa M, Doh SJ, Santosa SM, et al. Potential lymphangiogenesis therapies: learning from current antiangiogenesis therapies—a review. Med Res Rev. 2018; 38(6):1769–1798

[124] Weitman E, Cuzzone D, Mehrara BJ. Tissue engineering and regeneration of lymphatic structures. Future Oncol. 2013; 9(9): 1365–1374

[125] Hayashida K, Yoshida S, Yoshimoto H, et al. Adipose-derived stem cells and vascularized lymph node transfers successfully treat mouse hindlimb secondary lymphedema by early reconnection of the lymphatic system and lymphangiogenesis. Plast Reconstr Surg. 2017; 139(3):639–651

[126] Jeltsch M, Jha SK, Tvorogov D, et al. CCBE1 enhances lymphangiogenesis via A disintegrin and metalloprotease with thrombospondin motifs-3-mediated vascular endothelial growth factor-C activation. Circulation. 2014; 129(19):1962–1971

[127] Viitanen TP, Visuri MT, Sulo E, Saarikko AM, Hartiala P. Anti-inflammatory effects of flap and lymph node transfer. J Surg Res. 2015; 199(2):718–725

[128] Tian W, Rockson SG, Jiang X, et al. Leukotriene B_4 antagonism ameliorates experimental lymphedema. Sci Transl Med. 2017; 9 (389):389

[129] Schaupper M, Jeltsch M, Rohringer S, Redl H, Holnthoner W. Lymphatic vessels in regenerative medicine and tissue engineering. Tissue Eng Part B Rev. 2016; 22(5):395–407

Glossary

Autologous breast reconstruction
A procedure that uses perfused tissue (i.e., pedicled or microvascular flap) distant from the breast area to reconstruct it.

Immunomodulation
Regulatory adjustment of the immune system. This can be a part of the natural homeostasis of the immune system or the human-induced immunotherapy.

Indocyanine green
Fluorescent medical dye characterized by absorption in the infrared spectrum. It is frequently used for lymphatic imaging.

Lymph
Interstitial fluid rich in proteins and lipids. It returns macromolecules and excess interstitial fluid to the venous system and contributes to fat absorption and immunological processes (Latin *lympha* = water).

Lymphangion
A functional unit or segment of a collecting lymphatic vessel between two intraluminal lymphatic valves.

Lymphangiogenesis
Sprouting growth of lymphatic vessels from preexisting ones.

Lymphatic capillaries
Thin-walled and blind-ended microvessels composed of a single layer of overlapping lymphatic endothelial cells. Lymphatic capillaries lack an organized basement membrane and are deprived of pericytes. They facilitate a unidirectional flow of the lymph into the lymphatic capillary space.

Lymphatic endothelial cells
Endothelial cells with lymphatic differentiation lining the lymphatic vasculature in the tissue and lymph nodes.

Lymphatic (pre)collectors
Larger-diameter lymphatic vasculature lined with a basement membrane and tight zipper-like junctions that interconnect lymphatic endothelial cells. Collecting lymphatic vessels exhibit a layer of smooth muscle cells (with the exclusion of the valve area), allowing for contractions propelling the lymph toward a hydrostatic pressure gradient.

Lymphedema
Dysfunction of the lymphatic system leading to accumulation of lymph in the interstitial space. The clinical appearance may include swelling, limited motion, pain, and recurrent skin infections. Over time, lymphedema results in impaired immunity, chronic inflammation, and progressive fibro-adipose deposition.

Lymph node
Bean-shaped structure integrated in the lymphatic system and connected to one another by lymphatic vessels. Lymph nodes play a key role in the immune response and belong to the secondary lymphatic organs.

Lymphosome
Superficial collecting lymphatic vessel running in a straight path toward its corresponding lymph node dividing the skin into territories that correlate with their lymph basins.

Lymphvasculogenesis
De novo formation of lymphatic vessels from nonvenous-derived lymphatic endothelial progenitors.

Secondary lymphatic organs
Sites of lymphocyte activation following foreign antigen contact. These organs include the lymph nodes, the spleen, the tonsils, the Peyer's patches, and the mucosa-associated lymphoid tissue.

Suction-assisted lipectomy (distinct from "liposuction")
Suction-assisted lipectomy is an efficient surgical method to reduce excess subcutaneous tissue in patients with chronic lymphedema of the extremities following microsurgical reconstruction of the lymphatic outflow.

Index

Note: Page numbers set **bold** or *italic* indicate headings or figures, respectively.

T

U

V

W